D0973496

Contents

Contributors
and consultants

Lee (Haralee) Abramo, BSN, MSN
Director of Education
Los Robles Regional Medical Center
Thousand Oaks, Calif.
Part-time Nursing Faculty
California State University, Dominguez Hills
Carson

Ivy M. Alexander, PhD, CANP
Assistant Professor
Yale University
New Haven, Conn.

Deborah Bastien, RNC, BSN, MS
Professor of Nursing
College of the Mainland
Texas City, Tex.

Eric W. Bussear, MPH, PA-C
Assistant Professor
Nova Southeastern University
Fort Lauderdale, Fla.

Deborah Castellucci, RN, CRNP, PhD
Assistant Professor and Acting Chair
Millersville University of Pennsylvania
Geriatric Nurse Practitioner
Center for Urologic Care
Wyomissing, Pa.

Janie C. Choate, M.A.T., PA-C
Director, Physician Assistant Studies
University of the Sciences
Philadelphia

Wendy Tagan Conroy, MSN, FNP, BC
Advanced Practice Registered Nurse
Saint Francis Hospital and Medical Center
Hartford, Conn.

Sandra Davis, MSN, CRNP
Assistant Professor
Drexel University
Philadelphia

Ellen Digan, MA, MT(ASCP)
Professor of Biology, Coordinator MLT Program
Manchester (Conn.) Community College

Diane Dixon, PA-C, MA, MMSc
Assistant Professor
University of South Alabama
Mobile

Shelba Durston, RN, MSN, CCRN
Adjunct Faculty
San Joaquin Delta College
Stockton, Calif.
Staff Nurse
San Joaquin General Hospital
French Camp, Calif.

Ken W. Edmisson, RNC, ND, EdD, FNP
Associate Professor
Middle Tennessee State University
Murfreesboro

Carmel A. Esposito, RN, BSN, MSN, EdD
Consultant
Follansbee, W.Va.

Margaret Fried, RN, MA
Instructional Faculty
Pima Community College
Tucson, Ariz.

William F. Galvin, BA, MSEd, CRT, RRT, CPFT
Assistant Professor, School of Allied Health Professions
Program Director, Respiratory Care Program
Gwynedd Mercy College
Gwynedd Valley, Pa.

James J. Greco, MSN, ARNP-BC
Instructor
University of Florida
Gainesville

Teri Hamill, PhD
Fellow American Academy of Audiology
Associate Professor of Audiology
Nova Southeastern University
Fort Lauderdale, Fla.

Katherine Purgatorio Howard, RN, MS, BC
Instructor of Nursing
Charles E. Gregory School of Nursing
Raritan Bay Medical Center
Perth Amboy, N.J.

Nathan Kindig, BS, PA-C
Physician Assistant (Sports Medicine & Reconditioning
    Team)
Naval Medical Clinic
Pearl Harbor, Hawaii

Julie E. London, RN, MSN
Associate Professor of Nursing
Community College Allegheny County — Boyce Campus
Monroeville, Pa.

Cecilia Jane Maier, RN, MS, CCRN
Assistant Professor
Mount Carmel College of Nursing
Columbus, Ohio

Karen S. March, RN, MSN, CCRN, APRN-BC
Assistant Professor of Nursing
York College of Pennsylvania

Barbara Maxwell, RNC, MSN, CNS
Assistant Professor of Nursing
State University of New York at Ulster
Stone Ridge

Foreword

Diagnostic testing in health care continues to change at an exponential rate. At the same time, there are increased demands for diagnostic testing because it provides the basis for 80% of medical decisions. Many textbooks, journals, and other sources provide diagnostic testing information, but they're not easy to access and frequently lack all the pertinent information. Until now, it hasn't been easy to find a single resource that quickly and succinctly provides all the information nurses need about diagnostic testing.

Nurse's Quick Check: Diagnostic Tests is the resource that health care professionals — especially time-starved nurses — have been seeking. It's an exceptional guide to nearly 500 diagnostic tests. With easy-scan columns and concise bullets of information, the format of this handbook makes it a snap to find the answer to almost any question. For a nurse, the book is relevant in any type of work setting, providing streamlined information about the abnormal results of cardiac enzymes or lymphocyte assays or interfering factors that affect cerebrospinal fluid analysis, a lung perfusion scan, or thallium imaging. In the classroom, students will find the information easy to retrieve and always reliable.

This book is organized alphabetically with all the relevant information about a specific test usually contained on a single page. Each entry gives you all the information you need to grasp the intricacies of a specific diagnostic test and identifies key considerations associated with the test, including pretest and posttest care.

The alphabetical listings include tests about hematology and coagulation, blood chemistry, hormones, immunology, urine, system-specific specimens, cultures, biopsy, endoscopy, ultrasonography, radiography, computerized tomography and magnetic resonance imaging, nuclear medicine, monitoring and catheterization, and special functions, such as those pertaining to the eyes, ears, and kidneys. Each diagnostic test entry includes:
○ Background information with an overview of interesting, relevant facts
○ Purpose of the test
○ Test procedure, including steps for preparation, implementation, and complications
○ Key considerations for patient care

○ Normal test results
○ Abnormal test results and their implications
○ Factors that can interfere with giving the test or with test results.

Entries also contain logos to highlight certain special information:
○ *Alert* identifies critical information to ensure the patient's safety.
○ *Age aware* points out developmental concerns and age-related situations that may affect or be affected by the test.

Valuable appendices give information about normal and abnormal serum drug levels and key diagnostic findings in major disorders.

Practicing health care workers, especially nurses, and health care students must acquire a deep and broad knowledge of diagnostic tests — no easy task when new discoveries appear frequently and become more and more technically sophisticated. If you must stay abreast of new developments, techniques, and critical points of care, this handbook is the answer. It will become your companion and most reliable source of information.

Mary Jean Rutherford, MEd, MT(ASCP)SC, CLS(NCA)
Associate Professor
Clinical Laboratory Sciences Programs
Arkansas State University
Jonesboro

Nurse's
Quick
Check

Diagnostic
Tests

ABO blood typing

Overview

○ Classifies blood according to the presence of major antigens A and B on red blood cell (RBC) surfaces
○ Classifies blood according to serum antibodies anti-A and anti-B

Purpose

○ To establish a patient's blood group according to the ABO system
○ To check the compatibility of donor and recipient blood before a transfusion

Procedure

Preparation

○ Tell the patient that this test determines his blood group.
○ If the patient is to receive a transfusion, this test will determine the donor's blood type.
○ This test requires no food or fluid restriction.
○ Inform the patient that this test requires a venipuncture and blood sample.
○ Check the patient's history for recent administration of blood, dextran, or I.V. contrast media.

Implementation

○ Perform a venipuncture and collect the sample in a 10-ml tube without additives, following standard precautions.
○ Label the sample with the patient's name, the hospital or blood bank number, the date, and the phlebotomist's initials.
○ Handle the sample gently to prevent hemolysis and send it to the laboratory immediately with a properly completed laboratory request.

Patient care

○ Apply direct pressure to the venipuncture site until bleeding stops.

Complications

○ Hematoma at the venipuncture site

Interpretation

Normal results

○ In forward typing, if agglutination occurs when the patient's RBCs are mixed with anti-A serum, the A antigen is present, and the blood is type A.
○ In forward typing, if agglutination occurs when the patient's RBCs are mixed with anti-B serum, the B antigen is present, and blood is type B.

○ In forward typing, if agglutination occurs in both mixes, A and B antigens are present, and the blood is type AB.
○ In forward typing, if agglutination doesn't occur in either mix, no antigens are present, and the blood is type O.
○ In reverse typing, if agglutination occurs when B cells are mixed with the patient's serum, anti-B is present, and the blood is type A.
○ In reverse typing, if agglutination occurs when A cells are mixed, anti-A is present, and the blood is type B.
○ In reverse typing, if agglutination occurs when A and B cells are mixed, anti-A and anti-B are present, and the blood is typed O.
○ In reverse typing, if agglutination doesn't occur when A and B cells are mixed, neither anti-A nor anti-B is present, and the blood is type AB.

▽ ALERT *Donor blood is suitable for a transfusion only when ABO compatibility with the recipient's blood is definite; transfusion of blood containing either A or B antigens to a recipient whose RBCs lack these antigens can cause a potentially fatal reaction.*

Abnormal results

None known

Interfering factors

○ Recent administration of dextran or I.V. contrast media, causing cellular aggregation resembling antibody-mediated agglutination
○ Hemolysis from rough handling of the sample
○ Blood transfusion or pregnancy in the past 3 months (possibility of lingering antibodies)

Acetylcholine receptor antibodies

Overview

○ Most useful immunologic test for confirming acquired (autoimmune) myasthenia gravis
○ Two test methods: a binding assay and a blocking assay
○ Determines the relative concentration of acetylcholine receptor (AChR) antibodies in serum
○ Helps monitor immunosuppressive therapy for myasthenia gravis

Purpose

○ To confirm the diagnosis of myasthenia gravis
○ To monitor the effectiveness of immunosuppressive therapy for myasthenia gravis

Procedure

Preparation

○ Explain to the patient that this test helps confirm the diagnosis of myasthenia gravis.
○ Explain that the test assesses the effectiveness of treatment, if appropriate.
○ Inform the patient that he need not restrict food and fluids.
○ Tell the patient that the test requires a blood sample.
○ Check the patient's history for immunosuppressive drugs that may affect the test results and note such use on the laboratory request.

Implementation

○ Explain to the patient that he may experience slight discomfort from the tourniquet and the needle puncture.
○ Perform a venipuncture and collect the sample in a 7-ml tube without additives.
○ Keep the sample at room temperature and send it to the laboratory immediately.

Patient care

○ Because of the patient's compromised immune system, check the venipuncture site for infection and promptly report changes.
○ Keep a clean, dry bandage over the site for at least 24 hours.
○ Apply direct pressure to the venipuncture site until bleeding stops.

Complications

○ Hematoma at the venipuncture site

Interpretation

Normal results

○ Negative for AChR-binding antibodies and AChR-blocking antibodies

Abnormal results

○ Positive AChR antibodies in symptomatic adults confirm the diagnosis of myasthenia gravis.
○ Patients with ocular symptoms have lower antibody titers than those with generalized symptoms.

Interfering factors

○ Failure to maintain the sample at room temperature and failure to send the sample to the laboratory immediately
○ Thymectomy, thoracic duct drainage, immunosuppressive therapy, and plasmapheresis (possible decrease)
○ Amyotrophic lateral sclerosis (possible false-positive)

Acid mucopolysaccharides

Overview

○ Quantitative test that measures the urine level of acid mucopolysaccharides, a group of polysaccharides (carbohydrates)
○ Helps detect mucopolysaccharidosis, a rare disorder that may affect the skeleton, joints, liver, spleen, eye, ear, skin, teeth, and the cardiovascular, respiratory, and central nervous systems

Purpose

○ To diagnose mucopolysaccharidosis in infants with a family history of the disease

Procedure

Preparation

○ Explain to the infant's parents that the acid mucopolysaccharide test helps to determine the efficiency of carbohydrate metabolism.
○ Inform the parents that they need not restrict the child's food and fluids.
○ Tell the parents that the test requires urine collection for 24 hours, and instruct them on how to collect the specimen properly at home.
○ If the child is receiving therapy with heparin and must continue it, note this on the laboratory request.

Implementation

○ Collect the urine over a 24-hour period, discarding the first specimen and retaining the last.
○ Add 20 ml of toluene (as a preservative) to the collection container at the start of the collection.
○ Indicate the patient's age on the laboratory request.
○ Immediately after the 24-hour collection period, send the specimen to the laboratory.
○ Refrigerate the specimen or place it on ice during the collection period.

Patient care

○ Remove all of the urine collector adhesive from the infant's perineum.
○ Wash the area gently with soap and water; watch for irritation.

Complications

None known

Interpretation

Normal results

○ Value is expressed as milligrams of glucuronic acid divided by the amount of creatinine in the same spec-imen (which reflects glomerular filtration rate); this compensates for irregularities in the 24-hour urine collection.
○ Normal acid mucopolysaccharide values for adults are less than 13.3 µg glucuronic acid/mg creatinine/24 hours.
○ Child values vary with age.

Abnormal results

○ Elevated acid mucopolysaccharide levels reliably indicate mucopolysaccharidosis.
○ Supplementary quantitative analysis and detailed blood studies can identify the defective enzyme.

Interfering factors

○ Failure to collect all urine during the test period
○ Failure to properly store the specimen
○ Failure to send the specimen to the laboratory immediately after the collection is complete
○ Heparin (increase)

Acid perfusion (Bernstein) test

Overview

○ Helps to distinguish the pain caused by esophagitis (burning epigastric or retrosternal pain that radiates to the back or arms) from pain caused by angina pectoris or other disorders
○ Requires perfusion of saline and acidic solutions into the esophagus through a nasogastric (NG) tube

Purpose

○ To distinguish chest pain caused by esophagitis from chest pain caused by cardiac disorders

Procedure

Preparation

○ Tell the patient that the acid perfusion test helps distinguish heartburn from the pain caused by angina pectoris and other disorders.
○ Explain the following restrictions to the patient: no antacids for 24 hours before the test, no food for 12 hours before the test, and no fluids or smoking for 8 hours before the test.
○ Describe the test, including who will perform it, where it will take place, and how long it will last.
○ Explain to the patient that the test involves passing a tube through his nose into the esophagus and that he may experience some discomfort, a desire to cough, or a gagging sensation during tube passage.
○ Tell the patient that the liquid is slowly perfused through the tube into the esophagus and that he should immediately report pain or burning during perfusion.
○ Just before the test, check the patient's pulse rate and blood pressure. Ask him whether he's experiencing heartburn and, if so, to describe it.
○ Make sure that the patient or a responsible family member has signed an informed consent form.
○ The acid perfusion test is contraindicated in the patient with esophageal varices, heart failure, acute myocardial infarction, or other cardiac disorders.

Implementation

○ Mark an NG tube at 12″ (30.5 cm) from the tip.
○ After the patient is seated, insert the NG tube into his stomach. Attach a 20-ml syringe to the tube and aspirate the stomach contents. Withdraw the tube into the esophagus up to the 12″ mark.
○ Hang labeled containers of normal saline solution and a prescribed acidic solution (such as a mild hydrochloric acid) on an I.V. pole behind the patient, and then connect the NG tube to the I.V. tubing.

○ Open the line from the normal saline solution and infuse at a rate of 60 to 120 drops/minute. Continue perfusion for 5 to 10 minutes.
○ Ask the patient whether he's experiencing discomfort and record his response.
○ Without the patient's knowledge, close the line from the normal saline solution and open the line from the acidic solution. Infuse the acidic solution into the esophagus at the same rate used for the saline solution. Continue perfusion for 30 minutes.
○ Ask the patient again whether he's experiencing discomfort and record his response.
○ Assess the patient's pulse rate and rhythm to detect any arrhythmia that may develop.
○ If the patient experiences discomfort, close the line from the acidic solution immediately and open the line from the normal saline solution. Continue to perfuse this solution until the discomfort subsides.
○ If ordered, repeat perfusion of the acidic solution to verify the patient's response. If this isn't required or if the patient experiences no discomfort after perfusion of the acidic solution for 30 minutes, stop the solution and withdraw the NG tube.
○ Clamp the tube before removing it to prevent fluid aspiration into the lungs.

Patient care

○ If the patient complains of pain or burning, give him an antacid. If he complains of a sore throat, provide soothing lozenges or obtain an order for an ice collar.
○ Instruct the patient that he may resume his usual diet and medications.

Complications

○ Tube entering trachea instead of esophagus during intubation; withdraw the tube immediately if the patient develops cyanosis or paroxysmal coughing.

Interpretation

Normal results

○ Absence of pain or burning during perfusion of either solution indicates a healthy esophageal mucosa.

Abnormal results

○ In the patient with esophagitis, the acidic solution causes pain or burning, while the normal saline solution produces no adverse effects.
○ Occasionally, both solutions cause pain in the patient with esophagitis, but they may not cause pain in the patient with asymptomatic esophagitis.

Interfering factors

○ Failure to observe pretest restrictions
○ Beta blockers, anticholinergics, reserpine, corticosteroids, histamine-2 blockers, and acid pump inhibitors

Acid phosphatase

Overview

○ Measures total acid phosphatase and the prostatic fraction in serum
○ Prostatic isoenzyme more specific for prostate cancer than erythrocytic isoenzyme
○ Level more likely to be increased if cancer is widespread

Purpose

○ To detect prostate cancer
○ To monitor the patient's response to therapy for prostate cancer (successful treatment decreases acid phosphatase levels)

Procedure

Preparation

○ Explain to the patient that this test evaluates prostate function.
○ Tell the patient that the test requires a blood sample. Explain who will perform the venipuncture and when.
○ Explain to the patient that he may experience slight discomfort from the tourniquet and the needle puncture.
○ Inform the patient that he need not restrict food and fluids.
○ Notify the laboratory and physician of drugs the patient is taking that may affect test results; it may be necessary to restrict them.

Implementation

○ Perform a venipuncture and collect the sample in a 4-ml tube without additives.
○ Don't draw the sample within 48 hours of prostate manipulation (rectal examination).
○ Handle the sample gently to prevent hemolysis.
○ Send the sample to the laboratory immediately. Acid phosphatase levels decrease by 50% within 1 hour if the sample remains at room temperature without a preservative or if it isn't packed in ice.

Patient care

○ Apply direct pressure to the venipuncture site until bleeding stops.
○ Instruct the patient that he may resume medications stopped before the test.

Complications

○ Hematoma at the venipuncture site

Interpretation

Normal results

○ Serum values for total acid phosphatase depend on the assay method and range from 0 to 3.7 units/L (SI, 0 to 3.7 U/L).

Abnormal results

○ High prostatic acid phosphatase levels generally indicate the presence of a tumor that has spread beyond the prostatic capsule. If the tumor has metastasized to bone, high acid phosphatase levels are accompanied by high alkaline phosphatase (ALP) levels, reflecting increased osteoblastic activity.
○ Acid phosphatase levels rise moderately in prostatic infarction, Paget's disease (some cases), Gaucher's disease and, occasionally, other conditions such as multiple myeloma. High ALP levels can produce false results because acid phosphatase and ALP are similar, differing mainly in their optimum pH ranges.

Interfering factors

○ Hemolysis from rough handling of the sample or improper sample storage
○ Delayed delivery of the sample to the laboratory (possible false-low or false-normal)
○ Fluorides, phosphates, and oxalates (possible false-low)
○ Clofibrate (possible false-high)
○ Prostate massage, catheterization, or rectal examination within 48 hours of the test

Acid-fast stain

Overview

- Helps identify organisms of the genus *Mycobacterium*
- Because mycobacteria (including pathogens of tuberculosis and leprosy) are acid-fast, they retain carbolfuchsin stain after treatment with an acid-alcohol solution
- Particularly useful for identifying mycobacteria in sputum specimens, which may contain many different organisms

Purpose

- To examine a specimen for the presence of microorganisms, specifically mycobacteria, which include the bacteria that cause tuberculosis

Procedure

Preparation

- Explain to the patient or parent that preparation for the test depends on the type of specimen to be collected.
- Explain fully the type of test that he'll receive.
- Explain that in some cases a tissue biopsy or aspiration with a needle may be necessary.
- Explain that the amount of discomfort will depend on the type of sampling procedure.

Implementation

- Explain to the patient that blood, urine, stool, sputum, bone marrow, or tissue specimens may be collected, depending on the location of the suspected infection.
- After collecting the specimen, send it to the microbiology laboratory.

Patient care

- Check the site of specimen collection for signs of infection.
- Instruct the patient or parent to report adverse effects.

Complications

None known

Interpretation

Normal results

- Absence of acid-fast bacteria on the stained specimen

Abnormal results

- Presence of acid-fast bacteria, which can include those that cause tuberculosis, nontuberculous infections, and *Nocardia*

Interfering factors

None known

Acoustic admittance

Overview

○ Evaluates middle ear function by measuring the flow of sound energy into the ear (admittance)
○ Commonly measured by two tests: *tympanometry* and *acoustic reflex testing*

Purpose

○ Tympanometry: To assess the continuity and admittance of the middle ear and evaluate the status of the tympanic membrane
○ Acoustic reflex testing: To distinguish between cochlear and retrocochlear lesions; to differentiate eighth nerve or peripheral brain stem lesions from intra-axial brain stem lesions and locate seventh nerve lesions relative to stapedius muscle innervation; to confirm conductive hearing loss and help confirm nonorganic loss

Procedure

Preparation

○ Make sure that the ear is free of significant cerumen accumulation.
○ Describe the procedure to the patient and explain that acoustic admittance tests evaluate the condition of the middle ear.
○ Tell the patient that he'll feel pressure in the ear but that it won't be painful.
○ Ask the patient to remain still during testing, which takes just a few seconds.

Implementation

○ Tympanometry: An otoscopic examination is performed to verify whether impacted cerumen or other obstructions are in the ear canal.
○ The size and shape of the canal are checked to select the appropriate-sized probe tip, which is then attached to the probe.
○ The probe tip is inserted into the ear canal while the auricle is pulled upward and back to create a proper seal.
○ A graphic display of the tympanogram is obtained. If there's pressure in the middle ear, a clear peak will be present, and the pressure will print out with the test results.
○ If there's no change in admittance, the tympanogram results will appear flat. The possibility that the probe tip rested against the canal wall or that it was clogged with cerumen must be ruled out. A small ear canal (volume of 0.3 ml or less) is more likely to cause a flat tympanogram.
○ Acoustic reflex testing: The admittance probe is positioned in the ear (same as for tympanometry) but the probe is fixed to the patient's head to reduce the chance of other factors affecting the test results.

○ For threshold testing, stimuli of progressively louder levels are introduced until a reflex (if present) occurs.
○ Acoustic reflex decay testing presents a tone, 10 decibels (dB) above the reflex threshold, at one or more frequencies (1,000 hertz and below) for 10 seconds. The time the auditory system sustains the contraction at a level of half strength or greater is measured.
○ Reflexes and reflex decay can be measured ipsilaterally (the probe is in the same ear that receives the tone) or contralaterally (the probe is in the opposite ear from the ear that receives the tone).

Patient care

○ Obtain medical clearance before performing admittance tests in the patient who has head trauma, a possible labyrinthine fistula, or one who has had recent middle ear surgery.

Complications

None known

Interpretation

Normal results

○ Tympanometry: The four important measurements on a tympanogram are ear canal volume, peak compliance reading, peak pressure reading, and slope gradient. A type A tympanogram is a normal finding.
○ Acoustic reflex testing: Normal reflexes are present at an intensity of 65 to 100 dB hearing level. The sensation level of the reflex should also be 65 to 100 dB.

Abnormal results

○ Tympanometry: Evidence that doesn't reflect a type A tympanogram is considered abnormal.
○ Acoustic reflex testing: Ears that have conductive involvement commonly have absent reflexes. If the conductive loss is unilateral, presentation of the reflex tone to the involved ear, with measurement contralaterally, may reveal a reflex at an elevated hearing level.
○ If the cochlea is the site of a lesion, reflexes may be present at normal hearing levels, elevated, or absent. The more severe the hearing loss, the more likely the finding of an absent reflex.
○ Acoustic reflexes are present in most patients with mild to moderately severe hearing losses.
○ Absent acoustic reflexes raise the possibility of a retrocochlear lesion if conductive involvement or severe cochlear loss isn't present.
○ Acoustic reflex decay is an indicator of possible retrocochlear involvement.
○ Reflexes below the admitted threshold are an indicator of a nonorganic problem.

Interfering factors

○ Interpretation by audiologist of reflex findings in light of audiologic results
○ Patient movement resulting in false readings

Activated clotting time

Overview

- Measures whole blood clotting time
- Commonly performed during procedures that require extracorporeal circulation, such as cardiopulmonary bypass, ultrafiltration, hemodialysis, and extracorporeal membrane oxygenation (ECMO) and during invasive procedures, such as cardiac catheterization and percutaneous transluminal coronary angioplasty

Purpose

- To monitor the effect of heparin
- To monitor the effect of protamine sulfate in heparin neutralization
- To detect severe deficiencies in clotting factors (except factor VII)

Procedure

Preparation

- Explain to the patient that the activated clotting time test monitors the effect of heparin on the blood's ability to coagulate.
- Tell the patient that the test requires two blood samples, usually drawn from an existing vascular access site; therefore, no venipuncture will be necessary.
- Explain that the first blood sample will be discarded so that any heparin in the tubing won't interfere with the results.
- Explain who will perform the test and where it will occur — usually at the bedside.

Implementation

- If the sample is drawn from a line with a continuous infusion, stop the infusion before drawing the sample.
- Withdraw 5 to 10 ml of blood from the line and discard it.
- Withdraw a clean sample of blood into the special tube containing celite provided with the activated clotting time unit.
- Start the activated clotting time unit and wait for the signal before inserting the tube.
- Flush the vascular access site according to your facility's policy.

Patient care

- Instruct the patient to report discomfort at the site.
- Monitor the venipuncture site for signs of bleeding.

Complications

- Contamination with heparin if drawn from an access site containing heparin

Interpretation

Normal results

- In a non-anticoagulated patient, normal activated clotting time is 107 seconds, plus or minus 13 seconds (SI, 107 ± 13 s).
- During cardiopulmonary bypass, heparin is titrated to maintain an activated clotting time of 400 to 600 seconds (SI, 400 to 600 s).
- During ECMO, heparin is titrated to maintain the activated clotting time of 220 to 260 seconds (SI, 220 to 260 s).

Abnormal results

None known

Interfering factors

- Failure to fill the collection tube completely, to use proper anticoagulant, or to adequately mix the sample and the anticoagulant
- Failure to send the sample to the laboratory immediately or to place it on ice
- Hemolysis from rough handling of the sample or excessive probing at the venipuncture site
- Failure to draw at least 5 ml waste to avoid sample contamination when drawing the sample from a venous access device that's used for heparin infusion

Alanine aminotransferase

Overview

- Measures serum levels of alanine aminotransferase (ALT), one of two enzymes that catalyze a reversible amino group transfer reaction in the Krebs cycle
- Necessary for tissue energy production
- Found primarily in the liver, with lesser amounts in the kidneys, heart, and skeletal muscles (a sensitive indicator of acute hepatocellular disease)

Purpose

- To detect and evaluate treatment of acute hepatic disease, especially hepatitis and cirrhosis without jaundice
- To distinguish between myocardial and hepatic tissue damage (used with aspartate aminotransferase)
- To assess the hepatotoxicity of some drugs

Procedure

Preparation

- Explain to the patient that this test assesses liver function.
- Tell the patient that the test requires a blood sample. Explain who will perform the venipuncture and when.
- Explain to the patient that he may experience slight discomfort from the tourniquet and the needle puncture.
- Inform the patient that he need not restrict food and fluids.
- Notify the laboratory and physician of drugs the patient is taking that may affect test results; it may be necessary to restrict them.

Implementation

- Perform a venipuncture and collect the sample in a 4-ml tube without additives.
- Handle the sample gently to prevent hemolysis.
- ALT activity is stable in serum for up to 3 days at room temperature.

Patient care

- Apply direct pressure to the venipuncture site until bleeding stops.
- Instruct the patient that he may resume medications stopped before the test.

Complications

- Hematoma at the venipuncture site

Interpretation

Normal results

- 8 to 50 IU/L (SI, 0.14 to 0.85 µkat/L)

Abnormal results

- Very high ALT levels (up to 50 times normal) suggest viral or severe drug-induced hepatitis or other hepatic disease with extensive necrosis.
- Moderate to high levels may indicate infectious mononucleosis, chronic hepatitis, intrahepatic cholestasis or cholecystitis, early or improving acute viral hepatitis, or severe hepatic congestion from heart failure.
- Slight to moderate elevations of ALT may appear in any condition that produces acute hepatocellular injury, such as active cirrhosis and drug-induced or alcoholic hepatitis.
- Marginal elevations occasionally occur in acute myocardial infarction, reflecting secondary hepatic congestion or the release of small amounts of ALT from myocardial tissue.

Interfering factors

- Hemolysis from rough handling of the sample
- Barbiturates, griseofulvin, isoniazid, nitrofurantoin, methyldopa, phenothiazines, phenytoin, salicylates, tetracycline, chlorpromazine, para-aminosalicylic acid, and other drugs that cause hepatic injury by competitively interfering with cellular metabolism (false-high)
- Opioid analgesics, such as morphine, codeine, and meperidine (possible false-high from increased intrabiliary pressure)
- Ingestion of lead or exposure to carbon tetrachloride (sharp increase from direct injury to hepatic cells)

Albumin

Overview

- Measures the amount of albumin in serum
- Most abundant protein, composing almost 54% of plasma proteins

Purpose

- To help determine whether a patient has liver disease or kidney disease
- To determine whether enough protein is being absorbed by the body

Procedure

Preparation

- Tell the patient that there's no need for fluid restriction.
- Explain the venipuncture procedure.
- Explain that certain medications can increase albumin measurements. These include anabolic steroids, androgens, growth hormones, and insulin. The patient may need to stop these drugs prior to the test.

Implementation

- Explain to the patient that he may experience slight discomfort from the tourniquet and the needle puncture.
- Perform a venipuncture and collect 5 to 10 ml in a red-top tube.
- Follow standard precautions when collecting the sample.

Patient care

- Apply direct pressure to the venipuncture site until bleeding stops.
- Encourage the patient to eat a diet high in protein if not contraindicated.

Complications

- Hematoma at the venipuncture site

Interpretation

Normal results

- Adult: 3.4 to 5.4 g/dl
- Child: 4.0 to 5.8 g/dl
- Infant: 4.4 to 5.4 g/dl
- Neonate: 2.9 to 5.4 g/dl

Abnormal results

- A decreased level (hypoalbuminemia) may indicate cirrhosis, acute liver failure, severe burns, severe malnutrition, and ulcerative colitis.
- An elevated level (hyperalbuminemia) may indicate dehydration, severe vomiting, and severe diarrhea.

Interfering factors

- Penicillin, sulfonamides, aspirin, and ascorbic acid (decrease)
- Heparin (increase)

Aldosterone, serum

Overview

- Measures serum aldosterone levels by quantitative analysis and radioimmunoassay
- Regulates ion transport across cell membranes in the renal tubules to promote reabsorption of sodium and chloride in exchange for potassium and hydrogen ions
- Helps to maintain blood pressure and volume and to regulate fluid and electrolyte balance

Purpose

- To aid in the diagnosis of primary and secondary aldosteronism, adrenal hyperplasia, hypoaldosteronism, and salt-losing syndrome

Procedure

Preparation

- Explain to the patient that this test helps determine whether his symptoms are from improper hormonal secretion.
- Tell the patient that the test requires a blood sample.
- Explain to the patient that he may experience slight discomfort from the tourniquet and the needle puncture.
- Instruct the patient to maintain a low-carbohydrate, normal-sodium diet (135 mEq or 3 g/day) for at least 2 weeks or, preferably, for 30 days before the test.
- Withhold drugs that alter fluid, sodium, and potassium balance — especially diuretics, antihypertensives, steroids, hormonal contraceptives, and estrogens — for at least 2 weeks or, preferably, for 30 days before the test.
- Withhold all renin inhibitors for 1 week before the test. If the patient must continue them, note this on the laboratory request.
- Tell the patient to avoid licorice for at least 2 weeks before the test because it produces an aldosterone-like effect.

Implementation

- Perform a venipuncture while the patient is still supine after a night's rest.
- Collect the sample in a 7-ml clot-activator tube and send it to the laboratory immediately.
- Draw another sample 4 hours later, while the patient is standing and after he has been up and about, to evaluate the effect of postural change.
- Collect the second sample in a 7-ml clot-activator tube and send it to the laboratory immediately.
- Handle the sample gently to prevent hemolysis.
- Record on the laboratory request whether the patient was supine or standing during the venipuncture.

- If the patient is a premenopausal female, specify the phase of her menstrual cycle because aldosterone levels may fluctuate.

Patient care

- Apply direct pressure to the venipuncture site until bleeding stops.
- Instruct the patient that he may resume his usual diet and medications stopped before the test.

Complications

- Hematoma at the venipuncture site

Interpretation

Normal results

- Laboratory results vary with time of day and posture — upright postures have higher values.
- In people standing upright, normal results are 7 to 30 nanograms/dl (SI, 190 to 832 pmol/L).
- In supine people, normal results are 3 to 16 nanograms/dl (SI, 80 to 440 pmol/L).

Abnormal results

- Excessive aldosterone secretion may indicate a primary or secondary disease.
- Primary aldosteronism (Conn's syndrome) may result from adrenocortical adenoma or carcinoma or from bilateral adrenal hyperplasia.
- Secondary aldosteronism may result from renovascular hypertension, heart failure, cirrhosis of the liver, nephrotic syndrome, or idiopathic cyclic edema, and can occur during the third trimester of pregnancy.
- Low serum aldosterone levels may indicate primary hypoaldosteronism, salt-losing syndrome, eclampsia, or Addison's disease.

Interfering factors

- Failure to observe pretest restrictions
- Hemolysis from rough handling of the sample
- Some antihypertensives (possible decrease)
- Diuretics (possible increase)
- Some corticosteroids (possible decrease)
- Radioactive scan performed within 1 week before the test

Aldosterone, urine

Overview

○ Measures urine levels of aldosterone, the principal mineralocorticoid secreted by the adrenal cortex
○ Radioimmunoassay that's usually evaluated after measurement of serum electrolyte and renin levels

Purpose

○ To aid in the diagnosis of primary and secondary aldosteronism

Procedure

Preparation

○ Explain to the patient that the urine aldosterone test evaluates hormonal balance.
○ Instruct the patient to maintain a normal sodium diet (3 g/day) before the test and to avoid sodium-rich foods, such as bacon, barbecue sauce, corned beef, bouillon cubes or powder, pickles, snack foods (potato chips), and olives.
○ Advise the patient to avoid strenuous physical exercise and stressful situations during the collection period.
○ Tell the patient that the test requires the collection of urine during 24 hours, and teach him the proper collection technique.
○ Notify the laboratory and physician of drugs the patient is taking that may affect test results; it may be necessary to restrict them.

Implementation

○ Collect the patient's urine over a 24-hour period, discarding the first specimen and retaining the last. Use a bottle containing a preservative, such as boric acid, to keep the specimen at a pH of 4.0 to 4.5
○ Refrigerate the specimen or place it on ice during the collection period.
○ Send the specimen to the laboratory as soon as the collection is complete.

Patient care

○ Instruct the patient that he may resume his usual activities, diet, and medications.

Complications

None known

Interpretation

Normal results

○ 3 to 19 µg/24 hours (SI, 8 to 51 nmol/day)

Abnormal results

○ Elevated urine aldosterone levels suggest primary or secondary aldosteronism.
○ The primary form usually arises from an adenoma of the adrenal cortex that secretes aldosterone but may also result from adrenocortical hyperplasia.
○ Secondary aldosteronism, the more common form, results from external stimulation of the adrenal cortex such as that produced when hypertensive and edematous disorders activate the renin-angiotensin system.
○ Disorders that may result in secondary aldosteronism are malignant hypertension, heart failure, cirrhosis of the liver, nephrotic syndrome, and idiopathic cyclic edema.
○ Low urine aldosterone levels may result from Addison's disease, salt-losing syndrome, and toxemia of pregnancy. These levels normally rise during pregnancy but rapidly decline following parturition.

Interfering factors

○ Failure to maintain normal dietary sodium intake as well as excess intake of licorice or glucose
○ Failure to avoid strenuous physical exercise and emotional stress before the test (possible increase from stimulation of adrenocortical secretions)
○ Radioactive scan performed within 1 week before the test
○ Failure to collect all urine during the collection period, to properly store the specimen, or to send it to the laboratory immediately after the collection is complete
○ Antihypertensive drugs (possible decrease because of sodium and water retention)
○ Diuretics and most steroids (possible increase because of sodium excretion)
○ Some corticosteroids, such as fludrocortisone, which mimic mineralocorticoid activity (possible decrease)

Alkaline phosphatase

Overview

- Measures serum levels of alkaline phosphatase (ALP), an enzyme that influences bone calcification as well as lipid and metabolite transport
- Reflects the combined activity of several ALP isoenzymes found in the liver, bones, kidneys, intestinal lining, and placenta
- Is particularly sensitive to mild biliary obstruction and is a primary indicator of space-occupying hepatic lesions
- Is most useful for diagnosing metabolic bone disease

Purpose

- To detect and identify skeletal diseases primarily characterized by marked osteoblastic activity
- To detect focal hepatic lesions causing biliary obstruction, such as a tumor or an abscess
- To assess the patient's response to vitamin D in the treatment of rickets
- To supplement information from other liver function studies and GI enzyme tests

Procedure

Preparation

- Explain to the patient that this test assesses liver and bone function.
- Instruct the patient to fast for at least 8 hours before the test because fat intake stimulates intestinal ALP secretion.
- Tell the patient that this test requires a blood sample. Explain who will perform the venipuncture and when.
- Inform the patient that he may experience slight discomfort from the tourniquet and the needle puncture.

Implementation

- Perform a venipuncture and collect the sample in a 4-ml clot-activator tube.
- Apply direct pressure to the venipuncture site until bleeding stops.
- Handle the sample gently to prevent hemolysis.
- Send the sample to the laboratory immediately; ALP activity increases at room temperature because of a rise in pH.

Patient care

- Instruct the patient that he may resume his usual diet.

Complications

- Hematoma at the venipuncture site

Interpretation

Normal results

- 45 to 115 IU/ml (SI, 45 to 115 U/L)

Abnormal results

- Although significant ALP elevations are possible with diseases that affect many organs, they usually indicate skeletal disease or extrahepatic or intrahepatic biliary obstruction causing cholestasis.
- Many acute hepatic diseases cause ALP elevations before they affect serum bilirubin levels.
- Moderate increases in ALP levels may reflect acute biliary obstruction from hepatocellular inflammation in active cirrhosis, mononucleosis, or viral hepatitis.
- Moderate increases are also seen in osteomalacia and deficiency-induced rickets.
- Sharp elevations in ALP levels may indicate complete biliary obstruction by malignant or infectious infiltrations or fibrosis, most common in Paget's disease and, occasionally, in biliary obstruction, extensive bone metastasis, and hyperparathyroidism.
- Metastatic bone tumors resulting from pancreatic cancer raise ALP levels without a concomitant rise in serum alanine aminotransferase levels.
- Isoenzyme fractionation and additional enzyme tests (gamma glutamyl transferase, lactate dehydrogenase, 5'-nucleotidase, and leucine aminopeptidase) are sometimes performed when the cause of ALP elevations is in doubt.
- Rarely, low levels of serum ALP are linked to hypophosphatasia and protein or magnesium deficiency.

Interfering factors

- Hemolysis from rough handling of the sample
- Failure to analyze the sample within 4 hours
- Recent ingestion of vitamin D (possible increase because of the effect on osteoblastic activity)
- Recent infusion of albumin prepared from placental venous blood (marked increase)
- Drugs that influence liver function or cause cholestasis, such as barbiturates, chlorpropamide, hormonal contraceptives, isoniazid, methyldopa, phenothiazines, phenytoin, and rifampin (possible mild increase)
- Halothane sensitivity (possible drastic increase)
- Clofibrate (decrease)
- Healing long-bone fractures and the third trimester of pregnancy (possible increase)
- Age and sex (increase in infants, children, adolescents, and people over age 45)

Alpha$_1$-globulin

Overview

○ Roughly measures the various protein fractions in the serum portion of a blood sample

Purpose

○ To aid in ruling out inflammatory disease

Procedure

Preparation

○ Inform the patient that this test requires a venipuncture.

Implementation

○ Explain that the patient may experience slight discomfort from the tourniquet and the needle puncture.
○ Perform the venipuncture according to protocol.

Patient care

○ Apply direct pressure to the venipuncture site until bleeding stops.

Complications

○ Hematoma at the venipuncture site

Interpretation

Normal results

○ 0.1 to 0.3 g/dl

Abnormal results

○ Increased alpha$_1$-globulin proteins may indicate chronic inflammatory disease (for example, rheumatoid arthritis, systemic lupus erythematosus), acute inflammatory disease, or malignancy.
○ Decreased alpha$_1$-globulin proteins may indicate an alpha$_1$-antitrypsin deficiency.

Interfering factors

○ Drugs that can affect the measurement of total proteins, including chlorpromazine, corticosteroids, isoniazid, neomycin, phenacemide, salicylates, sulfonamides, and tolbutamide

Alpha$_2$-globulin

Overview

○ Roughly measures the various protein fractions in the serum portion of a blood sample

Purpose

○ To quantitate the alpha$_2$-globulin protein factor in the blood
○ To help detect the presence of inflammation

Procedure

Preparation

○ Inform the patient that this test requires a venipuncture.

Implementation

○ Explain that the patient may experience slight discomfort from the tourniquet and the needle puncture.
○ Perform the venipuncture according to protocol.

Patient care

○ Apply direct pressure to the venipuncture site until bleeding stops.

Complications

○ Hematoma at the venipuncture site

Interpretation

Normal results

○ 0.6 to 1.0 g/dl

Abnormal results

○ Increased alpha$_2$-globulin proteins may indicate acute or chronic inflammation.
○ Decreased alpha$_2$-globulin proteins may indicate hemolysis.

Interfering factors

○ Drugs that can affect the measurement of total proteins, including chlorpromazine, corticosteroids, isoniazid, neomycin, phenacemide, salicylates, sulfonamides, and tolbutamide

Alpha-fetoprotein

Overview

- Serum and amniotic fluid levels rise during fetal development
- Crosses the placenta and appears in maternal serum

Purpose

- To monitor the effectiveness of therapy in malignant conditions, such as hepatomas and germ cell tumors, and certain nonmalignant conditions such as ataxia-telangiectasia
- To screen those patients needing amniocentesis or high-resolution ultrasonography during pregnancy

Procedure

Preparation

- Explain that this test helps in monitoring fetal development, screens for a need for further testing, helps detect possible congenital defects in the fetus, and monitors the mother's response to therapy by measuring a specific blood protein, as appropriate.
- Inform the patient that she need not restrict food, fluids, or medications.
- Tell the patient that the test requires a blood sample. Explain who will perform the venipuncture and when.
- Explain to the patient that she may experience slight discomfort from the tourniquet and the needle puncture.

Implementation

- Perform a venipuncture and collect the sample in a 7-ml clot-activator tube.
- Record the patient's age, race, weight, and week of gestation on the laboratory request.
- Handle the sample gently to prevent hemolysis.

Patient care

- Apply direct pressure to the venipuncture site until bleeding stops.

Complications

- Hematoma at the venipuncture site

Interpretation

Normal results

- When tested by immunoassay, alpha-fetoprotein (AFP) values are less than 15 nanograms/ml (SI, < 15 mg/L) in men and nonpregnant women. Values in maternal serum are less than 2½ multiples of median for fetal gestational age.

Abnormal results

- Elevated maternal serum AFP levels may suggest neural tube defects or other tube anomalies. Maternal AFP levels rise sharply in the maternal blood of about 90% of women carrying a fetus with anencephaly and in 50% of those carrying a fetus with spina bifida.
- Definitive diagnosis requires ultrasonography and amniocentesis.
- High AFP levels may indicate intrauterine death. Sometimes, high levels indicate other anomalies, such as duodenal atresia, omphalocele, tetralogy of Fallot, and Turner's syndrome.
- Elevated serum AFP levels occur in 70% of nonpregnant patients with hepatocellular carcinoma.
- Elevated levels are also related to germ cell tumor of gonadal, retroperitoneal, or mediastinal origin.
- Serum AFP levels rise in ataxia-telangiectasia and sometimes in cancer of the pancreas, stomach, or biliary system and in nonseminiferous testicular tumors.
- Transient modest elevations can occur in nonneoplastic hepatocellular disease, such as alcoholic cirrhosis and acute or chronic hepatitis.
- Elevation of AFP levels after remission suggests tumor recurrence.
- In hepatocellular carcinoma, a gradual decrease in serum AFP levels indicates a favorable response to therapy. In germ cell tumors, serum AFP levels and serum human chorionic gonadotropin levels should be measured concurrently.

Interfering factors

- Hemolysis from rough handling of the sample
- Multiple pregnancies (possible false-positive)

Alpha-subunit of pituitary glycoprotein hormones

Overview

○ Measures the alpha-subunit of the pituitary glycoprotein hormones (alpha-PGH). These hormones (thyroid-stimulating hormone [TSH] and human chorionic gonadotropin) contain similar alpha-subunits but differ in their beta-subunits.

Purpose

○ To aid in the diagnosis of recurrent pituitary tumors in the patient who has undergone resection

Procedure

Preparation

○ Explain to the patient that this test helps assess pituitary function.
○ Inform the patient that he need not fast.
○ Tell the patient that the test requires a blood sample. Explain who will perform the venipuncture and when.
○ Explain to the patient that he may experience slight discomfort from the tourniquet and the needle puncture.

Implementation

○ Perform a venipuncture and collect the sample in a 5ml clot-activator tube.
○ Send the sample to the laboratory immediately.
○ Handle the sample gently to prevent hemolysis.
○ Indicate the patient's sex on the laboratory request.

Patient care

○ Apply direct pressure to the venipuncture site until bleeding stops.

Complications

○ Hematoma at the venipuncture site

Interpretation

Normal results

○ Less than or equal to 1.2 nanograms/ml (SI, 1.2 µg/L)

Abnormal results

○ Low levels of alpha-PGH appear in the patient with inadequate pituitary hormone production. Hypopituitarism results in reduced follicle-stimulating hormone, luteinizing hormone, and TSH levels.
○ Elevated alpha-PGH levels indicate recurrent pituitary tumors or ineffective treatment.

Interfering factors

○ Hemolysis from rough handling of the sample

Alveolar-to-arterial oxygen gradient

Overview

- Uses calculations based on the patient's laboratory values to help identify the cause of hypoxemia and intrapulmonary shunting by approximating the partial pressure of oxygenation of the alveoli and arteries
- May help differentiate the cause of ventilated alveoli but not perfusion, unventilated alveoli with perfusion, or collapse of the alveoli and capillaries

Purpose

- To evaluate the efficiency of gas exchange
- To assess the integrity of the ventilatory control system
- To monitor respiratory therapy

Procedure

Preparation

- Explain to the patient that the test evaluates how well the lungs are delivering oxygen to the blood and eliminating carbon dioxide.
- Tell the patient that the test requires a blood sample. Explain who will perform the arterial puncture and when.
- Inform the patient that he need not restrict food and fluids.
- Instruct the patient to breathe normally during the test, and warn him that he may experience cramping or throbbing pain at the puncture site.

Implementation

- Perform an arterial puncture or draw blood from an arterial line using a heparinized blood gas syringe.
- Eliminate all air from the sample and place it on ice immediately.
- Before sending the sample to the laboratory, note on the laboratory request whether the patient was breathing room air or receiving oxygen therapy when the sample was collected.
- If the patient was receiving oxygen therapy, note the flow rate and method of delivery. If he was on a ventilator, note the fraction of inspired oxygen, tidal volume, mode, respiratory rate, and positive end-expiratory pressure.
- Note the patient's rectal temperature.

Patient care

- Apply pressure to the puncture for 3 to 5 minutes or until bleeding has stopped.
- Place a gauze pad over the site and tape it in place, but don't tape the entire circumference.

- Monitor vital signs and observe for signs of circulatory impairment, such as swelling, discoloration, pain, numbness, and tingling in the bandaged arm or leg.

Complications

- Bleeding from the puncture site

Interpretation

Normal results

- Alveolar-to-arterial oxygen gradient ($A\text{-}aDo_2$) at rest in room air is < 10 mm Hg; at maximum exercise, 20 to 30 mm Hg.

Abnormal results

- Increased values may result from mucus plugs, bronchospasm, or airway collapse (asthma, bronchitis, emphysema).
- Hypoxemia results in increased $A\text{-}aDo_2$ and may result from arterial septal defects, pneumothorax, atelectasis, emboli, or edema.

Interfering factors

- Failure to heparinize the syringe, place the sample in an iced bag, or send the sample to the laboratory immediately
- Exposing the sample to air (increase or decrease)
- Age and increasing oxygen concentration (increase)

Ammonia, plasma

Overview

○ Measures plasma levels of ammonia, a nonprotein nitrogen compound that helps maintain acidbase balance
○ In such diseases as cirrhosis of the liver, ammonia can bypass the liver and accumulate in the blood
○ Plasma ammonia levels may help indicate the severity of hepatocellular damage

Purpose

○ To help monitor the progression of severe hepatic disease and the effectiveness of therapy
○ To recognize impending or established hepatic coma

Procedure

Preparation

○ Explain to the patient (or to a family member if the patient is comatose) that the plasma ammonia test is used to evaluate liver function.
○ Tell the patient that the test requires a blood sample. Explain who will perform the venipuncture and when.
○ Inform the patient that he may experience slight discomfort from the tourniquet and the needle puncture.
○ Notify the laboratory and physician of drugs the patient is taking that may affect the test results; it may be necessary to restrict them.

Implementation

○ Notify the laboratory before performing the venipuncture so that preliminary preparations can begin.
○ Perform a venipuncture and collect the sample in a 10-ml heparinized tube.
○ Handle the sample gently to prevent hemolysis, pack it in ice, and send it to the laboratory immediately.
○ Don't use a chilled container.

Patient care

○ Apply direct pressure to the venipuncture site until bleeding stops.

Complications

○ Hematoma at the venipuncture site
○ Signs of impending or established hepatic coma if plasma ammonia levels are high

Interpretation

Normal results

○ In adults, 15 to 45 μg/dl (SI, 11 to 32 μmol/L)

Abnormal results

○ Elevated plasma ammonia levels are common in severe hepatic disease, such as cirrhosis and acute hepatic necrosis, and can lead to hepatic coma.
○ Elevated levels may also occur in Reye's syndrome, severe heart failure, GI hemorrhage, and erythroblastosis fetalis.

Interfering factors

○ Hemolysis from rough handling of the sample
○ Delay in testing
○ Acetazolamide, thiazides, ammonium salts, and furosemide (increase)
○ Parenteral nutrition or a portacaval shunt (possible increase)
○ Lactulose, neomycin, and kanamycin (decrease)
○ Smoking, poor venipuncture technique, and exposure to ammonia cleaners in the laboratory (possible increase)

Amniotic fluid analysis

Overview

○ Indicated if the patient is over age 35; has a family history of genetic, chromosomal, or neural tube defects; or has had a miscarriage
○ Test repetition if test results are abnormal or tissue cultures fail to grow

Purpose

○ To detect fetal abnormalities, particularly chromosomal and neural tube defects
○ To detect hemolytic disease of the neonate
○ To diagnose metabolic disorders, amino acid disorders, and mucopolysaccharidosis
○ To determine fetal age and maturity
○ To assess fetal health by detecting the presence of meconium or blood or measuring amniotic levels of estriol and fetal thyroid hormone
○ To identify fetal gender when one or both parents are carriers of a sex-linked disorder

Procedure

Preparation

○ Explain procedure and answer patient's questions.
○ Inform the patient that she need not restrict food and fluids.
○ Explain to the patient that she'll feel a stinging sensation when the local anesthetic is injected.
○ Ask the patient to void just before the test to minimize the risk of puncturing the bladder.

Implementation

○ After determining fetal and placental position, a pool of amniotic fluid is located, usually through palpation and ultrasonic visualization.
○ The skin is prepared with antiseptic and alcohol, and 1 ml of 1% lidocaine is injected with a 25G needle, first intradermally and then subcutaneously.
○ A 20G spinal needle with a stylet is inserted into the amniotic cavity and the stylet is withdrawn.
○ A 10-ml syringe is attached to the needle; then the fluid is aspirated and placed in an amber or a foil-covered test tube.
○ The needle is withdrawn and an adhesive bandage placed over the needle insertion site.
○ The fetal heart rate and maternal vital signs are monitored every 15 minutes for at least 30 minutes.

Patient care

○ Before the patient is discharged, instruct her to immediately report abdominal pain or cramping, chills, fever, vaginal bleeding or leakage of serous vaginal fluid, or fetal hyperactivity or unusual fetal lethargy.

Complications

○ Spontaneous abortion, fetal or placental trauma, bleeding, premature labor, infection, and Rh sensitization from fetal bleeding into maternal circulation

Interpretation

Normal results

○ Normal amniotic fluid is clear but may contain white flecks of vernix caseosa when the fetus is near term.

Abnormal results

○ "Port wine" fluid may be a sign of abruptio placentae, and blood of fetal origin may indicate damage to the fetal, placental, or umbilical cord vessels by the amniocentesis needle.
○ Large amounts of bilirubin may indicate hemolytic disease of the neonate.
○ Meconium in the amniotic fluid produces a peak of 410 mµ on the spectrophotometric analysis. If meconium is present during labor, the neonate's nose and throat require thorough cleaning to prevent meconium aspiration.
○ High amniotic fluid levels indicate neural tube defects; the alpha-fetoprotein level (AFP) may remain normal if a defect is small and closed.
○ Elevated AFP levels may result from a multiple pregnancy; from an omphalocele, congenital nephrosis, esophageal or duodenal atresia, cystic fibrosis, exomphalos, Turner's syndrome, and fetal bladder neck obstruction with hydronephrosis; and from an impending fetal death.
○ Severe erythroblastosis fetalis, familial hyperuricemia, and Lesch-Nyhan syndrome tend to increase the uric acid level; severe erythroblastosis fetalis decreases the estriol level.
○ The lecithin-to-sphingomyelin (L/S) ratio confirms fetal pulmonary maturity (L/S ratio > 2) or suggests a risk of respiratory distress (L/S ratio < 2).
○ A glucose level greater than 45 mg/dl indicates poor maternal and fetal control.
○ Elevated acetylcholinesterase levels may occur with neural tube defects, exomphalos, and other serious malformations.

Interfering factors

○ Use of plastic disposable syringes (toxicity to amniotic fluid cells)
○ Failure to place the specimen in an appropriate amber or foil-covered tube (possible decrease in bilirubin)
○ Blood or meconium in the fluid (effect on L/S ratio)
○ Maternal blood in the fluid (possible decrease in creatinine)
○ Any amount of fetal blood in the fluid specimen (possible doubling of AFP concentrations)
○ Infectious mononucleosis, cirrhosis, hepatic cancer, teratoma, endodermal sinus tumor, gastric carcinoma, pancreatic carcinoma, and subacute hereditary tyrosinemia (possible increase in AFP)

Amsler's grid

Overview

- Easiest test for central field deficits caused by macular degeneration
- Composed of a central black dot and horizontal and vertical lines that form 5-mm squares, grid helps find central scotomas — blind or partially blind spots in the macular area of the retina
- Detects microscopic areas of macular or perimacular edema that cause visual distortions
- Only a screening test; must be supplemented by other tests, such as ophthalmoscopy, visual field testing, and fluorescein angiography, to determine the cause of abnormal vision

Purpose

- To detect central scotomas
- To evaluate the stability or progression of macular disease

Procedure

Preparation

- Explain to the patient that this test evaluates his central field of vision and takes 5 to 10 minutes to perform.
- If the patient normally wears corrective lenses, instruct him to keep them on during the test.

Implementation

- Occlude one of the patient's eyes and hold Amsler's grid at his customary reading distance, about 11″ to 12″ (28 to 30.5 cm) in front of the unoccluded eye.
- Tell the patient to stare at the central dot on the grid and then ask these questions: Can you see the black dot in the center? When you look directly at the dot, can you see all four sides of the grid? All of the little squares? Do all the lines appear ruler-straight? Is there any blurring, distortion, or movement?
- If the patient answers yes to any of these questions, ask him to elaborate.
- Give him a pencil and paper, and encourage him to outline and describe the specific areas that appear distorted.
- After recording the patient's observations, occlude the other eye and repeat the procedure.
- Remind the patient to keep his unoccluded eye fixed on the central black dot on the grid.
- Perform this test before dilating the patient's pupils and performing a funduscopic examination or the refraction test.

Patient care

- Support the patient throughout testing.

Complications

None known

Interpretation

Normal results

- Patient should be able to see the central black dot and, while staring at the dot, all four sides of the grid and all the small squares. All the lines should appear ruler-straight. He shouldn't see blurring, distortion, or missing squares. (See *Amsler's grid: Normal and abnormal views.*)

Abnormal results

- The inability to see the black dot in the center of the grid suggests a central scotoma.
- If any of the lines don't appear ruler-straight to the patient, metamorphopsia (distorted perception of objects) may be indicated.
- Blurring, distortion, or movement may signal an imminent scotoma.
- Further evaluation by ophthalmoscopy, visual field testing, and fluorescein angiography is needed for abnormal findings.

Interfering factors

- Inability to see grid because of poor eyesight, lack of cooperation, or failure to keep unoccluded eye fixed on central dot
- Bleaching of retina with bright light of retinoscope or ophthalmoscope before the test, impairing the ability to see the grid

Amsler's grid: Normal and abnormal views

The illustration on the left shows a normal view of Amsler's grid. The illustration on the right shows a grid as it might look to a patient with a central scotoma caused by a macular hole. The center dot is entirely absent, as are the lines around it. The lines of the periphery of the scotoma appear bowed asymmetrically.

NORMAL VIEW   ABNORMAL VIEW

Amylase, serum

Overview

○ Most important laboratory test in patients suspected of having acute pancreatic disease

Purpose

○ To diagnose acute pancreatitis
○ To distinguish between acute pancreatitis and other causes of abdominal pain that require immediate surgery
○ To evaluate possible pancreatic injury caused by abdominal trauma or surgery

Procedure

Preparation

○ Explain to the patient that this test assesses pancreatic function.
○ Tell the patient that this test requires a blood sample. Explain who will perform the venipuncture and when.
○ Inform the patient that he may experience slight discomfort from the tourniquet and the needle puncture.
○ Inform the patient that he need not fast before the test but must abstain from alcohol.
○ Notify the laboratory and physician of drugs the patient is taking that may affect test results; it may be necessary to restrict them.

Implementation

○ Perform a venipuncture and collect the sample in a 4-ml clot-activator tube.
○ If the patient has severe abdominal pain, draw the sample before diagnostic or therapeutic intervention. For accurate results, it's important to obtain an early sample.
○ Handle the sample gently to prevent hemolysis.

Patient care

○ Apply direct pressure to the venipuncture site until bleeding stops.
○ Instruct the patient that he may resume medications stopped before the test.

Complications

○ Hematoma at the venipuncture site

Interpretation

Normal results

○ 26 to 102 units/L (SI, 0.4 to 1.74 µkat/L) for adults ages 18 and older

Abnormal results

○ After the onset of acute pancreatitis, amylase levels begin to rise within 2 hours, peak within 12 to 48 hours, and return to normal within 3 to 4 days.
○ Determination of urine levels should follow normal serum amylase results to rule out pancreatitis.
○ Moderate serum elevations may accompany obstruction of the common bile duct, pancreatic duct, or ampulla of Vater; pancreatic injury from a perforated peptic ulcer; pancreatic cancer; and acute salivary gland disease.
○ Impaired kidney function may increase serum levels.
○ Levels may be slightly elevated in a patient who's asymptomatic or responding unusually to therapy.
○ Decreased levels can occur in patients with chronic pancreatitis, pancreatic cancer, cirrhosis, hepatitis, and toxemia of pregnancy.

Interfering factors

○ Hemolysis from rough handling of the sample
○ Ingestion of ethyl alcohol in large amounts (possible false-high)
○ Aminosalicylic acid, asparaginase, azathioprine, corticosteroids, cyproheptadine, narcotic analgesics, hormonal contraceptives, rifampin, sulfasalazine, and thiazide or loop diuretics (possible false-high)
○ Recent peripancreatic surgery, perforated ulcer or intestine, abscess, spasm of the sphincter of Oddi or, rarely, macroamylasemia (possible false-high)

Amylase, urine

Overview

○ Method for determining urine amylase levels; the dye-coupled starch method.

Purpose

○ To diagnose acute pancreatitis when serum amylase levels are normal or borderline
○ To aid in the diagnosis of chronic pancreatitis and salivary gland disorders

Procedure

Preparation

○ Explain to the patient that this test evaluates the function of the pancreas and the salivary glands.
○ Inform the patient that he need not restrict food and fluids.
○ Tell the patient that the test requires urine collection for 2, 6, 8, or 24 hours, and teach him how to collect a timed specimen.
○ Instruct the patient to empty his bladder and then begin timing the collection.
○ Notify the laboratory and physician of drugs the patient is taking that may affect test results; it may be necessary to restrict them.

Implementation

○ Collect the patient's urine during a 2-, 6-, 8-, or 24-hour period.
○ A 2-hour test is usually performed because collecting urine for a 2-hour period produces fewer errors than a more diagnostic 24-hour collection.
○ Cover and refrigerate the specimen during the collection period.
○ If the patient is catheterized, keep the collection bag on ice.
○ Send the specimen on ice to the laboratory as soon as the test is complete.

Patient care

○ Instruct the patient not to contaminate the specimen with toilet tissue or stool.

Complications

None known

Interpretation

Normal results

○ Urine amylase is reported in various units of measure, so values differ among laboratories. The Mayo Clinic reports normal urinary excretion of 1 to 17 units/hour (SI, 0.017 to 0.29 µkat/hour).

Abnormal results

○ Level increases in acute pancreatitis; obstruction of the pancreatic duct, intestines, or salivary duct; cancer of the head of the pancreas; mumps; acute injury of the spleen; renal disease, with impaired absorption; perforated peptic or duodenal ulcers; and gallbladder disease.
○ Level decreases in chronic pancreatitis, cachexia, alcoholism, liver cancer, cirrhosis, hepatitis, and hepatic abscess.

Interfering factors

○ Salivary amylase in the urine caused by coughing or talking over the sample (possible increase)
○ Failure to collect all urine during the test period, properly store the specimen, or send the specimen to the laboratory immediately after the collection is complete
○ High levels of bacterial contamination of the specimen or blood in the urine
○ Morphine, meperidine, codeine, pentazocine, bethanechol, thiazide diuretics, indomethacin, or alcohol within 24 hours of the test (possible increase)
○ Fluorides (possible decrease)

Androstenedione

Overview

○ Helps identify disorders related to altered hormone levels, such as female virilization syndromes and polycystic ovary (Stein-Leventhal) syndrome
○ Tumors of the ovaries or adrenal glands can secrete excessive amounts of androstenedione, which then converts to testosterone, resulting in virilizing symptoms, such as hirsutism and sterility

Purpose

○ To help determine the cause of gonadal dysfunction, menstrual or menopausal irregularities, virilizing symptoms, and premature sexual development

Procedure

Preparation

○ Explain to the patient that this test will help determine the cause of her symptoms.
○ Tell the patient that the test requires a blood sample. Explain who will perform the venipuncture and when.
○ Explain to the patient that she may experience slight discomfort from the tourniquet and the needle puncture.
○ Explain that the test should occur 1 week before or after her menstrual period and that it may be necessary to repeat it.
○ Withhold steroid and pituitary-based hormones. If the patient must continue them, note this on the laboratory request.

Implementation

○ Perform a venipuncture and collect a serum sample in a 7-ml clot-activator tube or collect a plasma sample in a green-top tube. If a plasma sample is taken, refrigerate it or place it on ice.
○ Label the sample appropriately and send it to the laboratory immediately.
○ Handle the sample gently to prevent hemolysis.
○ Record the patient's age, sex, and (if appropriate) phase of her menstrual cycle on the laboratory request.

Patient care

○ Apply direct pressure to the venipuncture site until bleeding stops.
○ Instruct the patient that she may resume medications stopped before the test.

Complications

○ Hematoma at the venipuncture site

Interpretation

Normal results

○ Females, 85 to 275 nanograms/dl (SI, 3.0 to 9.6 nmol/L)
○ Males, 75 to 205 nanograms/dl (SI, 2.6 to 7.2 nmol/L)

Abnormal results

○ Elevated androstenedione levels are linked to polycystic ovary (Stein-Leventhal) syndrome; Cushing's syndrome; ovarian, testicular, and adrenocortical tumors; ectopic corticotropin-producing tumors; late-onset congenital adrenal hyperplasia; and ovarian stromal hyperplasia.
○ Elevated levels result in increased estrone levels, causing premature sexual development in children; menstrual irregularities in premenopausal women; bleeding, endometriosis, and polycystic ovaries in postmenopausal women; and feminizing signs, such as gynecomastia, in men.
○ Decreased levels occur in patients with hypogonadism.

Interfering factors

○ Hemolysis from rough handling of the sample
○ Steroids and pituitary hormones (possible increase)

Angiotensin-converting enzyme

Overview

○ Measures serum levels of angiotensin-converting enzyme (ACE), which is found in lung capillaries and, in lesser concentrations, blood vessels and kidney tissue
○ Monitors response to treatment in sarcoidosis and helps confirm a diagnosis of Gaucher's disease or leprosy

Purpose

○ To aid diagnosis of sarcoidosis, especially pulmonary sarcoidosis
○ To monitor the patient's response to therapy in sarcoidosis
○ To help confirm Gaucher's disease or Hansen's disease

Procedure

Preparation

○ Inform the patient that he must fast for 12 hours before the test.
○ Explain to the patient that he may experience slight discomfort from the tourniquet and the needle puncture.
○ Note the patient's age on the laboratory request. If he's under age 20, the test may have to be postponed because a person under age 20 has variable ACE levels.

Implementation

○ Perform a venipuncture and collect the sample in a 7-ml clot-activator tube.
○ Avoid using a tube with ethylenediaminetetraacetic acid (EDTA) because this can decrease ACE levels, altering test results.
○ Handle the sample gently to prevent hemolysis.
○ Send the sample to the laboratory immediately or freeze it and place it on dry ice until the time of testing.

Patient care

○ Apply direct pressure to the venipuncture site until bleeding stops.

Complications

○ Hematoma at the venipuncture site

Interpretation

Normal results

○ In the colorimetric assay, normal results for serum ACE in patients age 20 and older range from 8 to 52 units/L (SI, 0.14 to 0.88 μkat/L).

Abnormal results

○ Elevated serum ACE levels may indicate sarcoidosis, Gaucher's disease, or Hansen's disease, but results must be correlated with the patient's clinical condition.
○ In some cases, elevated ACE levels may result from hyperthyroidism, diabetic retinopathy, or hepatic disease.
○ Serum ACE levels decline as the patient responds to steroid or prednisone therapy for sarcoidosis.

Interfering factors

○ Failure to fast before the test (may cause significant lipemia of the sample)
○ Use of a collection tube with EDTA (possible decrease)
○ Hemolysis from rough handling of the sample
○ Failure to send the sample to the laboratory at once or to freeze it and place it on dry ice (possible false-low from ACE degradation)

Anion gap

Overview

○ Cation and anion levels are usually equal, making serum electrically neutral. Measuring the gap between measured cation and anion levels provides information about the level of anions (including sulfate; phosphate; organic acids, such as ketone bodies and lactic acid; and proteins) that aren't routinely measured in laboratory tests.
○ In metabolic acidosis, test helps identify the type of acidosis and possible causes.
○ Determining the specific cause of metabolic acidosis usually requires further tests.

Purpose

○ To distinguish types of metabolic acidosis
○ To monitor renal function and total parenteral nutrition

Procedure

Preparation

○ Explain to the patient that the anion gap test determines the cause of acidosis.
○ Tell the patient that a blood sample is needed. Explain who will perform the venipuncture and when.
○ Tell the patient that he may experience slight discomfort from the tourniquet and the needle puncture.
○ Tell patient that he need not restrict food and fluids.
○ Notify the laboratory and physician of drugs the patient is taking that may affect test results; it may be necessary to restrict them.

Implementation

○ Perform a venipuncture and collect the sample in a 3- or 4-ml clot-activator tube.
○ Handle the sample gently to prevent hemolysis.

Patient care

○ Apply direct pressure to the venipuncture site until bleeding stops.
○ Instruct the patient to resume medications stopped before the test.

Complications

○ Hematoma at the venipuncture site

Interpretation

Normal results

○ 8 to 14 mEq/L (SI, 8 to 14 mmol/L)

Abnormal results

○ An increased anion gap indicates an increase in one or more of the unmeasured anions: sulfate; phos-

---

Anion gap and metabolic acidosis

Metabolic acidosis with a normal anion gap (8 to 14 mEq/L) occurs when bicarbonate is lost, such as:
● hypokalemic acidosis caused by renal tubular acidosis, diarrhea, or ureteral diversions
● hyperkalemic acidosis caused by acidifying agents (for example, ammonium chloride, hydrochloric acid), hydronephrosis, or sickle cell nephropathy.
Metabolic acidosis with an *increased anion gap* (greater than 14 mEq/L) occurs when organic acids, sulfates, or phosphates accumulate, such as:
● renal failure
● ketoacidosis caused by starvation, diabetes mellitus, or alcohol abuse
● lactic acidosis
● ingestion of toxins, such as salicylates, methanol, ethylene glycol (antifreeze), and paraldehyde.

---

phates; organic acids, such as ketone bodies and lactic acid; and proteins. This may occur with acidoses that are characterized by excessive organic or inorganic acids, such as lactic acidosis or ketoacidosis.
○ Acidosis from an accumulation of metabolic acids (for example, in lactic acidosis) increases the anion gap (> 14 mEq/L) because unmeasured anion level increases. Metabolic acidosis resulting from this accumulation is called *high anion gap acidosis.*
○ A decreased anion gap is rare but may occur with hypermagnesemia and paraproteinemic states, such as multiple myeloma and Waldenström's macroglobulinemia. (See *Anion gap and metabolic acidosis.*)

Interfering factors

○ Hemolysis from rough handling of the sample
○ Diuretics, lithium, chlorpropamide, and vasopressin (possible decrease from decreased sodium level)
○ Corticosteroids and antihypertensives (possible increase from increased sodium level)
○ Salicylates, paraldehyde, methicillin, dimercaprol, ammonium chloride, acetazolamide, ethylene glycol, and methyl alcohol (possible increase from decreased bicarbonate level)
○ Adrenocorticotropic hormone, cortisone, mercurial or chlorothiazide diuretics, and excessive ingestion of alkali or licorice (possible decrease from increased bicarbonate level)
○ Ammonium chloride, cholestyramine, boric acid, oxyphenbutazone, phenylbutazone, and excessive I.V. infusion of sodium chloride (possible decrease from increased chloride level)
○ Thiazide diuretics, ethacrynic acid, furosemide, bicarbonates, and prolonged I.V. infusion of dextrose 5% in water (possible increase from decreased chloride level)
○ Iodine absorption from povidone-iodine–packed wounds or from overuse of antacids containing magnesium, especially by patients with renal failure (possible false-low)

Antegrade pyelograph

Overview

○ Examines the upper collecting system when ureteral obstruction rules out retrograde ureteropyelography or when cystoscopy is contraindicated
○ Depends on percutaneous needle puncture for injection of contrast medium into the renal pelvis or calyces
○ Allows measurement of renal pressure
○ Collection of urine facilitates cultures, cytologic studies, and evaluation of the renal functional reserve before surgery

Purpose

○ To evaluate obstruction of the upper collecting system by stricture, calculus, clot, or tumor
○ To evaluate hydronephrosis revealed during excretory urography or ultrasonography and to enable placement of a percutaneous nephrostomy tube
○ To evaluate the function of the upper collecting system after ureteral surgery or urinary diversion
○ To assess renal functional reserve before surgery

Procedure

Preparation

○ Explain the procedure to the patient.
○ Tell the patient that he may need to fast for 6 to 8 hours before the test.
○ Explain that the test involves insertion of a needle into the kidney after the patient receives a sedative and local anesthetic. Explain that urine may be collected from the kidney for testing and that, if necessary, a tube will be left in the kidney for drainage.
○ Tell the patient that he may feel mild discomfort during injection of the local anesthetic and contrast medium and that he may also feel transient burning and flushing from the contrast medium.
○ Check the patient's history for hypersensitivity reactions to contrast media, iodine, or shellfish. Mark sensitivities clearly on the chart. Also check his history and recent coagulation studies for indications of bleeding disorders.
○ Give the patient a sedative just before the procedure, if needed, and check that pretest blood work has been performed, if ordered.

Implementation

○ The patient is placed in a prone position on the X-ray table. The skin over the kidney is cleaned with antiseptic solution and a local anesthetic injected.
○ Previous urographic films or ultrasound recordings are studied for anatomic landmarks. (If the kidney in question isn't in the normal position, the angle of needle entry may be adjusted during percutaneous puncture.)
○ Under guidance of fluoroscopy or ultrasonography, the percutaneous needle is inserted below the 12th rib at the level of the transverse process of the 2nd lumbar vertebra. Aspiration of urine confirms that the needle has reached the dilated collecting system; $2\frac{3}{4}''$ to $3\frac{1}{8}''$ (7 to 8 cm) below the skin surface in adults.
○ Flexible tubing is connected to the needle to prevent displacement during the procedure. If intrarenal pressure is to be measured, the manometer is connected to the tubing as soon as it's in place. Urine specimens are taken, if needed.
○ An amount of urine equal to the amount of contrast medium to be injected is withdrawn to prevent overdistention of the collecting system.
○ The contrast medium is injected under fluoroscopic guidance. Ureteral peristalsis is observed to evaluate obstruction.
○ A percutaneous nephrostomy tube is inserted if drainage is needed because of increased renal pressure, dilation, or intrarenal reflux.

Patient care

○ Check the patient's vital signs every 15 minutes for the first hour, every 30 minutes for the second hour, and then every 2 hours for the next 24 hours.
○ During each vital signs check, inspect the dressings for bleeding, hematoma, or urine leakage at the puncture site.
○ Report urine leakage or the patient's failure to void within 8 hours.
○ Monitor the patient's fluid intake and urine output for 24 hours.
○ Observe each specimen for hematuria. Report hematuria if it persists after the third voiding.
○ If a nephrostomy tube is inserted, make sure it's patent and draining well. Irrigate, to maintain patency.
○ Give prescribed antibiotics for several days after the procedure, along with prescribed analgesics.
○ If hydronephrosis is present, monitor intake and output, edema, hypertension, flank pain, acid-base status, and glucose level.

Complications

○ If bleeding occurs at the puncture site, apply pressure.
○ For a hematoma, apply warm soaks.
○ Watch for and report signs of sepsis or extravasation of contrast.

ALERT *Watch for and report signs that adjacent organs have been punctured, such as pain in the abdomen or flank or pneumothorax.*

○ Watch for signs of hypersensitivity to the contrast medium.

Interpretation

Normal results

○ The upper collecting system fills uniformly and appears normal in size and course. Normal structures are clearly outlined.

Abnormal results

○ Enlargements of the upper collecting system and parts of the ureteropelvic junction indicate obstruction.
○ In hydronephrosis, the ureteropelvic junction shows marked distention.
○ Intrarenal pressure greater than 20 cm H_2O indicates obstruction.

Interfering factors

○ Recent barium procedures; stool or gas in the bowel
○ An obese patient (possible difficulty in needle placement)

Antibody screening

Overview

- Also called the *indirect Coombs' test*
- Detects unexpected circulating antibodies
- Detects 95% to 99% of the circulating antibodies

Purpose

- To detect unexpected circulating antibodies to red blood cell (RBC) antigens in the recipient's or donor's serum before transfusion
- To determine the presence of anti-D antibody in maternal blood
- To evaluate the need for Rho(D) immune globulin
- To aid in the diagnosis of acquired hemolytic anemia

Procedure

Preparation

- Explain to the prospective blood recipient that the antibody screening test helps evaluate the possibility of a transfusion reaction or determines whether fetal antibodies are in the patient's blood and whether treatment is necessary.
- If the test is for a patient who's anemic, explain to him that it helps identify the type of anemia.
- Inform the patient that he need not restrict food and fluids.
- Tell the patient that the test requires a blood sample. Explain who will perform the venipuncture and when.
- Explain to the patient that he may experience slight discomfort from the tourniquet and the needle puncture.
- Check the patient's history for recent administration of blood, dextran, or I.V. contrast media.

Implementation

- Perform a venipuncture and collect the sample in two 10-ml tubes. If the antibody screen is positive, antibody identification is performed on the blood.
- Handle the sample gently to prevent hemolysis.
- Label the sample with the patient's name, the hospital or blood bank number, the date, and the phlebotomist's initials. Be sure to include on the laboratory request the patient's diagnosis and pregnancy status, history of transfusions, and current drug therapy.
- Send the sample to the laboratory immediately.

Patient care

- Apply direct pressure to the venipuncture site until bleeding stops.

Complications

- Hematoma at the venipuncture site

Interpretation

Normal results

- Agglutination doesn't occur, indicating that the patient's serum contains no circulating antibodies other than anti-A or anti-B.

Abnormal results

- A positive result indicates the presence of unexpected circulating antibodies to RBC antigens, which demonstrates donor and recipient incompatibility.
- A positive result in a pregnant patient with Rh-negative blood may indicate the presence of antibodies to the Rh factor from an earlier transfusion with incompatible blood or from a previous pregnancy with an Rh-positive fetus.

✺ *AGE AWARE A positive result indicates that the fetus may develop hemolytic disease of the newborn. As a result, repeated testing throughout the pregnancy is necessary to evaluate the development of circulating antibody levels.*

Interfering factors

- Previous administration of dextran or I.V. contrast media (causing aggregation resembling agglutination)
- Hemolysis from rough handling of the sample
- Blood transfusion or pregnancy within the past 3 months (possible presence of antibodies)

Anti-deoxyribonucleic acid antibodies

Overview

○ Serum anti–double-stranded deoxyribonucleic acid (dsDNA) levels are directly related to the extent of renal or vascular damage caused by the disease.
○ This test measures and differentiates these antibody levels in a serum sample, using radioimmunoassay, agglutination, complement fixation, or immunoelectrophoresis.
○ If antibodies are present, they combine with native DNA and form complexes that are too large to pass through a membrane filter. The test counts these oversized complexes.

Purpose

○ To confirm a diagnosis of systemic lupus erythematosus (SLE)
○ To monitor the SLE patient's response to therapy and determine his prognosis

Procedure

Preparation

○ Explain to the patient that this test helps diagnose and determine the appropriate therapy for SLE.
○ Inform the patient that he need not restrict food and fluids.
○ Tell the patient that the test requires a blood sample. Explain who will perform the venipuncture and when.
○ Explain to the patient that he may experience slight discomfort from the tourniquet and needle puncture.
○ Ask the patient if he has had a recent radioactive test; if so, note this on the laboratory request.

Implementation

○ Perform a venipuncture and collect the sample in a 7-ml tube without additives. Some laboratories may specify a tube with either ethylenediaminetetraacetic acid or sodium fluoride and potassium oxalate added.
○ Handle the sample gently to prevent hemolysis.

Patient care

○ Apply direct pressure to the venipuncture site until bleeding stops.

Complications

○ Hematoma at the venipuncture site

Interpretation

Normal results

○ An anti-dsDNA antibody level less than 25 IU/ml (SI, < 25 kIU/L) is considered negative for SLE.

Abnormal results

○ Elevated anti-dsDNA antibody levels may indicate SLE.
○ Values of 25 to 30 IU/ml (SI, 25 to 30 kIU/L) are considered borderline positive.
○ Values of 31 to 200 IU/ml (SI, 31 to 200 kIU/L) are positive, and those greater than 200 IU/ml (SI, > 200 kIU/L) are strongly positive.
○ Depressed levels may follow immunosuppressive therapy, demonstrating effective treatment of SLE.

Interfering factors

○ A radioactive scan performed within 1 week before sample collection
○ Hemolysis from rough handling of the sample

Antidiuretic hormone, serum

Overview

- Rare quantitative analysis of serum antidiuretic hormone (ADH) levels, may identify diabetes insipidus and other causes of severe homeostatic imbalance
- May be part of dehydration or hypertonic saline infusion testing to determine the body's response to hyperosmolality

Purpose

- To aid in the differential diagnosis of pituitary diabetes insipidus, nephrogenic diabetes insipidus (congenital or familial), and syndrome of inappropriate antidiuretic hormone (SIADH)

Procedure

Preparation

- Explain to the patient that this test, which measures hormonal secretion levels, may aid in identifying the cause of his symptoms.
- Instruct the patient to fast and limit physical activity for 10 to 12 hours before the test.
- Tell the patient that the test requires a blood sample. Explain who will perform the venipuncture and when.
- Explain to the patient that he may experience slight discomfort from the tourniquet and needle puncture.
- Withhold drugs that may cause SIADH before the test. If the patient must continue them, note this on the laboratory request.
- Make sure the patient is relaxed and recumbent for 30 minutes before the test.

Implementation

- Perform a venipuncture and collect the sample in a plastic collection tube (without additives) or a chilled ethylenediaminetetraacetic acid tube.
- Immediately send the sample to the laboratory, where serum must be separated from the clot within 10 minutes.
- Perform a serum osmolality test at the same time to help interpret the results.
- Make sure you use a syringe and collection tube made of plastic because the fragile ADH degrades on contact with glass.

Patient care

- Apply direct pressure to the venipuncture site until bleeding stops.
- Instruct the patient that he may resume his usual diet, activities, and medications that were stopped before the test.

Complications

- Hematoma at the venipuncture site

Interpretation

Normal results

- ADH values range from 1 to 5 pg/ml (SI, 1 to 5 mg/L).
- Level may also be evaluated in light of serum osmolality; if serum osmolality is less than 285 mOsm/kg, ADH is normally less than 2 pg/ml (SI, < 2 mg/L); if serum osmolality is greater than 290 mOsm/kg, ADH may range from 2 to 12 pg/ml (SI, 2 to 12 mg/L).

Abnormal results

- Absent or below-normal ADH levels indicate pituitary diabetes insipidus, resulting from a neurohypophyseal or hypothalamic tumor, viral infection, metastatic disease, sarcoidosis, tuberculosis, Hand-Schüller-Christian disease, syphilis, neurosurgical procedures, or head trauma.
- Normal ADH levels in the presence of signs of diabetes insipidus (such as polydipsia, polyuria, and hypotonic urine) may indicate the nephrogenic form of the disease, marked by renal tubular resistance to ADH; however, levels may rise if the pituitary gland tries to compensate.
- Elevated ADH levels may also indicate SIADH, possibly as a result of bronchogenic carcinoma, acute porphyria, hypothyroidism, Addison's disease, cirrhosis of the liver, infectious hepatitis, severe hemorrhage, or circulatory shock.

Interfering factors

- Failure to observe pretest restrictions
- Morphine, anesthetics, estrogen, oxytocin, chlorpropamide, vincristine, carbamazepine, cyclophosphamide, tranquilizers, hypnotics, lithium carbonate, and chlorothiazide (increase)
- Stress, pain, and positive-pressure ventilation (increase)
- Alcohol and negative-pressure ventilation (decrease)
- Radioactive scan performed within 1 week before the test
- Delay in sending sample to the laboratory

Anti-insulin antibodies

Overview

○ Detects insulin antibodies in the blood of a diabetic patient who takes insulin

Purpose

○ To determine insulin allergy
○ To confirm insulin resistance
○ To determine if hypoglycemia results from insulin overuse

Procedure

Preparation

○ Explain to the patient that this test determines the most appropriate treatment for his diabetes and determine whether he has insulin resistance or an allergy to insulin.
○ Tell the patient that the test requires a blood sample. Explain who will perform the venipuncture and when.
○ Explain to the patient that he may experience slight discomfort from the tourniquet and needle puncture.
○ Inform the patient that he need not restrict food and fluids.
○ Ask the patient if he has had a radioactive test recently; if so, note this on the laboratory request.

Implementation

○ Perform a venipuncture and collect the sample in a 7-ml tube without additives.
○ Handle the sample gently to prevent hemolysis.

Patient care

○ Apply direct pressure to the venipuncture site until bleeding stops.

Complications

○ Hematoma at the venipuncture site

Interpretation

Normal results

○ There should be less than 3% binding of the patient's serum with labeled beef, human, and pork insulin.

Abnormal results

○ Elevated levels may occur in insulin allergy or resistance and in factitious hypoglycemia.

Interfering factors

○ Radioactive test performed within 1 week before the test

Antimitochondrial antibodies

Overview

○ Detects antimitochondrial antibodies in serum by indirect immunofluorescence
○ Usually performed with the anti–smooth muscle antibodies test

Purpose

○ To aid in the diagnosis of primary biliary cirrhosis
○ To distinguish between extrahepatic jaundice and biliary cirrhosis

Procedure

Preparation

○ Explain to the patient that this test evaluates liver function.
○ Inform the patient that he need not restrict food and fluids.
○ Tell the patient that the test requires a blood sample. Explain who will perform the venipuncture and when.
○ Explain to the patient that he may experience slight discomfort from the tourniquet and needle puncture.
○ Check the patient's drug history for oxyphenisatin use and report it to the laboratory because it may produce antimitochondrial antibodies.

Implementation

○ Perform a venipuncture and collect the sample in a 7-ml tube with no additives.

Patient care

○ Because the patient with hepatic disease may bleed excessively, apply pressure to the venipuncture site until bleeding stops.

Complications

○ Hematoma at the venipuncture site

Interpretation

Normal results

○ Serum is normally negative for antimitochondrial antibodies.
○ Positive results are titered.

Abnormal results

○ Although antimitochondrial antibodies appear in 79% to 94% of patients with primary biliary cirrhosis, this test alone doesn't confirm the diagnosis. Further tests, such as serum alkaline phosphatase, serum bilirubin, aspartate aminotransferase, alanine aminotransferase and, possibly, liver biopsy or cholangiography, may also be necessary.
○ The autoantibodies also appear in some patients with chronic active hepatitis, drug-induced jaundice, and cryptogenic cirrhosis.
○ Antimitochondrial antibodies seldom appear in patients with extrahepatic biliary obstruction, and a positive test helps to rule out this condition.

Interfering factors

○ Confusion of antimitochondrial antibodies with heterophil antibodies, cardiolipin antibodies to syphilis, ribosomal antibodies, and microsomal hepatic or renal autoantibodies
○ Oxyphenisatin (possible false-positive results)

Antinuclear antibodies

Overview

○ Measures relative level of antinuclear antibodies (ANAs) in a serum sample through indirect immuno-fluorescence. Serial dilutions of serum are mixed with either Hep-2 or mouse kidney substrate.
○ If the serum contains ANAs, it forms antigen-antibody complexes with the substrate. After the preparation is mixed with fluorescein-labeled antihuman serum, it's examined under an ultraviolet microscope. If ANAs are present, the complex fluoresces.
○ Titer is taken at the greatest dilution that shows the reaction.

Purpose

○ To screen for systemic lupus erythematosus (SLE) (failure to detect ANAs essentially rules out active SLE)
○ To monitor the effectiveness of immunosuppressive therapy for SLE

Procedure

Preparation

○ Explain to the patient that this test evaluates the immune system and that further testing is usually required for diagnosis.
○ Inform the patient that it may be necessary to repeat the test to monitor his response to therapy.
○ Inform the patient that he need not restrict food and fluids.
○ Tell the patient that the test requires a blood sample. Explain who will perform the venipuncture and when.
○ Explain to the patient that he may experience slight discomfort from the tourniquet and needle puncture.
○ Check the patient's history for drugs that may affect test results, such as isoniazid and procainamide. Note findings on the laboratory request.

Implementation

○ Perform a venipuncture and collect the sample in a 7-ml tube without additives.

Patient care

○ Because a patient with an autoimmune disease has a compromised immune system, observe the venipuncture site for signs of infection, and report changes to the physician immediately.
○ Keep a clean, dry bandage over the site for at least 24 hours.
○ Apply direct pressure to the venipuncture site until bleeding stops.

Complications

○ Hematoma at the venipuncture site

Interpretation

Normal results

○ Test results are reported as positive (with pattern and serum titer noted) or negative.

Abnormal results

○ Low titers may occur in patients with viral diseases, chronic hepatic disease, collagen vascular disease, and autoimmune diseases and in some healthy adults; the incidence increases with age.
○ The higher the titer, the more specific the test is for SLE.
○ The pattern of nuclear fluorescence helps identify the type of immune disease present. A peripheral pattern almost exclusively indicates SLE because it shows the presence of anti-deoxyribonucleic acid (DNA) antibodies; sometimes anti-DNA antibodies are measured by radioimmunoassay if ANA titers are high or if a peripheral pattern occurs.
○ A homogeneous, or diffuse, pattern is also associated with SLE as well as with related connective tissue disorders; a nucleolar pattern, with scleroderma; and a speckled, irregular pattern, with infectious mononucleosis and mixed connective tissue disorders (for example, SLE and scleroderma).
○ A single serum sample, especially one collected from a patient with collagen vascular disease, may contain antibodies to several parts of the cell's nucleus.
○ In addition, as serum dilution increases, the fluorescent pattern may change because different antibodies are reactive at different titers.

Interfering factors

○ Most commonly isoniazid, hydralazine, and procainamide but also para-aminosalicylic acid, chlorpromazine, clofibrate, phenytoin, griseofulvin, ethosuximide, gold salts, methyldopa, hormonal contraceptives, penicillin, phenylbutazone, propylthiouracil, methysergide, streptomycin, sulfonamides, tetracyclines, mephenytoin, quinidine, primidone, reserpine, and trimethadione (possible production of a syndrome resembling SLE)

Anti–smooth muscle antibodies

Overview

○ Using indirect immunofluorescence, measures the relative level of anti–smooth muscle antibodies in serum; usually performed with the antimitochondrial antibodies test
○ The serum sample is exposed to a thin section of smooth muscle and incubated; then a fluorescent-labeled antiglobulin is added.
○ This antiglobulin binds only to antibodies that have complexed with smooth muscle and appear fluorescent when viewed through the microscope under ultraviolet light. (See *Serum antibodies in various disorders.*)

Purpose

○ To aid in the diagnosis of active chronic hepatitis and primary biliary cirrhosis

Procedure

Preparation

○ Explain to the patient that this test helps evaluate liver function.
○ Inform the patient that he need not restrict food and fluids.
○ Tell the patient that the test requires a blood sample. Explain who will perform the venipuncture and when.

○ Explain to the patient that he may experience slight discomfort from the tourniquet and needle puncture

Implementation

○ Perform a venipuncture and collect the sample in a 7-ml tube without additives.

Patient care

○ Because the patient with hepatic disease may bleed excessively, apply direct pressure to the venipuncture site until bleeding stops.

Complications

○ Hematoma at the venipuncture site

Interpretation

Normal results

○ A normal titer of anti-smooth-muscle antibodies is negative.
○ Positive results are titered.

Abnormal results

○ The test for anti–smooth muscle antibodies isn't specific; these antibodies appear in many patients with chronic active hepatitis and in fewer patients with primary biliary cirrhosis.
○ Anti–smooth muscle antibodies may also be present in patients with infectious mononucleosis, acute viral hepatitis, a malignant tumor of the liver, and intrinsic asthma.

Interfering factors

None significant

Serum antibodies in various disorders

This table shows the percentage of patients with certain disorders who have antimitochondrial or anti–smooth muscle antibodies in their serum. Patients with these antibodies in the serum need further testing to confirm the diagnosis. (Up to 1% of healthy people also show antimitochondrial antibodies.)

Disorder	Antimitochondrial antibodies	Anti–smooth muscle antibodies
Primary biliary cirrhosis	75% to 95%	0% to 50%*
Chronic active hepatitis	0% to 30%	50% to 80%
Extrahepatic biliary obstruction	0% to 5%	0%
Cryptogenic cirrhosis	0% to 25%	0% to 1%
Viral (infectious) hepatitis	0%	1% to 2%†
Drug-induced jaundice	50% to 80%	
Intrinsic asthma		20%
Rheumatoid arthritis and other collagen diseases	1% to 2%	
Systemic lupus erythematosus	3% to 5%††	0%

* In chronic disease, values fall at upper end of range.
† Much higher incidence occurs with hepatic damage.
†† Much higher incidence occurs with renal involvement.

Antistreptolysin-O

Overview

- Measures the relative levels of the antibody to streptolysin-O (ASO)
- Serum sample is diluted with a commercial preparation of ASO and incubated
- End point is read in Todd units, the reciprocal of the highest dilution (titer) that inhibits hemolysis

Purpose

- To confirm recent or ongoing streptococcal infection
- To help diagnose rheumatic fever and poststreptococcal glomerulonephritis in the presence of symptoms
- To distinguish between rheumatic fever and rheumatoid arthritis when joint pains are present

Procedure

Preparation

- Explain to the patient that this test detects an immunologic response to certain bacteria (streptococci).
- Inform the patient that he need not restrict food and fluids.
- Tell the patient that the test requires a blood sample. Explain who will perform the venipuncture and when.
- Explain to the patient that he may experience slight discomfort from the tourniquet and needle puncture.
- If the test is to be repeated at regular intervals to identify active and inactive states of rheumatic fever or to confirm acute glomerulonephritis, tell the patient that measuring the changes in antibody levels helps determine the effectiveness of therapy.
- Check the patient's history for drugs that may suppress the streptococcal antibody responses. If the patient must continue these drugs, note this on the laboratory request.

Implementation

- Perform a venipuncture and collect the sample in a 7-ml tube without additives.
- Handle the sample gently to prevent hemolysis.

Patient care

- Apply direct pressure to the venipuncture site until bleeding stops.

Complications

- Hematoma at the venipuncture site

Interpretation

Normal results

- Even healthy people have some detectable ASO titers from previous minor streptococcal infections.
- The normal ASO titers for school-age children is 170 Todd units/ml; for preschoolers and adults the normal titer is 85 Todd units/ml.

Abnormal results

- High ASO titers usually occur only after prolonged or recurrent infections.
- Generally, a titer higher than 166 Todd units/ml is considered a definite elevation.
- A low titer is good evidence of the absence of active rheumatic fever.
- A higher titer doesn't necessarily mean that rheumatic fever or glomerulonephritis is present; however, it does indicate the presence of a streptococcal infection.
- Serial titers, determined at 10- to 14-day intervals, provide more reliable information than a single titer. An increase in titer 2 to 5 weeks after the acute infection, which peaks 4 to 6 weeks after the initial increase, confirms poststreptococcal disease.

Interfering factors

- Streptococcal skin infections, seldom producing abnormal ASO titers even with poststreptococcal disease (probable false-negative)
- Antibiotic or corticosteroid therapy (possible suppression of the streptococcal antibody response)
- Hemolysis from rough handling of the sample

Antithyroid antibodies

Overview

○ Tanned red cell hemagglutination test detects antithyroglobulin and antimicrosomal antibodies.
○ Indirect immunofluorescence can also detect antimicrosomal antibodies.

Purpose

○ To detect circulating antithyroglobulin antibodies when clinical evidence indicates Hashimoto's thyroiditis, Graves' disease, or other thyroid diseases

Procedure

Preparation

○ Tell the patient that test evaluates thyroid function.
○ Inform the patient that he need not restrict food and fluids.
○ Tell patient that the test requires a blood sample. Explain who will perform the venipuncture and when.
○ Explain to the patient that he may experience slight discomfort from the tourniquet and needle puncture.

Implementation

○ Perform a venipuncture and collect the sample in a 7-ml tube without additives.

Patient care

○ Apply direct pressure to the venipuncture site until bleeding stops.

Complications

○ Hematoma at the venipuncture site

Interpretation

Normal results

○ The normal titer is less than 1:100 for antithyroglobulin and antimicrosomal antibodies.

Abnormal results

○ The presence of antithyroglobulin or antimicrosomal antibodies in serum can indicate subclinical autoimmune thyroid disease, Graves' disease, or idiopathic myxedema.
○ Titers of 1:400 or greater strongly suggest Hashimoto's thyroiditis.
○ Antithyroglobulin antibodies may also occur in some patients with other autoimmune disorders, such as systemic lupus erythematosus, rheumatoid arthritis, and autoimmune hemolytic anemia.

Interfering factors

None significant

Arginine

Overview

- Also known as *human growth hormone (hGH) stimulation test*
- Measures hGH levels after I.V. administration of arginine, an amino acid that normally stimulates hGH secretion
- Identifies pituitary dysfunction in infants and children with growth retardation and confirms hGH deficiency
- May be given with an insulin tolerance test or after administration of other hGH stimulants, such as glucagon, vasopressin, and levodopa

Purpose

- To aid diagnosis of pituitary tumors
- To confirm hGH deficiency in infants and children with low baseline levels

Procedure

Preparation

- Explain to the patient, or his parents, that this test identifies hGH deficiency.
- Instruct the patient to fast and limit physical activity for 10 to 12 hours before the test.
- Explain to the patient that this test requires I.V. infusion of a drug and collection of several blood samples. Tell him that the test takes at least 2 hours to perform.
- Withhold all steroid drugs, including pituitary-based hormones. If the patient must continue to take them, record this on the laboratory request.
- Tell the patient to lie down and relax for at least 90 minutes before the test.

Implementation

- Between 6 a.m. and 8 a.m., perform a venipuncture and collect 6 ml of blood (basal sample) in a clot-activator tube.
- Use an indwelling venous catheter to avoid repeated venipunctures. Start I.V. infusion of arginine (0.5 g/kg of body weight) in normal saline solution, and continue for 30 minutes.
- Stop the I.V. infusion, and then draw a total of three 6-ml samples at 30-minute intervals. Collect each sample in a clot-activator tube, and label it appropriately.
- Collect each sample at the scheduled time, and specify the collection time on the laboratory request.
- Send each sample to the laboratory immediately because hGH has a half-life of only 20 to 25 minutes.
- Handle the samples gently to prevent hemolysis.

Patient care

- Apply direct pressure to the venipuncture site until bleeding stops.

- Tell the patient that he may resume his usual diet, activities, and medications stopped before the test.

Complications

- Hematoma at the I.V. or venipuncture site

Interpretation

Normal results

- Arginine should raise hGH levels to more than 10 nanograms/ml (SI, > 10 µg/L) in men, more than 15 nanograms/ml (SI, > 15 µg/L) in women, and more than 48 nanograms/ml (SI, > 48 µg/L) in children. Such an increase may appear in the first sample collected 30 minutes after arginine infusion is stopped or in the samples collected 60 and 90 minutes afterward.

Abnormal results

- Levels that rise during fasting or during sleep help to rule out hGH deficiency.
- Failure of hGH levels to rise after arginine infusion indicates decreased anterior pituitary hGH reserve. In children, this deficiency causes dwarfism; in adults, it can indicate panhypopituitarism. When hGH levels fail to reach 10 nanograms/ml, retesting is required at the same time of day as the original test.

Interfering factors

- Failure to observe pretest restrictions
- Hemolysis from rough handling of the sample
- Radioactive scan performed within 1 week before the test

Arterial blood gas analysis

Overview

○ Measures the partial pressure of arterial oxygen (Pao_2), the partial pressure of arterial carbon dioxide ($Paco_2$), and the pH of an arterial sample
○ Measures oxygen content (O_2CT), arterial oxygen saturation (Sao_2), and bicarbonate (HCO_3^-) values
○ Pao_2: amount of oxygen the lungs deliver to the blood
○ $Paco_2$: how efficiently the lungs eliminate carbon dioxide
○ pH: acid-base level of the blood, or the hydrogen ion (H^+) level
○ Acidity indicates H^+ excess; alkalinity, H^+ deficit

Purpose

○ To evaluate the efficiency of pulmonary gas exchange
○ To assess the integrity of the ventilatory control system
○ To determine the acidbase level of the blood
○ To monitor respiratory therapy

Procedure

Preparation

○ Explain that arterial blood gas analysis evaluates how well the lungs are delivering oxygen to the blood and eliminating carbon dioxide.
○ Tell the patient that the test requires a blood sample. Explain who will perform the arterial puncture, when it will occur, and where the puncture site will be: radial, brachial, or femoral artery.
○ Inform the patient that he need not restrict food and fluids.
○ Instruct the patient to breathe normally during the test, and warn him that he may experience a brief cramping or throbbing pain at the puncture site.

Implementation

○ Wait at least 20 minutes before drawing arterial blood when starting, changing, or discontinuing oxygen therapy; after initiating or changing settings of mechanical ventilation; or after extubation.
○ Use a heparinized blood gas syringe to draw the sample.
○ Perform an arterial puncture or draw blood from an arterial line.
○ Eliminate air from the sample, place it on ice immediately, and prepare to transport it for analysis.
○ Before sending the sample to the laboratory, note on the laboratory request whether the patient was breathing room air or receiving oxygen therapy when the sample was collected.

○ Note the flow rate of oxygen therapy and method of delivery. If on a ventilator, note the fraction of inspired oxygen, tidal volume mode, respiratory rate, and positive-end expiratory pressure.
○ Note the patient's rectal temperature.

Patient care

○ After applying pressure to the puncture site for 3 to 5 minutes or until bleeding has stopped, tape a gauze pad firmly over it.
○ If the puncture site is on the arm, don't tape the entire circumference; this may restrict circulation.
○ If the patient is receiving anticoagulants or has a coagulopathy, apply pressure to the puncture site longer than 5 minutes if necessary.
○ Monitor vital signs and observe for signs of circulatory impairment, such as swelling, discoloration, pain, numbness, and tingling in the bandaged arm or leg.

Complications

○ Bleeding from the puncture site

Interpretation

Normal results

○ Pao_2: 80 to 100 mm Hg (SI, 10.6 to 13.3 kPa)
○ $Paco_2$: 35 to 45 mm Hg (SI, 4.7 to 5.3 kPa)
○ pH: 7.35 to 7.45 (SI, 7.35 to 7.45)
○ O_2CT: 15% to 23% (SI, 0.15 to 0.23)
○ Sao_2: 94% to 100% (SI, 0.94 to 1)
○ HCO_3^-: 22 to 25 mEq/L (SI, 22 to 25 mmol/L)

Abnormal results

○ Low Pao_2, O_2CT, and Sao_2 levels and a high $Paco_2$ may result from conditions that impair respiratory function, such as respiratory muscle weakness or paralysis, respiratory center inhibition (from head injury, brain tumor, or drug abuse), and airway obstruction (possibly from mucus plugs or a tumor).
○ Low readings may result from bronchiole obstruction caused by asthma or emphysema, from an abnormal ventilation-perfusion ratio caused by partially blocked alveoli or pulmonary capillaries, or from alveoli that are damaged or filled with fluid because of disease, hemorrhage, or near-drowning.
○ When inspired air contains insufficient oxygen, Pao_2, O_2CT, and Sao_2 decrease but $Paco_2$ may be normal. Such findings are common in pneumothorax, impaired diffusion between alveoli and blood (caused by interstitial fibrosis, for example), or an arteriovenous shunt that permits blood to bypass the lungs.
○ Low O_2CT — with normal Pao_2, Sao_2 and, possibly, $Paco_2$ values — may result from severe anemia, decreased blood volume, and reduced hemoglobin oxygen-carrying capacity.

Interfering factors

○ Failure to heparinize syringe, place sample in an iced bag, or send the sample to the laboratory immediately

○ Exposing the sample to air (increase or decrease in Pao_2 and $Paco_2$)

○ Venous blood in the sample (possible decrease in Pao_2 and increase in $Paco_2$)

○ HCO_3^-, ethacrynic acid, hydrocortisone, metolazone, prednisone, and thiazides (possible increase in $Paco_2$)

○ Acetazolamide, methicillin, nitrofurantoin, and tetracycline (possible decrease in $Paco_2$)

○ Fever (possible false-high Pao_2 and $Paco_2$)

Arterial-to-alveolar oxygen ratio

Overview

- Helps identify the cause of hypoxemia and intrapulmonary shunting by providing an approximation of the partial pressure of oxygenation of the alveoli and arteries
- May help differentiate the cause: ventilated alveoli but no perfusion, unventilated alveoli with perfusion, or collapse of the alveoli and capillaries

Purpose

- To evaluate the efficiency of gas exchange
- To assess the integrity of the ventilatory control system
- To monitor respiratory therapy

Procedure

Preparation

- Explain to the patient that the arterial-to-alveolar ratio test evaluates how well the lungs deliver oxygen to the blood and eliminate carbon dioxide.
- Tell the patient that the test requires a blood sample. Explain who will perform the arterial puncture and when.
- Inform the patient that he need not restrict food and fluids.
- Instruct the patient to breathe normally during the test, and warn him that he may experience cramping or throbbing pain at the puncture site.

Implementation

- Perform an arterial puncture or draw blood from an arterial line using a heparinized blood gas syringe.
- Eliminate all air from the sample and place it on ice immediately
- Before sending the sample to the laboratory, note on the laboratory request whether the patient was breathing room air or receiving oxygen therapy during the sample was collection.
- If the patient was receiving oxygen therapy, note the flow rate and method of delivery. If he was on a ventilator, note the fraction of inspired oxygen, tidal volume, mode, respiratory rate, and positive end-expiratory pressure.
- Note the patient's rectal temperature.

Patient care

- Apply pressure to the puncture site for 3 to 5 minutes or until bleeding stops.
- Place a gauze pad over the site and tape it in place, but don't tape the entire circumference.
- Monitor vital signs and observe for signs of circulatory impairment, such as swelling, discoloration, pain, numbness, and tingling in the bandaged arm or leg.

Complications

- Bleeding from the puncture site

Interpretation

Normal results

- A normal arterial-to-alveolar ratio is 75%.

Abnormal results

- Increased values may result from mucus plugs, bronchospasm, or airway collapse (asthma, bronchitis, emphysema).
- Hypoxemia results in increased alveolar-to-arterial oxygen gradient and may result from arterial septal defects, pneumothorax, atelectasis, emboli, or edema.

Interfering factors

- Failure to heparinize the syringe, place the sample in an iced bag, or send the sample to the laboratory immediately
- Exposing the sample to air (increase or decrease)
- Age and increasing oxygen concentration (increase)

Arthrocentesis

Overview

- Synovial fluid aspiration
- Fluid specimen obtained by insertion of a needle into a joint space, most commonly the knee, under sterile conditions
- Indicated in undiagnosed articular disease and symptomatic joint effusion

Purpose

- To analyze synovial fluid
- To aid in the differential diagnosis of arthritis, especially septic or crystal-induced arthritis
- To identify the cause or nature of joint effusion
- To relieve pain and distention from joint effusion
- To give local drug such as corticosteroid

Procedure

Preparation

- Explain the purpose of the procedure, describing how it's done, who will perform it, and where it will occur. Tell the patient that the test takes less than 15 minutes.
- Make sure the patient has signed a consent form.
- Note and report allergies.
- If glucose testing of synovial fluid is ordered, advise fasting for 6 to 12 hours before the test; otherwise, there's no need to restrict food and fluids before the test.
- Inform the patient that failure to adhere to dietary restrictions can affect glucose levels.
- Warn the patient that transient pain may occur when the needle penetrates the joint capsule.
- Give the patient a sedative.

Implementation

- Test shouldn't be performed near skin or wound infections.
- Strict sterile technique used during aspiration prevents contamination of joint space or synovial fluid specimen.
- The patient is positioned properly and told to maintain this position during the procedure.
- Skin over puncture site is cleaned and prepared.
- A local anesthetic is given; an aspirating needle is inserted quickly through the skin, subcutaneous tissue, and synovial membrane into the joint space.
- As much fluid as possible, preferably at least 15 ml, is aspirated into the syringe.
- The joint (except the area around the puncture site) is bandaged to compress the free fluid into this portion of the sac, ensuring maximal collection of fluid.
- If a corticosteroid is injected, the syringe is detached, leaving the needle in the joint. The syringe

containing the steroid is attached to the needle, and the steroid is injected.
- The needle is withdrawn and pressure applied to the puncture site until bleeding stops.
- The puncture site is cleaned and sterile dressing applied.
- If measuring synovial fluid glucose, a venipuncture is performed to get a blood glucose analysis specimen.
- Send the properly labeled specimens to the laboratory immediately. If a white blood cell (WBC) count is ordered, clearly label the specimen "Synovial fluid" and "Caution: Don't use acid diluents," because these can alter the count.

Patient care

- Apply cold to the affected joint for 24 to 36 hours after aspiration to decrease pain and swelling.
- Use pillows to support the joint.
- If a large quantity of fluid was aspirated, apply an elastic bandage to prevent fluid from accumulating again.
- If the patient's condition permits, resume the patient's normal activities and diet immediately after the procedure.
- Warn the patient to avoid excessive use of the joint for a few days after the test, even if pain and swelling have subsided.
- Excessive use can cause transient pain, swelling, and stiffness.
- Watch for and immediately report increased pain and fever, which could indicate joint infection.

Complications

- Joint infection
- Hemorrhage
- Hemarthrosis

Interpretation

Normal results

- Color: colorless to pale yellow
- Clarity: clear
- Quantity (in knee): 0.3 to 3.5 ml
- pH: 7.2 to 7.4
- Mucin clot: good

Abnormal results

- Inflammatory disease (systemic lupus erythematosus, rheumatic fever, pseudogout, gout, and rheumatoid arthritis), noninflammatory disease (traumatic arthritis and osteoarthritis), and septic disease (tuberculous and septic arthritis)

Interfering factors

- Failure to adhere to dietary restrictions
- Specimen contamination
- Acid diluents added to the specimen for WBC count
- Failure to adequately mix specimen and anticoagulant or to send specimen to the laboratory immediately

Arthrography

Overview

○ Radiographic examination of a joint after injection of a radiopaque dye, air, or both (double-contrast arthrography)
○ Contraindicated in pregnancy and in patients with active arthritis, joint infection, and previous hypersensitivity to iodinated contrast media

Purpose

○ To outline joint contour and soft-tissue structures
○ To evaluate persistent unexplained joint discomfort or pain
○ To identify acute or chronic abnormalities of the joint capsule or supporting ligaments of the knee, shoulder, ankle, hip, or wrist
○ To detect internal joint derangements
○ To locate synovial cysts
○ To evaluate damage from recurrent dislocations

Procedure

Preparation

○ Make sure the patient has signed an appropriate consent form.
○ Explain the purpose of the study, how it's done, who will perform the study and where. Tell the patient that the study takes about 45 minutes
○ Note and report all allergies.
○ Inform the patient that restriction of food or fluids isn't necessary.
○ Warn the patient that a tingling sensation, burning, or pressure in the joint may occur with the contrast injection.
○ Explain to the patient that some swelling, discomfort, or crepitant noises may occur in the joint after the study and that these usually disappear after 1 to 2 days. Tell the patient to contact his physician if symptoms persist.

Implementation

○ Clean the skin around the puncture site with an antiseptic solution and inject with a local anesthetic.
○ A needle is then inserted into the joint space.
○ Fluid may be aspirated and sent to the laboratory for analysis.
○ When fluoroscopic examination shows correct needle placement, a contrast medium is injected into the joint space.
○ The needle is removed, and the puncture site is covered with a sterile dressing.
○ The joint is put through its range of motion to distribute the contrast medium within the joint space.
○ A series of radiographs is rapidly taken before the joint tissue can absorb the contrast medium.

Patient care

○ Tell the patient to rest the joint for 6 to 12 hours.
○ Wrap the knee in an elastic bandage for several days if a knee arthrography was performed.
○ Apply ice to the joint for swelling.
○ Give the patient an analgesic.
○ Ask the patient to report signs and symptoms of infection.

Complications

○ Hypersensitivity reactions to contrast medium
○ Persistent joint swelling, pain, or crepitus
○ Infection

Interpretation

Normal results

○ A knee arthrogram shows a characteristic wedge-shaped shadow pointed toward the interior of the joint, indicating a normal medial meniscus.
○ A shoulder arthrogram shows the bicipital tendon sheath, redundant inferior joint capsule, and intact subscapular bursa.

Abnormal results

○ Structural abnormalities of the knee commonly suggest tears and lacerations of the meniscus.
○ Extrameniscal lesions may suggest osteochondral fractures, cartilaginous abnormalities, synovial abnormalities, cruciate ligament tears, and joint capsule and collateral ligament disruptions.
○ Shoulder abnormalities may suggest adhesive capsulitis, bicipital tenosynovitis or rupture, and rotator cuff tears.

Interfering factors

○ Incomplete aspiration of joint effusion dilutes the contrast medium and diminishes film quality

Arthroscopy

Overview

- Visual examination of the interior of a joint using a fiber-optic endoscope
- Most commonly used to examine the knee joint
- Permits concurrent surgery or biopsy using triangulation, in which instruments are passed through a separate cannula
- Usually an outpatient procedure
- Contraindicated in patients with fibrous ankylosis with flexion of less than 50 degrees and patients with local skin or wound infections

Purpose

- To evaluate suspected or confirmed joint disease
- To provide a safe, convenient alternative to open surgery (arthrotomy) and separate biopsy
- To detect, diagnose, treat, and monitor therapy for meniscal, patellar, condylar, extrasynovial, and synovial diseases

Procedure

Preparation

- Explain the purpose of the study, how it's done, who will perform the study and where. Tell the patient that the study takes about 1 hour.
- Make sure the patient has signed a consent form.
- Note and report all allergies.
- Tell the patient to fast after midnight before the procedure.
- Warn the patient that he may feel discomfort from injection of the anesthetic and tourniquet pressure.
- Explain that patient may feel a thumping sensation as the cannula is inserted into the joint.
- Advise the patient to avoid tub baths until after the postoperative visit, although showers are allowed 48 hours after the study.

Implementation

- Arthroscopic techniques vary depending on the surgeon and the type of arthroscope used.
- Shave and prepare an area 5″ (12.7 cm) above and below the joint.
- Give the patient a sedative.
- A local or regional anesthesia is given; general anesthesia is for more extensive surgery.
- As much blood as possible is usually drained from the leg by wrapping it in an elastic bandage and elevating it.
- A mixture of lidocaine, epinephrine, and sterile normal saline solution may be injected to distend the knee, reduce bleeding, and provide a better view.
- A cannula is passed through a small incision and positioned in the joint cavity.
- The arthroscope is inserted through the cannula.

- The knee structures are visually examined.
- Photographs are taken for further study, if indicated.
- A synovial biopsy or appropriate surgery is performed, if indicated.
- The arthroscope is removed and the joint is irrigated.
- An adhesive strip and compression bandage are applied to the site.

Patient care

- Give analgesics.
- Elevate the leg and apply ice for the first 24 hours.
- Report fever, bleeding, drainage, or increased swelling or pain in the joint.
- Limit weight bearing by using a walker, cane, or crutches for 48 hours.
- Apply an immobilizer if ordered.
- Resume the patient's usual diet.
- Monitor the site for localized inflammation and neurovascular status of the extremity.

Complications

- Infection
- Hematoma
- Thrombophlebitis
- Joint injury

Interpretation

Normal results

- Diarthrodial joint surrounded by muscles, ligaments, cartilage, tendons; lined with synovial membrane.

❊ *AGE AWARE In a child, the menisci are smooth and opaque, with their thick outer edges attached to the joint capsule and their inner edges lying snugly against the condylar surfaces, unattached.*

- Articular cartilage appears smooth and white.
- Ligaments and tendons appear cablelike and silvery.
- The synovium is smooth and marked by a fine vascular network.
- Degenerative changes begin during adolescence.

Abnormal results

- Meniscal abnormalities may suggest a torn meniscus.
- Patellar abnormalities may suggest chondromalacia, dislocation, subluxation, fracture, or parapatellar synovitis.
- Condylar abnormalities may suggest degenerative articular cartilage, osteochondritis dissecans, or loose bodies.
- Extrasynovial abnormalities may suggest torn anterior cruciate or tibial collateral ligaments, Baker's cyst, or ganglion cyst.
- Synovial abnormalities may suggest synovitis, rheumatoid arthritis, or degenerative arthritis.
- Foreign bodies may suggest gout, pseudogout, and osteochondromatosis.

Interfering factors

None known

Arylsulfatase

Overview

- Measures urine arylsulfatase (ARSA) level by colorimetric or kinetic techniques
- Level rises in transitional bladder cancer, colorectal cancer, and leukemia
- Unknown whether elevated level provokes malignancies or is an enzymatic response to these growths

Purpose

- To aid in the diagnosis of bladder, colon, or rectal cancer; myeloid (granulocytic) leukemia; and metachromatic leukodystrophy (an inherited lipid storage disease)

Procedure

Preparation

- Tell the patient that this test measures an enzyme that's present throughout the body.
- Advise the patient that he need not restrict food and fluids.
- Tell the patient that the test requires urine collection over a 24-hour period, and teach him how to collect a timed specimen.

Implementation

- Collect the patient's urine over a 24-hour period, discarding the first sample and retaining the last sample in the appropriate container.
- If a female patient is menstruating, anticipate possible test rescheduling.
- Keep the collection container refrigerated or on ice during the collection period.
- Send the specimen to the laboratory as soon as the collection period has ended.
- If the patient has an indwelling urinary catheter in place, keep the collection bag on ice for the duration of the test.
- Begin the test period with a new, unused continuous urinary drainage apparatus.

Patient care

- Tell the patient not to contaminate the urine specimen with toilet tissue or stool.

Complications

None known

Interpretation

Normal results

- Normally, random values are 1.6 to 42 units/g creatinine; 24-hour urine values are 0.37 to 3.60 units/day creatinine; 1-hour test values are 2 to 19 units/hour (SI, 2 to 19 U/h); 2-hour test values are 4 to 37 units/2 hours (SI, 4 to 37 U/2 h); 24-hour test values are 170 to 2,000 units/24 hours (SI, 2.89 to 34.0 µkat/ L).

Abnormal results

- Elevated ARSA levels may result from cancer of the bladder, colon, or rectum or from myeloid leukemia.
- Depressed ARSA levels can result from metachromatic leukodystrophy. In a patient with this condition, urine studies show metachromatic granules in the urinary sediment.

Interfering factors

- Failure to collect all urine during the test period, to properly store the specimen, or to send the specimen to the laboratory immediately after the collection is complete
- Contamination of the specimen with toilet tissue, stool, or menstrual blood
- Surgery within 1 week before the test (possible increase)

Aspartate aminotransferase

Overview

○ Found in the cytoplasm and mitochondria of many cells, primarily in the liver, heart, skeletal muscles, kidneys, pancreas, and red blood cells; also released into serum in response to cellular damage
○ High correlation between myocardial infarction (MI) and elevated AST levels, but test is sometimes superfluous for diagnosing an MI because it isn't specifically for the heart; it doesn't differentiate between acute MI and the effects of hepatic congestion caused by heart failure.

Purpose

○ To aid detection and differential diagnosis of acute hepatic disease
○ To monitor patient progress and prognosis in cardiac and hepatic diseases
○ To aid diagnosis of an MI in correlation with creatine kinase and lactate dehydrogenase levels

Procedure

Preparation

○ Explain to the patient that this test assesses heart and liver function.
○ Inform the patient that the test usually requires three venipunctures (one on admission and one each day for the next 2 days).
○ Tell the patient that he need not restrict food and fluids.
○ Explain to the patient that he may experience slight discomfort from the tourniquet and needle puncture.
○ Notify the laboratory and physician of drugs the patient is taking that may affect test results; it may be necessary to restrict them.

Implementation

○ Perform a venipuncture and collect the sample in a 4-ml clot-activator tube.
○ To avoid missing peak AST levels, draw serum samples at the same time each day.
○ Handle the sample gently to prevent hemolysis and send it to the laboratory immediately.

Patient care

○ Apply direct pressure to the venipuncture site until bleeding stops.
○ Instruct the patient that he may resume medications stopped before the test.

Complications

○ Hematoma at the venipuncture site

Interpretation

Normal results

○ 12 to 31 units/L (SI, 0.14 to 0.78 µkat/L)

 AGE AWARE Normal results for infants are typically higher.

Abnormal results

○ AST levels fluctuate in response to the extent of cellular necrosis, being transiently and minimally increased early in the disease process and extremely increased during the most acute phase. Depending on when the initial sample is drawn, AST levels may increase, indicating increasing disease severity and tissue damage, or decrease, indicating disease resolution and tissue repair.
○ Maximum elevations (more than 20 times normal) may indicate acute viral hepatitis, severe skeletal muscle trauma, extensive surgery, drug-induced hepatic injury, or severe passive liver congestion.
○ High levels (10 to 20 times normal) may indicate a severe MI, severe infectious mononucleosis, or alcoholic cirrhosis.
○ High levels also occur during the prodromal or resolving stages of conditions that cause maximum elevations.
○ Moderate to high levels (5 to 10 times normal) may indicate dermatomyositis, Duchenne's muscular dystrophy, or chronic hepatitis.
○ Moderate to high levels also occur during prodromal and resolving stages of diseases that cause high elevations.
○ Low to moderate levels (2 to 5 times normal) occur at some time during the preceding conditions or may indicate hemolytic anemia, metastatic hepatic tumors, acute pancreatitis, pulmonary emboli, delirium tremens, or fatty liver. AST levels rise slightly after the first few days of biliary duct obstruction.

Interfering factors

○ Hemolysis from rough handling of the sample
○ Failure to draw the sample as scheduled (may miss peak)
○ Chlorpropamide, opioids, methyldopa, erythromycin, sulfonamides, pyridoxine, dicumarol, and antitubercular agents; large doses of acetaminophen, salicylates, or vitamin A; and many other drugs known to affect the liver (increase)
○ Strenuous exercise and muscle trauma caused by I.M. injections (increase)

Atrial natriuretic factor, plasma

Overview

○ Radioimmunoassay that measures the plasma level of atrial natriuretic peptides or atriopeptin
○ May provide a marker for early asymptomatic left ventricular dysfunction and increased cardiac volume

Purpose

○ To confirm heart failure
○ To identify asymptomatic cardiac volume overload

Procedure

Preparation

○ As appropriate, explain the purpose of the test to the patient.
○ Inform the patient that he must fast for 12 hours before the test.
○ Tell the patient the test requires a blood sample. Explain who will perform the venipuncture and when.
○ Explain to the patient that he may experience slight discomfort from the tourniquet and needle puncture.
○ Explain that the test results will be available within 4 days.
○ Check the patient's history for drugs that can influence test results.
○ Withhold beta blockers, calcium antagonists, diuretics, vasodilators, and cardiac glycosides for 24 hours before collection.

Implementation

○ Perform a venipuncture and collect the sample in a prechilled potassium ethylenediaminetetraacetic acid (EDTA) tube.
○ After chilled centrifugation, promptly freeze the EDTA plasma and send it to the laboratory.
○ Handle the sample gently to prevent hemolysis.

Patient care

○ Apply direct pressure to the venipuncture site until bleeding stops.
○ Instruct the patient that he may resume his usual diet and medications stopped before the test.

Complications

○ Hematoma at the venipuncture site

Interpretation

Normal results

○ 20 to 77 pg/ml

Abnormal results

○ Increased level may indicate heart failure and elevated cardiac filling pressure.

Interfering factors

○ Cardiovascular drugs, including beta blockers, calcium antagonists, diuretics, vasodilators, and cardiac glycosides
○ Pancreatic and gastric hormone tests

Auditory brain stem evoked-response testing

Overview

○ Auditory brain stem evoked-response (ABR) is also called *brain stem auditory evoked response*
○ Most common form of auditory evoked potentials testing
○ Traces are analyzed to determine if a response is present, and characteristics are analyzed

Purpose

○ To screen neonatal hearing, the goal being to provide amplification by age 6 months
○ To estimate or confirm the extent of hearing loss in infants and toddlers
○ To estimate the threshold in other difficult-to-test patients, such as those with developmental disabilities and those suspected of nonorganic hearing loss
○ To evaluate cranial nerve (CN) VIII and lower brain stem auditory synchronization, which will be abnormal if lesions exist in this area or if auditory neuropathy is present (auditory dyssynchronization)

Procedure

Preparation

○ Clean ear canals are required for this test and are particularly important when referring for electrocochleography.

✸ AGE AWARE *Depending on a child's age, sedation may be necessary, in which case a health care facility must perform it. In other facilities, a child may have to undergo sleep deprivation to make sure he sleeps during testing.*

○ Advise the patient to dress comfortably and to avoid wearing foundation make-up. Inform the patient that, although the test is painless, electrodes will be applied to the skin and the test will require 1 to 1½ hours to complete.

Implementation

○ Electrodes are connected to a physiologic amplifier and signal-averaging computer.
○ Threshold estimation is conducted by an audiologist. The intensity of the signal is varied until the response threshold is obtained. The response threshold is slightly above the hearing threshold, but estimation is possible if the patient has normal hearing.
○ In testing for CN VIII and auditory brain stem response, make click signals that are clearly audible and occur at different rates. Rapid clicks may reveal a pathology more readily. A click stimulus is presented at a supra-threshold level. The time at which wave V occurs in each ear, the time difference between the evoked waves I and V in each ear, and the time difference between both of these measures is used to indicate the probability of retrocochlear pathology.
○ Assessment of central auditory processing ability involves assessing brain stem potentials and one or more of the potentials generated by the neural structures superior to the brain stem.

Patient care

○ If the patient was sedated, monitor him until he completely recovers.

Complications

○ Skin abrasion from electrode placement causes irritation and minor allergic reactions.

Interpretation

Normal results

○ ABR wave latencies occur at predictable times for the patient who has normal hearing or who has cochlear loss but hears signals that are above the hearing threshold. The latency between waves I and V is about 4.0 milliseconds. The interaural latency difference of wave V and the I-V interaural latency differences is small, generally less than 0.3 or 0.4 millisecond.
○ The threshold of the ABR is about 10 to 20 decibels (dB) normal hearing level (nHL) for click or high-frequency stimuli, and 20 or 30 dB nHL for lower-frequency stimuli.

Abnormal results

○ Cochlear loss increases the threshold of the ABR response.
○ The time between waves I and V is unaffected or shortens with cochlear loss; establishing wave I may be more difficult.
○ Prolonged I-V interpeak latency is an indicator of CN VIII or lower brain stem pathology.
○ Asymmetry of the I-V interpeak interval between ears is also a strong sign of a retrocochlear disorder.

Interfering factors

○ Hearing loss developed after birth, such as from maternal cytomegalovirus infection and some genetic hearing losses or progressive hearing loss

Barium enema

Overview

- Radiographic examination of the large intestine after rectal instillation of barium sulfate (single-contrast technique) or barium sulfate and air (double-contrast technique)
- Single-contrast technique provides a profile view of the large intestine
- Double-contrast technique provides profile and frontal views

Purpose

- To aid in the diagnosis of colorectal cancer and inflammatory disease
- To detect polyps, diverticula, and structural changes in the large intestine

Procedure

Preparation

- Explain that the test permits examination of the large intestine through X-rays taken after a barium enema.
- Accurate test results depend on the patient's cooperation with prescribed dietary restrictions and bowel preparation.
- Common bowel preparation includes restricted intake of dairy products and maintenance of a liquid diet for 24 hours before the test. The patient is encouraged to drink five 8-oz glasses of water or clear liquids 12 to 24 hours before the test.
- A GoLYTELY preparation isn't recommended because it leaves the bowel too wet for the barium to coat the walls of the bowel.
- Advise the patient to give himself enemas until the return is clear.
- Tell the patient not to eat breakfast before the procedure; if the test is scheduled for late afternoon, he may have clear liquids.
- The patient may experience cramping pains or the urge to defecate as the barium or air is introduced into the intestine. Instruct him to breathe deeply and slowly through his mouth to ease the discomfort.
- The patient must contract his anal sphincter tightly against the rectal tube.
- Stress the importance of retaining the barium.

Implementation

- After the patient is in a supine position on a tilting X-ray table, spot films of the abdomen are taken.
- Patient is assisted to Sims' position; a well-lubricated rectal tube is inserted through the anus. For anal sphincter atony or severe mental or physical debilitation, a rectal tube with a retaining balloon is inserted.
- The barium is given slowly. The filling process is monitored fluoroscopically. To aid filling, the table is tilted or the patient assisted to supine, prone, and lateral decubitus positions.
- As barium flow is observed, significant spot films are taken.
- The rectal tube is withdrawn and the patient escorted to a toilet or given a bedpan to expel as much barium as possible.
- After evacuation, additional overhead film is taken to record mucosal pattern and evaluate the efficiency of colonic emptying.
- A double-contrast barium enema may directly follow the examination or may occur separately. If performed immediately, a thin film of barium remains in the intestine, coating the mucosa, and air is carefully injected to distend the bowel lumen.
- If a double-contrast technique is performed separately, instill a colloidal barium suspension, filling the intestine to either the splenic flexure or the middle of the transverse colon. The suspension is then aspirated, and air is forcefully injected into the intestine. If filling the intestine to the lower descending colon, forcefully inject air without first aspirating the suspension.
- The patient is assisted to erect, prone, supine, and lateral decubitus positions in sequence. Filling is monitored fluoroscopically, and spot films are taken of significant findings.
- After films are taken, the patient is escorted to a toilet or provided with a bedpan.

Patient care

- Make sure that the patient isn't to have further studies before allowing him to have food and fluids. Encourage him to take extra fluids because the bowel preparation and test itself can cause dehydration.
- Encourage the patient to rest because the bowel preparation and test are exhausting.
- Barium retention can cause an intestinal obstruction or fecal impaction. If this happens, give a mild cathartic or enema. The patient's stool will be light colored for 24 to 72 hours. Record and describe stools.

Complications

- Perforation of the colon, water intoxication, barium granulomas, intraperitoneal and extraperitoneal extravasation of barium, and barium embolism

Interpretation

Normal results

- *Single-contrast enema:* Barium uniformly fills the intestine, and colonic haustral markings are clearly apparent. The intestinal walls collapse as the patient expels the barium, and the mucosa has a regular, feathery appearance on the post-evacuation film.
- *Double-contrast enema:* The intestines uniformly distend with air and have a thin layer of barium, providing excellent detail of the mucosal pattern.

Abnormal results

- An adenocarcinoma or sarcoma occurring higher in the intestine
- A carcinoma, either as a localized filling defect with a sharp transition between normal and necrotic mucosa or circumferential with an "apple-core" appearance (characteristics that help distinguish a carcinoma from the more diffuse lesions of inflammatory disease)
- Inflammatory disease, such as diverticulitis, ulcerative colitis, and granulomatous colitis
- Saccular adenomatous polyps, broad-based villous polyps, structural changes in the intestine (such as intussusception, telescoping of the bowel, sigmoid volvulus, sigmoid torsion, gastroenteritis, irritable colon, vascular injury)

Interfering factors

- Inadequate bowel preparation (possible poor imaging)
- Barium retained from previous studies (possible poor imaging)
- Patient's inability to retain barium

Barium swallow

Overview

○ Examination of the pharynx and esophagus after ingesting thick and thin mixtures of barium sulfate
○ Usually part of the upper GI series; indicated in patients with histories of dysphagia and regurgitation

Purpose

○ To diagnose hiatal hernia, diverticula, and varices
○ To detect strictures, ulcers, tumors, polyps, and motility disorders

Procedure

Preparation

○ Explain that the test evaluates the function of the pharynx and esophagus.
○ Instruct the patient to fast after midnight the night before the test. (For an infant, delay feeding to ensure complete digestion of the barium.)
○ The patient may be given a restricted diet for 2 to 3 days before test.
○ Describe the test, who will perform it, and where it will take place.
○ Describe the milk shake consistency and chalky taste of the barium preparation. Although flavored, it may be unpleasant to swallow.
○ The patient will first receive a thick mixture, then a thin one; he must drink 12 to 14 oz (355 to 414 ml) during the examination.
○ Inform the patient that he'll be placed in various positions on a tilting X-ray table and that X-rays will be taken.
○ Reassure him about safety precautions.
○ Withhold antacids, histamine-2 blockers, and proton pump inhibitors, if gastric reflux is suspected
○ Instruct the patient to put on a gown without snap closures and to remove jewelry, dentures, hair clips, or other radiopaque objects.

Implementation

○ The patient is placed in an upright position behind the fluoroscopic screen, and his heart, lungs, and abdomen are examined.
○ The patient is instructed to take one swallow of the thick barium mixture; pharyngeal action is recorded using cineradiography.
○ The patient is instructed to take several swallows of the thin barium mixture. Passage of the barium is examined fluoroscopically; spot films of the esophageal region are taken from lateral angles and from right and left posteroanterior angles.
○ To accentuate small strictures or demonstrate dysphagia, the patient may be asked to swallow a "barium marshmallow" (soft white bread soaked in barium) or a barium pill.

○ The patient is then secured to the X-ray table and rotated to Trendelenburg position to evaluate esophageal peristalsis or demonstrate hiatal hernia and gastric reflux.
○ The patient is instructed to take several swallows of barium while the esophagus is examined fluoroscopically; spot films are taken.
○ After the table is rotated to a horizontal position, the patient takes several swallows of barium so that the esophagogastric junction and peristalsis may be evaluated.
○ Passage of the barium is fluoroscopically observed, and spot films are taken with the patient in the supine and prone positions.
○ During fluoroscopic examination of the esophagus, the stomach and duodenum are also carefully studied because neoplasms in these areas may invade the esophagus and cause obstruction.

Patient care

○ Check that additional films and fluoroscopic evaluation haven't been ordered before allowing the patient to resume his usual diet.
○ Instruct the patient to drink plenty of fluids, unless contraindicated, to help eliminate the barium.
○ Give a cathartic if prescribed. Tell the patient to notify the physician if he fails to expel the barium in 2 or 3 days.
○ Inform the patient that stools will be chalky and light-colored for 24 to 72 hours.

Complications

○ Barium retained in the intestine may harden, causing obstruction or fecal impaction
○ Abdominal distention and absent bowel sounds, which may indicate constipation and suggest barium impaction

Interpretation

Normal results

○ The swallowed barium bolus pours over the base of the tongue into the pharynx.
○ A peristaltic wave propels the bolus through the entire length of the esophagus in about 2 seconds.
○ When the wave reaches the base of the esophagus, the cardiac sphincter opens, allowing the bolus to enter the stomach. After passage of the bolus, the cardiac sphincter closes.
○ The bolus evenly fills and distends the lumen of the pharynx and esophagus, and the mucosa appears smooth and regular.

Abnormal results

○ Hiatal hernia, diverticula, varices; lung aspiration
○ Strictures, tumors, polyps, ulcers, and motility disorders (definitive diagnosis requires further testing)

Interfering factors

○ Poor swallowing reflex

Basal gastric secretion

Overview

- Measures basal secretion during fasting by aspirating stomach contents through a nasogastric (NG) tube
- Indicated in the patient with obscure epigastric pain, anorexia, and weight loss

Purpose

- To determine gastric output while the patient is fasting

Procedure

Preparation

- Explain to the patient that the test measures the stomach's secretion of acid.
- Instruct the patient to restrict food for 12 hours, and fluids and smoking for 8 hours before the test.
- Tell the patient who will perform the test. Tell him the procedure takes about 1¼ hours (or 2¼ hours, if followed by the gastric acid stimulation test).
- Inform the patient that the test requires insertion of a tube through his nose and into his stomach, that he may initially experience discomfort, and that he may cough or gag.
- To prevent contamination of the specimens with saliva, instruct the patient to expectorate excess saliva.
- Notify the laboratory and physician of drugs the patient is taking that may affect test results; it may be necessary to restrict them. If the patient must continue these drugs, note this on the laboratory request.
- Check the patient's pulse rate and blood pressure just before the test.
- Encourage the patient to relax.

Implementation

- Insert the NG tube after seating the patient comfortably.
- Attach a 20-ml syringe to it and aspirate the stomach contents.
- Ensure complete emptying of the stomach by asking the patient to assume three positions in sequence — supine and right and left lateral decubitus — while aspirating the stomach contents.
- Label the specimen container RESIDUAL CONTENTS.
- Connect the NG tube to the suction machine. Aspirate the gastric contents by continuous low suction for 1 hour. It's also possible to perform aspiration manually with a syringe.
- Collect a specimen every 15 minutes, but discard the first two; this eliminates the specimens that could be affected by the stress of intubation.
- Record the color and odor of each specimen and note the presence of food, mucus, bile, or blood.
- Label these specimens BASAL CONTENTS, and number them 1 through 4.
- Measure secretion volume and acid concentration.

Patient care

- Monitor the patient's vital signs during the intubation and observe for arrhythmias.
- If the NG tube is to remain in place, clamp it or attach it to low intermittent suction.
- Provide soothing lozenges for a sore throat.
- Instruct the patient that he may resume his usual diet and medications, unless the gastric acid stimulation test will also be performed.

Complications

- Nausea, vomiting, and abdominal distention or pain, after removal of the NG tube
- NG tube entering the trachea and not the esophagus during insertion; remove NG tube immediately if the patient develops cyanosis or paroxysmal coughing

Interpretation

Normal results

- In males, 1 to 5 mEq/hour
- In females, 0.2 to 3.3 mEq/hour

Abnormal results

- Abnormal findings are nonspecific and must be considered with the results of the gastric acid stimulation test.
- Elevated secretion may suggest a duodenal or jejunal ulcer (after partial gastrectomy); markedly elevated secretion suggests Zollinger-Ellison syndrome.
- Depressed secretion may indicate gastric carcinoma or a benign gastric ulcer.
- Absence of secretion may indicate pernicious anemia.

Interfering factors

- Failure to observe pretest restrictions (increase)
- Psychological stress (possible increase)
- Cholinergics, reserpine, alcohol, adrenergic-receptor blockers, and adrenocorticosteroids (possible increase)
- Antacids, anticholinergics, histamine-2 blockers, and proton pump inhibitors (possible decrease)

Basophils

Overview

○ Number of basophils increases during infection; basophils accumulate at the site of infection or inflammation.

Purpose

○ To determine the number of basophils in a peripheral blood smear
○ To aid in determining specific conditions related to basophil counts such as myeloproliferative disease

Procedure

Preparation

○ Explain the purpose of testing to the patient.
○ Explain that the testing involves a venipuncture.
○ Explain to the patient that he may experience discomfort from the tourniquet and the needle puncture.

Implementation

○ Perform a venipuncture to collect the sample.

Patient care

○ Apply direct pressure at the venipuncture site.

Complications

○ Hematoma at venipuncture site

Interpretation

Normal results

○ A normal peripheral blood smear contains infrequent basophils.

Abnormal results

○ Basophilic leukocytosis is linked to myeloproliferative disease (myelofibrosis; agnogenic myeloid metaplasia, and polycythemia vera).
○ A rapid decrease in basophils is linked to an anaphylactic reaction.

Interfering factors

None known

Beta globulin

Overview

○ Beta globulins include low-density substances involved in fat transport (lipoproteins), iron transport (transferrin), and blood clotting (plasminogen and complement).

Purpose

○ To evaluate, diagnose, and monitor a variety of diseases and conditions such as cancer, intestinal or kidney protein-wasting syndromes, disorders of the immune system, liver dysfunction, impaired nutrition, and chronic fluid-retaining conditions

Procedure

Preparation

○ Explain the procedure to the patient.
○ Explain that the serum test requires a blood sample and that he may experience discomfort from the tourniquet and the needle puncture.
○ Inform the patient that he need not restrict fluids or food.

Implementation

○ Collect the sample according to facility policy.

Patient care

○ Apply pressure at the venipuncture site.

Complications

○ Hematoma at venipuncture site

Interpretation

Normal results

○ 0.5 to 1 g/dl

Abnormal results

○ Increased in conditions of high cholesterol levels (hypercholesterolemia) and iron deficiency anemia
○ Decreased in malnutrition

Interfering factors

None known

Beta-hydroxybutyrate assay

Overview

○ Measures serum levels of beta-hydroxybutyric acid (beta-hydroxybutyrate), one of the three ketone bodies
○ Other two ketone bodies: acetoacetate and acetone
○ Accumulation of all three ketone bodies is *ketosis*; excessive formation of ketone bodies in the blood is *ketonemia*

Purpose

○ To diagnose carbohydrate deprivation, which may result from starvation, digestive disturbances, dietary imbalances, or frequent vomiting
○ To aid in the diagnosis of diabetes mellitus resulting from decreased carbohydrate intake
○ To aid in the diagnosis of glycogen storage diseases, specifically von Gierke's disease
○ To diagnose or monitor the treatment of metabolic disorders, such as diabetic ketoacidosis or lactic acidosis

Procedure

Preparation

○ Explain to the patient that this test evaluates ketones in the blood.
○ Tell the patient that the test requires a blood sample. Explain who will perform the venipuncture and when.
○ Explain to the patient that he may experience slight discomfort from the tourniquet and the needle puncture.
○ Inform the patient that he need not restrict food and fluids.

Implementation

○ Perform a venipuncture and collect the sample in a 5-ml clot-activator tube.
○ Allow the sample to clot.
○ Centrifuge the sample and remove the serum.
○ If an acetone level is requested, have this analysis performed first.
○ Keep in mind that serum beta-hydroxybutyrate remains stable for at least 1 week at 25.6° to 46.4° F (−3.6° to 8° C). Plasma is also an acceptable sample for beta-hydroxybutyrate analysis.
○ Send the sample to the laboratory immediately.

Patient care

○ Apply direct pressure to the venipuncture site until bleeding stops.

Complications

○ Hematoma at the venipuncture site

Interpretation

Normal results

○ Less than 0.4 mmol/L (SI, < 0.4 mmol/L)

Abnormal results

○ Increased levels may suggest worsening ketosis. If the reference values are greater than 2 mmol/L (SI, > 2 mmol/L), report this to the patient's physician immediately.

Interfering factors

○ Presence of high levels of lactate dehydrogenase and lactic acid at levels greater than 10 mmol/L (SI, > 10 mmol/L) (possible increase)
○ Increased sodium fluoride levels (possible decrease)
○ Fasting (increase with extended fasting time)

Bilirubin, serum, direct and indirect

Overview

- Measures serum levels of bilirubin, the predominant pigment in bile
- Especially significant in neonates because elevated unconjugated bilirubin can accumulate in the brain, causing irreparable damage

Purpose

- To evaluate liver function
- To aid in the differential diagnosis of jaundice and monitor its progress
- To aid in the diagnosis of biliary obstruction and hemolytic anemia
- To determine whether a neonate requires an exchange transfusion or phototherapy because of dangerously high unconjugated bilirubin levels

Procedure

Preparation

- Explain to the patient that the bilirubin test evaluates liver function and the condition of red blood cells.
- Tell the patient that the test requires a blood sample. Explain who will perform the venipuncture and when.

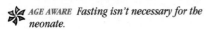 *AGE AWARE If the patient is an infant, tell the parents that a small amount of blood will be drawn from his heel. Tell them who will be performing the heel stick and when.*

- Explain to the patient that he may experience slight discomfort from the tourniquet and the needle puncture.
- Inform the adult patient that he need not restrict fluids but should fast for at least 4 hours before the test.

AGE AWARE Fasting isn't necessary for the neonate.

Implementation

- If the patient is an adult, perform a venipuncture and collect the sample in a 3- or 4-ml clot-activator tube.

AGE AWARE If the patient is an infant, perform a heel stick and fill the microcapillary tube to the designated level with blood.

- Protect the sample from strong sunlight and ultraviolet light.
- Handle the sample gently and send it to the laboratory immediately.

Patient care

- Apply direct pressure to the venipuncture site until bleeding stops.

Complications

- Hematoma at the venipuncture or heel stick site

Interpretation

Normal results

- In adults, normal indirect serum bilirubin levels are 1.1 mg/dl (SI, 19 µmol/L), and direct serum bilirubin levels are less than 0.5 mg/dl (SI, < 6.8 µmol/L).
- In neonates, total serum bilirubin levels are 2 to 12 mg/dl (SI, 34 to 205 µmol/L).

Abnormal results

- Elevated indirect serum bilirubin levels usually indicate hepatic damage.
- High levels of indirect bilirubin are also likely in severe hemolytic anemia.
- If hemolysis continues, direct and indirect bilirubin levels may rise.
- Other causes of elevated indirect bilirubin levels include congenital enzyme deficiencies such as Gilbert syndrome.
- Elevated direct serum bilirubin levels usually indicate biliary obstruction.
- If obstruction continues, direct and indirect bilirubin levels may rise.
- In severe chronic hepatic damage, direct bilirubin concentrations may return to normal or near-normal levels, but indirect bilirubin levels remain elevated.
- In neonates, total bilirubin levels of 15 mg/dl (SI, 257 µmol/L) or more indicate the need for an exchange transfusion.

Interfering factors

- Exposure of the sample to direct sunlight or ultraviolet light (possible decrease)
- Hemolysis from rough handling of the sample

Bilirubin, urine

Overview

○ Based on a color reaction with a specific reagent, detects water-soluble direct (conjugated) bilirubin in the urine
○ When combined with urobilinogen measurements, helps identify disorders that can cause jaundice
○ Can take place at the bedside, using a bilirubin reagent strip, or in the laboratory

Purpose

○ To help identify the cause of jaundice
○ To compare urine and serum bilirubin levels and other liver enzyme tests

Procedure

Preparation

○ Explain to the patient that the urine bilirubin test helps determine the cause of jaundice.
○ Inform the patient that he need not restrict food and fluids.
○ Tell the patient that the test requires a random urine specimen.
○ Advise the patient that testing of the specimen will occur at the bedside or in the laboratory.
○ Notify the laboratory and physician of drugs the patient is taking that may affect test results; it may be necessary to restrict them.

Implementation

○ Collect a random urine specimen in the container provided.
○ For bedside analysis using the dip-strip procedure: Dip the reagent strip into the specimen and remove it immediately. Compare the strip color with the color standards after 20 seconds.
○ Record the test results on the patient's chart.
○ For bedside analysis using the Ictotest procedure: Place five drops of urine on the asbestos-cellulose test mat. If bilirubin is present, the mat will absorb it. Put a reagent tablet on the wet area of the mat and place two drops of water on the tablet. If bilirubin is present, a blue to purple stain will develop on the mat. Pink or red indicates the absence of bilirubin.
○ Use only a freshly voided specimen. Bilirubin disintegrates after 30 minutes of exposure to room temperature or light.
○ If the laboratory will be analyzing the specimen, send it there immediately.
○ If testing will occur at the bedside, make sure 20 seconds elapse before interpreting the color change on the dip-strip. Make sure enough light is available to see the color.

Patient care

○ Instruct the patient that he may resume his usual medications.

Complications

None known

Interpretation

Normal results

○ Bilirubin isn't found in urine during a routine screening test.

Abnormal results

○ High concentrations of direct bilirubin in the urine may be evident from the specimen's appearance (dark, with yellow foam).
○ To diagnose jaundice, correlate the presence or absence of direct bilirubin in the urine with serum test results and with urine and fecal urobilinogen levels.

Interfering factors

○ Failure to test the specimen promptly or to send it to the laboratory immediately
○ Phenazopyridine and phenothiazine derivatives (chlorpromazine and acetophenazine maleate) (false-positive)
○ Large amounts of ascorbic acid and nitrite (false-negative if using dipstick testing, such as Chemstrip or NMultistix)
○ Exposure of specimen to room temperature or light (decrease because of bilirubin degradation)

Bleeding time

Overview

○ Measures the duration of bleeding after a measured skin incision
○ Three methods of measuring bleeding: template, Ivy, or Duke
○ Template method the most common and the most accurate because the incision size is standardized
○ Depends on the elasticity of the blood vessel wall and on the number and functional capacity of platelets
○ Although usually for the patient with a personal or family history of bleeding disorders, also useful for preoperative screening
○ Usually not recommended for the patient with a platelet count of less than $75 \times 10^3/\mu l$ (SI, $75 \times 10^9/L$)

Purpose

○ To assess overall hemostatic function (platelet response to injury and functional capacity of vasoconstriction)
○ To detect platelet function disorders

Procedure

Preparation

○ Explain to the patient that the bleeding time test measures the time it takes to form a clot and stop bleeding.
○ Tell the patient who will perform the test and when it will take place.
○ Inform the patient that he need not restrict food and fluids.
○ Inform the patient that he may feel some discomfort from the incisions, the antiseptic, and the tightness of the blood pressure cuff.
○ Inform the patient that, depending on the method used, incisions or punctures may leave tiny scars that should be barely visible when healed.
○ Notify the laboratory and physician of drugs the patient is taking that may affect test results; it may be necessary to restrict them.

Implementation

○ *Template method:* Wrap the pressure cuff around the upper arm and inflate the cuff to 40 mm Hg. Select an area on the patient's forearm with no superficial veins; clean it with antiseptic. Allow the skin to dry completely before making the incision. Apply the appropriate template lengthwise onto the forearm. Use a lancet to make two incisions 1 mm deep and 9 mm long. Start the stopwatch. Without touching the cuts, gently blot the drops of blood with filter paper every 30 seconds until the bleeding stops in both cuts. Average the bleeding time of the two cuts and record the result.

○ *Ivy method:* After applying the blood pressure cuff and preparing the test site, make three small punctures with a disposable lancet. Start the stopwatch immediately. Taking care not to touch the punctures, blot each site with filter paper every 30 seconds until the bleeding stops. Average the bleeding time of the three punctures and record the result.
○ *Duke method:* Drape the patient's shoulder with a towel. Clean the earlobe and let it air-dry. Make a puncture wound 2 to 4 mm deep on the earlobe with a disposable lancet. Start the stopwatch. Being careful not to touch the ear, blot the site with filter paper every 30 seconds until the bleeding stops. Record the bleeding time.
○ Be sure to maintain the cuff pressure at 40 mm Hg throughout the test.

Patient care

○ In a patient with a bleeding tendency (hemophilia), maintain a pressure bandage over the incision for 24 to 48 hours to prevent further bleeding. Check the test area frequently; keep the edges of the cuts aligned to minimize scarring.
○ If bleeding hasn't slowed after 15 minutes, stop the test and apply direct pressure to the test site.
○ In other patients, a piece of gauze held in place by an adhesive bandage is sufficient.
○ Instruct the patient that he may resume medications stopped before the test.

Complications

○ Bleeding that doesn't slow after 15 minutes

Interpretation

Normal results

○ 3 to 6 minutes (SI, 3 to 6 min) in the template method; 3 to 6 minutes in the Ivy method; and 1 to 3 minutes (SI, 1 to 3 min) in the Duke method.

Abnormal results

○ Prolonged bleeding time may indicate disorders linked to thrombocytopenia, such as Hodgkin's disease, acute leukemia, disseminated intravascular coagulation, hemolytic disease of the newborn, Schönlein-Henoch purpura, severe hepatic disease (cirrhosis, for example), or severe deficiency of factors I, II, V, VII, VIII, IX, and XI.
○ Prolonged bleeding time in a patient with a normal platelet count suggests a platelet function disorder (thrombasthenia, thrombocytopathia) and requires further investigation with clot retraction, prothrombin consumption, and platelet aggregation tests.

Interfering factors

○ Sulfonamides, thiazide diuretics, antineoplastics, anticoagulants, nonsteroidal anti-inflammatory drugs, vitamin E supplementation, aspirin and aspirin compounds, and some nonopioid analgesics (prolonged bleeding time)

Blood culture

Overview

- Involves inoculating a culture medium with a blood sample and incubating it for isolation and identification of the causative pathogens in bacteremia and septicemia
- Identifies about 67% of pathogens within 24 hours, and up to 90% within 72 hours
- Timing of the specimen collection dependent on type of suspected bacteremia and if drug therapy needs to restart regardless of test results

Purpose

- To confirm bacteremia
- To identify the causative organism in bacteremia and septicemia
- To determine the cause of fever with an unknown origin

Procedure

Preparation

- Inform the patient he need not restrict food and fluids.
- Explain that he may feel transient discomfort from the tourniquet and needle punctures.
- Explain the purpose of the test, who will perform it, and how many samples will be necessary.
- Explain that the study usually takes less than 5 minutes.

Implementation

- Clean the venipuncture site first with an alcohol swab and then with a povidone-iodine swab, starting at the site and working outward in a circular motion.
- Wait at least 1 minute for the skin to dry.
- Perform a venipuncture and draw 10 to 20 ml of blood for an adult, or 2 to 6 ml for a child.
- Clean the diaphragm tops of the culture bottles with alcohol or iodine and change the needle on the syringe.
- If using broth, add blood to each bottle until achieving a 1:5 or 1:10 dilution. For example, add 10 ml of blood to a 100-ml bottle. Note that the size of the bottle may vary depending on hospital protocol.
- If using a special resin, add blood to the resin in the bottles according to facility protocol, and invert gently to mix it.
- Draw the blood directly into a special collection-processing tube if using the lysis-centrifugation technique (Isolator).
- Document the tentative diagnosis and current or recent antimicrobial therapy on the laboratory request.
- Send each sample to the laboratory immediately.
- Collect blood cultures before giving antimicrobial agents whenever possible because previous or current antimicrobial therapy may give false-negative results.
- To detect most causative agents, it's best to perform the blood cultures on 2 consecutive days.

Patient care

- Use alcohol to remove the iodine from the venipuncture site.
- Monitor the venipuncture site for bleeding and signs of infection.

Complications

- Hematoma at the venipuncture site

Interpretation

Normal results

- Blood cultures are normally sterile.
- For negative specimens, make reports at 24 hours, 48 hours, and 1 week of incubation.

Abnormal results

- Positive blood cultures don't necessarily confirm pathologic septicemia.
- Mild, transient bacteremia may occur during the course of many infectious diseases or may complicate other disorders.
- Persistent, continuous, or recurrent bacteremia reliably confirms the presence of serious infection.
- Although 2% to 3% of cultured blood samples are contaminated by skin bacteria, such as *Staphylococcus epidermidis,* diphtheroids, and propionibacterium, these organisms may be clinically significant when isolated from multiple cultures or from immunocompromised patients.
- Debilitated or immunocompromised patients may have isolates of *Candida albicans.*

Interfering factors

- Improper collection techniques contaminating the sample
- Removal of culture bottle caps preventing anaerobic growth
- Use of incorrect bottle and media preventing aerobic growth and also resulting in rejection of the specimen by the laboratory

Blood urea nitrogen

Overview

○ Measures the nitrogen fraction of urea, the chief end product of protein metabolism
○ Formed in the liver from ammonia and excreted by the kidneys, urea constitutes 40% to 50% of the blood's nonprotein nitrogen
○ Reflects protein intake and renal excretory capacity but is a less reliable indicator of uremia than the serum creatinine level

Purpose

○ To evaluate kidney function and aid in the diagnosis of renal disease
○ To aid in the assessment of hydration

Procedure

Preparation

○ Tell the patient that this test is used to evaluate kidney function.
○ Inform the patient that he need not restrict food and fluids but should avoid a diet high in meat.
○ Tell the patient that the test requires a blood sample. Explain who will perform the venipuncture and when.
○ Explain to the patient that he may experience slight discomfort from the tourniquet and the needle puncture.
○ Notify the laboratory and physician of drugs the patient is taking that may affect test results; they may need to be restricted.

Implementation

○ Perform a venipuncture and collect the sample in a 3- to 4-ml clot-activator tube.
○ Handle the sample gently to prevent hemolysis.

Patient care

○ Apply direct pressure to the venipuncture site until bleeding stops.
○ Inform the patient that he may resume taking his usual medications stopped before the test.

Complications

○ Hematoma at the venipuncture site

Interpretation

Normal results

○ 8 to 20 mg/dl (SI, 2.9 to 7.5 mmol/L)

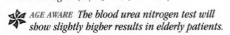 AGE AWARE *The blood urea nitrogen test will show slightly higher results in elderly patients.*

Abnormal results

○ *Elevated levels:* Renal disease, reduced renal blood flow (caused by dehydration, for example), urinary tract obstruction, and increased protein catabolism (such as burns)
○ *Low levels:* Severe hepatic damage, malnutrition, and overhydration

Interfering factors

○ Hemolysis from rough handling of the sample
○ Chloramphenicol (possible decrease)
○ Aminoglycosides, amphotericin B, and methicillin (increase caused by nephrotoxicity)

Bone biopsy

Overview

- Removal of a piece or a core of bone for histologic examination
- Performed using a special drill needle under local anesthesia (drill biopsy) or by surgical excision under general anesthesia (open biopsy)
- Excision provides a larger specimen than a drill biopsy and permits immediate surgical treatment if rapid histologic analysis of the specimen reveals a malignant tumor
- Indicated in patients with bone pain and tenderness who have a bone scan, computed tomography scan, radiographs, or arteriography that reveals a mass or deformity

Purpose

- To distinguish between benign and malignant bone tumors

Procedure

Preparation

- Make sure the patient has signed a consent form.
- Note and report allergies. Check the patient's history for hypersensitivity to the anesthetic.
- For drill biopsy, food and fluid restriction isn't usually necessary.
- For open biopsy, patient must fast overnight before the test.
- Give a local anesthetic before a drill biopsy.
- Warn the patient that he'll experience some discomfort and pressure when the biopsy needle enters the bone during a drill biopsy.
- Inform the patient that the test should take about 30 minutes.

Implementation

Drill biopsy

- The biopsy site is shaved and prepared. After a local anesthetic is given, a small incision (usually about 3 mm) is made.
- The biopsy needle is pushed into the bone using firm, even pressure. The needle is engaged in the bone and rotated about 180 degrees while maintaining steady pressure. When the bone core is obtained, the trocar is withdrawn by reversing the drilling motion.
- The biopsy specimen is placed in a properly labeled container with 10% formalin solution or Zenker's acetic acid solution.

Open biopsy

- After patient is anesthetized, the biopsy site is shaved and prepared. An incision is made and a piece of bone is removed and sent to the laboratory for immediate histologic analysis.
- The incision is closed and a sterile dressing applied.

Patient care

- Pressure is applied to the drill biopsy site with a sterile gauze pad until bleeding stops.
- A sterile dressing is applied for drill and open biopsy sites.
- Notify the physician of excessive drainage or bleeding at the biopsy site.
- Give the patient an analgesic.
- Resume the patient's usual diet after he fully recovers from anesthesia.
- Monitor the patient's vital signs and the biopsy site for signs and symptoms of infection.

Complications

- For several days after the biopsy, watch for indications of bone infection, including fever, headache, pain on movement, and tissue redness or abscess at or near the biopsy site. Notify the physician if these symptoms develop.
- Bone biopsy is performed cautiously in patients with uncorrected coagulopathy.
- Bone fracture, damage to surrounding tissue, and infection (osteomyelitis) can occur.

Interpretation

Normal results

- Bone tissue is one of two histologic types: compact or cancellous.
- Compact bone has dense, concentric layers of mineral deposits, or lamellae.
- Cancellous bone has widely spaced lamellae with osteocytes and red and yellow marrow between them.

Abnormal results

- Well-circumscribed and nonmetastasizing lesions suggest benign tumors, such as osteoid osteoma, osteoblastoma, osteochondroma, unicameral bone cyst, benign giant cell tumor, and fibroma.
- Irregularly and rapidly spreading lesions suggest malignant tumors, such as multiple myeloma and osteosarcoma.

Interfering factors

- Failure to obtain a representative bone specimen or to use the proper fixative may alter test results

Bone densitometry

Overview

- Noninvasive means to measure bone mass
- Uses a radiography tube and computer-analyzed images to measure bone mineral density
- Exposes the patient to minimal radiation
- Also called *dual energy X-ray absorptiometry*

Purpose

- To determine bone mineral density
- To identify patients at risk for osteoporosis
- To evaluate clinical response to therapy aimed at reducing the rate of bone loss

Procedure

Preparation

- Remove all metal objects from the area to be scanned.
- Explain to the patient who will perform the test and where it will occur.
- Explain the purpose of the test and how it's done.
- Explain that the test is painless and exposure to radiation is minimal.
- Explain that the test takes from 10 minutes to 1 hour, depending on the areas scanned.

Implementation

- The patient is positioned on a table under the scanning device, with the radiation source below him and the detector above.
- The lumbar spine and the proximal femur, two sites at high risk for fracture, may be scanned.
- The distal forearm may be scanned; research shows a high correlation between the bone mineral density of this area and bone mineral density of the spine and femur.
- Bone size, thickness, and volumetric density are calculated to determine potential resistance to mechanical stress.
- The detector measures the bone's absorption of radiation and registers a digital readout.

Patient care

- Make sure the patient is comfortable after the test.

Complications

None known

Interpretation

Normal results

- T-score above −1.

Abnormal results

- T-score between −1 and −2.5 may suggest osteopenia.
- T-score at or below −2.5 may suggest osteoporosis.

Interfering factors

- Osteoarthritis, fractures, size of the region to be scanned, and fat tissue distribution influencing accuracy of the test results

Bone marrow aspiration and biopsy

Overview

○ Collection of a soft tissue specimen from the medullary canals of long bone and interstices of cancellous bone for histologic and hematologic examination
○ Performed by aspiration or needle biopsy under local anesthesia
○ *Aspiration biopsy:* Removal of a fluid specimen from the bone marrow
○ *Needle biopsy:* Removal of a core of marrow cells
○ Common to perform both methods at the same time to obtain the best possible specimens

Purpose

○ To diagnose thrombocytopenia, leukemias, granulomas, anemias, and primary and metastatic tumors
○ To determine causes of infection
○ To help stage diseases such as with Hodgkin's disease
○ To evaluate chemotherapy
○ To monitor myelosuppression

Procedure

Preparation

○ Make sure the patient has signed a consent form.
○ Note all allergies.
○ Explain that collection of a blood sample is necessary before the biopsy for laboratory testing.
○ Explain to the patient that he'll feel pressure on insertion of the biopsy needle and a brief, pulling pain on removal of the marrow.
○ Give a mild sedative 1 hour before the test.
○ Explain that the test usually takes only 5 to 10 minutes.
○ Explain which bone site (sternum, anterior or posterior iliac crest, vertebral spinous process, rib, or tibia) will receive the test.

Implementation

○ The patient is positioned and instructed to remain as still as possible.

Aspiration biopsy
○ The biopsy site is prepared and draped and a local anesthetic is injected. The marrow aspiration needle is inserted through the skin, subcutaneous tissue, and bone cortex, using a twisting motion.
○ The stylet is removed from the aspiration needle, and a 10- to 20-ml syringe is attached. From 0.2 to 0.5 ml of marrow is aspirated and the needle withdrawn.
○ If the aspiration specimen is inadequate, the needle may be repositioned within the marrow cavity or removed and reinserted in another anesthetized site. If the second attempt fails, a needle biopsy may be necessary.

Needle biopsy
○ The biopsy site is prepared and draped. The skin is marked at the site with an indelible pencil or marking pen. A local anesthetic is injected intradermally, subcutaneously, and at the surface of the bone.
○ The biopsy needle is inserted into the periosteum and the needle guard set as indicated. Rotating the inner needle alternately clockwise and counterclockwise directs the needle into the marrow cavity.
○ A tissue plug is removed and the needle assembly withdrawn. The marrow is expelled into a labeled bottle containing a special fixative.

Patient care

○ While the marrow slides are being prepared, apply pressure to the biopsy site until bleeding stops.
○ Clean the biopsy site and apply a sterile dressing.
○ Monitor the patient's vital signs and the biopsy site for signs and symptoms of infection.

Complications

○ Hemorrhage and infection
○ Puncture of the mediastinum (sternum)

Interpretation

Normal results

○ Yellow marrow contains fat cells and connective tissue.
○ Red marrow contains hematopoietic cells, fat cells, and connective tissue.
○ The iron stain, which measures hemosiderin (storage iron), has a +2 level.
○ The Sudan black B stain, which shows granulocytes, is negative.
○ The periodic acid–Schiff (PAS) stain, which detects glycogen reactions, is negative.

Abnormal results

○ Decreased hemosiderin levels in an iron stain may indicate a true iron deficiency.
○ Increased hemosiderin levels may suggest other types of anemias or blood disorders.
○ A positive stain can differentiate acute myelogenous leukemia from acute lymphoblastic leukemia (negative stain).
○ A positive stain may also suggest granulation in myeloblasts.
○ A positive PAS stain may suggest acute or chronic lymphocytic leukemia, amyloidosis, thalassemia, lymphoma, infectious mononucleosis, iron-deficiency anemia, or sideroblastic anemia.

Interfering factors

○ Failure to obtain a representative specimen, to use a fixative for histologic analysis, or to immediately send the specimen to the laboratory

Bone scan

Overview

- Imaging of the skeleton with a scanning camera after I.V. injection of a radioactive tracer compound (radioactive technetium diphosphonate).
- Increased concentrations of the tracer collect in bone tissue at sites of abnormal metabolism; when scanned, these sites appear as hot spots (commonly detectable months before radiography reveals a lesion).
- May be performed with a gallium scan to detect lesions at an early stage.
- Primary indications for the test include patients with symptoms of metastatic bone disease, patients with bone trauma, and those with known degenerative disorders that require monitoring.

Purpose

- To detect malignant bone lesions when radiographic findings are normal but cancer is confirmed or suspected
- To rule out suspected bone lesions
- To detect occult bone trauma associated with pathologic fractures
- To monitor degenerative bone disorders
- To detect infection
- To evaluate unexplained bone pain
- To assist in staging cancer

Procedure

Preparation

- Make sure the patient has signed an appropriate consent form, if required.
- Note all allergies.
- Inform the patient that there are no dietary restrictions.
- Instruct the patient to drink fluids to maintain hydration and to reduce the radiation dose to the bladder after the tracer injection and before scanning.
- Explain the importance of holding still during scanning.
- Explain that the scan is painless and takes about 1 hour and that the radioactive isotope emits less radiation than a standard radiograph machine.
- Explain that the patient will receive analgesics for positional discomfort.

Implementation

- The I.V. tracer and imaging agent are given 3 hours before the scan.
- Encourage increased fluid intake for the next 1 to 3 hours to facilitate the renal clearance of circulating free tracer that isn't picked up by bone.

- Instruct the patient to urinate immediately before the procedure, or insert a urinary catheter to empty the bladder.
- The patient is positioned on the scanner table.
- As the scanner moves over the patient's body, it detects low-level radiation emitted by the skeleton and translates this into a two-dimensional picture.
- The scanner takes as many views as needed to cover the specified area.
- The patient may be repositioned as needed during the test to obtain adequate views.

🌟 *AGE AWARE It may be necessary to sedate children who are unable to hold still for the scan.*

Patient care

- Instruct the patient to drink additional fluids and to empty his bladder frequently for the next 24 to 48 hours.
- Monitor the patient for signs and symptoms of infection at the injection site.
- Monitor intake and output.
- Avoid scheduling additional radionuclide tests for the next 24 to 48 hours.

Complications

- Infection at the injection site
- Allergic reactions to radionuclide (rare)

Interpretation

Normal results

- Uptake of the tracer is symmetrical and uniform.
- The tracer concentrates at sites of new bone formation or increased metabolism.
- The epiphyses of growing bone are normal sites of high concentration or hot spots.

Abnormal results

- Increased uptake of tracer where bone formation is occurring faster than in surrounding bone may suggest all types of bone cancer, infection, fracture or additional disorders when used in conjunction with the patient's medical and surgical history, radiographic findings, and laboratory test results.

Interfering factors

- Antihypertensives
- A distended bladder obscuring pelvic detail
- Improper injection technique allowing the tracer to seep into muscle tissue, producing erroneous hot spots

Breast biopsy

Overview

- Allows histologic examination of breast tissue to confirm or rule out cancer.
- Needle biopsy or fine-needle biopsy: Obtains a core of tissue or a fluid aspirate; provide only limited diagnostic values because it may obtain small and unrepresentative specimens.
- Open biopsy: Provides a complete tissue specimen, which allows sectioning of the specimen and a more accurate evaluation.
- Breast tissue analysis usually includes an estrogen and progesterone receptor assay to aid in selecting therapy if a mass is malignant.
- Indications for the test include palpable masses, suspicious areas on mammography, bloody discharge from the nipples, persistently encrusted, inflamed, or eczematoid breast lesions.

Purpose

- To differentiate between benign and malignant breast tumors

Procedure

Preparation

- Make sure the patient has signed a consent form.
- Note and report all allergies.
- If the patient is to receive local anesthesia, tell her she need not restrict food or fluids.
- If the patient is to have general anesthesia, tell her she is to have nothing by mouth after midnight before the procedure.
- Obtain and report abnormal results of prebiopsy studies, such as blood tests, urine tests, and radiographs of the chest.
- Explain that the test takes 15 to 30 minutes.

Implementation

Needle biopsy
- The site is prepared and draped, and the patient is given a local anesthetic.
- The syringe is introduced into the lesion. Aspirated fluid is placed into a labeled, heparinized tube.
- The aspiration procedure is both diagnostic and therapeutic if cyst fluid is clear yellow and the mass disappears. In this case, the aspirate is discarded.
- If cyst aspiration yields no fluid or if the lesion recurs two or three times, an open biopsy is appropriate.
- The tissue is placed in a labeled specimen bottle containing normal saline solution or formalin.
- With fine-needle aspiration, a slide is made for cytology and viewed immediately under a microscope.

Open biopsy
- The site is prepared and draped, and the patient is given a local or general anesthetic.
- An incision is made in the breast to expose the mass. A portion of tissue or the entire mass is excised.
- Benign-appearing masses smaller than ¾″ (2 cm) in diameter are usually excised.
- The specimens are placed in properly labeled specimen bottles containing 10% formalin solution.
- The malignant-appearing tissue is sent for frozen section and receptor assays.

Patient care

- Tell the patient to wear a support bra at all times after the test until healing is complete.
- Apply pressure to the biopsy site until bleeding stops.
- For a needle biopsy, apply a sterile dressing.
- After an open biopsy, the site is sutured and a sterile dressing applied.
- Give the patient an analgesic.
- Apply an ice bag to the site for discomfort.
- Provide emotional support.
- Monitor the patient's vital signs and the site for bleeding.
- Monitor the patient for signs and symptoms of infection at the biopsy site.

Complications

- Bleeding and infection

Interpretation

Normal results

- Breast tissue consists of cellular and noncellular connective tissue, fat lobules, and various lactiferous ducts.
- Breast tissue is pink, more fatty than fibrous, and shows no abnormal development of cells or tissue elements.

Abnormal results

- Benign tumors may suggest fibrocystic disease, adenofibroma, intraductal papilloma, mammary fat necrosis, or plasma cell mastitis.
- Malignant tumors may suggest adenocarcinoma, cystosarcoma, intraductal or infiltrating carcinoma, inflammatory carcinoma, medullary or circumscribed carcinoma, colloid carcinoma, lobular carcinoma, sarcoma, or Paget's disease.

Interfering factors

- Failure to obtain an adequate tissue specimen or to place the specimen in the proper solution container interfering with test results

Bronchography

Overview

- X-ray examination of the tracheobronchial tree after instillation of a radiopaque iodine contrast agent through a catheter into the lumens of the trachea and bronchi.
- Contrast agent coats the bronchial tree, permitting visualization of anatomic deviations.
- Bronchography of a localized lung area is possible by instilling contrast dye through a fiber-optic bronchoscope.

Purpose

- To help detect bronchiectasis and map its location for surgical resection
- To detect bronchial obstruction, pulmonary tumors, cysts, and cavities; to help pinpoint the cause of hemoptysis
- To provide permanent films of pathologic findings
- To guide procedures such as bronchoscopy

Procedure

Preparation

- Explain to the patient that bronchography helps evaluate abnormalities of the bronchial structures.
- Instruct the patient to fast for 12 hours before the test.
- Tell the patient to perform good oral hygiene the night before and the morning of the test.
- Make sure the patient or a responsible family member has signed an informed consent form.
- Check the patient's history for hypersensitivity to anesthetics, iodine, or contrast media.
- If the patient has a productive cough, give a prescribed expectorant and perform postural drainage 1 to 3 days before the test.
- If the procedure will involve a local anesthetic, tell the patient that he'll receive a sedative to help him relax and to suppress the gag reflex. Prepare him for the unpleasant taste of the anesthetic spray.
- Warn the patient that he may experience some difficulty breathing during the procedure, but reassure him that his airway won't be blocked and that he'll receive enough oxygen. Tell him the catheter or bronchoscope will pass more easily if he relaxes.
- If bronchography is to occur under a general anesthetic, inform the patient that he'll receive a sedative before the test to help him relax.
- Just before the test, instruct the patient to remove his dentures (if present) and to void.

Implementation

- After a local anesthetic is sprayed into the patient's mouth and throat, a bronchoscope or catheter is passed into the trachea and the anesthetic and contrast medium are instilled.
- The patient is placed in various positions during the test to promote movement of the contrast medium into different areas of the bronchial tree. After X-rays are taken, the contrast medium is removed through postural drainage and by having the patient cough it up.

Patient care

- Withhold food, fluids, and oral drugs until the gag reflex returns (usually in 2 hours). Fluid intake before the gag reflex returns may cause aspiration.
- Encourage gentle coughing and postural drainage to facilitate clearing of the contrast medium. A post-drainage film is usually done in 24 to 48 hours.
- If the patient has a sore throat, reassure him that it's only temporary and provide throat lozenges or a liquid gargle when his gag reflex returns.
- Advise the outpatient not to resume his usual activities until the next day.

Complications

- Laryngeal spasm (dyspnea) or edema (hoarseness, dyspnea, laryngeal stridor) because of traumatic intubation
- Allergic reaction to the contrast medium or anesthetic, causing itching, dyspnea, tachycardia, palpitations, excitation, hypotension, hypertension, or euphoria
- Chemical or secondary bacterial pneumonia — with fever, dyspnea, crackles, or rhonchi — caused by incomplete expectoration of the contrast medium
- Laryngeal spasm (dyspnea) because of the instillation of the contrast medium, in patients with asthma
- Airway occlusion secondary to the instillation of the contrast medium, in patients with chronic obstructive pulmonary disease

Interpretation

Normal results

- The right mainstem bronchus is shorter, wider, and more vertical than the left bronchus. Successive branches of the bronchi become smaller in diameter and are free from obstruction or lesions.

Abnormal results

- Bronchiectasis or bronchial obstruction caused by tumors, cysts, cavities, or foreign objects.

Interfering factors

- Presence of secretions or improper patient positioning (possible poor imaging because of inadequate filling of bronchial tree)
- Inability to suppress coughing (interferes with bronchial filling and retention of the contrast medium)

Bronchoscopy

Overview

- Direct visualization of the larynx, trachea, and bronchi using a rigid or fiber-optic bronchoscope
- Flexible fiber-optic bronchoscope: allows a better view of the segmental and subsegmental bronchi with less risk of trauma
- Large, rigid bronchoscope: Removes foreign objects, excises endobronchial lesions, and controls massive hemoptysis; requires general anesthesia
- Brush, biopsy forceps, or catheter may be passed through the bronchoscope to obtain specimens for cytologic or microbiologic examination

Purpose

- To allow visual examination of tumors, obstructions, secretions, or foreign bodies in the tracheobronchial tree
- To diagnose bronchogenic carcinoma, tuberculosis, interstitial pulmonary disease, and fungal or parasitic pulmonary infections
- To obtain specimens for microbiological and cytologic examination
- To locate bleeding sites in the tracheobronchial tree
- To remove foreign bodies, malignant or benign tumors, mucous plugs, and excessive secretions from the tracheobronchial tree

Procedure

Preparation

- Make sure the patient has signed an appropriate consent form.
- Note allergies.
- Instruct the patient to fast for 6 to 12 hours before the test.
- Obtain results of preprocedure studies; report abnormal results.
- Obtain baseline vital signs.
- An I.V. sedative may be given.
- Remove the patient's dentures.
- Explain to the patient that the test takes 45 to 60 minutes.
- Inform the patient that blocking of the airway won't occur and that hoarseness, loss of voice, hemoptysis, and sore throat may occur.

Implementation

- Position the patient properly.
- Give the patient supplemental oxygen by nasal cannula, if ordered.
- Monitor the patient's pulse oximetry, vital signs, and cardiac rhythm.
- Local anesthetic is sprayed into the patient's mouth and throat to suppress the gag reflex.
- The bronchoscope is inserted through the mouth or nose; a bite block is placed in the mouth if using the oral approach.
- When the bronchoscope is just above the vocal cords, about 3 to 4 ml of 2% to 4% lidocaine is flushed through the inner channel of the scope to the vocal cords to anesthetize deeper areas.
- A fiber-optic camera is used to take photographs for documentation.
- Tissue specimens are obtained from suspect areas.
- A suction apparatus may remove foreign bodies or mucous plugs.
- Bronchoalveolar lavage may remove thickened secretions or may diagnose infectious causes of infiltrates.
- Specimens are prepared properly and immediately sent to the laboratory.

Patient care

- Position a conscious patient in semi-Fowler's position.
- Position an unconscious patient on one side, with the head of the bed slightly elevated to prevent aspiration.
- Instruct the patient to spit out saliva rather than swallow it.
- Observe the patient for bleeding.
- Resume the patient's usual diet, beginning with sips of clear liquid or ice chips, when the gag reflex returns.
- Provide lozenges or a soothing liquid gargle to ease discomfort when the gag reflex returns.
- Check the follow-up chest X-ray for pneumothorax.
- Monitor the patient's vital signs, characteristics of sputum, and respiratory status.

Complications

- Subcutaneous crepitus around the patient's face, neck, or chest, which may indicate tracheal or bronchial perforation or pneumothorax
- Symptoms of respiratory difficulty from laryngeal edema or laryngospasm, such as laryngeal stridor and dyspnea
- Hypoxemia, cardiac arrhythmias, bleeding, infection, bronchospasm, and laryngeal edema

Interpretation

Normal results

- The bronchi appear structurally similar to the trachea.
- The right bronchus is slightly larger and more vertical than the left.
- Smaller segmental bronchi branch off from the main bronchi.

Abnormal results

- Structural abnormalities of the bronchial wall indicating inflammation, ulceration, tumors, and enlargement of submucosal lymph nodes

- Structural abnormalities of endotracheal origin suggesting stenosis, compression, ectasia, and diverticula
- Structural abnormalities of the trachea or bronchi suggesting calculi, foreign bodies, masses, and paralyzed vocal cords
- Tissue and cell study abnormalities suggesting interstitial pulmonary disease, infection, carcinoma, and tuberculosis

Interfering factors

- Failure to observe pretest dietary restrictions, possibly causing aspiration
- Failure to place the specimens in the appropriate containers or to send them to the laboratory immediately, which may interfere with accurate test results

B-type natriuretic peptide assay

Overview

○ B-type natriuretic peptide (BNP) is a neurohormone produced predominantly by the heart ventricle.
○ Heart releases BNP in response to blood volume expansion or pressure overload.
○ Plasma BNP increases with the severity of heart failure. (The heart is the major source of circulating BNP.)

Purpose

○ To aid in the diagnosis and severity of heart failure

Procedure

Preparation

○ Explain to the patient that the BNP assay is used to identify the presence and severity of heart failure.
○ Tell the patient that the assay requires a blood sample. Explain who will perform the venipuncture and when.
○ Explain to the patient that he may experience slight discomfort from the tourniquet and the needle puncture.

○ Inform the patient that he need not restrict food and fluids.

Implementation

○ Perform a venipuncture and collect the sample in a 3.5-ml ethylenediaminetetraacetic acid tube.
○ Handle the sample gently to prevent hemolysis.

Patient care

○ Apply direct pressure to the venipuncture site until bleeding stops.

Complications

○ Hematoma at the venipuncture site

Interpretation

Normal results

○ Less than 100 pg/ml

Abnormal results

○ Blood levels greater than 100 pg/ml are an accurate predictor of heart failure.
○ The level of BNP in the blood is related to the severity of heart failure.
○ The higher the level, the worse the symptoms of heart failure. (See *Linking BNP levels to severity of heart failure symptoms.*)

Interfering factors

○ Hemolysis from rough handling of the sample

Linking BNP levels to severity of heart failure symptoms

This table shows B-type natriuretic peptide (BNP) levels and the correlation with symptoms of heart failure. The higher the level of BNP, the more severe the symptoms.

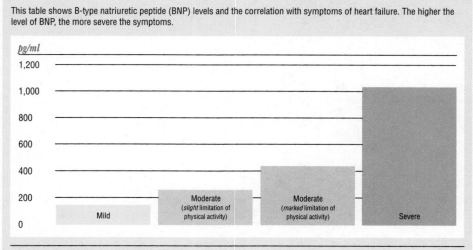

Adapted with permission of Biosite Diagnostics. © 2001 Biosite Diagnostics.

Calcium, ionized

Overview

○ Measures the fraction of serum calcium that's in the ionized form

Purpose

○ To screen for or monitor diseases of the bone or calcium-regulation disorders (that is, diseases of the parathyroid gland or kidneys)

Procedure

Preparation

○ Explain to the patient that the test requires a blood sample.
○ Explain the reason for testing.
○ Inform the patient that some drugs can increase ionized calcium measurements. These include calcium salts (found in nutritional supplements or antacids), hydralazine, lithium, thiazide diuretics, and thyroxine.
○ Instruct the patient to fast for 6 hours before the test.

Implementation

○ Perform a venipuncture and collect 5 to 10 ml of venous blood in a red-top tube.

Patient care

○ Apply a pressure dressing to the venipuncture site.

Complications

○ Hematoma at the venipuncture site

Interpretation

Normal results

○ In adults, 4.4 to 5.3 mg/dl
○ In children, 4.4 to 6 mg/dl

Abnormal results

○ Decreased levels (from many possible causes) may lead to neuromuscular irritability or tetany symptoms.
○ Diarrhea, malabsorption of calcium, burns, alcoholism, pancreatitis, and chronic renal failure may cause decreased levels.
○ Malignant neoplasm of the bone, lung, breast, bladder, or kidney may cause increased levels.

Interfering factors

○ Antibiotics, magnesium products, laxatives, and heparin (decrease)
○ Alkaline antacids, calcium salts, and vitamin D (increase)
○ Excessive ingestion of milk (increase)

Calcium, serum

Overview

○ Measures the total amount of calcium in the blood

Purpose

○ To evaluate endocrine function, calcium metabolism, and acid-base balance
○ To guide therapy in patients with renal failure, renal transplant, endocrine disorders, malignancies, cardiac disease, and skeletal disorders

Procedure

Preparation

○ Explain to the patient that the serum calcium test determines blood calcium levels.
○ Tell the patient that the test requires a blood sample. Explain who will perform the venipuncture and when.
○ Explain to the patient that he may experience slight discomfort from the tourniquet and the needle puncture.
○ Inform the patient that he need not restrict food and fluids.

Implementation

○ Perform a venipuncture (without a tourniquet if possible) and collect the sample in a 3- or 4-ml clot-activator tube.

Patient care

○ Apply direct pressure to the venipuncture site until bleeding stops.

Complications

○ Hematoma at the venipuncture site

Interpretation

Normal results

○ In adults, 8.2 to 10.2 mg/dl (SI, 2.05 to 2.54 mmol/L)
○ In children, 8.6 to 11.2 mg/dl (SI, 2.15 to 2.79 mmol/L)

Abnormal results

○ Abnormally high serum calcium levels (hypercalcemia) may occur in hyperparathyroidism and parathyroid tumors, Paget's disease of the bone, multiple myeloma, metastatic carcinoma, multiple fractures, and prolonged immobilization.
○ Elevated levels may also result from inadequate excretion of calcium, such as adrenal insufficiency and renal disease; from excessive calcium ingestion; and from overuse of antacids such as calcium carbonate.

○ Observe the patient with hypercalcemia for deep bone pain, flank pain caused by renal calculi, and muscle hypotonicity. Hypercalcemic crisis begins with nausea, vomiting, and dehydration, leading to stupor and coma, and can end in cardiac arrest.
○ Low calcium levels (hypocalcemia) may result from hypoparathyroidism, total parathyroidectomy, and malabsorption.
○ Decreased serum calcium levels may also occur with Cushing's syndrome, renal failure, acute pancreatitis, peritonitis, malnutrition with hypoalbuminemia, and blood transfusions (caused by citrate).
○ In the patient with hypocalcemia, be alert for circumoral and peripheral numbness and tingling, muscle twitching, Chvostek's sign (facial muscle spasm), tetany, muscle cramping, Trousseau's sign (carpopedal spasm), seizures, arrhythmias, laryngeal spasm, decreased cardiac output, prolonged bleeding time, fractures, and prolonged QT interval.

Interfering factors

○ Venous stasis from prolonged tourniquet application (false-high)
○ Excessive ingestion of vitamin D or its derivatives (dihydrotachysterol, calcitriol) or use of androgens, calciferol-activated calcium salts, progestins-estrogens, and thiazide diuretics (increase)
○ Acetazolamide, corticosteroids, plicamycin, chronic laxative use, and excessive transfusions of citrated blood (increase or decrease)

Calcium, urine

Overview

○ Measures the level of calcium in the urine; generally parallels serum level

Purpose

○ To evaluate calcium metabolism and excretion
○ To monitor treatment of calcium deficiency

Procedure

Preparation

○ Explain to the patient that the urine calcium test measures the amount of calcium in the urine.
○ Encourage the patient to be as active as possible before the test.
○ Tell the patient that the test requires urine collection over 24 hours. If the patient is to collect the specimen, teach him the proper technique.
○ Provide a diet that contains about 130 mg of calcium/24 hours for 3 days before the test or provide information about the diet for the patient to follow at home.
○ Notify the laboratory and physician of drugs the patient is taking that may affect test results; it may be necessary to restrict them.

Implementation

○ Collect the patient's urine over 24 hours, discarding the first specimen and retaining the last.
○ Tell the patient not to contaminate the specimen with toilet tissue or stool.

Patient care

○ Observe the patient with low urine calcium levels for tetany.
○ Inform the patient that he may resume his usual diet, activities, and medications.

Complications

None known

Interpretation

Normal results

○ For a normal diet, urine calcium levels in 24 hours 100 to 300 mg/24 hours (SI, 2.5 to 7.5 mmol/day)

Abnormal results

○ Many disorders may affect calcium levels. (See *Disorders that affect urine calcium and urine phosphorus levels.*)

Interfering factors

○ Failure to collect all urine during the test period
○ Parathyroid hormones (decrease calcium)
○ Thiazide diuretics (decrease)
○ Prolonged inactivity and ingestion of corticosteroids, sodium phosphate, calcitonin (increase)

Disorders that affect urine calcium and urine phosphorus levels

Disorder	Urine calcium level	Urine phosphate level
Acute nephritis	Suppressed	Suppressed
Acute nephrosis	Suppressed	Suppressed or normal
Chronic nephrosis	Suppressed	Suppressed
Hyperparathyroidism	Elevated	Elevated
Hypoparathyroidism	Suppressed	Suppressed
Metastatic carcinoma	Elevated	Normal
Milk-alkali syndrome	Suppressed or normal	Suppressed or normal
Multiple myeloma	Elevated or normal	Elevated or normal
Osteomalacia	Suppressed	Suppressed
Paget's disease	Normal	Normal
Renal insufficiency	Suppressed	Suppressed
Renal tubular acidosis	Elevated	Elevated
Sarcoidosis	Elevated	Suppressed
Steatorrhea	Suppressed	Suppressed
Vitamin D intoxication	Elevated	Suppressed

Capillary fragility

Overview

○ Also called the *positive-pressure test*, the *tourniquet test*, and the *Rumpel-Leede test*, the capillary fragility test is a nonspecific method for evaluating bleeding tendencies
○ Measures the ability of capillaries to remain intact under increased intracapillary pressure

Purpose

○ To assess the fragility of capillary walls
○ To identify a platelet deficiency (thrombocytopenia)

Procedure

Preparation

○ Explain to the patient that the capillary fragility test identifies abnormal bleeding tendencies.
○ Tell the patient who will be performing the procedure and when.
○ Inform the patient that he need not restrict food and fluids.
○ Explain to the patient that he may feel discomfort from the pressure of the blood pressure cuff.

Implementation

○ The patient's skin temperature and the room temperature should be normal to ensure accurate results.
○ Select and mark a 2″ (5-cm) space on the patient's forearm. Ideally, the site should be free from petechiae; otherwise, record the number of petechiae before starting the test.
○ Fasten the cuff around the arm and raise the pressure to a point midway between the systolic and diastolic blood pressures.
○ Maintain this pressure for 5 minutes; then release the cuff.
○ Count the number of petechiae that appear in the 2″ space.
○ Record the test results.

Patient care

○ Encourage the patient to open and close his hand a few times to hasten the return of blood to the forearm.
○ Don't repeat this test on the same arm within 1 week.

Complications

○ Contraindicated in patients with disseminated intravascular coagulation (DIC) or other bleeding disorders and in those with significant petechiae already present.

Interpretation

Normal results

○ A few petechiae may normally be present before the test. Fewer than 10 petechiae on the forearm 5 minutes (SI, 5 minutes) after the test is considered normal, or a negative result; more than 10 petechiae is considered a positive result.

Abnormal results

○ A positive result (more than 10 petechiae, or a score of 2+ to 4+) indicates weakness of the capillary walls (vascular purpura) or a platelet defect. It may occur in such conditions as thrombocytopenia, thrombasthenia, purpura senilis, scurvy, DIC, von Willebrand's disease, vitamin K deficiency, dysproteinemia, polycythemia vera, and in severe deficiencies of factor VII, fibrinogen, or prothrombin. Conditions unrelated to bleeding defects, such as scarlet fever, measles, influenza, chronic renal disease, hypertension, and diabetes with coexisting vascular disease, may increase capillary fragility.
○ An abnormal number of petechiae sometimes appear before menstruation and at other times in some healthy persons, especially in women over age 40.

Interfering factors

○ Decreasing estrogen levels in postmenopausal women (increase)
○ Glucocorticoids (decrease)
○ Repeating the test on the same arm within 1 week, causing errors in counting the number of petechiae

Carcinoembryonic antigen

Overview

○ Stages and monitors treatment of certain cancers

Purpose

○ To monitor the effectiveness of cancer therapy
○ To assist in preoperative staging of colorectal cancers, assess the adequacy of surgical resection, and test for recurrence of colorectal cancers

Procedure

Preparation

○ Explain to the patient that this test detects and measures a special protein that isn't normally present in adults.
○ Inform the patient that it may be necessary to repeat the test to monitor the effectiveness of therapy.
○ Inform the patient that he need not restrict food, fluids, or drugs.
○ Tell the patient that the test requires a blood sample.
○ Explain to the patient that he may experience slight discomfort from the tourniquet and the needle puncture.

Implementation

○ Perform a venipuncture and collect the sample in a 7-ml tube without additives.
○ Handle the sample gently to prevent hemolysis.
○ Send the sample to the laboratory immediately.

Patient care

○ Apply direct pressure to the venipuncture site until bleeding stops.

Complications

○ Hematoma at the venipuncture site

Interpretation

Normal results

○ Less than 5 nanograms/ml

Abnormal results

○ Persistent elevations suggest residual or recurrent tumor.
○ High levels are characteristic in various malignant conditions, particularly endodermally derived neoplasms of the GI organs and lungs, and in certain nonmalignant conditions, such as benign hepatic disease, hepatic cirrhosis, alcoholic pancreatitis, and inflammatory bowel disease.
○ Elevated levels may occur in nonendodermal carcinomas, such as breast and ovarian cancers.

Interfering factors

○ Chronic cigarette smoking (increase)
○ Rough handling of the sample (hemolysis)

Cardiac blood pool imaging

Overview

○ Evaluates regional and global ventricular performance after I.V. injection of human serum albumin or red blood cells (RBCs) tagged with the isotope technetium 99m (^{99m}Tc) pertechnetate

○ In first-pass imaging, a scintillation camera records the radioactivity emitted by the isotope in its initial pass through the left ventricle

○ Higher counts of radioactivity occur during diastole because there's more blood in the ventricle; lower counts occur during systole as the blood is ejected

○ It's possible to calculate the portion of isotope ejected during each heartbeat to determine the ejection fraction and to determine the presence and size of intracardiac shunts

○ More accurate and involves less risk to the patient than left ventriculography in assessing cardiac function

Purpose

○ To evaluate left ventricular function

○ To detect aneurysms of the left ventricle and other motion abnormalities of the myocardial wall (areas of akinesia or dyskinesia)

○ To detect intracardiac shunting

Procedure

Preparation

○ Explain to the patient that cardiac blood pooling imaging permits assessment of the heart's left ventricle.

○ Describe the test, including who will perform it, where it will take place, and its expected duration.

○ Tell the patient that he need not restrict food and fluids.

○ Explain to the patient that he'll receive an I.V. injection of a radioactive tracer and that a detector positioned above his chest will record the circulation of this tracer through his heart.

○ Reassure the patient that the tracer poses no radiation hazard and rarely produces adverse effects.

○ Inform the patient that he may experience slight discomfort from the needle puncture but that the imaging itself is painless.

○ Instruct the patient to remain silent and motionless during imaging, unless otherwise instructed.

○ Make sure that the patient or a responsible family member has signed an informed consent form.

Implementation

○ The patient is placed in a supine position beneath the detector of a scintillation camera and 15 to 20 milli-curies of albumin or RBCs tagged with ^{99m}Tc pertechnetate is injected I.V.

○ For the next minute, the scintillation camera records the first pass of the isotope through the heart to locate the aortic and mitral valves.

○ Then, using an electrocardiogram, the camera is gated for selected 60-millisecond intervals, representing end-systole and end-diastole, and 500 to 1,000 cardiac cycles are recorded on X-ray or Polaroid film.

○ To observe septal and posterior wall motion, the patient may be assisted to a modified left anterior oblique position or he may be assisted to a right anterior oblique position and given 0.4 mg of nitroglycerin sublingually. The scintillation camera then records additional gated images to evaluate abnormal contraction in the left ventricle.

○ The patient may be asked to exercise as the scintillation camera records gated images.

▽ *AGE AWARE If the patient is elderly or physically compromised, assist him to a sitting position and make sure he isn't dizzy. Then assist him in getting off the examination table.*

Patient care

○ Monitor the patient's vital signs and response to the testing.

○ Answer the patient's questions about the test.

Complications

○ Contraindicated during pregnancy

Interpretation

Normal results

○ The left ventricle contracts symmetrically, and the isotope appears evenly distributed in the scans. Normal ejection fraction is 55% to 65%.

Abnormal results

○ The patient with coronary artery disease usually has asymmetrical blood distribution to the myocardium, which produces segmental abnormalities of ventricular wall motion; such abnormalities may also result from pre-existing conditions such as myocarditis.

○ The patient with a cardiomyopathy shows globally reduced ejection fractions.

○ In the patient with a left-to-right shunt, the recirculating radioisotope prolongs the down slope of the curve of scintigraphic data; early arrival of activity in the left ventricle or aorta signifies a right-to-left shunt.

Interfering factors

None known

Cardiac catheterization

Overview

○ Involves passage of a catheter into the right, left, or both sides of the heart
○ Measures pressure in chambers of the heart; records films of the ventricles (contrast ventriculography) and arteries (coronary arteriography)
○ Left-sided heart catheterization: Assesses patency of the coronary arteries and function of left ventricle
○ Right-sided heart catheterization: Assesses pulmonary artery pressures

Purpose

○ To evaluate valvular insufficiency or stenosis, septal defects, congenital anomalies, myocardial function, myocardial blood supply, and cardiac wall motion
○ To aid in diagnosing left ventricular enlargement, aortic root enlargement, ventricular aneurysms, and intracardiac shunts

Procedure

Preparation

○ Make sure the patient has signed a consent form.
○ Notify the physician of hypersensitivity to shellfish, iodine, or contrast media.
○ Stop anticoagulant as ordered to reduce complications of bleeding.
○ Restrict food and fluids for at least 6 hours before the test.
○ Explain that if a mild sedative is given, the patient remains conscious.
○ Warn the patient that a transient hot, flushing sensation or nausea may occur.
○ Tell the patient that the test will take 1 to 2 hours.

Implementation

○ The patient is placed supine on a padded table and his heart rate and rhythm, respiratory status, and blood pressure are monitored throughout the procedure.
○ An I.V. line is started, if not already in place, and a local anesthetic is injected at the insertion site.
○ A small incision is made into the artery or vein, depending on whether the test is for the left or right.
○ The catheter is passed through the sheath into the vessel and guided using fluoroscopy.
○ In right-sided heart catheterization, the catheter is inserted into the antecubital or femoral vein and advanced through the vena cavae into the right side of the heart and into the pulmonary artery.
○ In left-sided heart catheterization, the catheter is inserted into the brachial or femoral artery and advanced retrograde through the aorta into the coronary artery ostium and left ventricle.

○ When the catheter is in place, contrast medium is injected to make visible the cardiac vessels and structures.
○ Nitroglycerin is given to eliminate catheter-induced spasm or watch its effect on the coronary arteries.
○ After the catheter is removed, direct pressure is applied to the incision site until bleeding stops, and a sterile dressing is applied.

Patient care

○ Reinforce the dressing as needed.
○ Enforce bed rest for 8 hours.
○ If the femoral route was used for catheter insertion, keep the leg straight at the hip for 6 to 8 hours.
○ If the antecubital fossa route was used, keep the arm straight at the elbow for at least 3 hours.
○ Resume medications and give analgesics.
○ Encourage fluid intake.
○ Monitor patient's vital signs, intake and output, cardiac rhythm, neurologic and respiratory status, and peripheral vascular status distal to the puncture site.
○ Check the catheter insertion site and dressings for signs and symptoms of infection.

Complications

○ Infective endocarditis in a patient with valvular heart disease (administer prophylactic antibiotics)
○ Left- or right-sided heart catheterization: Myocardial infarction, arrhythmias, cardiac tamponade, infection, hypovolemia, pulmonary edema, hematoma, blood loss, adverse reaction to contrast media, and vasovagal response
○ Left-sided heart catheterization: Arterial thrombus or embolism, and stroke
○ Right-sided heart catheterization: Thrombophlebitis and pulmonary embolism

Interpretation

Normal results

○ No abnormalities of heart valves, chamber size, pressures, configuration, wall motion or thickness, and blood flow.
○ Coronary arteries have a smooth and regular outline.

Abnormal results

○ Coronary artery narrowing greater than 70% suggests significant coronary artery disease.
○ Narrowing of the left main coronary artery and occlusion or narrowing high in the left anterior descending artery suggests the need for revascularization surgery.
○ Impaired wall motion suggests myocardial incompetence.
○ A pressure gradient indicates valvular heart disease.
○ Retrograde flow of the contrast medium across a valve during systole indicates valvular incompetence.

Interfering factors

None known

Cardiac magnetic resonance imaging

Overview

○ Magnetic resonance imaging (MRI) — a noninvasive procedure providing cross-sectional images of bone and delineation of fluid-filled soft tissue in great detail; produces images of organs and vessels in motion
○ Most commonly relies on the magnetic properties of hydrogen, the most abundant and magnetically sensitive of the body's atoms
○ Cardiac MRI: Involves placing the patient in a magnetic field, obtaining cross-sectional images of the heart and related structures in multiple planes, and making a permanent record
○ Magnetic fields and radiofrequency (RF) energy are imperceptible; no harmful effects have been documented
○ There are optimal magnetic fields and RF waves for each type of tissue under investigation

Purpose

○ To identify anatomic sequelae related to myocardial infarction, such as formation of ventricular aneurysm and mural thrombus
○ To detect and evaluate cardiomyopathy
○ To detect and evaluate pericardial disease
○ To identify paracardiac or intracardiac masses
○ To detect and evaluate congenital heart disease, such as atrial or ventricular septal defects and malposition of the great vessels
○ To identify vascular disease, such as thoracic aortic aneurysm and dissection
○ To assess the structure of the pulmonary vasculature

Procedure

Preparation

○ Make sure the patient has signed an appropriate consent form.
○ Note and report allergies.
○ Explain to the patient that restriction of food and fluids isn't necessary.
○ Have the patient remove all metal objects.
○ Make sure the patient doesn't have a pacemaker or surgically implanted joints, pins, clips, valves, or pumps containing metal that could be attracted to the strong MRI magnet.
○ Ask if the patient has ever worked with metals.
○ Explain that MRI is painless, but that remaining still inside a small space during the test may make the patient feel uncomfortable.
○ The patient may wear earplugs because the scanner makes clicking, whirring, and thumping noises as it moves.

○ Provide reassurance to the patient that he'll be able to communicate with the technician at all times; tell him the procedure will be stopped if he feels claustrophobic.
○ Give a sedative if ordered, especially for a claustrophobic patient.
○ Explain that the test takes up to 90 minutes.
○ Unstable patients need an I.V. access without metal components, and all equipment must be MRI-compatible.

Implementation

○ Check the patient for metal objects; no metal can enter the testing area because the MRI works through a powerful magnetic field.
○ The patient is placed in a supine position on a narrow, padded, nonmetallic bed that slides to the desired position inside the scanner.
○ During the procedure the patient is asked to remain still.
○ The patient's response to the enclosed environment is assessed; reassurance and sedation is provided if necessary.
○ RF energy is directed at the patient's chest.
○ Resulting images are displayed on a monitor and recorded for permanent storage.
○ Verbal contact with a conscious patient should be maintained.

Patient care

○ No specific care is necessary unless the patient received sedation.
○ Monitor a sedated patient's hemodynamic, cardiac, respiratory, and mental status until the effects of the sedative have worn off.

Complications

○ Panic attacks related to claustrophobia
○ Adverse reactions to sedation

Interpretation

Normal results

○ No cardiovascular abnormalities are present.

Abnormal results

○ Cardiovascular abnormalities may suggest cardiomyopathy and pericardial disease, atrial or ventricular septal defects, congenital defects, paracardiac or intracardiac masses, pericardiac or vascular disease.

Interfering factors

○ Patients with pacemakers, intracranial aneurysm clips, or other ferrous metal implants (can't be done)
○ Ventilators, I.V. infusion pumps, and other metallic or computer-based equipment
○ Excessive patient movement (blurred images)

Cardiac positron emission tomography

Overview

○ Combines elements of both computed tomography (CT) scanning and conventional radionuclide imaging
○ Measures the particle emissions of injected radioisotopes, called *positrons*, and converts them to tomographic images
○ Uses radioisotopes of biologically important elements, such as oxygen, nitrogen, carbon, and fluorine
○ Positron emitters can be chemically tagged to biologically active molecules, such as carbon monoxide, neurotransmitters, hormones, and metabolites (particularly glucose), allowing study of their uptake and distribution in tissue
○ Radiation is 25% of that received from a CT scan
○ Costly because of short half-lives of the radioisotopes, which must be produced at an on-site cyclotron and attached quickly to the desired tracer molecules
○ Also known as *PET scanning*

Purpose

○ To detect coronary artery disease
○ To evaluate myocardial metabolism
○ To distinguish viable from infarcted cardiac tissue, especially during early stages of myocardial infarction

Procedure

Preparation

○ Make sure the patient has signed an appropriate consent form.
○ Note and report allergies.
○ Carefully screen female patients of childbearing age because the radioisotope can harm a fetus.
○ Provide reassurance that the test is painless, other than minor discomfort if the patient receives an I.V. access insertion.
○ Inform the patient that he may need to fast after midnight the night before the test.
○ Inform the patient that he may need to abstain from caffeinated beverages, alcohol, and tobacco products for 24 hours before the test.
○ Stress the importance of remaining still during the study.

Implementation

○ The patient is placed in a supine position with his arms above his head.
○ An attenuation scan, lasting about 30 minutes, is performed.
○ The appropriate positron emitter is given and scanning is completed.
○ A different positron emitter may be given if comparative studies are needed.

Patient care

○ Instruct the patient to move slowly immediately after the procedure to avoid orthostatic hypotension.
○ Encourage the patient to drink liquids to help flush the radioisotope from the bladder.

Complications

○ Orthostatic hypotension

Interpretation

Normal results

○ No areas of ischemic tissue are present.
○ If the patient receives two tracers, the flow and distribution should match.

Abnormal results

○ Reduced blood flow with increased glucose use indicates ischemia.
○ Reduced blood flow with decreased glucose use indicates necrotic, scarred tissue.

Interfering factors

○ Failure of the patient to maintain proper positioning, preventing accurate imaging

Cardiolipin antibodies

Overview

- Measures serum levels of immunoglobulin (Ig) G and IgM antibodies in relation to the phospholipid cardiolipin
- Appear in some patients with systemic lupus erythematosus (SLE) whose serum also contains a coagulation inhibitor (lupus anticoagulant)
- Also appear in some patients who don't fulfill all the diagnostic criteria for SLE but who experience recurrent episodes of spontaneous thrombosis, fetal loss, or thrombocytopenia
- Serum levels measured by enzyme-linked immunosorbent assay

Purpose
- To aid in the diagnosis of cardiolipin antibody syndrome in the patient with or without SLE who experiences recurrent episodes of spontaneous thrombosis, fetal loss, or thrombocytopenia

Procedure

Preparation
- Tell the patient that this test helps diagnose cardiolipin antibody syndrome and SLE.
- Inform the patient that he need not restrict food and fluids.
- Tell the patient that the test requires a blood sample. Explain who will perform the venipuncture and when.
- Explain to the patient that he may experience slight discomfort from the tourniquet and needle puncture.

Implementation
- Perform a venipuncture and collect the sample in a 5-ml tube without additives.
- Handle the sample gently to prevent hemolysis and send it to the laboratory immediately.

Patient care
- Apply direct pressure to the venipuncture site until bleeding stops.

Complications
- Hematoma at the venipuncture site

Interpretation

Normal results
- Cardiolipin antibody results are reported as negative or positive.
- A positive result is titered.

Abnormal results
- A positive result along with a history of recurrent spontaneous thrombosis, fetal loss, or thrombocytopenia suggests cardiolipin antibody syndrome.
- Treatment may involve anticoagulant or platelet inhibitor therapy.

Interfering factors
- Rough handling of the sample (hemolysis)
- Failure to send the sample to the laboratory immediately

Catecholamines, urine

Overview

○ Measures urine levels of the major catecholamines using spectrophotofluorometry
○ Catecholamines help regulate metabolism and prepare the body for the fight-or-flight response to stress (Certain tumors can also secrete catecholamines.)
○ A 24-hour urine specimen preferred because catecholamine secretion fluctuates diurnally and in response to various stimuli, conditions, and drugs
○ A random specimen may be useful for evaluating catecholamine levels after a hypertensive episode.
○ For a complete diagnostic workup of catecholamine secretion, urine levels of catecholamine metabolites must be measured. (Metabolites appear in the urine in greater quantities than catecholamines.)

Purpose

○ To aid in the diagnosis of pheochromocytoma in a patient with unexplained hypertension
○ To aid in the diagnosis of neuroblastoma, ganglioneuroma, and dysautonomia

Procedure

Preparation

○ Explain to the patient that the urine catecholamine test evaluates adrenal function.
○ Tell the patient to avoid chocolate, coffee, and bananas for 7 hours before the test and to avoid stressful situations and excessive physical activity during the collection period.
○ Tell the patient that the test requires collection of urine over 24 hours or a random specimen; explain the collection procedure.
○ Notify the laboratory and physician of drugs the patient is taking that may affect test results; it may be necessary to restrict them.

Implementation

○ Collect the patient's urine over a 24-hour period. Use a bottle containing a preservative to keep the specimen acidified to a pH of 3.0 or less.
○ Refrigerate a 24-hour specimen or place it on ice during the collection period.
○ If a random specimen is ordered, collect it immediately after a hypertensive episode.
○ Send the specimen to the laboratory as soon as the collection is complete.

Patient care

○ Instruct the patient that he may resume his usual activities, diet, and medications.

Complications

None known

Interpretation

Normal results

○ Values for catecholamine fractionalization range as follows: epinephrine: 0 to 20 µg/24 hours (SI, 0 to 109 nmol/24 hours); norepinephrine: 15 to 80 µg/24 hours (SI, 89 to 473 nmol/24 hours); dopamine: 65 to 400 µg/24 hours (SI, 425 to 2,610 hours)

Abnormal results

○ In a patient with undiagnosed hypertension, elevated urine catecholamine levels after a hypertensive episode usually indicate a pheochromocytoma.
○ If tests indicate a pheochromocytoma, the patient may undergo a test for multiple endocrine neoplasias.
○ With the exception of homovanillic acid (HVA) — a dopamine metabolite — catecholamine metabolites may also be elevated.
○ High HVA levels rule out a pheochromocytoma because this tumor secretes mainly epinephrine; its primary metabolite is vanillylmandelic acid, not HVA.
○ Elevated catecholamine levels, without marked hypertension, may be caused by a neuroblastoma or a ganglioneuroma, although HVA levels reflect these conditions more accurately.
○ Elevated levels occur in severe systemic conditions (burns, peritonitis, shock, and septicemia), cor pulmonale, manic-depressive disorders, or depressive neurosis.
○ Myasthenia gravis and progressive muscular dystrophy commonly cause urine catecholamine levels to rise above normal, but use of this test is rare for diagnosing these disorders.
○ Consistently low-normal catecholamine levels may indicate dysautonomia marked by orthostatic hypotension.

Interfering factors

○ Failure to comply with medication restrictions, to collect all urine during the collection period, or to store the specimen properly
○ Excessive physical exercise or emotional stress (increase)
○ Caffeine, insulin, nitroglycerin, aminophylline, sympathomimetics, methyldopa, tricyclic antidepressants, chloral hydrate, quinidine, quinine, tetracycline, B-complex vitamins, isoproterenol, levodopa, and monoamine oxidase inhibitors (increase)
○ Clonidine, guanethidine, reserpine, and iodine-containing contrast media (decrease)
○ Phenothiazines, erythromycin, and methenamine compounds (increase or decrease)

Celiac and mesenteric arteriography

Overview

- Radiographic examination of abdominal vasculature after intra-arterial injection of a contrast medium through a catheter.
- Catheter passes through the femoral artery into the abdominal aorta and is positioned in the celiac, superior mesenteric, or inferior mesenteric artery using fluoroscopic guidance.

Purpose

- To locate the source of and control GI bleeding when other measures fail
- To distinguish benign from malignant neoplasms
- To evaluate cirrhosis and portal hypertension
- To evaluate vascular damage after abdominal trauma
- To detect vascular abnormalities

Procedure

Preparation

- Make sure the patient has signed a consent form.
- Check the patient's history for hypersensitivity to iodine, shellfish, or contrast media.
- Obtain results of preprocedure tests and report abnormal results.
- Require fasting for 8 hours before the test.
- Tell the patient that he'll receive an I.V. conscious sedation and a local anesthetic.
- Warn that transient burning may be felt as the contrast is injected.
- Give a sedative if ordered.
- Tell the patient that the test can take 30 minutes to 3 hours, depending on the number of vessels studied.

Implementation

- The patient is placed in a supine position on the radiography table and an I.V. infusion is started.
- The puncture site, usually the right groin, is cleaned and prepared.
- A local anesthetic is injected.
- The needle is inserted into the femoral artery.
- A guide wire is passed through the needle into the aorta and the needle is removed.
- A catheter is inserted over the guide wire and andvanced into the artery. The guide wire is removed.
- A series of films is taken as contrast is injected through the catheter.
- The catheter is withdrawn and firm pressure applied.
- The site is cleaned and a sterile dressing is applied.

Patient care

- Maintain bed rest and keep the affected leg straight for 4 to 6 hours.
- Raise the head of the bed 30 degrees.
- Assist the patient in rolling side to side.
- Encourage fluid intake.
- Monitor the patient's vital signs, along with intake and output.
- Monitor the patient's peripheral pulses, color, temperature, and sensation in leg used for the test. Immediately notify the physician of changes.
- Check puncture site for bleeding or expanding hematoma. If either develops, apply direct manual pressure to the site and notify physician immediately.

Complications

- Reactions to the contrast medium
- Hemorrhage, thrombosis, and emboli
- Cardiac arrhythmias and infection

Interpretation

Normal results

- The arteries taper in size.
- The contrast medium spreads evenly within the sinusoids (it empties from the intestine into the superior mesenteric vein and into the portal vein).

Abnormal results

- Extravasation of contrast from damaged vessels suggests GI hemorrhage.
- Findings suggesting abdominal neoplasm: Invasion, encasement, distortion, or displacement of blood vessels; areas of necrosis appearing as puddles of contrast; a tumor blush or stain produced by contrast remaining longer in the neoplasm; and arteriovenous (AV) shunting, depending on tumor size and location.
- Findings suggesting cirrhosis: Diminished portal venous flow, dilated and tortuous collateral veins, and reversed portal venous flow.
- Findings suggesting splenic injury: Displaced intrasplenic arterial branches, contrast leakage from splenic arteries into splenic pulp, displaced splenic arteries and veins by enlarged spleen, and stretched intrasplenic arteries and compressed splenic pulp by an avascular mass indicating a subcapsular hematoma.
- Findings suggesting hepatic injury: Vascular distortion, displaced and stretched intrahepatic arteries by intrahepatic and subcapsular hematomas, and AV fistulas between the hepatic artery and portal vein.
- Narrowed or occluded arterial lumens suggest atherosclerotic plaque, vessel spasm, or emboli.

Interfering factors

- Gas, stool, or barium from a previous procedure
- Atherosclerotic lesions preventing passage of the catheter

Cerebral angiography

Overview

○ Radiographic examination of the cerebral vasculature after injection of intra-arterial contrast medium
○ Most common approach: femoral artery
○ Other approaches: direct carotid or vertebral artery puncture or the brachial, axillary, or subclavian artery
○ Usually performed on patients with suspected abnormalities of the cerebral vasculature, which have been suggested by other imaging studies

Purpose

○ To detect cerebrovascular abnormalities, such as aneurysm or arteriovenous malformation, thrombosis, narrowing, or occlusion
○ To evaluate vascular displacement caused by tumor, hematoma, edema, herniation, vasospasm, increased intracranial pressure, or hydrocephalus
○ To locate clips applied to blood vessels during surgery and to evaluate the postoperative status of such vessels
○ To evaluate the presence and degree of carotid artery disease

Procedure

Preparation

○ Make sure the patient has signed a consent form.
○ Note and report allergies.
○ Have the patient fast for 8 to 10 hours before the test.
○ Tell the patient that his head will be immobilized and he'll need to lie still.
○ Explain to the patient that he'll receive a local anesthetic.
○ Warn the patient that nausea, warmth, or burning may occur with the contrast injection.
○ Initiate an I.V. access and give I.V. fluids.
○ Give a sedative.
○ Explain to the patient that the test takes 2 to 4 hours.

Implementation

○ The patient is placed in a supine position on a radiographic table.
○ The access site is prepared and draped and a local anesthetic is injected.
○ The artery is punctured with the appropriate needle and catheterized under fluoroscopic guidance.
○ Catheter placement is verified by fluoroscopy and a contrast medium is injected.
○ A series of radiographs is taken and reviewed.
○ Arterial catheter patency is maintained by continuous or periodic flushing.
○ The patient's vital signs and neurologic status are monitored continuously.

○ The catheter is removed, firm pressure is applied to the access site until bleeding stops, and a pressure dressing is applied.

Patient care

○ Enforce bed rest and apply an ice bag.
○ If active bleeding or expanding hematoma occurs, apply firm pressure to the puncture site and inform the physician immediately.
○ Ensure adequate hydration.
○ Provide analgesia.
○ Monitor the patient's vital signs, along with intake and output.
○ Monitor the neurovascular status of the extremity distal to the access site.
○ If the femoral approach was used, keep the involved leg straight at the hip and check pulses distal to the site (dorsalis pedis, posterior tibial, and popliteal).
○ If the carotid artery was used as the access site, watch for dysphagia or respiratory distress, which can result from hematoma or edema. Also watch for disorientation, weakness, or numbness in the extremities (signs of neurovascular compromise) and for arterial spasms, which produce symptoms of transient ischemic attacks (TIAs). Notify the physician immediately if abnormal signs develop.
○ If the brachial artery was used, keep the arm straight at the elbow and assess distal pulses (radial and ulnar). Avoid venipuncture and blood pressures in the affected arm. Observe the extremity for changes in color, temperature, or sensation. If it becomes pale, cool, or numb, notify the physician immediately.

Complications

○ Adverse reaction to contrast media
○ Embolism, bleeding, hematoma, and infection
○ Vasospasm, thrombosis, TIA, or stroke

Interpretation

Normal results

○ Cerebral vasculature is normal.
○ During the arterial phase of perfusion, the contrast medium fills and opacifies superficial and deep arteries and arterioles.
○ During the venous phase, the contrast medium opacifies superficial and deep veins.

Abnormal results

○ Changes in the caliber of vessel lumina suggest vascular disease.
○ Vessel displacement suggests a possible tumor.

Interfering factors

○ Head movement affecting the clarity of the angiographic images

Cerebrospinal fluid analysis

Overview

○ Most commonly obtained by lumbar puncture (usually between the third and fourth lumbar vertebrae) and, rarely, by cisternal or ventricular puncture (for qualitative analysis)
○ May also be obtained during other neurologic tests such as myelography

Purpose

○ To measure cerebrospinal fluid (CSF) pressure as an aid in detecting an obstruction of CSF circulation
○ To aid in the diagnosis of viral or bacterial meningitis, subarachnoid or intracranial hemorrhage, tumors, and brain abscesses
○ To aid in the diagnosis of neurosyphilis and chronic central nervous system infections
○ To check for Alzheimer's disease

Procedure

Preparation

○ Describe the procedure to the patient and explain that this test analyzes the fluid around the spinal cord.
○ Inform the patient that he need not restrict food and fluids.
○ Advise the patient that a headache is the most common adverse effect of a lumbar puncture, but reassure him that his cooperation during the test helps minimize this effect.
○ Make sure that the patient or a responsible family member has signed an informed consent form.
○ If the patient is unusually anxious, assess and report his vital signs.

Implementation

○ During the procedure, observe closely for adverse reactions, such as elevated pulse rate, pallor, or clammy skin. Report any significant changes immediately.
○ Position the patient on his side at the edge of the bed with his knees drawn up to his abdomen and his chin on his chest. Provide pillows to support the spine on a horizontal plane. This position allows full flexion of the spine and easy access to the lumbar subarachnoid space. Help him maintain this position by placing one arm around his knees and the other arm around his neck.
○ If the sitting position is preferable, have the patient sit up and bend his chest and head toward his knees. Help him maintain this position throughout the procedure.

○ The skin is prepared for injection and the area is draped.
○ Tell the patient that when the spinal needle is inserted, he may feel slight local pain as the needle transverses the dura mater.
○ Ask the patient to report pain or sensations that differ from or continue after this expected discomfort because such sensations may indicate irritation or puncture of a nerve root, requiring needle repositioning.
○ Instruct the patient to remain still and breathe normally; movement and hyperventilation can alter pressure readings or cause injury.
○ The anesthetic is injected, and the spinal needle is inserted in the midline, between the spinous processes of the vertebrae (usually between the third and fourth lumbar vertebra). At this point, initial (or opening) CSF pressure is measured and a specimen is obtained.
○ After the specimen is collected, label the containers in the order in which they were filled.
○ Record the collection time on the test request form. Send the labeled specimens to the laboratory immediately after collection.
○ A final pressure reading is taken, and the needle is removed.
○ The puncture site is cleaned with a local antiseptic, such as povidone-iodine solution, and a small adhesive bandage is applied.

Patient care

○ Check whether the patient must lie flat or if the head of his bed may be slightly elevated. In most cases, instruct the patient to keep lying flat for 8 hours after the lumbar puncture. Sometimes, a 30-degree elevation at the head of the bed is allowed. Remind the patient that although he must not raise his head, he can turn from side to side.
○ Encourage the patient to drink fluids. Provide a flexible straw.
○ Check the puncture site for redness, swelling, and drainage every hour for the first 4 hours, and then every 4 hours for the first 24 hours.
○ If CSF pressure is elevated, assess the patient's neurologic status every 15 minutes for 4 hours. If he's stable, assess him every hour for 2 hours and then every 4 hours or according to the pretest schedule.

Complications

○ Reaction to the anesthetic, meningitis, bleeding into the spinal canal, cerebellar tonsillar herniation, and medullary compression
○ Signs of meningitis: Fever, neck rigidity, and irritability
○ Signs of herniation: Decreased level of consciousness, changes in pupil size and equality, altered vital signs, and respiratory failure

Interpretation

Normal results

○ Clear, colorless fluid
○ Cell count: No red blood cells (RBCs); 0 to 5 white blood cells (WBCs)
○ Gram stain: No organisms
○ Pressure: 50 to 180 mm H_2O

Abnormal results

○ Cloudy, bloody, brown, orange, or yellow fluid
○ Cell count: RBCs present; increased WBCs
○ Gram stain: Gram positive or gram-negative organisms
○ Pressure: Increased or decreased

Interfering factors

○ Patient position and activity (possible increase or decrease in CSF pressure)
○ Crying, coughing, or straining
○ Delay between collection time and laboratory testing
○ Infection at the puncture site contraindicates removal of CSF

Ceruloplasmin

Overview

○ Used to measure serum levels of ceruloplasmin, an alpha$_2$-globulin that binds about 95% of serum copper, usually in the liver
○ Thought to regulate iron uptake by transferrin, making iron available to reticulocytes for heme synthesis

Purpose

○ To aid in the diagnosis of Wilson's disease, Menkes' syndrome, and copper deficiency

Procedure

Preparation

○ Explain to the patient that this test determines the copper content of blood.
○ Tell the patient that the test requires a blood sample. Explain who will perform the venipuncture and when.
○ Explain to the patient that he may experience slight discomfort from the tourniquet and the needle puncture.
○ Notify the laboratory and physician of drugs the patient is taking that may affect test results; it may be necessary to restrict them.

Implementation

○ Perform a venipuncture and collect the sample in a 7-ml clot-activator tube.
○ Send the sample to the laboratory immediately.

Patient care

○ Apply direct pressure to the venipuncture site until bleeding stops.
○ Instruct the patient to resume medications discontinued before the test.

Complications

○ Hematoma at the venipuncture site

Interpretation

Normal results

○ 22.9 to 43.1 g/dl (SI, 0.22 to 0.43 g/L)

Abnormal results

○ Decreased levels usually indicate Wilson's disease.
○ Decreased levels may also occur in Menkes' syndrome, nephrotic syndrome, and hypocupremia caused by total parenteral nutrition.
○ Increased levels may indicate certain hepatic diseases and infections.

Interfering factors

○ Estrogen, methadone, phenytoin, and pregnancy (possible increase)

Cervical punch biopsy

Overview

- Involves excision by sharp forceps of a tissue specimen from the cervix for histologic examination
- Usual to obtain multiple biopsies from all areas with abnormal tissue
- Occurs when the cervix is least vascular (usually 1 week after menses)
- Biopsy site selection is by direct visualization of the cervix with a colposcope (the most accurate method) and by Schiller's test (normal squamous epithelium stains dark mahogany while abnormal tissue fails to change color)

Purpose

- To evaluate suspicious cervical lesions
- To diagnose cervical cancer

Procedure

Preparation

- Make sure the patient has signed a consent form.
- Note and report allergies.
- Just before the biopsy, ask the patient to void.
- Inform the patient that the test takes about 15 minutes.
- Tell her that she may experience mild discomfort during and after the biopsy.
- Inform the patient that she should have someone accompany her home after the biopsy.

Implementation

- Assist the patient into the lithotomy position.
- A nonlubricated speculum is inserted.
- For direct visualization, the colposcope is inserted through the speculum.
- The biopsy site is located, and the cervix is cleaned with a swab soaked in 3% acetic acid solution.
- Biopsy forceps are inserted through the speculum or the colposcope.
- Tissue from the lesion or selected sites is removed, starting from the posterior lip to avoid obscuring other sites with blood.
- Each specimen is immediately placed in 10% formalin solution in a labeled bottle.
- The cervix is swabbed with 5% silver nitrate solution (cautery or sutures may be used instead) to control bleeding.
- The examiner may insert a tampon if bleeding persists.
- For Schiller's test, an applicator stick saturated with iodine solution is inserted through the speculum. This stains the cervix to identify lesions for biopsy.

Patient care

- Instruct the patient to avoid strenuous exercise for 8 to 24 hours.
- Encourage the outpatient to rest briefly before leaving the office.
- Tell the patient to leave the tampon (if used) in place for 8 to 24 hours.
- Inform the patient that some bleeding may occur, but to report heavy bleeding (heavier than menstrual) to the physician.
- Warn the patient to avoid using additional tampons, which can irritate the cervix and provoke bleeding, according to her physician's directions.
- Tell the patient to avoid douching.
- Tell the patient to refrain from sexual intercourse for up to 2 weeks, or as directed, if the procedure involved cryotherapy or laser treatment.
- Inform the patient that a foul-smelling, gray-green vaginal discharge is normal for several days after the biopsy and may persist for 3 weeks.

Complications

- Bleeding
- Infection

Interpretation

Normal results

- No dysplasia and abnormal cell growth are present.
- Normal cervical tissue is composed of columnar and squamous epithelial cells, loose connective tissue, and smooth-muscle fibers.

Abnormal results

- Dysplasia or abnormal cell growth on histologic examination of a cervical tissue specimen may suggest intraepithelial neoplasia or invasive cancer.

Interfering factors

- Failure to obtain representative specimens or to immediately place them in the preservative

Chest radiography

Overview

○ Noninvasive and relatively inexpensive study
○ X-ray beams penetrate the chest and react on specially sensitized film; air is radiolucent, so thoracic structures appear as different densities on the film
○ Commonly known as *chest X-ray*

Purpose

○ To establish a baseline for future comparison
○ To detect pulmonary disorders such as pneumonia
○ To detect mediastinal abnormalities such as tumors
○ To verify correct placement of pulmonary artery catheters, endotracheal (ET) tubes, and chest tubes
○ To determine location of swallowed or aspirated radiopaque foreign bodies
○ To determine location and size of lesions
○ To evaluate response to interventions such as diuretic therapy

Procedure

Preparation

○ Make sure the patient has signed an appropriate consent form.
○ The patient need not restrict food and fluids.
○ Move cardiac monitoring cables, oxygen tubing, I.V. tubing, pulmonary artery catheter lines, and other equipment out of the radiographic field.
○ Explain that the patient will be asked to take a deep breath and hold it momentarily during the X-ray.
○ Explain that the test takes less than 5 minutes.

Implementation

○ The patient is instructed to stand or sit in front of a stationary radiography machine.
○ Posteroanterior and left lateral views are obtained.
○ A portable radiography machine is used at the patient's bedside if he can't travel to radiology.
○ Because an upright chest radiograph is preferable, move the patient to the head of the bed if he can tolerate this position.
○ Elevate the head of the bed for maximum upright positioning.

Patient care

○ Check that no tubes have been dislodged during positioning.
○ Whenever possible, place a lead apron over the patient's abdomen to protect the gonads.
○ To avoid radiation exposure, leave the area or wear lead shielding while the films are being taken.

Complications

○ Potential for dislodging tubes or wires, such as the ET tube or pacemaker wires, during positioning

Interpretation

Normal results

○ The trachea is visible midline in the anterior mediastinal cavity, appearing translucent and tubelike.
○ The heart is visible in the anterior left mediastinal cavity, appearing solid because of its blood content.
○ The aortic knob is visible as water density.
○ The mediastinum (mediastinal shadow) is visible as the space between the lungs, appearing shadowy and widened at the hilum.
○ The ribs are visible as a thoracic cavity encasement.
○ The spine has a visible midline in the posterior chest that's most visible on a lateral view.
○ The clavicles are visible in the upper thorax. They're intact and equidistant in properly centered films.
○ The hila (lung roots) are visible above the heart and exist where pulmonary vessels, bronchi, and lymph nodes join the lungs. They appear as small, white, bilateral branching densities.
○ The mainstem bronchus is visible as part of the hila. It has a translucent, tubelike appearance.
○ The bronchi aren't usually visible.
○ The lung fields aren't usually visible, except for blood vessels.
○ The hemidiaphragm is rounded and visible. The right side is ⅜″ to ¾″ (1 to 2 cm) higher than the left side.

Abnormal results

○ Deviation of the trachea from midline suggests possible tension pneumothorax or pleural effusion.
○ Right side of the heart hypertrophy suggests possible cor pulmonale or heart failure.
○ A tortuous aortic knob suggests atherosclerosis.
○ Gross widening of the mediastinum suggests neoplasm or aortic aneurysm.
○ A break or misalignment of bones suggests fracture.
○ Visible bronchi suggest bronchial pneumonia.
○ Flattening of the diaphragm suggests emphysema or asthma.
○ Irregular, patchy infiltrates in the lung fields suggest pneumonia.

Interfering factors

○ Portable films (less reliable than stationary radiographs)
○ Inability to take a full inspiration (decrease in quality)

Chloride, serum

Overview

- Measures the serum levels of chloride, the major extracellular fluid anion
- Chloride helps maintain osmotic pressure of blood and, therefore, helps regulate blood volume and arterial pressure
- Chloride levels also affect the acid-base balance
- Chloride is absorbed in the intestines and excreted primarily by the kidneys

Purpose

- To detect acid-base imbalance (acidosis or alkalosis) and to aid evaluation of fluid status and extracellular cation-anion balance

Procedure

Preparation

- Explain to the patient that the serum chloride test evaluates the chloride content of blood.
- Tell the patient that the test requires a blood sample. Explain who will perform the venipuncture and when.
- Explain to the patient that he may experience slight discomfort from the tourniquet and the needle puncture.
- Inform the patient that he need not restrict food and fluids.
- Notify the laboratory and physician of drugs the patient is taking that may affect test results; it may be necessary to restrict them.

Implementation

- Perform a venipuncture and collect the sample in a 3- or 4-ml clot-activator tube.
- Handle the sample gently to prevent hemolysis.

Patient care

- Apply direct pressure to the venipuncture site until bleeding stops.
- Instruct the patient to resume medications discontinued before the test.

Complications

- Hematoma at the venipuncture site
- Hypochloremia: Hypertonicity of muscles, tetany, depressed respirations, and decreased blood pressure with dehydration
- Hyperchloremia: Stupor, rapid deep breathing, and weakness, which may lead to coma

Interpretation

Normal results

- In adults, 100 to 108 mEq/L (SI, 100 to 108 mmol/L)

Abnormal results

- Chloride levels are inversely related to bicarbonate levels, reflecting acidbase balance.
- Excessive loss of gastric juices or other secretions containing chloride may cause hypochloremic metabolic alkalosis; excessive chloride retention or ingestion may lead to hyperchloremic metabolic acidosis.
- An increase in chloride levels may be evident in severe dehydration, complete renal shutdown, head injury (producing neurogenic hyperventilation), and primary aldosteronism.
- Decreased levels of chloride may result from low sodium and potassium levels due to prolonged vomiting, gastric suctioning, intestinal fistula, chronic renal failure, and Addison's disease. Heart failure or edema resulting in excess extracellular fluid can cause dilutional hypochloremia.

Interfering factors

- Hemolysis from rough handling of the sample
- Use of ammonium chloride, cholestyramine, boric acid, oxyphenbutazone, or phenylbutazone and excessive I.V. infusion of sodium chloride (possible increase)
- Use of thiazide diuretics, ethacrynic acid, furosemide, or bicarbonates and prolonged I.V. infusion of dextrose 5% in water (decrease)

Chloride, urine

Overview

○ Measures urine sodium and chloride concentrations, evaluates renal conservation of these two electrolytes, and confirms serum sodium and chloride values

Purpose

○ To help evaluate fluid and electrolyte imbalance
○ To monitor the effects of a low-sodium diet
○ To help evaluate renal and adrenal disorders

Procedure

Preparation

○ Explain to the patient that the urine sodium and chloride test helps determine the balance of salt and water in the body.
○ Advise the patient that no special restrictions are necessary.
○ Tell the patient that the test requires urine collection over a 24-hour period.
○ If the patient will be collecting the specimen at home, instruct him on proper collection technique.
○ Notify the laboratory and physician of drugs the patient is taking that may affect test results; it may be necessary to restrict them.

Implementation

○ Collect the patient's urine over a 24-hour period, discarding the first specimen and retaining the last.
○ Tell the patient not to contaminate the specimen with toilet tissue or stool.
○ Tell the patient not to use a metallic bedpan for specimen collection.

Patient care

○ Instruct the patient that he may resume his usual medications.

Complications

None known

Interpretation

Normal results

○ In adults, 110 to 250 nmol/24 hours (SI, 110 to 250 mmol/d)
○ In children, 15 to 40 nmol/24 hours (SI, 15 to 40 mmol/d)
○ In infants, 2 to 10 mmol/24 hours (SI, 2 to 10 mmol/)

Abnormal results

○ Typically, urine sodium and urine chloride levels are parallel, rising and falling in tandem. Abnormal levels of both minerals may indicate the need for more specific testing.
○ Elevated urine chloride levels may result from water-deficient dehydration, salicylate toxicity, diabetic ketoacidosis, adrenocortical insufficiency (Addison's disease), or salt-losing renal disease.
○ Decreased levels may result from excessive diaphoresis, heart failure, hypochloremic metabolic alkalosis, or prolonged vomiting or gastric suctioning.

Interfering factors

○ Failure to collect all urine during the test period
○ Ammonium chloride and potassium chloride (increase in chloride)

Cholangiography, postoperative

Overview

○ Radiographic and fluoroscopic examination of the biliary ducts after injection of a contrast medium
○ Performed through a T-shaped rubber tube inserted into the common bile duct, immediately after cholecystectomy or common bile duct exploration, to facilitate drainage
○ Also known as *T-tube cholangiography*

Purpose

○ To assess size and patency of the biliary ducts
○ To detect obstructions overlooked during surgery
○ To detect calculi, strictures, neoplasms, and fistulae in the biliary ducts

Procedure

Preparation

○ Make sure the patient has signed an appropriate consent form.
○ Check the patient's history for hypersensitivity to iodine, seafood, or contrast media.
○ Note and report allergies.
○ Clamp the T-tube the day before the procedure if ordered.
○ Withhold the meal preceding the test.
○ Give an enema about 1 hour before the procedure if ordered.
○ Warn the patient that he may feel a bloating sensation in the right upper quadrant during injection of the contrast medium.
○ Explain that the test takes about 15 minutes.

Implementation

○ The patient is placed in a supine position on the radiograph table.
○ The injection area of the T tube is cleaned.
○ A needle attached to a long transparent catheter is inserted into the end of the T tube.
○ Injecting air into the biliary tree is avoided because air bubbles may affect the clarity of the radiograph films.
○ A contrast medium is injected under fluoroscopic guidance.
○ A series of radiographs is taken.
○ The T tube is clamped and additional films are taken in the erect position (to distinguish air bubbles from calculi).
○ Final films are taken to record emptying of contrast-laden bile into the duodenum.

Patient care

○ Reattach the T tube to the drainage system.
○ Have the patient resume a normal diet.
○ Monitor the patient's vital signs, intake and output, and T-tube drainage.

Complications

○ Adverse reaction to the contrast medium
○ Infection

Interpretation

Normal results

○ Filling of the bile ducts with contrast medium is homogeneous.
○ The diameter of the biliary ducts is normal.
○ The flow of contrast into the duodenum is unimpeded.

Abnormal results

○ Biliary duct filling defects, associated with dilation, suggest calculi or neoplasms.
○ Abnormal channels of contrast medium from biliary ducts suggest possible fistulae.

Interfering factors

○ Marked gas overlying the biliary ducts

Cholecystography, oral

Overview

○ Radiographic examination of the gallbladder after administration of a contrast medium
○ Indicated for patients with symptoms of biliary tract disease
○ Commonly performed to confirm gallbladder disease

Purpose

○ To detect gallstones
○ To aid diagnosis of inflammatory disease and tumors of the gallbladder

Procedure

Preparation

○ Make sure the patient has signed an appropriate consent form.
○ Note and report allergies.
○ Instruct the patient to eat a meal containing fat at noon the day before the test, to stimulate release of bile from the gallbladder.
○ Instruct the patient to eat a fat-free meal in the evening, to inhibit gallbladder contraction and to promote bile accumulation.
○ The patient may have nothing to eat or drink, except water, after the evening meal.
○ Give the patient an oral contrast agent (usually tablets), 2 to 3 hours after the evening meal.
○ Examine vomitus or diarrhea for undigested tablets. If noted, notify the physician and the radiography department.
○ Give an enema the morning of the test if ordered.
○ Explain to the patient that the test usually takes 30 to 45 minutes.

Implementation

○ A fluoroscopic examination is performed to evaluate gallbladder opacification.
○ Various positions are used to detect filling defects.
○ A fat stimulus, such as a high-fat meal or a synthetic fat-containing agent may be given.
○ The emptying of the gallbladder is observed in response to the fat stimulus and spot films are taken to show the common bile duct.
○ If the gallbladder empties slowly or not at all, delayed films are taken.

Patient care

○ If the test results are normal, the patient may resume his usual diet.
○ If gallstones are present, the patient needs an appropriate diet, usually fat-restricted, to help prevent acute attacks.

○ Before repeating oral cholecystography, the patient must continue a low-fat diet until a definitive diagnosis can be made.

Complications

○ Adverse reaction to contrast medium

Interpretation

Normal results

○ Opacification of the gallbladder
○ Pear-shaped gallbladder with smooth, thin walls

Abnormal results

○ Filling defects may indicate gallstones.
○ Fixed defects may indicate polyps or a benign tumor.
○ Failed or faint opacification may indicate inflammatory disease, such as cholecystitis, with or without gallstones.
○ Failure of the gallbladder to contract following stimulation by a fatty meal may indicate cholecystitis or common bile duct obstruction.

Interfering factors

○ Should precede barium studies to prevent retained barium from interfering with subsequent radiograph films

Cholinesterase

Overview

○ Measures the amounts of two similar enzymes that hydrolyze acetylcholine: acetylcholinesterase and pseudocholinesterase.
○ Acetylcholinesterase is present in nerve tissue, red cells of the spleen, and the gray matter of the brain. It inactivates acetylcholine at nerve junctions and helps transmit impulses across nerve endings to muscle fibers.
○ Pseudocholinesterase produced primarily in the liver and appears in small amounts in the pancreas, intestines, heart, and white matter of the brain.
○ Although pseudocholinesterase has no known function, its measurement is significant because certain chemicals that inactivate acetylcholinesterase also affect pseudocholinesterase.
○ In suspected poisoning by an organophosphate, testing can measure either cholinesterase. (For technical reasons, pseudocholinesterase is generally tested, although this analysis is less sensitive than for acetylcholinesterase.)
○ In suspected poisoning by muscle relaxants, the patient lacks adequate pseudocholinesterase, which usually inactivates the muscle relaxant. (In this case, measurement of pseudocholinesterase is required.)

Purpose

○ To evaluate before surgery or electroconvulsive therapy the patient's potential response to succinylcholine, which is hydrolyzed by cholinesterase
○ To screen for adverse reactions to muscle relaxants
○ To assess overexposure to insecticides containing organophosphate compounds
○ To assess liver function and aid diagnosis of hepatic disease (a rare purpose)

Procedure

Preparation

○ Explain to the patient that this test assesses muscle function or the extent of poisoning.
○ Tell the patient that the test requires a blood sample. Explain who will perform the venipuncture and when.
○ Explain to the patient that he may experience slight discomfort from the tourniquet and the needle puncture.
○ Inform the patient that he need not restrict food and fluids.
○ Notify the laboratory and physician of drugs the patient is taking that may affect test results; it may be necessary to restrict them.

Implementation

○ Perform a venipuncture and collect the sample in a 7-ml clot-activator tube.
○ Handle the sample gently to prevent hemolysis.
○ Send the sample to the laboratory within 6 hours after being drawn. If this isn't possible, refrigerate it.

Patient care

○ Apply direct pressure to the venipuncture site until bleeding stops.
○ Instruct the patient that he may resume medications discontinued before the test.

Complications

○ Hematoma at the venipuncture site

Interpretation

Normal results

○ Pseudocholinesterase levels range from 204 to 532 IU/dl (SI, 2.04 to 5.32 kU/L).

Abnormal results

○ Severely decreased pseudocholinesterase levels suggest a congenital deficiency or organophosphate insecticide poisoning; levels near zero necessitate emergency treatment.
○ Pseudocholinesterase levels are usually normal in early extrahepatic obstruction and variably decreased in hepatocellular diseases, such as hepatitis and cirrhosis (especially cirrhosis with ascites and jaundice).
○ Levels also drop in acute infections, chronic malnutrition, anemia, myocardial infarction, obstructive jaundice, and metastasis.

Interfering factors

○ Hemolysis from rough handling of the sample
○ Pregnancy or recent surgery
○ Cyclophosphamide, echothiophate iodide, monoamine oxidase inhibitors, succinylcholine, neostigmine, quinine, quinidine, chloroquine, caffeine, theophylline, epinephrine, ether, barbiturates, atropine, morphine, codeine, phenothiazines, vitamin K, and folic acid (possible false-low)

Chorionic villi sampling

Overview

- Prenatal test for quick detection of fetal chromosomal and biochemical disorders
- Performed during the first trimester
- Fingerlike projections that surround the embryonic membrane and eventually give rise to the placenta

Purpose

- To analyze for fetal abnormalities

Procedure

Preparation

- Explain to the patient that samples are best obtained between the 8th and 10th weeks of pregnancy.

Implementation

- Assist the patient into the lithotomy position.
- The physician checks placement of the patient's uterus bimanually and then inserts a Graves speculum and swabs the cervix with an antiseptic solution.
- If necessary, a tenaculum is used to straighten an acutely flexed uterus, permitting cannula insertion.
- Guided by ultrasound and possibly endoscopy, the catheter is directed through the cannula to the villi.
- Suction is applied to the catheter to remove about 30 mg of tissue from the villi.
- A specimen is withdrawn and placed in a Petri dish. It's examined with a dissecting microscope. Part of the specimen is then cultured for further testing. (See *Chorionic villi sampling*.)

Patient care

- Monitor the patient closely for adverse effects.

Complications

- Slight risk of spontaneous abortion, cramps, infection, and bleeding

Interpretation

Normal results

- No abnormalities are found.

Abnormal results

- The test can detect about 200 diseases prenatally, including chromosome disorders, hemoglobinopathies, and Tay-Sachs disease.

Interfering factors

- Sample contains too few cells, or cells fail to grow in the culture

Chorionic villi sampling

Chorionic villi sampling is a prenatal test for quick detection of fetal chromosomal and biochemical disorders that's performed during the first trimester of pregnancy.

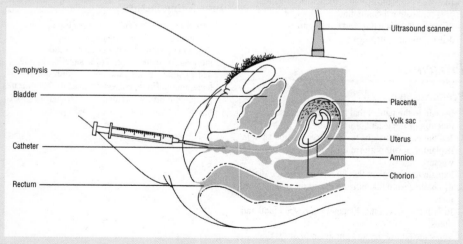

Chromosome analysis

Overview

○ Studies the relationship between the microscopic appearance of chromosomes and an individual's phenotype — the expression of the genes in physical, biochemical, or physiologic traits.
○ Specimen required (blood, bone marrow, amniotic fluid, skin, or placental tissue) and specific procedure determined by reason for test.
○ Umbilical cord sampling allows chromosome analysis.

Purpose

○ To identify chromosomal abnormalities, such as hypoploidy or hyperploidy, as the underlying cause of malformation, maldevelopment, or disease

Procedure

Preparation

○ Explain to the patient or his parents, if appropriate, the purpose of the chromosome analysis.
○ Tell the patient who will perform the test and the type of specimen required.
○ Inform the patient when results will be available, according to the specimen required.

Implementation

○ Collect a blood sample (in a 5- to 10-ml heparinized tube), a tissue specimen, 1 ml of bone marrow, or at least 20 ml of amniotic fluid.
○ Keep specimens sterile, especially those requiring a tissue culture.
○ To facilitate interpretation of test results, send the specimen to the laboratory immediately after collection, with a brief patient history and the indication for the test.
○ Refrigerate the specimen if transport is delayed, but *never* freeze it.

Patient care

○ Provide appropriate care after the test, depending on the type of procedure.
○ Explain to the patient or his parents, if he's a child, the test results and their implications if a chromosomal abnormality is present.
○ Recommend appropriate genetic or other counseling and follow-up care if necessary, such as an infant stimulation program for a patient with Down syndrome.

Complications

None known

Interpretation

Normal results

○ 46 chromosomes: 22 pairs of nonsex chromosomes (autosomes) and 1 pair of sex chromosomes (Y for the male-determining chromosome, X for the female-determining chromosome). On a karyotype, chromosomes are arranged according to size and the location of their primary constrictions, or centromeres.
○ The centromere may be medial (metacentric), slightly to one end of the chromosome (submetacentric), or entirely to one end (acrocentric).
○ The largest chromosomes are displayed first; the others are arranged in order of decreasing size, with the two sex chromosomes traditionally placed last. By convention, the centromere is always placed at the top in a karyotype. If the two pairs of chromosomal arms are of unequal length, the arm above the centromere will be shorter. The letter "p" designates the short arm; the letter "q," the long arm.
○ Special stains identify individual chromosomes and locate and enumerate portions of chromosomes.

Abnormal results

○ Chromosomal abnormalities may be numerical or structural.
○ Any numerical deviation from the norm of 46 chromosomes is called *aneuploidy.*
○ Fewer than 46 chromosomes is called *hypoploidy;* more than 46, *hyperploidy.*
○ Special designations exist for whole multiples of the haploid number 23; for example, *diploidy* for the normal somatic number of 46, *triploidy* for 69, and *tetraploidy* for 92.
○ Aneuploidy usually follows failure of the chromosomal pair to separate (nondisjunction) in anaphase.
○ If nondisjunction or anaphase lag occurs during meiosis, the cells of the zygote will all be the same.
○ Errors in mitotic division after zygote formation will produce more than one cell line (mosaicism).
○ Structural chromosomal abnormalities result from chromosome breakage.
○ Intrachromosomal rearrangement occurs within a single chromosome in *deletion* — loss of an end (terminal) or middle (interstitial) portion of a chromosome; *inversion* — end-to-end reversal of a chromosome segment; *ring chromosome formation* — breakage of both ends of a chromosome and reunion of the ends; or *isochromosome formation* — abnormal splitting of the centromere in a transverse rather than a longitudinal plane. Interchromosomal rearrangements also occur.

Interfering factors

○ Chemotherapy
○ Contaminated tissue by a bacterium, fungus, or virus
○ Inclusion of maternal cells in a specimen obtained by amniocentesis, with subsequent culturing

Cold agglutinins

Overview

- Antibodies, usually of the immunoglobulin M type, that cause red blood cells (RBCs) to aggregate at low temperatures
- May occur in small amounts in healthy people
- Transient elevations of these antibodies develop during certain infectious diseases, notably primary atypical pneumonia
- Reliably detects such pneumonia within 1 to 2 weeks after its onset
- Patients with high titers, such as those with primary atypical pneumonia, may develop acute transient hemolytic anemia after repeated exposure to cold; patients with persistently high titers may develop chronic hemolytic anemia

Purpose

- To help confirm primary atypical pneumonia
- To provide additional diagnostic evidence for cold agglutinin disease associated with many viral infections and lymphoreticular cancer
- To detect cold agglutinins in the patient with suspected cold agglutinin disease

Procedure

Preparation

- Explain to the patient that this test detects antibodies in the blood that attack RBCs after exposure to low temperatures.
- Tell the patient that the test will be repeated to monitor his response to therapy, if appropriate.
- Tell the patient that he need not restrict food and fluids.
- Tell the patient that the test requires a blood sample. Explain who will perform the venipuncture and when.
- Explain to the patient that he may experience slight discomfort from the tourniquet and the needle puncture.
- If the patient is receiving antimicrobial drugs, note this on the laboratory request because the use of such drugs may interfere with the development of cold agglutinins.

Implementation

- Perform a venipuncture and collect the sample in a 7-ml tube without additives that has been prewarmed to 98.6° F (37° C).
- Handle the sample gently to prevent hemolysis and send it to the laboratory immediately.
- Don't refrigerate the sample; cold agglutinins will coat the RBCs, leaving none in the serum for testing.

Patient care

- If cold agglutinin disease is suspected, keep the patient warm. If he's exposed to low temperatures, agglutination may occur within peripheral vessels, possibly leading to frostbite, anemia, Raynaud's phenomenon and, rarely, focal gangrene.
- Watch for signs of vascular abnormalities, such as mottled skin, purpura, jaundice, pallor, pain or swelling of extremities, and cramping of fingers and toes. Hemoglobinuria may result from severe intravascular hemolysis on exposure to severe cold.
- Apply direct pressure to the venipuncture site until bleeding stops.

Complications

- Hematoma at the venipuncture site

Interpretation

Normal results

- Results are reported as negative or positive.
- A positive result, indicating the presence of cold agglutinin, is titered.
- A normal titer is less than 1:64.

Abnormal results

- High titers may occur as primary phenomena or secondary to infections or lymphoreticular cancer.
- High titers may be present in infectious mononucleosis, cytomegalovirus infection, hemolytic anemia, multiple myeloma, scleroderma, malaria, cirrhosis of the liver, congenital syphilis, peripheral vascular disease, pulmonary embolism, trypanosomiasis, tonsillitis, staphylococcemia, scarlatina, influenza and, occasionally, pregnancy.
- Chronically elevated titers are most commonly associated with pneumonia and lymphoreticular cancer; an acute transient elevation typically accompanies many viral infections.
- In primary atypical pneumonia, cold agglutinins appear in serum in one-half to two-thirds of all patients during the first week of acute infection, even before antimycoplasmal antibodies are detectable by complement fixation or metabolic inhibition tests. Titers usually become positive at 7 days, peak above 1:32 in 4 weeks, and disappear rapidly after 6 weeks. Sequential titers verifying this pattern and symptoms of pneumonia confirm the diagnosis.
- Titers exceeding 1:2,000 can occur with idiopathic cold agglutinin disease that precedes lymphoma. Patients with titers this high are susceptible to intravascular agglutination.

Interfering factors

- Hemolysis from rough handling of the sample (possible false-low titer)
- Refrigeration of the sample before serum is separated from RBCs (possible false-low titer)
- Antimicrobial drugs

Cold stimulation test for Raynaud's disease

Overview

○ Demonstrates Raynaud's disease by recording temperature changes in the patient's fingers before and after submersion in ice water
○ Digital blood pressure recording or examination of the arteries in the arm and palmar arch should precede this test to rule out arterial occlusive disease
○ Contraindicated in the patient with gangrenous fingers or open, infected wounds

Purpose

○ To detect Raynaud's disease, an arteriospastic disorder characterized by intense vasospasm of the small cutaneous arteries and arterioles of the hands after exposure to cold or stress

Procedure

Preparation

○ Explain to the patient that the cold stimulation test for Raynaud's disease detects vascular disorders.
○ Tell the patient that he need not restrict food and fluids.
○ Describe the test, including who will perform it, where it will take place, and how long it will last.
○ Explain to the patient that he may experience discomfort when his hands are briefly immersed in ice water.
○ Have the patient remove his watch and other jewelry and encourage him to relax.
○ To minimize extraneous environmental stimuli, make sure the test room is neither too warm nor too cold.

Implementation

○ Tape a thermistor to each of the patient's fingers and record the temperature.
○ Have the patient submerge his hands in an ice-water bath for 20 seconds.
○ When the patient removes his hands from the water, record the temperature of his fingers immediately and every 5 minutes thereafter until it returns to the baseline temperature.

Patient care

○ After the procedure, monitor the patient.

Complications

None known

Interpretation

Normal results

○ Normally, digital temperature returns to baseline levels within 15 minutes.

Abnormal results

○ If digital temperature takes longer than 20 minutes to return to the baseline level, Raynaud's disease is indicated.
○ Its benign form requires no specific treatment and has no serious sequelae.
○ Its more serious form, Raynaud's phenomenon, involves connective tissue disorders that may not be clinically apparent for several years, such as scleroderma, systemic lupus erythematosus, and rheumatoid arthritis. Distinguishing between Raynaud's phenomenon and Raynaud's disease is difficult.

Interfering factors

○ Excessively warm or cold test environment

Colonoscopy

Overview

- Flexible fiber-optic video endoscope permits visual examination of the lining of the large intestine
- Indicated for patients with a history of constipation or diarrhea, persistent rectal bleeding, and lower abdominal pain when the results of proctosigmoidoscopy and a barium enema test are negative or inconclusive

Purpose

- To detect or evaluate inflammatory and ulcerative bowel disease
- To locate the origin of lower GI bleeding
- To aid in the diagnosis of colonic strictures and benign or malignant lesions
- To evaluate postoperatively for recurrence of polyps and malignant lesions

Procedure

Preparation

- Check the patient's medical history for allergies, medications, and information pertinent to the current complaint.
- Tell the patient to maintain a clear liquid diet for 24 to 48 hours before the test and to take nothing by mouth after midnight the night before.
- Instruct the patient regarding the appropriate bowel prep.
- Inform the patient that he'll receive an I.V. line and I.V. sedation before the procedure.
- Tell the patient that the colonoscope is well lubricated to ease insertion and initially feels cool.
- Explain that he may feel an urge to defecate when it's inserted and advanced.
- Inform him that air may be introduced through the colonoscope to distend the intestinal wall and to facilitate viewing the lining and advancing the instrument.

Implementation

- The patient is assisted onto his left side with knees flexed. Cover him with a drape.
- Baseline vital signs are obtained; vital signs and electrocardiogram are monitored during the procedure.
- Continuous or periodic pulse oximetry is advisable.
- The physician palpates the mucosa of the anus and rectum and inserts the lubricated colonoscope through the patient's anus into the sigmoid colon under direct vision.
- A small amount of air is insufflated to locate the bowel lumen and then advance the scope through the rectum.
- Abdominal palpation or fluoroscopy may be used to help guide the colonoscope through the large intestine.
- Suction may be used to remove blood and secretions that obscure vision.
- Biopsy forceps or a cytology brush may be passed through the colonoscope to obtain specimens for histologic or cytologic examination; an electrocautery snare may be used to remove polyps.
- Tissue specimens are immediately placed in a specimen bottle containing 10% formalin and cytology smears in a Coplin jar containing 95% ethyl alcohol.
- Specimens are sent to the laboratory immediately.

Patient care

- The patient is observed closely for signs of bowel perforation.
- Check the patient's vital signs and document them accordingly.
- Watch the patient closely for adverse effects of the sedative.
- After recovery from sedation, he may resume his usual diet unless the physician orders otherwise.
- The patient may pass large amounts of flatus after insufflation.
- After polyp removal, the stool may contain some blood. Report excessive bleeding immediately.
- If a polyp is removed, but not retrieved, give enemas and strain the stools to retrieve it.

Complications

- Perforation of the large intestine, excessive bleeding, and retroperitoneal emphysema

Interpretation

Normal results

- The mucosa of the large intestine beyond the sigmoid colon appears light pink-orange and is marked by semilunar folds and deep tubular pits.
- Blood vessels are visible beneath the intestinal mucosa.

Abnormal results

- Proctitis, granulomatous or ulcerative colitis, Crohn's disease, and malignant or benign lesions
- Diverticular disease or lower GI bleeding

Interfering factors

- Fixation of the sigmoid colon from inflammatory bowel disease, surgery, or radiation therapy
- Blood from acute colonic hemorrhage (hinders visualization)
- Insufficient bowel preparation or barium retained in the intestine
- Failure to place histologic or cytologic specimens in the appropriate preservative or to send the specimens to the laboratory immediately

Color vision

Overview

- Tests assess the ability to recognize differences in color.
- A common use is to evaluate patients with suspected retinal disease or with a family history of color vision deficiency.
- Tests also screen applicants for jobs in which accurate color perception is vital, such as in the military and electronics fields.
- Most common color vision tests use pseudoisochromatic plates made up of dot patterns of the primary colors superimposed on backgrounds of randomly mixed colors. (A patient with normal color vision can identify the dot pattern; a patient with a color vision deficiency can't distinguish between the pattern and the background.)
- Basic color vision tests merely indicate the presence of a deficiency; more sophisticated tests can determine the degree of deficiency.

Purpose

- To detect color vision deficiency

Procedure

Preparation

- Explain to the patient that this test evaluates color perception, takes only a few minutes, and causes no pain.
- If the patient normally wears glasses or contact lenses, tell him to wear them during the test.

Implementation

- After seating the patient comfortably, occlude one of his eyes.
- Hold the test book about 14″ (35.5 cm) in front of his unoccluded eye and give him the pointer.
- Explain to the patient what patterns or symbols he may see.
- Show him the sample plates and tell him that you will ask him to identify the symbols and then to trace them with the pointer. Inform him that some symbols are more difficult to see than others.
- Conduct the test, eliciting immediate responses from the patient.
- Record the responses according to the instructions included with the test kit.
- When testing the other eye (or repeating the test, if necessary), rotate the plates 90 to 180 degrees to minimize recall.
- To prevent discoloration of the plates, keep the test book closed when it's not in use and turn the pages by their edges.

Patient care

- Assess the patient's response to testing.

Complications

None known

Interpretation

Normal results

- A person with normal color vision — a trichromat — can identify all of the patterns or symbols.

Abnormal results

- A patient with deficit color vision — an anomalous trichromat — can't identify all the patterns or symbols.
- A more precise diagnosis is possible by noting the combinations of colors that elicit incorrect responses.
- Protanopia is a deficiency of the retinal cone pigment that's sensitive to red. A patient with protanopia has difficulty discriminating red from green and blue from green.
- A patient with deuteranopia, a deficiency of the retinal pigment sensitive to green, can't distinguish between green-purple and red-purple.
- Tritanopia, a deficiency of the pigment sensitive to blue, causes the patient to have difficulty discriminating between blue-green and yellow-green.
- Achromatopsia — true color blindness — is a rare disease inherited as a Mendelian autosomal dominant or autosomal recessive trait. Patients with achromatopsia, called *monochromats*, see all colors as shades of gray. These patients may also have impaired visual acuity, nystagmus, and photophobia from reduced or absent cone function.
- Inherited color deficiency affects both eyes; acquired deficiency may affect only one eye. The patient with an acquired deficiency may complain of an inability to recognize colors that were formerly recognizable.
- Abnormalities of the ocular media, retina, or optic nerve can cause deficient color vision. For this reason, a patient with an acquired color vision deficiency or an inherited deficiency accompanied by a loss of visual acuity should be referred for a complete ophthalmologic examination to determine the source of the deficiency.

Interfering factors

- Failure to cooperate, an inability to see the plates because of reduced visual acuity or failure to wear glasses, or improper lighting
- Errors in the testing procedure, such as inaccurately recording the patient's responses or allowing too much time for a response

Colposcopy

Overview

○ Visual examination of the cervix and vagina by means of a colposcope, an instrument with a magnifying lens and light source

Purpose

○ To confirm cervical intraepithelial neoplasia or invasive carcinoma after an abnormal Papanicolaou (Pap) test
○ To evaluate vaginal or cervical lesions
○ To monitor conservatively treated cervical intraepithelial neoplasia
○ To monitor patients whose mothers received diethylstilbestrol during pregnancy

Procedure

Preparation

○ Make sure the patient has signed an appropriate consent form.
○ Note and report allergies.
○ Restriction of food and fluids is unnecessary.
○ Instruct the patient not to douche, use tampons or vaginal medication, or have sexual intercourse for 2 days before the study.
○ Explain that the test is safe and painless and takes 10 to 15 minutes.
○ Explain that the procedure is similar to a routine pelvic examination, except the practitioner looks through the colposcope.
○ Explain that the patient may experience minimal bleeding and mild cramping with biopsy and endocervical curettage, if performed.

Implementation

○ Assist the patient into the lithotomy position.
○ A speculum is inserted into the vagina.
○ A Pap test is performed, if indicated.
○ A small amount of dilute vinegar solution is applied to the cervix to aid in differentiating the cell types; it makes abnormal areas more readily visible.
○ The cervix and vagina are visually examined.
○ A biopsy is performed on areas that appear abnormal.
○ Endocervical curettage to sample the cells just inside the cervical canal is then performed.
○ Bleeding is controlled by applying pressure or hemostatic solutions or by cautery.

Patient care

○ After a biopsy, instruct the patient to abstain from sexual intercourse until the biopsy site heals (about 10 days).
○ Instruct the patient to avoid inserting anything into the vagina (such as tampons) until the biopsy site heals.
○ Inform the patient to expect a watery vaginal discharge, which is normal during healing.

Complications

○ Bleeding (especially in pregnant patient)
○ Infection

Interpretation

Normal results

○ Surface contour of the cervical vessels is smooth and pink.
○ Columnar epithelium appears grapelike.
○ Different tissue types are sharply demarcated.

Abnormal results

○ White epithelium or punctuation and mosaic patterns may indicate underlying cervical intraepithelial neoplasia.
○ Keratinization in the transformation zone may indicate cervical intraepithelial neoplasia or invasive carcinoma.
○ Atypical vessels may indicate invasive carcinoma.
○ Inflammatory changes suggest possible infection.
○ Condyloma suggests human papillomavirus.

Interfering factors

○ Failure to clean the cervix of foreign materials, such as creams and medications (impairs visibility)
○ Hormonal contraceptives

Complement assays

Overview

○ Complement deficiency can increase susceptibility to infection and can predispose a person to other diseases.
○ Complement assays are performed in patients who may have an immune-mediated disease or those who repeatedly respond abnormally to infection.
○ Various laboratory methods evaluate and measure total complement and its components; hemolytic assay, laser nephelometry, and radial immunodiffusion are the most common.
○ Although complement assays provide valuable information about the patient's immune system, the results must be considered in light of serum immunoglobulin and autoantibody tests for a definitive diagnosis of immune-mediated disease or an abnormal response to infection.
○ Complement components are designated as C1 through C9, with C1 having three subcomponents: C1q, C1r, and C1s. (These complements constitute 3% to 4% of total serum globulins and play a key role in antibody-mediated immune reactions.)

Purpose

○ To help detect immune-mediated disease and genetic complement deficiency
○ To monitor the effectiveness of therapy

Procedure

Preparation

○ Explain to the patient that this test measures a group of proteins that fight infection.
○ Inform the patient that he need not restrict food and fluids.
○ Tell the patient that the test requires a blood sample. Explain who will perform the venipuncture and when.
○ Explain to the patient that he may experience slight discomfort from the tourniquet and the needle puncture.
○ If the patient is scheduled for a C1q assay, check his history for recent heparin therapy. Report such therapy to the laboratory.

Implementation

○ Perform a venipuncture and collect the sample in a 7-ml tube without additives.
○ Handle the sample gently to prevent hemolysis.
○ Send the sample to the laboratory immediately because the complement is heat labile and deteriorates rapidly.

Patient care

○ Because many patients with complement defects have a compromised immune system, keep the venipuncture site clean and dry.
○ Apply direct pressure to the venipuncture site until bleeding stops.

Complications

○ Hematoma at the venipuncture site

Interpretation

Normal results

○ Total complement: 25 to 110 units/ml (SI, 0.25 to 1.1 g/L)
○ C3: 70 to 150 mg/dl (SI, 0.7 to 1.5 g/L)
○ C4: 15 to 45 mg/dl (SI, 0.15 to 0.45 g/L)

Abnormal results

○ Complement abnormalities may be genetic or acquired; acquired abnormalities are most common.
○ Depressed total complement levels (which are clinically more significant than elevations) may result from excessive formation of antigen-antibody complexes, insufficient complement synthesis, inhibitor formation, or increased complement catabolism and are characteristic in such conditions as systemic lupus erythematosus (SLE), acute poststreptococcal glomerulonephritis, and acute serum sickness.
○ Low levels may also occur in some patients with advanced cirrhosis of the liver, multiple myeloma, hypogammaglobulinemia, or rapidly rejecting allografts.
○ Elevated total complement may occur in obstructive jaundice, thyroiditis, acute rheumatic fever, rheumatoid arthritis, acute myocardial infarction, ulcerative colitis, and diabetes.
○ C1 esterase inhibitor deficiency is characteristic in hereditary angioedema, the most common genetic abnormality associated with complement.
○ C3 deficiency is characteristic in recurrent pyogenic infection and disease activation in SLE.
○ C4 deficiency is characteristic in SLE and rheumatoid arthritis. C4 is increased in autoimmune hemolytic anemia.

Interfering factors

○ Hemolysis from rough handling of the sample
○ Failure to send the sample to the laboratory immediately
○ Recent heparin therapy

Computed tomography

Overview

○ Combines radiologic and computer technology to produce cross-sectional images of various layers of tissue, called computed tomography (CT)
○ Reconstructs cross-sectional, horizontal, sagittal, and coronal plane images
○ Accentuates tissue density differences through use of I.V. or oral contrast medium accentuates
○ Also known as a *CT scan*

Purpose

○ To produce tissue images not readily seen on standard radiographs

Procedure

Preparation

○ Make sure the patient has signed an appropriate consent form.
○ Note and report allergies.
○ A CT scan usually isn't recommended during pregnancy because of potential risk to the fetus.
○ Check the patient's history for hypersensitivity to shellfish, iodine, or iodinated contrast media, and document such reactions on the patient's chart.
○ The specific type of CT scan dictates the need for an oral or I.V. contrast medium.
○ Warn the patient about transient discomfort from the needle puncture and a warm or flushed feeling from an I.V. contrast medium, if used.
○ Instruct the patient to remain still during the test because movement can limit the accuracy of results.
○ Tell the patient he may experience minimal discomfort because of lying still.
○ Tell the patient to immediately report feelings of nausea, vomiting, dizziness, headache, itching, or hives. Check the patient's history for hypersensitivity to iodine or contrast media used in other diagnostic tests.
○ Tell the patient that the study takes from 5 minutes to 1 hour depending on the type of CT and his ability to remain still.

Implementation

○ The patient is positioned on an adjustable table inside a scanning gantry.
○ A series of transverse radiographs is taken and recorded.
○ The information is reconstructed by a computer and selected images are photographed.
○ After the images are reviewed, an I.V. contrast enhancement may be ordered.
○ Additional images are obtained after the I.V. contrast injection.
○ The patient is observed carefully for adverse reactions to the contrast medium.

Patient care

○ Normal diet and activities may resume, unless otherwise ordered.

Complications

○ Adverse reaction to iodinated contrast media

Interpretation

Normal results

○ The specific type of CT scan dictates normal findings.
○ Structures are evaluated according to their density, size, shape, and position.
○ Tissue densities appear as black, white, or shades of gray on the CT image. Bone, the densest tissue, appears white. Cerebrospinal fluid, the least dense, appears black.

Abnormal results

○ See specific types of CT.

Interfering factors

○ Oral or I.V. contrast media use in previous diagnostic tests (obscure the images)

Computed tomography of the abdomen and pelvis

Overview

○ Combines radiologic and computer technology to produce cross-sectional images of various layers of tissue
○ For computed tomography (CT) of the abdomen, includes the area between the dome of the diaphragm and iliac crests
○ CT scan of the abdomen may be performed with or without a CT scan of the pelvis
○ For pelvic CT, includes the area between the iliac crests and the perineum; in men, includes the bladder and prostate, in women, the bladder and adnexa
○ May include spiral CT scans of the abdomen and pelvis

Purpose

○ To evaluate soft tissue and organs of the abdomen, pelvis, and retroperitoneal space
○ To evaluate inflammatory disease
○ To aid staging of neoplasms
○ To evaluate trauma
○ To detect tumors, cysts, hemorrhage, or edema
○ To evaluate response to chemotherapy

Procedure

Preparation

○ Make sure the patient has signed an appropriate consent form.
○ Note and report allergies.
○ CT scanning of the abdomen and pelvis usually isn't recommended during pregnancy because of potential risk to the fetus.
○ Check the patient's history for hypersensitivity to shellfish, iodine, or iodinated contrast media and document such reactions on the patient's chart.
○ Inform the physician of any sensitivity so that prophylactic medications may be ordered; the physician may choose not to use the contrast.
○ If the patient won't receive a contrast medium, tell him that he need not restrict food and fluids.
○ If the patient will receive a contrast medium, instruct him to fast for 4 hours before the test.
○ Stress to the patient the need to remain still during testing because movement can limit the test's accuracy. The patient may experience minimal discomfort because of lying still.
○ Warn about transient discomfort from the needle puncture and a warm or flushed feeling or metallic taste if an I.V. contrast medium is used.
○ Inform the patient that he'll hear clacking sounds as the table moves into the scanner.
○ Explain that the test takes about 35 to 40 minutes.

Implementation

○ Usually, the test requires oral contrast material to outline the intestines.
○ The patient is assisted into a supine position with his arms above his head.
○ I.V. contrast agent may be injected into a vein to help define certain tissues.
○ The table will advance slightly between each scan.
○ Cross-sectional images are obtained and reviewed.

Patient care

○ The patient may resume his normal diet and activities unless otherwise ordered.

Complications

○ Adverse reaction to iodinated contrast medium

Interpretation

Normal results

○ The organs are normal in size and position.
○ There are no masses or other abnormalities.

Abnormal results

○ Well-circumscribed or poorly defined areas of slightly lower density than normal parenchyma suggest possible primary and metastatic neoplasms.
○ Relatively low-density, homogeneous areas, usually with well-defined borders suggest possible abscesses.
○ Sharply defined round or oval structures, with densities less than that of abscesses and neoplasms, suggest cysts.
○ Dilatation of the biliary ducts suggests obstructive disease from a tumor or calculi.

Interfering factors

None known

Computed tomography of the bone

Overview

- Series of tomograms, translated by a computer and displayed on a monitor, representing cross-sectional images of various layers (or slices) of bone
- Can reconstruct cross-sectional, horizontal, sagittal, and coronal plane images
- By taking collimated (parallel) radiographs, increases the number of radiation density calculations the computer makes and improving the degree of resolution, specificity, and accuracy
- Combines hundreds of thousands of readings of radiation levels absorbed by tissues to depict anatomic slices of varying thicknesses

Purpose

- To determine the existence and extent of primary bone tumors, skeletal metastases, soft-tissue tumors, injuries to ligaments or tendons, and fractures
- To diagnose joint abnormalities that are difficult to detect by other methods

Procedure

Preparation

- Explain to the patient that a skeletal computed tomography (CT) scan allows imaging of bones and joints.
- If the patient won't receive a contrast medium, tell him that he need not restrict food and fluids.
- If the patient will receive a contrast medium, instruct him to fast for 4 hours before the test.
- Check the patient's history for hypersensitivity reactions to iodine, shellfish, or contrast media. Mark such reactions in the chart and notify the physician, who may order prophylactic medications or choose not to use a contrast medium.
- Explain to the patient that he'll lie on an X-ray table inside a CT scanner and be asked to lie still; the computer-controlled scanner will revolve around him taking multiple scans.
- Stress that he should lie as still as possible.
- If the patient is to receive a contrast medium, tell him that he may feel flushed and warm and may experience a transient headache, a salty or metallic taste, and nausea or vomiting after its injection.
- Instruct the patient to remove all metal objects and jewelry in the X-ray field.
- If the patient appears restless or apprehensive about the procedure, a mild sedative may be prescribed.
- For the patient with significant bone or joint pain, give analgesics so that he can lie comfortably during the scan.

Implementation

- The patient is assisted into a supine position on an X-ray table and ask him to lie as still as possible.
- The table is slid into the circular opening of the CT scanner. The scanner revolves around the patient, taking radiographs at preselected intervals.
- After the first set of scans is taken, the patient is removed from the scanner and a contrast medium is given, if necessary.
- Observe the patient for signs and symptoms of a hypersensitivity reaction, including pruritus, rash, and respiratory difficulty, for 30 minutes after injection of the contrast medium.
- After the contrast medium I.V. injection, the patient is moved back into the scanner and another series of scans is taken. The images obtained from the scan are displayed on a monitor during the procedure and stored on magnetic tape to create a permanent record for subsequent study.

Patient care

- If contrast medium is used, observe the patient for a delayed allergic reaction and treat as necessary. (Diphenhydramine is the drug of choice.)
- Encourage fluids to assist in eliminating the contrast medium.
- Tell the patient that he may resume his usual diet and activities, if appropriate.
- Provide comfort measures and pain medication because of prolonged positioning on the table.

Complications

- The patient may experience strong feelings of claustrophobia or anxiety when inside the CT body scanner. In this case, a mild sedative may be ordered to help reduce anxiety.

Interpretation

Normal results

- No pathology in the bones or joints
- Crisp images of the structure while blurring or eliminating details of surrounding structures

Abnormal results

- Differentiation of tissues, showing primary bone tumors, soft-tissue tumors, and skeletal metastasis
- Details of bone fractures visible
- Different characteristics of tissues and organs, revealing other abnormalities
- Joint abnormalities (hard to detect by other methods)

Interfering factors

- Claustrophobia (possible interference with the patient's ability to lie in the scanner for long periods)
- Excessive patient movement
- Failure to remove metallic objects from the examination field (possible poor imaging)

Computed tomography of the brain

Overview

○ Series of tomograms, translated by a computer and displayed on an oscilloscope screen, usually using a contrast medium
○ Provides layers of cross-sectional images of the brain
○ Reconstructs cross-sectional, horizontal, sagittal, and coronal-plane images
○ Also known as *intracranial computed tomography*.

Purpose

○ To diagnose intracranial lesions and abnormalities
○ To monitor the effects of surgery, radiotherapy, or chemotherapy in treatment of intracranial tumors
○ To guide cranial surgery
○ To assess focal neurologic abnormalities
○ To evaluate suspected head injury such as subdural hematoma

Procedure

Preparation

○ Make sure the patient has signed an appropriate consent form.
○ Note and report allergies.
○ If the patient won't receive a contrast medium, tell him that he need not restrict food and fluids.
○ If the patient will receive a contrast medium, instruct him to fast for 4 hours before the test.
○ Stress that the patient must remain still during the test because movement can limit accuracy of the test.
○ Warn the patient that he may experience minimal discomfort because of lying still and immobilizing his head.
○ Warn about transient discomfort from the needle puncture and a warm or flushed feeling if an I.V. contrast medium is used.
○ Caution that the patient will hear clacking sounds as the head of the table moves into the scanner, which rotates around the patient's head.
○ Explain that the test takes 15 to 30 minutes.

Implementation

○ The patient is assisted into a supine position on a radiographic table.
○ The patient's head is immobilized with straps and he is asked to lie still.
○ The head of the table is moved into the scanner, which rotates around the patient's head, taking radiographs.
○ When the initial series of radiographs is complete, the contrast enhancement is given if ordered.
○ Usually, 50 to 100 ml of contrast medium is injected by I.V. bolus or infusion.

○ The patient is observed for hypersensitivity reactions.
○ Another series of scans is taken.
○ Selected views are taken for further study.

Patient care

○ If the patient received a contrast medium, watch for delayed adverse reactions.
○ Have him resume his usual diet and medications unless otherwise ordered.

Complications

○ Adverse reaction to iodinated contrast medium

Interpretation

Normal results

○ Brain matter appears in shades of gray.
○ Ventricular and subarachnoid cerebrospinal fluid appears black.

Abnormal results

○ Enlarged ventricles with large sulci suggest cerebral atrophy.

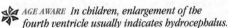 *AGE AWARE In children, enlargement of the fourth ventricle usually indicates hydrocephalus.*

○ Areas of marked generalized lucency suggest cerebral edema.
○ Cerebral vessels appearing with slightly increased density suggest possible arteriovenous malformation.
○ Areas of altered density or displaced vasculature or other structures may indicate intracranial tumors, intracranial hematoma, cerebral atrophy, infarction, edema, and congenital anomalies such as hydrocephalus.

Interfering factors

○ Claustrophobia (possible interference with the patient's ability to lie in the scanner for long periods)
○ Excessive patient movement
○ Failure to remove all metal objects (possible poor imaging)

Computed tomography of the ear

Overview

○ Combines radiologic and computer technology to produce cross-sectional images of various layers of tissue
○ Uses high-resolution computed tomography (HRCT) to evaluate patients for cochlear implants, differentiate osseous changes involving the external auditory canal and middle ear, differentiate the osseous structures of the temporal bone and petrous bone, and provide differential diagnoses for middle ear and inner ear problems
○ Evaluates cholesteatomas, establishes surgical and other therapeutic approaches for the patient, and evaluates the postsurgical management of a patient with a middle or inner ear disorder

Purpose

○ To investigate the cause of bilateral hearing loss
○ To confirm cochlear abnormalities
○ To differentiate chronic inflammation from cholesteatoma
○ To evaluate ossification of the cochlea coils before cochlear implantation
○ To depict osseous changes involving the temporal and petrous bone contained in the inner ear
○ To accurately define appropriate surgical and therapeutic approaches for patients with middle ear and inner ear disorders
○ To assess postsurgical management of patients with middle ear and inner ear disorders

Procedure

Preparation

○ Describe the procedure to the patient. Tell him to remove any metal objects such as jewelry.
○ Explain to the patient that he'll be secured to the scanner table to eliminate movement.
○ Check the patient for allergies to iodine products if a contrast medium is to be used. Tell him that he'll receive the contrast medium I.V.
○ If the patient will receive a contrast medium I.V., instruct him to fast from food and fluids for 4 hours before the test.
○ A contrast medium isn't required for evaluating ossification of the cochlea coils or studying the petrous portion of the temporal bone.
○ If the patient won't receive a contrast medium, tell him that he need not restrict food and fluids.
○ Inform the patient that his body and head will be moved into the scanner, which is an air-conditioned chamber that resembles a giant doughnut. The technician will remain present and communicate with the patient throughout the test, which will last from 15 to 20 minutes.
○ Warn the patient that he'll hear a humming sound while the machine records the images.
○ Ask the patient about feelings of claustrophobia. He may require preprocedure medication to alleviate his fears.

Implementation

○ The protocol for each HRCT depends on the purpose of the test, with most HRCT studies focused on the axial and coronal planes.
○ In the radiology department, the patient is placed on the scanner table with his head toward the machine. The mobile scanner table allows for easy transfer and accurate positioning in the machine.
○ A trained technician conducts the study under the supervision of a radiologist.
○ The technician explains the details of the procedure to the patient to reassure him and gain his cooperation.
○ Numerous low-dose X-ray beams pass through the patient's body at different angles for a fraction of a second as the scanner rotates around him.
○ Detectors in the scanner record the number of X-rays absorbed by different tissues, and a computer transforms these data into an image, which is interpreted by the radiologist.
○ The temporal bones are imaged separately in the axial and coronal planes. Because contrast already exists between bone, air, and soft tissue, the use of a contrast medium isn't necessary in most cases.

Patient care

○ The patient may resume his normal diet and activities unless otherwise ordered.

Complications

None known

Interpretation

Normal results

○ Normal anatomic structures should be easy to identify.

Abnormal results

○ Tympanosclerosis and osseous changes of the external auditory canal and middle and inner ear structures
○ Cochlear abnormalities

Interfering factors

○ Patient's inability to lie still during the scan
○ Failure to remove all metal objects
○ Allergies to iodine if a contrast medium was used

Computed tomography of the kidneys

Overview

- Combines radiologic and computer technology to produce cross-sectional images of layers of tissue
- Reveals masses and other lesions by measuring the amount of radiation the kidney tissue absorbs
- Highly accurate test to investigate diseases found by other tests such as excretory urography

Purpose

- To detect and evaluate renal abnormalities, such as tumor, obstruction, calculi, polycystic disease, congenital anomalies, and abnormal fluid accumulation
- To evaluate the retroperitoneum

Procedure

Preparation

- Make sure the patient signs a consent form.
- Check the patient's history for hypersensitivity to shellfish, iodine, or contrast media.
- Instruct the patient to put on a gown and remove metallic objects that could interfere with the scan.
- Give prescribed sedatives.
- Tell the patient that this computed tomography (CT) scan will examine his kidneys.
- If the patient is to receive a contrast medium, instruct him to fast for 4 hours before the test.
- Inform the patient that he'll lie on an X-ray table and that he'll need to be secured to the table with straps while a scanner takes films of his kidneys.
- Warn the patient that the scanner may make loud, clacking sounds as it rotates around his body.
- Tell the patient side effects include flushing, metallic taste, and headache after contrast medium injection.

Implementation

- The patient is assisted into the supine position on the X-ray table and secure him with straps.
- The table is moved into the scanner.
- The patient is instructed to lie still.
- The scanner rotates around the patient, taking multiple images at different angles within each cross-sectional slice.
- When one series of tomograms is complete, the I.V. contrast enhancement may be performed. Another series of tomograms is then taken.
- After the I.V. contrast medium is given, the patient is monitored for allergic reactions, such as respiratory difficulty, urticaria, or skin eruptions.
- Information from the scan is stored on a disk or magnetic tape, fed into a computer, and converted into an image for display on a monitor. Radiographs and photographs are taken of selected views.

Patient care

- If the procedure used contrast enhancement, watch for hypersensitivity to the contrast medium.
- After the test, tell the patient to resume his usual diet.
- If calculi are present, strain the urine, hydrate the patient, and discuss nutritional adaptations.
- Support the patient and his family if surgery is indicated for a neoplasm.
- Monitor patient's vital signs if he received a sedative.

Complications

- Hypersensitivity to the contrast medium

Interpretation

Normal results

- Renal parenchyma density higher than hepatic but less than bone, which appears white on a CT scan.
- The density of the collecting system is generally low (black), unless a contrast medium enhances it to a higher density (whiter).
- Evaluating kidney position depends on the surrounding structures; counting cuts between the superior and inferior poles and following the contour of the kidneys' outline gives size and shape.

Abnormal results

- Renal masses appear as areas of different density than normal parenchyma, possibly altering the kidneys' shape or projecting beyond their margins.
- Renal cysts appear as smooth, sharply defined masses with thin walls and a lower density than normal parenchyma.
- Tumors such as renal cell carcinoma, however, usually aren't as well delineated; they have thick walls and nonuniform density.
- With contrast enhancement, solid tumors show a higher density than renal cysts but a lower density than normal parenchyma.
- Tumors with hemorrhage, calcification, or necrosis show higher densities.
- Vascular tumors are more clearly defined with contrast enhancement.
- Adrenal tumors are confined masses, usually detached from the kidneys and from other retroperitoneal organs.
- Obstructions, calculi, polycystic kidney disease, congenital anomalies, and abnormal accumulations of fluid around the kidneys, such as hematomas, lymphoceles, and abscesses can also be identified.
- The kidney may be abnormally large or small, may appear damaged, or may be infected.
- After nephrectomy, scanning can detect abnormal masses such as recurrent tumors in a renal fossa that should be empty.

Interfering factors

- Patient's inability to remain still
- Presence of contrast media from other recent tests or of foreign bodies, such as catheters or surgical clips

Computed tomography of the liver and biliary tract

Overview

○ Combines radiologic and computer technology to produce cross-sectional images of various layers of tissue
○ Penetrates the upper abdomen with multiple X-rays, while a detector records the differences in tissue attenuation, displayed as an image on a screen
○ Distinguishes the biliary tract and the liver if the ducts are large through a series of cross-sectional views
○ Performed in patients who are obese and in those with livers positioned high under the rib cage because excessive fat and bone hinder ultrasound transmission

Purpose

○ To distinguish between obstructive and nonobstructive jaundice
○ To detect intrahepatic tumors and abscesses, subphrenic and subhepatic abscesses, cysts, and hematomas

Procedure

Preparation

○ Explain to the patient that computed tomography (CT) scanning helps detect biliary tract and liver disease.
○ Check the patient's history for hypersensitivity to iodine, seafood, or the contrast media used in other diagnostic tests.
○ If ordered, give the patient the oral contrast medium supplied by the radiology department. Tell the patient that he'll drink a contrast medium and then fast until after the examination. If I.V. contrast medium isn't ordered, fasting isn't necessary.
○ If the patient will receive I.V. contrast, he'll need to fast from food and fluids for 4 hours before the test.
○ Tell the patient to immediately report nausea, vomiting, dizziness, headache, and hives.
○ If the test will involve an I.V. contrast medium, tell the patient that he may experience transient discomfort from the needle puncture and a localized feeling of warmth on injection, as well as a salty or metallic taste.
○ Inform the patient that he'll lie on an adjustable table inside a scanning gantry.
○ Tell the patient that he'll need to remain still during the test and periodically hold his breath. Stress the importance of remaining still during the test because

movement can cause artifacts, thereby prolonging the test and limiting its accuracy.

Implementation

○ The patient is placed in the supine position on an X-ray table, and the table is positioned within the opening in the scanning gantry.
○ A series of transverse X-rays is taken and recorded on magnetic tape.
○ This information is reconstructed by a computer and appears as images on a television screen.
○ When the first series of X-rays is completed, the images are reviewed.
○ If contrast enhancement is ordered, the contrast medium is injected. A second series of X-rays is taken. The patient is observed carefully for an allergic reaction.

Patient care

○ Monitor the patient for adverse effects to the contrast medium.

Complications

○ Adverse effects from contrast medium

Interpretation

Normal results

○ The liver has a uniform density that's slightly greater than that of the pancreas, kidneys, and spleen.
○ Linear and circular areas of slightly lower density, representing hepatic vascular structures, may interrupt this uniform appearance.
○ The portal vein is usually visible; the hepatic artery usually isn't.
○ I.V. contrast medium enhances the isodensity of vascular structures and liver parenchyma.
○ Intrahepatic biliary radicles aren't visible, but the common hepatic and bile ducts may be visible as low-density structures.
○ Because bile has the same density as water, use of an I.V. contrast medium improves demarcation of the biliary tract by enhancing the surrounding parenchyma and vascular structures.
○ Like the biliary ducts, the gallbladder is visible as a round or elliptic low-density structure.

Abnormal results

○ Most focal hepatic defects appear less dense than the normal parenchyma, and CT scans can detect small lesions.
○ Use of rapid-sequence scanning with an I.V. contrast medium helps distinguish between the two because the normal parenchyma shows greater enhancement than focal defects.
○ Primary and metastatic neoplasms may appear as well-circumscribed or poorly defined areas of slightly lower density than the normal parenchyma.
○ Some lesions have the same density as the liver parenchyma and may be undetectable.

○ Especially large neoplasms may distort the liver's contour.
○ Hepatic abscesses appear as relatively low-density, homogeneous areas, usually with well-defined borders.
○ Hepatic cysts appear as sharply defined round or oval structures and have a density lower than abscesses and neoplasms.
○ Density of a hepatic hematoma varies with its age.
○ Subcapsular hematomas are usually crescent-shaped and compress the liver away from the capsule.
○ Absence of dilation indicates nonobstructive jaundice.
○ Biliary duct dilation indicates obstructive jaundice.
○ Dilated intrahepatic bile ducts appear as low-density linear and circular branching structures.
○ Dilation of the common hepatic duct, common bile duct, and gallbladder may also be apparent, depending on the site and severity of obstruction.
○ Usually, CT scanning can identify the cause of obstruction.

Interfering factors

○ Presence of oral or I.V. contrast media, including barium, in the bile duct from earlier tests (possible poor imaging)

Computed tomography of the pancreas

Overview

○ Combines radiologic and computer technology to produce cross-sectional images of various layers of tissue
○ Penetrates the upper abdomen with multiple X-rays, while a detector records the differences in tissue attenuation, displayed as an image on a screen
○ Provides a detailed look at the pancreas through a series of cross-sectional views
○ Accurately distinguishes the pancreas and surrounding organs and vessels if enough fat is present between the structures
○ Goes beyond ultrasonography by showing the general swelling that accompanies acute inflammation of the gland (in retroperitoneal disorders, specifically when pancreatitis is suspected)
○ Easily detects calcium deposits commonly missed by simple radiography, particularly in obese patients (in chronic cases)

Purpose

○ To detect pancreatic carcinoma or pseudocysts
○ To detect or evaluate pancreatitis
○ To distinguish between pancreatic disorders and disorders of the retroperitoneum

Procedure

Preparation

○ Explain to the patient that computed tomography scanning helps detect disorders of the pancreas.
○ Check the patient's history for recent barium studies and for hypersensitivity to iodine, seafood, or contrast media used in previous tests.
○ Tell the patient that he may receive an I.V. contrast medium, oral contrast medium, or both to enhance visualization of the pancreas.
○ Give the oral contrast medium if ordered.
○ Instruct the patient to fast after administration of the oral contrast medium.
○ If the patient will receive I.V. contrast, tell him to fast from food and fluids for 4 hours before the test.
○ Describe possible adverse reactions to the medium, such as nausea, flushing, dizziness, and sweating, and tell him to report these symptoms.
○ Tell the patient that he'll lie on an adjustable table that's positioned inside a scanning gantry. Assure him that the procedure is painless.
○ Explain to the patient that he'll need to remain still during the test and periodically hold his breath.

Implementation

○ The patient is helped into the supine position on the X-ray table and the table is positioned within the opening in the scanning gantry.
○ A series of transverse X-rays is taken and recorded on magnetic tape. The images are studied, and selected ones are photographed.
○ After the first series of X-rays is complete, the images are reviewed. Contrast enhancement may be ordered.
○ After the contrast medium is given, another series of X-rays is taken. The patient is observed for an allergic reaction, such as itching, hypotension, hypertension, diaphoresis, or dyspnea.

Patient care

○ After the procedure, tell the patient he may resume his usual diet.

Complications

○ Delayed allergic reaction to the contrast dye, such as urticaria, headache, and vomiting

Interpretation

Normal results

○ The pancreatic parenchyma displays a uniform density, especially when an I.V. contrast medium is used.
○ The gland thickens from tail to head and has a smooth surface.

Abnormal results

○ Because the tissue density of pancreatic carcinoma resembles that of the normal parenchyma, changes in pancreatic size and shape help demonstrate carcinoma and pseudocysts.
○ Usually, a carcinoma first appears as a localized swelling of the head, body, or tail of the pancreas and may spread to obliterate the fat plane, dilate the main pancreatic duct and common bile duct by obstructing them, and produce low-density focal lesions in the liver from metastasis.
○ Use of an I.V. contrast medium helps detect metastases by opacifying the pancreatic and hepatic parenchyma.
○ Adenocarcinoma and islet cell tumors are the most common carcinomas of the pancreas.
○ Cystadenomas and cystadenocarcinoma, usually multilocular, occur most frequently in the body and tail of the pancreas and appear as low-density focal lesions marked by internal septa.
○ Acute pancreatitis, either edematous (interstitial) or necrotizing (hemorrhagic), produces diffuse enlargement of the pancreas.
○ In acute edematous pancreatitis, parenchyma density is uniformly decreased.
○ In acute necrotizing pancreatitis, the density is nonuniform because of the presence of necrosis and hemorrhage. The areas of tissue necrosis have diminished density.

- In acute pancreatitis, inflammation typically spreads into the peripancreatic fat, causes stranding in the mesenteric fat, and blurs the gland margin.
- Abscesses, within or outside the pancreas, appear as low-density areas and are most readily detected when they contain gas.
- Pseudocysts, which may be unilocal or multilocal, appear as sharply circumscribed, low-density areas that may contain debris.
- Ascites and pleural effusion may also be apparent in acute pancreatitis.
- In chronic pancreatitis, the pancreas may appear normal, enlarged, or atrophic, depending on disease severity.

Interfering factors

- Barium or other contrast media in the GI tract from earlier tests
- Excessive peristalsis or excessive patient movement

Computed tomography of the spine

Overview

○ Provides detailed high-resolution images in the cross-sectional, longitudinal, sagittal, and lateral planes.
○ Multiple X-ray beams from a computerized body scanner are directed at the spine from different angles; these pass through the body and strike radiation detectors, producing electrical impulses.
○ A computer converts these impulses into digital information, which appears as a three-dimensional image on a monitor.
○ Storage of the digital information allows electronic recreation and manipulation of the image, creating a permanent record of the images to enable reexamination without repeating the procedure.
○ Images are helpful in defining the lesions causing spinal cord compression.
○ Metastatic disease and discogenic disease with osteophyte formation and calcification are examples of pathologic processes diagnosed by computed tomography (CT) scans.

Purpose

○ To diagnose spinal lesions and abnormalities
○ To monitor the effects of spinal surgery or therapy

Procedure

Preparation

○ Explain that spinal CT allows imaging of the spine.
○ If the patient won't receive a contrast medium, tell him that he need not restrict food and fluids.
○ If the patient will receive a contrast medium, instruct him to fast for 4 hours before the test.
○ Explain to the patient that he'll lie on an X-ray table inside a CT body scanning unit and be asked to lie still because movement during the procedure may cause distorted images.
○ The computer-controlled scanner will revolve around him, taking multiple scans.
○ If he'll receive a contrast medium, tell him that he may feel flushed and warm and may experience a transient headache, a salty taste, and nausea or vomiting after the injection. Reassure him that these reactions are normal.
○ Instruct the patient to wear a radiologic examining gown and to remove all metal objects and jewelry.
○ Check the patient's history for hypersensitivity reactions to iodine, shellfish, or contrast media. Note them in the chart and notify the physician who may order prophylactic medications or choose not to use contrast enhancement.

○ If the patient appears restless or apprehensive about the procedure, a mild sedative may be prescribed.
○ For the patient with significant back pain, give prescribed analgesics before the scan.

Implementation

○ The patient is assisted into the supine position on an X-ray table and asked to lie as still as possible.
○ The table slides into the circular opening of the CT scanner and the scanner revolves around the patient, taking radiographs at preselected intervals.
○ After the first set of scans is taken, the patient is removed from the scanner. Contrast medium may be given.
○ The patient is observed for signs and symptoms of a hypersensitivity reaction, including pruritus, rash, and respiratory difficulty, for 30 minutes after the contrast medium injection.
○ After the contrast medium injection, the patient is moved back into the scanner, and another series of scans is taken.

Patient care

○ After testing with contrast enhancement, observe the patient for residual effects, such as headache, nausea, and vomiting.
○ Have the patient resume his usual diet.
○ If the patient becomes claustrophobic or anxious inside the CT body scanner, a mild sedative may be given to help relieve these symptoms.

Complications

○ Claustrophobia or anxiety when inside the CT body scanner

Interpretation

Normal results

○ Spinal tissue appears white, black, or gray, depending on its density.
○ Vertebrae, the densest tissues, are white; cerebrospinal fluid is black; soft tissues appear in shades of gray.

Abnormal results

○ Spinal lesions and other abnormalities are visualized on the scan.
○ Tumors appear as masses varying in density. Measuring this density and noting the configuration and location relative to the spinal cord can usually identify the type of tumor. For example, a neurinoma (schwannoma) appears as a spherical mass dorsal to the cord. A darker, wider mass lying more lateral or ventral to the cord may be a meningioma.
○ Degenerative processes and structural changes show in detail.
○ A herniated nucleus pulposus shows as an obvious herniation of disk material with unilateral or bilateral nerve root compression; if the herniation is midline, spinal cord compression will be evident.

- Cervical spondylosis shows as cervical cord compression; lumbar stenosis, as hypertrophy of the lumbar vertebrae.
- Facet disorders show as soft-tissue changes, bony overgrowth, and spurring of the vertebrae.
- Fluid-filled arachnoidal and other paraspinal cysts show as dark masses displacing the spinal cord.
- Vascular malformations, evident after contrast, show as masses or clusters, usually on the dorsal aspect of the spinal cord.
- Congenital spinal malformations show as abnormally large, dark gaps between the white vertebrae.

Interfering factors

- Excessive patient movement
- Failure to remove metallic objects from the scan area

Computed tomography of the thorax

Overview

○ Provides cross-sectional views of the chest by passing an X-ray beam from a computerized scanner through the body at different angles
○ Provides a three-dimensional image and is especially useful in detecting small differences in tissue density
○ May replace mediastinoscopy in the diagnosis of mediastinal masses and Hodgkin's disease; its value in the evaluation of pulmonary pathology is proven

Purpose

○ To locate suspected neoplasms (such as in Hodgkin's disease), especially with mediastinal involvement
○ To differentiate coin-sized calcified lesions (indicating tuberculosis) from tumors
○ To differentiate emphysema or bronchopleural fistula from lung abscess
○ To distinguish tumors adjacent to the aorta from aortic aneurysms
○ To detect the invasion of a neck mass in the thorax
○ To evaluate primary malignancy that may metastasize to the lungs, especially in the patient with a primary bone tumor, soft-tissue sarcoma, or melanoma
○ To evaluate the mediastinal lymph nodes
○ To evaluate the severity of lung disease such as emphysema
○ To detect a dissection or leak of an aortic aneurysm or aortic arch aneurysm
○ To plan radiation treatment

Procedure

Preparation

○ Explain that the thoracic computed tomography (CT) provides cross-sectional views of the chest and distinguishes small differences in tissue density.
○ If the patient won't receive a contrast medium, tell him that he need not restrict food and fluids.
○ If the patient will receive a contrast medium, instruct him to fast for 4 hours before the test.
○ Inform the patient that he'll lie on an X-ray table that moves into the center of a large ring-shaped piece of X-ray equipment and that the equipment may be noisy.
○ Inform the patient that a contrast medium may be injected into a vein in his arm. If so, he may experience nausea, warmth, flushing of the face, and a salty or metallic taste. Reassure him that these symptoms are normal and that radiation exposure is minimal.
○ Tell the patient that he must remain still during the test, breathing normally until told to follow specific breathing instructions.

○ Ask him to remove all jewelry and metallic objects in the X-ray field.
○ Check the patient's history for hypersensitivity to iodine, shellfish, or contrast media.
○ Make sure that the patient or a responsible family member has signed an informed consent form, if required.

Implementation

○ The patient is assisted into the supine position on the X-ray table and the contrast medium is injected. The machine scans the patient at different angles while the computer calculates small differences in densities of various tissues, water, fat, bone, and air.
○ Information is displayed as a printout of numerical values and a projection on a monitor. Images may be recorded for further study.

Patient care

○ Watch the patient for signs of delayed hypersensitivity to the contrast medium (itching, hypotension or hypertension, or respiratory distress).
○ After the test, encourage the patient to drink lots of fluids.

Complications

○ Adverse effects from contrast medium

Interpretation

Normal results

○ Black and white areas on a thoracic CT scan refer, respectively, to air and bone densities.
○ Shades of gray correspond to water, fat, and soft-tissue densities.

Abnormal results

○ Tumors, nodules, cysts, aortic aneurysms, enlarged lymph nodes, pleural effusion, and accumulations of blood, fluid, or fat

Interfering factors

○ Failure to remove all metallic objects from the scanning field
○ Patient's inability to remain still during the procedure
○ An obese patient, who may be too heavy for the scanning table

Concentration and dilution, urine

Overview

- Kidneys normally concentrate or dilute urine according to fluid intake. When such intake is excessive, the kidneys excrete more water in the urine; when intake is limited, they excrete less
- Evaluates renal capacity to concentrate urine in response to fluid deprivation or to dilute it in response to fluid overload
- Also known as the *water loading* or *water deprivation test*

Purpose

- To evaluate renal tubular function
- To detect renal impairment
- To diagnose disorders such as diabetes insipidus

Procedure

Preparation

- Explain to the patient that this test evaluates kidney function.
- Tell him the test requires multiple urine specimens. Explain how many specimens will be collected and at what intervals.
- Instruct him to discard urine voided for a specific time, according to laboratory protocol, such as all urine collected during the night.
- Withhold diuretics as needed.
- For several days before the concentration test, the patient should eat a normal diet. He may receive special instructions about water loading or water deprivation.
- The night before the test, the patient should eat a high-protein meal and only 200 ml of fluid. Afterwards, the patient should restrict food and fluid for at least 14 hours before the test. (Some concentration tests prohibit water for 24 hours but permit relatively normal food intake.)
- For a concentration test, the patient must also limit salt intake at the evening meal to prevent excessive thirst.
- For the dilution test, preparation is the same as for the concentration test and necessitates no additional patient preparation. If it's performed alone, simply withhold breakfast.

Implementation

- *Concentration test:* Collect urine specimens at 6 a.m., 8 a.m., and 10 a.m.
- *Dilution test:* Instruct the patient to void and discard the first urine sample. Give the patient 1,500 ml of water to drink within a 30-minute period. Collect urine specimens every half hour or every hour for 4 hours thereafter.
- For both tests provide a balanced meal or a snack after collecting the final specimen. Make sure the patient voids within 8 hours after the catheter is removed.
- Send each specimen to the laboratory immediately after collection.

Patient care

- Provide the patient with a clean bedpan, urinal, or toilet specimen pan if he's unable to urinate into the specimen containers.
- If the patient is catheterized, empty the drainage bag before the test. Obtain the specimens from the catheter and clamp the catheter between collections.

Complications

None known

Interpretation

Normal results

- Normal specific gravity ranges from 1.005 to 1.035; osmolality normally ranges from 300 to 900 mOsm/kg.
- *Concentration test:* Specific gravity ranges from 1.025 to 1.032, and osmolality rises above 800 mOsm/kg of water (SI, > 800 mmol/kg) in the patient with normal renal function.
- *Dilution test:* Specific gravity falls below 1.003 and osmolality below 100 mOsm/kg for at least one specimen; 80% or more of the ingested water is eliminated in 4 hours.

Abnormal results

- Decreased renal capacity to concentrate urine in response to fluid deprivation, or to dilute urine in response to fluid overload, may indicate tubular epithelial damage, decreased renal blood flow, loss of functional nephrons, or pituitary or cardiac dysfunction.

 AGE AWARE In an elderly person, depressed values may indicate normal renal function.

Interfering factors

- Failure to observe pretest restrictions
- Use of radiographic contrast agents within 7 days of test (possible increase in osmolality)
- Diuretics and nephrotoxic drugs (possible increase or decrease in specific gravity and osmolality)
- Glycosuria

Contraction stress test

Overview

○ Measures fetal heart rate in response to uterine contractions
○ Usually, the heart rate of a healthy fetus won't slow down when contractions begin and after they end
○ Generally occurs weekly until delivery

Purpose

○ To measure fetal heart rate in response to contractions

Procedure

Preparation

○ Explain testing procedure to the patient.
○ Explain that the test generally lasts for 30 to 40 minutes.

Implementation

○ After the patient lies down, place two belts around the abdomen with transducers positioned over the fetal heartbeat and over the uterus for contractions.
○ Connect the belts to an external fetal monitor.
○ Record the fetal heart rate and contractions on the monitor and on a paper printout.
○ If the patient isn't having contractions, ask her to stimulate one of her nipples for a brief time, until contractions begin.
○ In some cases, oxytocin is given I.V. to stimulate contractions.
○ Give a diluted solution of oxytocin at a rate of 1 mU/minute, increasing the oxytocin rate until the patient experiences three contractions within 10 minutes, each lasting longer than 45 seconds.
○ If no decelerations occur during three contractions, the patient may be discharged. Late decelerations during any of the contractions require notification of the physician and further tests.

Patient care

○ Monitor the patient closely.

Complications

None known

Interpretation

Normal results

○ Normal results occur when 3 contractions occur in a 10-minute period with no slowing (or late decelerations) of the fetal heart rate in response to contractions.

Abnormal results

○ Abnormal results occur when late decelerations of the fetal heart rate occur in response to the contractions. This may indicate a problem that requires further testing or delivery.

Interfering factors

None known

Corneal staining

Overview

- Allows a detailed view of the anterior part of the eye that isn't ordinarily visible during slit-lamp examination with fluorescein dye
- Special attachment during the slit-lamp examination enhances visibility

Purpose

- To detect the depth and pattern of injuries to the corneal surface of the eye
- To diagnose corneal injuries

Procedure

Preparation

- Describe the procedure to the patient. Explain that corneal staining evaluates the eye surface and is painless.
- Tell the patient who will perform the test and where it will take place.
- Ask the patient for a detailed history of the eye injury and the symptoms associated with the injury.
- Ask the patient to remove his glasses or contact lenses before the test.

Implementation

- The patient is seated in the examination chair.
- The patient's eye surface is stained with the fluorescein dye by touching the tip of the fluorescein strip to the lower conjunctival sac.
- The patient is asked to close his eye to help spread the dye over the corneal surface.
- The patient is asked to sit properly in the examination chair with his forehead placed against the bar apparatus.
- The patient is instructed to look straight ahead while his eyes are examined with the slit lamp.
- Defects are recorded while the eye is being examined with a bright light.
- The patient is informed that any blurring of vision will gradually disappear within 2 hours.

Patient care

- Monitor the patient for allergic reaction to the fluorescein dye.
- Because the dye used in this test causes blurred vision, make sure that the patient has a responsible person to take him home.

Complications

None known

Interpretation

Normal results

- The normal cornea is convex in shape and has a smooth, shiny appearance.
- There are no scratches or indentations.

Abnormal results

- Corneal scratches, abrasions, ulcerations, and keratitis

Interfering factors

- Patient's inability to remain still during the examination
- Allergy to the fluorescein dye

Corticotropin, plasma

Overview

- Measures the plasma levels of corticotropin by radioimmunoassay.
- Corticotropin levels vary diurnally, peaking between 6 and 8 a.m. and ebbing between 6 and 11 p.m.
- Emotional and physical stress (pain, surgery, insulin-induced hypoglycemia) stimulate secretion and can override the effects of plasma cortisol levels.
- May be ordered for a patient with signs of adrenal hypofunction (insufficiency) or hyperfunction (Cushing's syndrome).
- Corticotropin suppression or stimulation testing usually necessary to confirm the diagnosis.

Purpose

- To facilitate a differential diagnosis of primary and secondary adrenal hypofunction
- To aid a differential diagnosis of Cushing's syndrome

Procedure

Preparation

- Explain to the patient that this test helps determine if his hormonal secretion is normal.
- Advise the patient that he must fast and limit his physical activity for 10 to 12 hours before the test.
- Tell the patient that the test requires a blood sample. Explain who will perform the venipuncture and when.
- Explain that the patient may experience slight discomfort from the tourniquet and the needle puncture.
- Check the patient's history for medications that may affect the accuracy of the test results. Withhold these medications for 48 hours or longer before the test. If the patient must continue them, note this on the laboratory request.

Implementation

- For a patient with suspected adrenal hypofunction, perform the venipuncture for a baseline level between 6 a.m. and 8 a.m. (peak secretion).
- For a patient with suspected Cushing's syndrome, perform the venipuncture between 6 p.m. and 11 p.m. (low secretion).
- Collect the sample in a plastic EDTA tube (corticotropin may adhere to glass). The tube must be full because excess anticoagulant will affect results.
- Pack the sample in ice and send it to the laboratory immediately, where plasma must be rapidly separated from blood cells at 39.2° F (4° C). The collection technique may vary, depending on the laboratory.

Patient care

- Apply direct pressure to the venipuncture site until bleeding stops.
- Tell the patient he may resume his usual diet, activities, and medications stopped before the test.

Complications

- Hematoma at the venipuncture site

Interpretation

Normal results

- Mayo Medical Laboratories sets baseline values at less than 120 pg/ml (SI, < 26.4 pmol/L at 6 a.m. to 8 a.m.), but these may vary with each laboratory.

Abnormal results

- A higher-than-normal corticotropin level may indicate primary adrenal hypofunction (Addison's disease), in which the pituitary gland attempts to compensate for the unresponsiveness of the target organ by releasing excessive corticotropin.
- The underlying cause of adrenocortical hypofunction may be idiopathic atrophy of the adrenal cortex or partial destruction of the gland by granuloma, neoplasm, amyloidosis, or inflammatory necrosis.
- A low-normal corticotropin level suggests secondary adrenal hypofunction resulting from pituitary or hypothalamic dysfunction.
- The primary determinant may be panhypopituitarism, absence of corticotropin-releasing hormone in the hypothalamus, or chronic blunting of corticotropin levels by long-term corticosteroid therapy.
- In suspected Cushing's syndrome, an elevated corticotropin level suggests Cushing's disease, in which pituitary dysfunction (from adenoma) causes continuous hypersecretion of corticotropin and, consequently, continuously elevated cortisol levels without diurnal variations.
- Moderately elevated corticotropin levels suggest pituitary-dependent adrenal hyperplasia and nonadrenal tumors such as oat cell carcinoma of the lungs.
- A low-normal corticotropin level implies adrenal hyperfunction due to adrenocortical tumor or hyperplasia.

Interfering factors

- Failure to observe pretest restrictions
- Corticosteroids, including cortisone and its analogues (decrease)
- Drugs that increase endogenous cortisol secretion, such as estrogens, calcium gluconate, amphetamines, spironolactone, and ethanol (decrease)
- Lithium carbonate (decreases cortisol levels and may interfere with corticotropin secretion)
- Menstrual cycle and pregnancy
- Radioactive scan performed within 1 week before the test
- Acute stress (including hospitalization and surgery) and depression (increase)

C-peptide

Overview

○ Biologically inactive chain formed during the proteolytic conversion of proinsulin to insulin in the pancreatic beta cells
○ As insulin enters the bloodstream, the C-peptide chain splits off from the hormone

Purpose

○ To determine the cause of hypoglycemia
○ To indirectly measure insulin secretion in the presence of circulating insulin antibodies
○ To detect residual tissue after total pancreatectomy for carcinoma
○ To determine beta-cell function in the patient with diabetes mellitus

Procedure

Preparation

○ Explain to the patient that this test helps to evaluate pancreatic function and to determine the cause of hypoglycemia.
○ Instruct the patient to fast for 8 to 12 hours before testing; he need not restrict water.
○ Tell the patient that the test requires a blood sample.
○ Explain to the patient that he may experience slight discomfort from the tourniquet and the needle puncture.
○ If the patient is to receive radioisotope testing, it should take place after blood is drawn for C-peptide levels.
○ Blood glucose levels are usually drawn at the same time as C-peptide levels.
○ If the patient receives a C-peptide stimulation test, give I.V. glucagon after a baseline blood sample is drawn.
○ Withhold medications that may interfere with test results. If the patient must continue them, note this on the laboratory request.

Implementation

○ Perform a venipuncture and collect a 1-ml sample in a chilled clot-activator tube. The blood is separated and frozen to be tested later.
○ Collect a sample for testing glucose level in a tube with sodium fluoride and potassium oxalate, if ordered.
○ Pack the sample in ice and send it immediately, along with the glucose sample, to the laboratory.
○ Handle the samples gently to prevent hemolysis.

Patient care

○ Apply direct pressure to the venipuncture site until bleeding stops.
○ Instruct the patient that he may resume his usual activities, diet, and medications discontinued before the test.

Complications

○ Hematoma at the venipuncture site

Interpretation

Normal results

○ Serum C-peptide levels generally parallel those of insulin.
○ Normal fasting values range between 0.78 and 1.89 nanograms/ml (SI, 0.26 to 0.63 mmol/L).
○ An insulin: C-peptide ratio may be performed to differentiate insulinoma from factitious hypoglycemia.
○ A ratio of 1.0 or less indicates increased, endogenous insulin secretion; a ratio of 1.0 or more indicates exogenous insulin.

Abnormal results

○ Elevated levels may indicate endogenous hyperinsulinism (insulinemia), oral hypoglycemic drug ingestion, pancreas or B-cell transplantation, renal failure, or type 2 diabetes mellitus.
○ Decreased levels may indicate factitious hypoglycemia (surreptitious insulin administration), radical pancreatectomy, or type 1 diabetes.

Interfering factors

○ Failure to observe pretest restrictions
○ Hemolysis from rough handling of the sample
○ Failure to pack the sample in ice and send it to the laboratory

Creatine kinase and isoforms

Overview

○ Fractionation and measurement of three distinct creatine kinase (CK) isoenzymes — CK-BB, CK-MB, and CK-MM — have replaced total CK levels to accurately localize the site of increased tissue destruction
○ CK-BB most commonly found in brain tissue.
○ CK-MM and CK-MB found primarily in skeletal and heart muscle
○ Subunits of CK-MB and CK-MM, called *isoforms* or *isoenzymes*, can be assayed to increase the sensitivity of the test

Purpose

○ To detect and diagnose acute myocardial infarction (MI)
○ To evaluate possible causes of chest pain and to monitor the severity of myocardial ischemia
○ To detect early dermatomyositis and musculoskeletal disorders that aren't neurogenic in origin

Procedure

Preparation

○ Explain to the patient that he may have slight discomfort from the tourniquet and needle puncture.
○ If the patient is to receive a test for musculoskeletal disorders, advise him to avoid exercising for 24 hours before the test.
○ Notify the laboratory and physician of drugs the patient is taking that may affect test results; it may be necessary to restrict them.

Implementation

○ Perform a venipuncture and collect the sample in a 4-ml tube without additives.
○ Draw the sample before giving I.M. injections or 1 hour after giving them because muscle trauma increases the total CK level.
○ Note on the laboratory request the time the sample was drawn.
○ Handle the sample gently to prevent hemolysis.
○ Send the sample to the laboratory immediately because CK activity diminishes significantly after 2 hours at room temperature.

Patient care

○ Apply direct pressure to the venipuncture site until bleeding stops.
○ Instruct the patient that he may resume exercise and medications discontinued before the test.

Complications

○ Hematoma at the venipuncture site

Interpretation

Normal results

○ Total CK values determined by ultraviolet or kinetic measurement range from 55 to 170 units/L (SI, 0.94 to 2.89 µkat/L) for men and from 30 to 135 units/L (SI, 0.51 to 2.3 µkat/L) for women.
○ CK levels may be significantly higher in muscular people.
○ Infants up to age 1 have levels two to four times higher than adult levels, possibly reflecting birth trauma and striated muscle development.
○ Normal ranges for isoenzyme levels: CK-BB, undetectable; CK-MB, < 5% (SI, < 0.05); CK-MM, 90% to 100% (SI, 0.9 to 1.0).

Abnormal results

○ Detectable CK-BB isoenzyme may suggest without confirming brain tissue injury, widespread malignant tumors, severe shock, or renal failure.
○ CK-MB levels greater than 5% of the total CK level indicate an MI, especially if the lactate dehydrogenase (LD) isoenzyme ratio is more than 1 (flipped LD).
○ In acute MI and after cardiac surgery, CK-MB begins to increase within 2 to 4 hours, peaks within 12 to 24 hours, and usually returns to normal within 24 to 48 hours; persistent elevations and increasing levels indicate ongoing myocardial damage. Total CK follows similar pattern increases slightly later.
○ Serious skeletal muscle injury that occurs in certain muscular dystrophies, polymyositis, and severe myoglobinuria may produce a mild CK-MB increase because a small amount of this isoenzyme is present in some skeletal muscles.
○ Increasing CK-MM values follow skeletal muscle damage from trauma, such as surgery and I.M. injections, and from diseases, such as dermatomyositis and muscular dystrophy
○ Moderately increasing CK-MM levels develop in a patient with hypothyroidism; sharp increases occur with muscle activity caused by agitation such as during an acute psychotic episode.
○ Total CK levels may increase in patients with severe hypokalemia, carbon monoxide poisoning, malignant hyperthermia, alcoholic cardiomyopathy, after seizures, and in patients who have suffered pulmonary or cerebral infarctions.

Interfering factors

○ Hemolysis from rough handling of the sample
○ Failure to send the sample to the laboratory immediately or to refrigerate the serum if testing won't occur for more than 2 hours
○ Failure to draw the samples at the scheduled time
○ Halothane and succinylcholine, alcohol, lithium, large doses of aminocaproic acid, I.M. injections, cardioversion, invasive diagnostic procedures, recent vigorous exercise or muscle massage, severe coughing, and trauma (increase in total CK)

Creatinine, serum

Overview

- Provides a more sensitive measure of renal damage than blood urea nitrogen levels
- Nonprotein end product of creatine metabolism that appears in serum in amounts proportional to the body's muscle mass

Purpose

- To assess glomerular filtration
- To screen for renal damage

Procedure

Preparation

- Explain to the patient that the serum creatinine test evaluates kidney function.
- Tell the patient that the test requires a blood sample. Explain who will perform the venipuncture and when.
- Explain to the patient that he may experience slight discomfort from the tourniquet and needle puncture.
- Instruct the patient that he need not restrict food and fluids.
- Notify the laboratory and physician of drugs the patient is taking that may affect test results; it may be necessary to restrict them.

Implementation

- Perform a venipuncture and collect the sample in a 3- or 4-ml clot-activator tube.
- Handle the sample gently to prevent hemolysis.
- Send the sample to the laboratory immediately.

Patient care

- Apply direct pressure to the venipuncture site until bleeding stops.
- Inform the patient that he may resume his usual medications discontinued before the test.

Complications

- Hematoma at the venipuncture site

Interpretation

Normal results

- In men, 0.8 to 1.2 mg/dl (SI, 62 to 115 µmol/L)
- In women, 0.6 to 0.9 mg/dl (SI, 53 to 97 µmol/L)

Abnormal results

- Elevated levels generally indicate renal disease that has seriously damaged 50% or more of the nephrons.
- Elevated levels may also indicate gigantism and acromegaly.

Interfering factors

- Ascorbic acid, barbiturates, and diuretics (possible increase)
- Exceptionally large muscle mass, such as that found in athletes (possible increase despite normal renal function)
- Hemolysis from rough handling of the sample
- Phenolsulfonphthalein (given within the previous 24 hours can elevate creatinine levels if the test is based on the Jaffé reaction)

Creatinine clearance

Overview

- Excellent diagnostic indicator of renal function, determines how efficiently the kidneys are clearing creatinine from the blood
- Rate of clearance is expressed in terms of the volume of blood (in milliliters) that can be cleared of creatinine in 1 minute
- Creatinine levels become abnormal when more than 50% of the nephrons have been damaged

Purpose

- To assess renal function (primarily glomerular filtration)
- To monitor progression of renal insufficiency

Procedure

Preparation

- Explain to the patient that the test assesses kidney function.
- Inform the patient that he may need to avoid meat, poultry, fish, tea, or coffee for 6 hours before the test.
- Advise the patient to avoid strenuous physical exercise during the collection period.
- Tell the patient that the test requires a timed urine specimen and at least one blood sample.
- Tell the patient how the urine specimen will be collected. Also inform him who will perform the venipuncture and when. Tell him that he may feel some discomfort from the needle puncture.
- Explain that more than one venipuncture may be necessary.
- Notify the laboratory and physician of drugs the patient is taking that may affect test results; it may be necessary to restrict them.
- Refrigerate the urine specimen or keep it on ice during the collection period.
- Send the specimen to the laboratory as soon as the collection is complete.

Implementation

- Collect a timed urine specimen at 2, 6, 12, or 24 hours in a bottle containing a preservative to prevent creatinine degradation.
- Perform a venipuncture anytime during the collection period and collect the sample in a 7-ml tube without additives.

Patient care

- Apply direct pressure to the venipuncture site until bleeding stops.
- Instruct the patient that he may resume his usual activities, diet, and medications.

Complications

- Hematoma at the venipuncture site

Interpretation

Normal results

- Varies with age: in males, it ranges from 94 to 140 ml/minute/1.73 m² (SI, 0.91 to 1.35 ml/s/m²); in females, 72 to 110 ml/minute/1.73 m² (SI, 0.69 to 1.06 ml/s/m²)

Abnormal results

- Low creatinine clearance may result from reduced renal blood flow (associated with shock or renal artery obstruction), acute tubular necrosis, acute or chronic glomerulonephritis, advanced bilateral chronic pyelonephritis, advanced bilateral renal lesions (which may occur in polycystic kidney disease, renal tuberculosis, and cancer), nephrosclerosis, heart failure, or severe dehydration.
- High creatinine clearance can suggest poor hydration.

Interfering factors

- Failure to observe restrictions, to collect all urine during the test period, to properly store the specimen, or to send the sample to the laboratory immediately after the collection is completed
- Amphotericin B, thiazide diuretics, furosemide, and aminoglycosides (possible decrease)
- High-protein diet or strenuous exercise (increase)

Creatinine, urine

Overview

- Measures urine levels of creatinine, the chief metabolite of creatine.
- Produced in amounts proportional to total body muscle mass, creatinine is removed from the plasma primarily by glomerular filtration and is excreted in the urine.
- Because the body doesn't recycle it, creatinine has a relatively high, constant clearance rate, making it an efficient indicator of renal function.
- The creatinine clearance test, which measures urine and plasma creatinine clearance, is a more precise index than this test.
- A standard method for determining urine creatinine levels is based on Jaffé's reaction, in which creatinine treated with an alkaline picrate solution yields a bright orange-red complex.

Purpose

- To help assess glomerular filtration
- To check the accuracy of 24-hour urine collection, based on the relatively constant levels of creatinine excretion

Procedure

Preparation

- Explain to the patient that the urine creatinine test helps evaluate kidney function.
- Inform the patient that he need not restrict fluids, but that he shouldn't eat an excessive amount of meat before the test.
- Advise the patient that he should avoid strenuous physical exercise during the collection period.
- Tell the patient that the test usually requires urine collection over a 24-hour period, and teach him the proper collection technique.
- Notify the laboratory and physician of drugs the patient is taking that may affect test results; it may be necessary to restrict them.

Implementation

- Collect the patient's urine during a 24-hour period, discarding the first specimen and retaining the last. Use a specimen bottle that contains a preservative to prevent creatinine degradation.
- Refrigerate the specimen or keep it on ice during the collection period.
- Send the specimen to the laboratory immediately after the collection is complete.

Patient care

- Instruct the patient that he may resume his usual activities, diet, and medications.

Complications

None known

Interpretation

Normal results

- In males, 14 to 26 mg/kg body weight/24 hours (SI, 124 to 230 µmol/kg body weight/d)
- In females, 11 to 20 mg/kg body weight/24 hours (SI, 97 to 177 µmol/kg body weight/d)

Abnormal results

- Decreased urine creatinine levels may result from impaired renal perfusion (associated with shock, for example) or from renal disease due to urinary tract obstruction.
- Chronic bilateral pyelonephritis, acute or chronic glomerulonephritis, and polycystic kidney disease may also depress creatinine levels.
- Increased levels generally have little diagnostic significance.

Interfering factors

- Failure to observe restrictions, to collect all urine during the test period, to properly store the specimen, or to send the specimen to the laboratory immediately after the collection is complete
- Corticosteroids, gentamicin, tetracyclines, diuretics, and amphotericin B (possible decrease)

Crossmatching

Overview

○ Also known as *compatibility testing*; establishes compatibility or incompatibility of a donor's and a recipient's blood.
○ Best antibody detection test available for avoiding lethal transfusion reactions.
○ After the donor's and the recipient's ABO and Rh-factor type are determined, major crossmatching determines compatibility between the donor's red blood cells (RBCs) and the recipient's serum.
○ Minor crossmatching determines compatibility between the donor's serum and the recipient's RBCs. (Because all blood donors routinely receive the antibody-screening test, minor crossmatching is commonly omitted.)
○ Because a complete crossmatch may take from 45 minutes to 2 hours, an incomplete (10-minute) crossmatch may be performed in an emergency such as severe blood loss due to trauma.
○ In an emergency, transfusion can begin with limited amounts of group O packed RBCs while crossmatching is completed.
○ Incomplete typing and crossmatching increase the risk of complications.
○ After crossmatching, compatible units of blood are labeled and a compatibility record is completed.

Purpose
○ To serve as the final check for compatibility between a donor's and a recipient's blood

Procedure

Preparation
○ Explain to the patient that this test ensures that the blood he receives matches his own to prevent a transfusion reaction.
○ Inform the patient that he need not restrict food and fluids.
○ Tell the patient that the test requires a blood sample. Explain who will perform the venipuncture and when.
○ Explain to the patient that he may experience slight discomfort from the tourniquet and needle puncture.
○ Check the patient's history for recent administration of blood, dextran, or I.V. contrast media.
○ If more than 72 hours have elapsed since an earlier transfusion, previously crossmatched donor blood must be crossmatched again with a new recipient serum sample to detect newly acquired incompatibilities.
○ If the patient is scheduled for surgery and has received blood during the past three months, be aware that his blood needs to be crossmatched again if his surgery is rescheduled to detect recently acquired incompatibilities.

Implementation
○ Perform a venipuncture and collect the sample in a 10-ml tube without additives or EDTA. ABO typing, Rh typing, and crossmatching all occur together.
○ Handle the sample gently to prevent hemolysis, which can mask hemolysis of the donor's RBCs.
○ Label the sample with the patient's name, the hospital or blood bank number, the date, and the phlebotomist's initials.
○ Indicate on the laboratory request the amount and type of blood component needed.
○ Send the sample to the laboratory immediately.

Patient care
○ Apply direct pressure to the venipuncture site until bleeding stops.

Complications
○ Hematoma at the venipuncture site

Interpretation

Normal results
○ Absence of agglutination indicates compatibility between the donor's and the recipient's blood, which means that the transfusion of donor blood can proceed. Note that this doesn't guarantee a safe transfusion.

Abnormal results
○ A positive crossmatch indicates incompatibility between the donor's blood and the recipient's blood, which means that the donor's blood can't be transfused to the recipient.
○ The sign of a positive crossmatch is agglutination, or clumping, when the donor's RBCs and the recipient's serum are correctly mixed and incubated. Agglutination indicates an undesirable antigen-antibody reaction.
○ The donor's blood must be withheld and the crossmatch continued to determine the cause of the incompatibility and identify the antibody.

Interfering factors
○ Recent administration of dextran or I.V. contrast media (causing cellular aggregation resembling antibody-mediated agglutination)
○ Previous blood transfusion (possibility of new antibodies to donor blood)
○ Hemolysis from rough handling of the sample
○ Delay of testing for more than 72 hours after sample collection

Cryoglobulins

Overview

○ The presence of cryoglobulins in the blood (cryo-globulinemia) usually indicates immunologic disease but can also occur without known immunopathology.
○ If patients with cryoglobulinemia are subjected to cold, they may experience Raynaud-like symptoms (pain, cyanosis, and cold fingers and toes), which generally result from cryoglobulin precipitation in cooler parts of the body.
○ Involves refrigerating a serum sample at 33.8° F (1° C) for 24 hours and observing it for formation of a heat-reversible precipitate.
○ Such a precipitate requires further study by immuno-electrophoresis or double diffusion to identify cryo-globulin components.

Purpose

○ To detect cryoglobulinemia in the patient with Raynaud-like vascular symptoms

Procedure

Preparation

○ Explain to the patient that this test detects antibodies in blood that may cause sensitivity to low temperatures.
○ Instruct the patient to fast for 4 to 6 hours before the test.
○ Tell the patient that the test requires a blood sample.
○ Explain to the patient that he may experience slight discomfort from the tourniquet and needle puncture.

Implementation

○ Perform a venipuncture and collect the sample in a prewarmed 10-ml tube without additives.
○ Warm the syringe and collection tube to 98.6° F (37° C) before venipuncture and keep the tube at that temperature to prevent cryoglobulin loss.
○ Send the sample to the laboratory immediately.

Patient care

○ Instruct the patient that he may resume his usual diet.
○ Tell the patient to avoid cold temperatures or contact with cold objects if the test is positive for cryoglobu-lins.
○ Apply direct pressure to the venipuncture site until bleeding stops.

Complications

○ Hematoma at the venipuncture site
○ Intravascular coagulation, with such signs as de-creased color and temperature in fingers and toes and increased pain

Interpretation

Normal results

○ Normally, serum is negative for cryoglobulins.
○ Positive results are reported as a percentage based on the amount of sample cryoprecipitation.

Abnormal results

○ The presence of cryoglobulins in the blood confirms cryoglobulinemia. This finding doesn't always indi-cate the presence of clinical disease.

Interfering factors

○ Failure to adhere to dietary restrictions
○ Failure to keep the sample at 98.6° F before centrifu-gation (possible loss of cryoglobulins)
○ Reading the sample before the 72-hour precipitation period ends (possible incorrect analysis of results because some cryoglobulins take several days to pre-cipitate)

Culture for chlamydia

Overview

- Identification of this parasite requires cultivation in the laboratory.
- After incubation, *Chlamydia*-infected cells can be detected by fluorescein isothiocyanate-conjugated monoclonal antibodies or by iodine stain.
- Detection in cell cultures of *C. psittaci* and *C. pneumoniae* requires specific technical manipulations and reagents; deoxyribonucleic acid detection may also be performed in women who may be susceptible to the infections, whether they have symptoms or not.
- Is the detection method of choice, but rapid noncultural (antigen detection) procedures are also available.

Purpose

- To confirm infections caused by *C. trachomatis*

Procedure

Preparation

- Explain the purpose of the test to the patient.
- Describe the procedure for collecting a specimen for culture.
- If the specimen will be collected from the patient's genital tract, instruct him not to urinate for 3 to 4 hours before the specimen is taken.
- Tell a female patient not to douche for 24 hours before the test.
- Tell a male patient that he may experience some burning and pressure during the collection procedure but that the discomfort will subside after a few minutes.

Implementation

- Obtain a specimen of the epithelial cells from the infected site. In adults, these sites may include the eye, urethra (rather than from the purulent exudate that may be present), endocervix, and rectum.
- Obtain a urethral specimen by inserting a cotton-tipped applicator ¾" to 2" (2 to 5 cm) into the urethra.
- To collect a specimen from the endocervix, use a microbiologic transport swab or Cytobrush.
- Extract the specimen into an appropriate transport medium.
- Extract specimens from the throat, eye, and nasopharynx, and aspirates from infants into an appropriate transport medium. Send specimens to the laboratory at 39.2° F (4° C).
- If the anticipated time between specimen collection and inoculation into cell culture is more than 24 hours, freeze the transport medium and send it to the laboratory with dry ice.

- In the patient suspected of being sexually abused, be sure to process the specimen by culture rather than by antigen detection methods.
- Advise the patient to avoid all sexual contact until after the test results are available.
- If the culture confirms infection, provide counseling for the patient regarding treatment of sexual partners.
- Assist the male patient into a supine position to prevent him from falling if vasovagal syncope occurs when the cotton swab or wire loop enters the urethra. Observe the patient for profound hypotension, bradycardia, pallor, and sweating.
- Wear gloves when performing the procedures and handling the specimens.
- Collect a urethral specimen at least 1 hour after the patient has voided to prevent loss of urethral secretions.
- After collecting the specimens, carefully dispose of gloves, swabs, and speculum to prevent staff exposure.

Patient care

- Answer the patient's questions about testing.
- Monitor the patient for adverse effects.

Complications

- Hypotension
- Bradycardia
- Pallor
- Diaphoresis

Interpretation

Normal results

- No *C. trachomatis* in the culture

Abnormal results

- A positive culture confirms *C. trachomatis* infection.

Interfering factors

- Using an antimicrobial drug within a few days before specimen collection (possible inability to recover *C. trachomatis*)
- In males, voiding within 1 hour of specimen collection
- In females, douching within 24 hours of specimen collection (fewer organisms available for culture)
- Failure to use the proper collection technique
- Contamination of the specimen due to fecal material in a rectal culture

Culture for gonorrhea

Overview

- Stained smear of genital exudate can confirm gonorrhea in 90% of men with characteristic symptoms, but a culture is usually necessary in women, especially those who are asymptomatic
- Possible culture sites include the urethra (usual site in men), endocervix (usual site in women), anal canal, and oropharynx

Purpose

- To confirm gonorrhea

Procedure

Preparation

- Describe procedure and explain tests to patient.
- Instruct woman not to douche for 24 hours pre-test.
- Tell a man not to void during the hour preceding the test. Warn him that men sometimes experience nausea, sweating, weakness, and fainting from stress or discomfort when the cotton swab or wire loop enters the urethra.

Implementation

- *Endocervical culture:* Place the patient in the lithotomy position, drape her appropriately.
  - To obtain a culture, use gloved hands and insert a vaginal speculum that has been lubricated only with warm water. Clean mucus from the cervix, using cotton balls in a ring forceps.
  - Next, insert a dry, sterile cotton swab into the endocervical canal and rotate it from side to side. Leave the swab in place for several seconds for optimum absorption of organisms.
  - In cases of deep pelvic inflammatory disease, it may be necessary to take cultures of the endometrium or aspirations by laparoscopy or culdoscopy.
- *Urethral culture:* Place the patient in a supine position and drape him appropriately.
  - Clean the urethral meatus with sterile gauze or a cotton swab and then insert a thin urogenital alginate swab or a wire bacteriologic loop ⅜" to ¾" (1 to 2 cm) into the urethra, and rotate the swab or loop from side to side. Leave it in place for several seconds for optimum absorption of organisms.
- *Rectal culture:* After obtaining an endocervical or a urethral specimen insert a sterile cotton swab into the anal canal about 1" (2.5 cm), move the swab from side to side, and leave it in place for several seconds for optimum absorption.
  - If the rectal swab is contaminated with stool, discard it and repeat the procedure with a clean swab.
- *Throat culture:* Position the patient with his head tilted back.
  - Check his throat for inflamed areas using a tongue blade. Rub a sterile swab from side to side over the tonsillar areas, including inflamed or purulent sites.
- *After specimen collection:* Roll the swab in a Z pattern in a plate containing modified Thayer-Martin medium. Then cross-streak the medium with a sterile wire loop or the tip of the swab and cover the plate.
  - Label the specimen with the appropriate information.
  - Make direct smears of obtained material immediately to prepare the Gram stain. Quickly inoculate remaining material into selective culture media or into a transport system.
  - Use a Culturette transport tube or a swab transport medium containing charcoal. Charcoal helps neutralize toxic materials in the specimen.
  - If laboratory facilities aren't readily available, uncap the Transgrow medium specimen bottle just before inserting the swab of test material into the bottle. Keep the bottle upright to minimize loss of carbon dioxide. With the swab, absorb the excess moisture within the bottle and then roll the swab across the Transgrow medium. Discard the swab. Place the lid on the bottle and label it appropriately.

Patient care

- Advise the patient to avoid all sexual contact until test results are available.
- Explain that treatment usually begins after confirming a positive culture, except in a person who has symptoms of gonorrhea or who has had intercourse with someone known to have gonorrhea.
- Advise the patient that a repeat culture is necessary 1 week after completion of treatment to evaluate the effectiveness of therapy.
- Inform the patient that positive culture findings must be reported to the local health department.

Complications

- Vasovagal response in men

Interpretation

Normal results

- No *Neisseria gonorrhoeae* in the culture

Abnormal results

- A positive culture confirms gonorrhea.

Interfering factors

- Pretest antimicrobial therapy
- Contamination from fecal material in a rectal culture
- Failure to use the proper collection technique
- In men, voiding within 1 hour of specimen collection; in women, douching within 24 hours of specimen collection (fewer organisms available for culture)

Culture for herpes simplex virus

Overview

- The herpes virus group includes Epstein-Barr virus, cytomegalovirus (CMV), varicella-zoster virus (VZV), human herpesvirus-6, herpesvirus-7, herpesvirus-8, and the two closely related serotypes of herpes simplex virus (HSV) — types 1 and 2.
- Only CMV, VZV, and HSV replicate in the standard cell cultures of diagnostic laboratories.
- About 50% of HSV strains are detectable by characteristic cytopathic effects within 24 hours after the laboratory receives the specimen; 5 to 7 days are required to detect the remaining HSV strains. (Alternatively, early HSV antigens can be detected by monoclonal antibodies in shell vial cell cultures within 16 hours after receipt of the specimen with the same sensitivity and specificity as standard tube cell cultures.)

Purpose

- To confirm diagnosis of HSV infection by culturing the virus from specimens

Procedure

Preparation

- Explain to the patient that this test detects HSV infection.
- Explain to the patient that specimens will be collected from suspected lesions during the prodromal and acute stages of clinical infection.

Implementation

- Collect a specimen for culture in the appropriate collection device.
- Obtain vesicle fluid with a 27G needle or a tuberculin syringe. If the fluid is scant, scrape the base of the ulcer with a swab to remove cells.
- For the throat, skin, eye, or genital area, use a microbiologic transport swab.
- For body fluids or other respiratory specimens (washings, lavage), use a sterile screw-capped jar.
- Transport the specimen to the laboratory as soon as possible after collection. If the anticipated time between collection and inoculation of cell cultures is more than 3 hours, the specimen should be stored and transported at 39.2° F (4° C).
- Wear gloves when obtaining and handling all specimens.
- Don't allow the specimen to dry up.

Patient care

- Answer the patient's questions about testing procedures.

Complications

- None known

Interpretation

Normal results

- HSV is seldom recovered from an immunocompetent patient who shows no overt signs of the disease.

Abnormal results

- Detectable HSV in specimens taken from dermal lesions, the eye, or cerebrospinal fluid is highly significant.
- Specimens from the upper respiratory tract may be associated with intermittent shedding of the virus, particularly in an immunocompromised patient.
- Like other herpesviruses, HSV can be shed from the immunocompromised patient intermittently in the absence of apparent disease.
- For epidemiologic purposes, HSV detected by characteristic cytopathic effects in standard tube cell cultures is confirmed and identified as type 1 or 2.

Interfering factors

- Administration of antiviral drugs before specimen collection

Cyclic adenosine monophosphate

Overview

○ The nucleotide cyclic adenosine monophosphate (cAMP) influences the protein synthesis rate within cells.
○ Measurement of the urinary excretion of cAMP after an I.V. infusion of a standard dose of parathyroid hormone (PTH) can show renal tubular resistance in a patient with hypoparathyroid symptoms and high levels of PTH.
○ Such findings suggest type I pseudohypoparathyroidism, a rare inherited disorder.
○ Urinary cAMP levels respond normally with type II pseudohypoparathyroidism because the defect is beyond the level of cAMP generation.

Purpose

○ To aid in the differential diagnosis of hypoparathyroidism and pseudohypoparathyroidism

Procedure

Preparation

○ Explain to the patient that this test evaluates parathyroid function.
○ Tell the patient that the test requires a 15-minute I.V. infusion of PTH and a 3- to 4-hour urine specimen collection.
○ Perform a skin test to detect an allergy to PTH; keep epinephrine or a histamine-1 receptor antagonist, such as diphenhydramine or glucocorticoids (methylprednisolone), readily available in case of an adverse reaction.
○ Just before performing the procedure, instruct the patient not to touch the I.V. line or exert pressure on the arm receiving the infusion.
○ Tell the patient that he may experience discomfort from the needle puncture. Ask him to notify you if he feels severe burning or if the site becomes inflamed or swollen.
○ Tell the patient to avoid contaminating the urine specimen with toilet tissue or stool.

Implementation

○ Instruct the patient to empty his bladder.
○ If the patient has an indwelling urinary catheter in place, replace the collection apparatus with an unused one.
○ Send this specimen to the laboratory if ordered; otherwise, discard it.
○ Prepare the PTH for infusion, as directed, using sterile water for dilution.

○ Start the infusion with dextrose 5% in water, and infuse the PTH over 15 minutes. Record the start of the infusion as time zero.
○ Collect a urine specimen 3 to 4 hours after the infusion.
○ Stop the I.V. infusion.
○ Send the specimen to the laboratory immediately after the collection is completed; if transport is delayed, refrigerate the specimen.
○ Keep the collection bag on ice if the patient has a catheter in place.

Patient care

○ Observe the patient for symptoms of hypercalcemia, including lethargy, anorexia, nausea, vomiting, vertigo, and abdominal cramps.

Complications

○ Hematoma or irritation at the venipuncture site
○ Contraindicated in patients with a positive PTH test result and in those with high calcium levels
○ Use cautiously in patients receiving a cardiac glycoside and in those with sarcoidosis or renal or cardiac disease

Interpretation

Normal results

○ Levels of cAMP are normally 0.3 to 3.6 mg/day (SI, 100 to 723 nmol/d) or 0.29 to 2.1 mg/g creatinine (SI, 100 to 723 nmol/d creatinine).

Abnormal results

○ Failure to respond to PTH, indicated by normal urinary excretion of cAMP, suggests type I pseudohypoparathyroidism.

Interfering factors

○ Contamination or improper storage of the specimen or failure to acidify the urine with hydrochloric acid

Cystometry

Overview

○ Measures pressure and volume of fluid in the bladder during filling, storing, and voiding
○ Assesses neuromuscular function of the bladder

Purpose

○ To evaluate detrusor muscle function and tonicity
○ To determine the cause of bladder dysfunction
○ To measure bladder reaction to thermal stimulation
○ To detect the cause of involuntary bladder contractions and incontinence

Procedure

Preparation

○ Note and report allergies.
○ Check the medication history for medications that may affect test results such as antihistamines.
○ Ask the patient to urinate before the test.
○ Assess for signs and symptoms of urinary tract infection.
○ Tell the patient he may feel a strong urge to urinate during the test.
○ Warn the patient that the procedure may cause embarrassment and be uncomfortable.
○ Explain that the test takes about 40 minutes.

Implementation

○ The patient is assisted into the supine position on an examination table.
○ A catheter is passed into the bladder to measure residual urine.
○ To test the response to thermal sensation, 30 ml of room-temperature normal saline solution or sterile water is instilled into the bladder.
○ An equal volume of warm fluid (110° to 115° F [43.3° to 46.1° C]) is then instilled.
○ The patient is asked to report the need to urinate, nausea, or a flushed feeling.
○ Fluid is drained from the bladder and the catheter is connected to the cystometer.
○ Normal saline solution, sterile water, or gas (usually carbon dioxide) is slowly introduced into the bladder.
○ The patient is asked to indicate when he feels an urge to void.
○ Related pressures and volumes are automatically plotted on a graph.
○ When the bladder reaches its full capacity, the patient is asked to urinate.
○ Maximal intravesical voiding pressure is recorded.
○ The bladder is drained.
○ If abnormal bladder function is the result of muscle incompetence or disrupted innervation, anticholinergic or cholinergic medication may be injected and the study repeated in 20 to 30 minutes.

Patient care

○ Give a sitz bath or warm tub bath for discomfort.
○ Encourage oral fluid intake (unless contraindicated) to relieve dysuria.
○ Notify the physician if hematuria persists after the third voiding.
○ Give the patient a prescribed antibiotic.
○ Monitor the patient's vital signs, intake and output, and signs of infection.

Complications

○ Infection, bleeding

Interpretation

Normal results

○ Ability to start and stop micturition, no residual urine
○ Positive vesical sensation
○ First urge to void at 150 to 200 ml
○ Bladder capacity: 400 to 500 ml
○ No bladder contractions, low intravesical pressure
○ Positive bulbocavernosus reflex, positive saddle sensation test
○ Positive ice water test, positive anal reflex
○ Positive heat sensation and pain

Abnormal results

○ Inability to stop micturition, early first urge to void, decreased bladder capacity, bladder contractions, increased intravesical pressure, and positive bethanechol sensitivity test suggest inhibited neurogenic bladder.
○ Inability to start and stop micturition, residual urine, absent vesical sensation, absent first urge to void, decreased bladder capacity, bladder contractions, increased intravesical pressure, increased bulbocavernosus reflex, negative saddle sensation test, and absent heat sensation and pain suggest reflex neurogenic bladder.
○ Inability to start and stop micturition, residual urine, absent vesical sensation, increased bladder capacity, decreased intravesical pressure, absent bulbocavernosus reflex, negative saddle sensation test, negative ice water test, absent anal reflex and heat sensation, and pain, suggest autonomous neurogenic bladder.
○ Residual urine, absent vesical sensation, delayed first urge to void, increased bladder capacity, decreased intravesical pressure, negative ice water test, variable anal reflex, and absent heat sensation and pain suggest sensory paralytic bladder.
○ Inability to start and stop micturition, residual urine, negative ice water test, and variable anal reflex suggest motor paralytic bladder.

Interfering factors

○ Straining with urination
○ Drugs such as antihistamines
○ Inability to urinate supine
○ Test performed within 6 to 8 weeks after surgery for a spinal cord injury

Cystourethroscopy

Overview

- Allows visual examination of the bladder, urethra, ureter orifice, ureters, and prostate in males
- Combines two endoscopic techniques: Cystoscopy and urethroscopy
- Cystoscope examines the bladder
- Urethroscope, or panendoscope, examines bladder neck and urethra
- Cystoscope and urethroscope pass through a common sheath inserted into the urethra to obtain the desired view
- Usually preceded by kidney-ureter-bladder radiography, excretory urography, and the bladder tumor antigen urine test

Purpose

- To diagnose and evaluate urinary tract disorders by direct visualization of urinary structures
- To facilitate biopsy, lesion resection, removal of calculi, dilatation of a constricted urethra, and catheterization of the renal pelvis for pyelography

Procedure

Preparation

- Make sure the patient has signed a consent form.
- Note and report allergies.
- Give a sedative if ordered.
- Instruct the patient to urinate.
- Restriction of food and fluids is unnecessary unless general anesthesia will be used.
- If only local anesthesia is used, the patient may complain of a burning sensation when the instrument enters the urethra and an urgent need to urinate as the bladder fills with irrigating solution.
- The patient may experience some discomfort after the procedure, including a slight burning during urination. Explain that the test takes about 20 to 30 minutes.

Implementation

- General or regional anesthesia is given.
- The patient is assisted into the lithotomy position on a cystoscopic table.
- The genitalia are cleaned with an antiseptic solution and the patient is draped.
- The urethra is examined with a urethroscope.
- The urethroscope is removed and a cystoscope is inserted into the bladder.
- The bladder is filled with irrigating solution and the entire bladder surface wall and ureteral orifices are examined.
- The cystoscope is removed and the urethroscope reinserted.
- The bladder neck and various portions of the urethra, including the internal and external sphincters, are examined as the urethroscope is withdrawn.
- A urine specimen is taken from the bladder for culture and sensitivity testing.
- Residual urine volume is measured.
- Urine is taken for a cytologic examination if a tumor is suspected.
- If a tumor is found, it may be necessary to perform a biopsy.
- If a urethral stricture is present, urethral dilatation may be necessary before cystourethroscopy.

Patient care

- Give postoperative general anesthesia care.
- Encourage oral fluid intake and give I.V. fluids.
- Give the patient analgesics.
- Give the patient antibiotics.
- Report flank or abdominal pain, chills, fever, an elevated white blood cell count, or low urine output to the physician immediately.
- Notify the physician if the patient doesn't void within 8 hours after the test or if bright red blood persists after three voidings.
- Instruct the patient to abstain from alcohol for 48 hours.
- Apply heat to the lower abdomen to relieve pain and muscle spasm (if ordered).
- Give a warm sitz bath.
- Monitor the patient's vital signs, intake and output, and bleeding.
- Monitor the patient for hematuria and signs and symptoms of infection.
- Watch for bladder distention.

Complications

- Sepsis
- Infection
- Bleeding

Interpretation

Normal results

- Urethra, bladder, and ureteral orifices appear normal in size, shape, and position.
- Mucosal lining of the lower urinary tract appears smooth and shiny.
- No erythema, cysts, or other abnormalities.
- There are no obstructions, tumors, or calculi in the bladder.

Abnormal results

- Structural abnormalities suggest various disorders, including enlarged prostate gland in older men, urethral strictures, calculi, tumors, diverticula, ulcers and polyps.

Interfering factors

- Patient's inability to cooperate

Cytomegalovirus antibody screen

Overview

○ Antibodies to cytomegalovirus (CMV) are detectable with several methods, including passive hemagglutination, latex agglutination, enzyme immunoassay, and indirect immunofluorescence.
○ The complement fixation test is only 60% sensitive compared with other assays and shouldn't be used to screen for CMV antibodies.
○ Screening tests for CMV antibodies are qualitative; they detect the presence of an antibody at a single low dilution. (In quantitative methods, several dilutions of the serum sample are tested to indicate acute CMV infection.)

Purpose

○ To detect CMV infection in donors and recipients of organs and blood and in immunocompromised patients
○ To screen for CMV infection in infants who require blood transfusions or tissue transplants

Procedure

Preparation

○ Explain the purpose of the test to the patient or the parents of an infant, as appropriate.
○ Tell the patient that the test requires a blood sample. Explain who will perform the venipuncture and when.
○ Explain to the patient that he may experience slight discomfort from the tourniquet and needle puncture.

Implementation

○ Perform a venipuncture and collect the sample in a 5-ml tube designated by the laboratory.
○ Allow the blood to clot for at least 1 hour at room temperature.
○ Handle the sample gently to prevent hemolysis.
○ Transfer the serum to a sterile tube or vial and send it to the laboratory.
○ If transfer must be delayed, store the serum at 39.2° F (4° C) for 1 to 2 days or at −4° F (−20° C) for longer periods to avoid contamination.

Patient care

○ Apply direct pressure to the venipuncture site until bleeding stops.
○ Because the patient may have a compromised immune system, keep the venipuncture site clean and dry.

Complications

○ Hematoma at the venipuncture site

Interpretation

Normal results

○ The patient who has never been infected with CMV has no detectable antibodies to the virus.
○ Immunoglobulin (Ig) G and IgM are normally negative.

Abnormal results

○ A serum sample collected early during the acute phase or late in the convalescent stage may not contain detectable IgG or IgM antibodies to CMV. Therefore, a negative result doesn't preclude recent infection. More than a single sample is needed to ensure accurate results.
○ A serum sample that tests positive for antibodies at this single dilution indicates that the patient has been infected with CMV and that his white blood cells contain latent virus capable of being reactivated in an immunocompromised host.
○ An immunosupressed patient lacking CMV antibodies should receive blood products or organ transplants from a donor who is also seronegative.
○ A patient with CMV antibodies doesn't need seronegative blood products.

Interfering factors

○ Hemolysis from rough handling of the sample

D-dimer

Overview

○ An asymmetrical carbon compound fragment formed after thrombin converts fibrinogen to fibrin, factor XIIIa stabilizes it into a clot, and plasma acts on the cross-linked, or clotted, fibrin.
○ Specific for fibrinolysis because test confirms the presence of fibrin-split products.

Purpose

○ To diagnose disseminated intravascular coagulation (DIC)
○ To differentiate subarachnoid hemorrhage from a traumatic lumbar puncture in spinal fluid analysis

Procedure

Preparation

○ Obtain the patient's history of hematologic diseases, recent surgery, and the results of other tests.
○ Explain to the patient that the test determines whether blood is clotting normally.
○ Tell the patient that the test requires a blood sample. Explain who will perform the venipuncture and when.
○ Explain to the patient that he may feel slight discomfort from the tourniquet and needle puncture.

Implementation

○ Perform a venipuncture and collect the sample in a 4.5-ml tube with sodium citrate added.
○ For a spinal fluid analysis, the sample is collected during a lumbar puncture and placed in a plastic vial.
○ Completely fill the collection tube, invert it gently several times, and send it to the laboratory immediately.

Patient care

○ Apply pressure to the venipuncture site for 5 minutes or until bleeding stops.
○ For a patient with coagulation problems, you may need to apply additional pressure at the venipuncture site to control bleeding.

Complications

○ Hematoma at the venipuncture site

Interpretation

Normal results

○ Collection yields less than 250 µg/L (SI, < 1.37 nmol/L).

Abnormal results

○ A level greater than 250 µg/L (SI, > 1.37 nmol/L) may indicate DIC, pulmonary embolism, arterial or venous thrombosis, neoplastic disease, pregnancy (late and postpartum), surgery occurring up to 2 days before testing, subarachnoid hemorrhage (spinal fluid only), or secondary fibrinolysis.

Interfering factors

○ Failure to fill the collection tube completely or to send the sample to the laboratory immediately
○ Hemolysis from rough handling of the sample
○ High rheumatoid factor titers or increased CA-125 levels (possible false-positive)
○ Spinal fluid analysis in an infant under age 6 months (possible false-negative).

Delayed-type hypersensitivity skin tests

Overview

○ Skin testing for delayed-type hypersensitivity (DTH) is an important method for evaluating T-cell mediated immune response in a patient.
○ Positive reactions don't indicate protection against the antigen.
○ Accurate test response requires previous exposure to the antigen and an intact immune system.
○ Most commonly used recall antigen is *Mycobacterium tuberculosis* (purified protein derivative Mantoux test).
○ Other antigens used in the clinical setting include *Candida, Trichophyton*, and mumps (some antigens previously used for DTH testing, such as fungi and streptococci, are no longer available or recommended).
○ Assesses status of an individual's immune system in severe infection, cancer, pretransplantation, and malnutrition; antigens used for this testing must be antigens the patient has been exposed to previously.
○ Limited value in infants because of their immature immune system and lack of previous sensitization.
○ Involves applying antigenic material to the skin; helps confirm allergic contact sensitization and isolate the causative agent.

Purpose

○ To assess for exposure to or activation of certain diseases, most commonly tuberculosis (TB)
○ To assess the status of a patient's immune system during illness
○ To evaluate sensitivity to environmental antigens in the patient with persistent symptoms

Procedure

Preparation

○ Explain to the patient that a small amount of antigenic material will be injected superficially or applied to the skin.
○ Inform the patient that testing takes only a few minutes for each antigen. Reactions will be evaluated 48 to 72 hours later.
○ The test may be repeated in 2 to 3 weeks if the first result is negative. The first test "reminds" the body that it was previously exposed to the antigen, and a response is noted on retesting. This is common procedure for TB testing and is called the *two-step test.*
○ Ask the patient about sensitivity to the test antigens, whether he has had previous skin testing, and what the outcomes of that testing were.

○ Ask the patient if he has had TB or been exposed to it and if he has had bacille Calmette-Guérin vaccination.

Implementation

○ Inject each antigen being tested intradermally, using a separate tuberculin syringe, on the patient's forearm.
○ Inject the control allergy diluent on the other forearm.
○ Inspect the injection sites for reactivity after 48 to 72 hours.
○ Record induration and erythema in millimeters.
○ Confirm a negative test result at the first concentration of antigen by using a higher concentration.
○ If appropriate, store antigens in lyophilized (freeze-dried) form at 39.2° F (4° C) and protect from light. Reconstitute shortly before use and check expiration dates. If the patient may be hypersensitive to the antigens, apply them initially in low concentrations.
○ If the patient's forearms aren't disease-free (for example, if he has atopic dermatitis), use other sites such as the back.

Patient care

○ Watch closely for severe local reactions that may occur at the test site, such as pain, blistering, swelling, induration, itching, and ulceration. Scarring or hyperpigmentation may also result.
○ Observe for swelling and tenderness in lymph nodes at the elbow or axillary region. Check for tachycardia and fever, although these rarely occur. Symptoms typically appear in 15 to 30 minutes.
○ Tell the patient who experiences hypersensitivity that steroids will control the reaction; skin lesions may persist for 10 to 14 days.
○ Advise the patient to avoid scratching or otherwise disturbing the affected area.
○ If signs or symptoms of anaphylactic shock develop, give epinephrine and notify the physician immediately.

Complications

○ Anaphylactic shock

Interpretation

Normal results

○ The test result is positive (at least 5 mm of induration at the test site, appearing 48 hours after injection).

Abnormal results

○ Diminished DTH is demonstrated by a positive response to fewer than two of the test antigens, a persistent unresponsiveness to intradermal injection of higher-strength antigens, or a generalized diminished reaction (causing < 10 mm combined induration).
○ Diminished DTH can result from Hodgkin's disease; sarcoidosis; liver disease; congenital immunodeficiency disease, such as ataxia-telangiectasia, Di-

George's syndrome, and Wiskott-Aldrich syndrome; uremia; acute leukemia; viral diseases, such as influenza, infectious mononucleosis, measles, mumps, and rubella; fungal diseases, such as coccidioidomycosis and cryptococcosis; bacterial diseases, such as leprosy and TB; terminal cancer; and immunosuppressive or steroid therapy or viral vaccination.

Interfering factors

○ Use of antigens that have expired or that have been exposed to heat and light or to bacterial contamination
○ Poor injection technique
○ Inaccurate dilution of antigens or an error in reading or timing test results
○ A strong immediate reaction to the antigen at the injection site
○ Use of hormonal contraceptives

Dexamethasone suppression test

Overview

- Requires administration of dexamethasone, an oral steroid
- Suppresses the levels of circulating adrenal steroid hormones in healthy people but fails to suppress them in patients with Cushing's syndrome and some forms of clinical depression

Purpose

- To diagnose Cushing's syndrome
- To aid in the diagnosis of clinical depression

Procedure

Preparation

- Explain to the patient the purpose of the dexamethasone suppression test.
- Restrict food and fluids for 10 to 12 hours before the test.
- Inform the patient that the test requires two blood samples drawn after he receives dexamethasone. Explain who will perform the venipunctures and when.
- Explain to the patient that he may feel slight discomfort from the tourniquet and needle puncture.

Implementation

- On the first day, give the patient 1 mg of dexamethasone at 11 p.m.
- On the next day, collect blood samples at 4 p.m. and 11 p.m.

Patient care

- Apply pressure to venipuncture site.
- Observe the site for complications.

Complications

- Hematoma at the venipuncture site

Interpretation

Normal results

- Failure of dexamethasone suppression is indicated by a cortisol level of 5 g/dl (140 nmol/L) or greater.
- A normal test result doesn't rule out major depression.

Abnormal results

- If test result isn't normal, abnormal secretion of cortisol is likely (Cushing's syndrome).
- An abnormal test result strengthens a clinically based diagnosis of major depression.

Interfering factors

- Diabetes mellitus, pregnancy, and severe stress, such as trauma, severe weight loss, dehydration, and acute alcohol withdrawal (possible false-positive)
- Many drugs, including corticosteroids, hormonal contraceptives, lithium, methadone, aspirin, diuretics, morphine, and monoamine oxidase inhibitors (if possible, restrict use of these drugs for 24 to 48 hours before the test)
- Caffeine consumed after midnight the night before the test (possible false-positive)

Digital subtraction angiography, cerebral

Overview

- Sophisticated radiographic technique using video equipment and computer-assisted image enhancement to provide a high-contrast view of blood vessels without interfering images or shadows of bone and soft tissue
- Superior image quality and I.V., rather than intra-arterial, administration of contrast media
- Has been used to study peripheral and renal vascular disease but is most useful to evaluate cerebrovascular disorders

Purpose

- To show extracranial and intracranial cerebral blood flow
- To detect and evaluate cerebrovascular abnormalities
- To aid postoperative evaluation of cerebrovascular surgery

Procedure

Preparation

- Make sure the patient has signed an appropriate consent form.
- Check the patient's history for any allergies, including hypersensitivity to iodine, iodine-containing substances such as shellfish, and contrast media.
- Note previous hypersensitivity on the patient's medical record and tell the physician.
- Instruct the patient to fast for 4 hours before the test. Tell him that he need not restrict fluids.
- Stress the importance of lying still during the procedure; even swallowing can interfere with imaging. The patient will need to hold his breath for 10-second intervals at various times during the study.
- Warn the patient that he may experience warmth, headache, metallic taste, nausea, or vomiting after injection of the contrast medium.
- Explain to the patient that the test may take 1 to 2 hours.

Implementation

- The patient is assisted into the supine position on a radiography table with his arms at his sides.
- An initial series of fluoroscopic pictures (mask images) is taken.
- The access site is shaved and prepared (a vein or artery may be used).
- The patient is given a local anesthetic.
- The patient is given an I.V. sedative.
- The vessel is cannulated and a catheter inserted and advanced to the area to be studied.

- The contrast medium is injected and films are taken in various views.
- The patient's vital signs and neurologic status are monitored. The patient is observed for signs of a hypersensitivity reaction, such as urticaria, pruritus, and respiratory distress.

Patient care

- The patient should drink at least 1 qt (1 L) of fluid on the day of the procedure because contrast medium acts as a diuretic. Extra fluid intake also aids excretion of the contrast medium.
- Instruct him to resume a normal diet.
- Monitor vital signs, intake and output, puncture site, neurologic status, and signs and symptoms of infection.
- Monitor the patient for a delayed hypersensitivity reaction to the contrast medium and thrombotic events.
- If bleeding occurs, apply firm pressure to the puncture site and tell the physician immediately.

Complications

- Infection
- Thrombotic and embolic events
- Bleeding

Interpretation

Normal results

- The contrast medium fills and opacifies all superficial and deep arteries, arterioles, and veins.

Abnormal results

- Vascular filling defects may indicate arteriovenous occlusion or stenosis.
- Outpouchings in vessel lumina may reflect aneurysms.
- Vessel displacement or vascular masses may indicate a tumor.

Interfering factors

- Patient movement
- Radiopaque objects in the fluoroscopic field

Direct antiglobulin

Overview

○ Detects immunoglobulins (antibodies) on the surface of red blood cells (RBCs); immunoglobulins coat RBCs when they've become sensitized to an antigen such as the Rh factor.
○ Antiglobulin (Coombs') serum added to saline-washed RBCs results in agglutination if immunoglobulins or complement is present (considered direct because it requires only one step — the addition of Coombs' serum to washed cells).

Purpose

○ To diagnose hemolytic disease of the newborn (HDN)
○ To investigate hemolytic transfusion reactions
○ To aid in the differential diagnosis of hemolytic anemias, which may be congenital or may result from an autoimmune reaction or use of certain drugs

Procedure

Preparation

○ If the patient is suspected of having hemolytic anemia, explain that the test determines whether the condition results from an abnormality in the body's immune system, the use of certain drugs, or some unknown cause.
○ Inform the adult patient that he need not restrict food and fluids.

✷ AGE AWARE *If the patient is a neonate, explain to the parents that this test helps diagnose HDN. Tell the neonate's parents that the test requires taking a blood sample.*

○ Tell the patient that the test requires a blood sample. Explain who will perform the venipuncture and when.
○ Explain to the patient that he may feel slight discomfort from the tourniquet and needle puncture.
○ Withhold drugs that may interfere with test results, including cephalosporins, chlorpromazine, diphenylhydantoin, ethosuximide, hydralazine, isoniazid, levodopa, mefenamic acid, melphalan, methyldopa, penicillin, quinidine, procainamide, rifampin, streptomycin, sulfonamides, and tetracyclines.

Implementation

○ For an adult, perform a venipuncture and collect the sample in two 5-ml ethylenediaminetetraacetic acid (EDTA) tubes.
○ For a neonate, draw 5 ml of cord blood into a tube with EDTA or additives after the cord is clamped and cut.
○ Handle samples gently to prevent hemolysis.

○ Label the sample with the patient's full name, the facility or blood bank number, the date, and the phlebotomist's initials.
○ Send the sample to the laboratory immediately.

Patient care

○ Apply direct pressure to the venipuncture site until bleeding stops.
○ Instruct the patient that he may resume medications stopped before the test.
○ Tell the patient or the parents of the neonate with HDN that further tests will be necessary to monitor anemia.

Complications

○ Hematoma at the venipuncture site

Interpretation

Normal results

○ Neither antibodies nor complement appears on the RBCs.

Abnormal results

○ In neonates, a positive test result on umbilical cord blood indicates that maternal antibodies have crossed the placenta and coated fetal RBCs, causing HDN. Transfusion of compatible blood lacking the antigens to these maternal antibodies may be necessary to prevent anemia.
○ In other patients, a positive test result may indicate hemolytic anemia and help differentiate between autoimmune and secondary hemolytic anemia, which can be drug-induced or associated with an underlying disease. A positive test result can also indicate sepsis.
○ A weakly positive test result may suggest a transfusion reaction in which the patient's antibodies react with transfused RBCs containing the corresponding antigen.

Interfering factors

○ Hemolysis from rough handling of the sample
○ Cephalosporins, chlorpromazine, diphenylhydantoin, ethosuximide, hydralazine, isoniazid, levodopa, mefenamic acid, melphalan, methyldopa, penicillin, procainamide, quinidine, rifampin, streptomycin, sulfonamides, and tetracyclines (positive test results, possibly from immune hemolysis)

Doppler ultrasound

Overview

- Noninvasive test to evaluate blood flow in the major veins and arteries of the arms and legs and in the extracranial cerebrovascular system.
- Handheld transducer directs high-frequency sound waves to an artery or vein; the transducer amplifies the sound waves to permit direct listening and graphic recording of blood flow.
- Measurement of systolic pressure helps to detect the presence, location, and extent of peripheral arterial occlusive disease.
- Accuracy rate 95% in detecting arteriovenous disease that impairs at least 50% of blood flow.

Purpose

- To aid the diagnosis of venous insufficiency, superficial and deep vein thromboses, and peripheral artery disease and arterial occlusion
- To monitor patients who have had arterial reconstruction and bypass grafts
- To detect abnormalities of carotid artery blood
- To evaluate arterial trauma

Procedure

Preparation

- Make sure the patient has signed a consent form.
- Note and report all allergies.
- Tell the patient the test takes about 20 minutes.
- Explain that test doesn't involve risk or discomfort.

Implementation

- Doppler ultrasonography is performed bilaterally.
- The patient is assisted into the supine position on the examination table with his arms at his sides.

Peripheral arterial evaluation

- For peripheral arterial evaluation in the leg, the usual test sites are the common and superficial femoral, popliteal, posterior tibial, and dorsalis pedis arteries.
- For peripheral arterial evaluation in the arm, the usual test sites are the subclavian, brachial, radial, and ulnar arteries.
- Brachial blood pressure is measured, and the transducer is placed at various points along the test arteries.
- The signals are monitored, and the waveforms are recorded for later analysis.
- The blood flow velocity is monitored and recorded over the test artery.
- Segmental limb blood pressures are obtained to localize arterial occlusive disease.

Peripheral venous evaluation

- For peripheral venous evaluation in the leg, the usual test sites are the popliteal, superficial and common femoral veins, and posterior tibial vein.

- For extracranial cerebrovascular evaluation, usual test sites are the supraorbital artery; the common, external, and internal carotid arteries; the vertebral arteries; and the brachial, axillary, subclavian, and jugular veins.
- The transducer is placed over the appropriate vessel, waveforms are recorded, and respiratory modulations are noted.
- Proximal limb compression maneuvers are performed.
- Augmentation after release of compression is noted to evaluate venous valve competency.
- For tests involving the legs and feet, the patient is asked to perform Valsalva's maneuver, and venous blood flow is recorded.

Patient care

- Remove the conductive jelly from the patient's skin.

Complications

- Bradyarrhythmia (if probe placed near carotid sinus)

Interpretation

Normal results

- Arterial waveforms of the arms and legs are multiphasic, with a prominent systolic component and one or more diastolic sounds.
- Arm pressure is unchanged despite postural changes.
- Proximal thigh pressure is normally 20 to 30 mm Hg greater than arm pressure.
- Venous blood flow velocity is phasic with respiration, with a lower pitch than arterial flow.
- Blood flow velocity increases with distal compression or release of proximal limb compression.
- Valsalva's maneuver interrupts venous flow velocity.
- In cerebrovascular testing, a strong velocity signal is present.
- In the common carotid artery, blood flow velocity increases during diastole.
- Periorbital arterial flow is normally anterograde out of the orbit.
- Ankle-brachial index (ABI) is > 0.9.

Abnormal results

- Diminished blood flow velocity signal suggests arterial stenosis or occlusion.
- Absent velocity signals suggest complete occlusion and lack of collateral circulation.
- ABI 0.5 to 0.9 indicates claudication; ABI < 0.5, resting ischemic pain; ABI < 0.2, gangrenous foot or leg.
- Venous blood flow velocity unchanged by respirations, not increased with compression or Valsalva's maneuver, or absent indicates venous thrombosis.
- A reversed flow velocity signal may indicate chronic venous insufficiency and varicose veins.
- Absent Doppler signals during cerebrovascular examination implies total arterial occlusion.

Interfering factors

None known

Duodenal contents culture

Overview

○ Duodenal tube insertion, aspiration of duodenal contents, and cultivation of microbes to isolate and identify pathogens that may cause duodenitis, cholecystitis, and cholangitis.
○ Specimen obtained during surgery.
○ Duodenal contents (pancreatic and duodenal enzymes and bile) normally almost sterile; subject to infection by many pathogens, such as *Escherichia coli, Staphylococcus aureus,* and *Salmonella,* resulting in duodenitis, cholecystitis, or cholangitis.
○ Contraindicated in pregnancy; acute pancreatitis or cholecystitis; esophageal varices, stenosis, and diverticular malignant neoplasms; recent severe gastric hemorrhage; aortic aneurysm; heart failure; and myocardial infarction.

Purpose

○ To detect bacterial infection of the biliary tract and duodenum
○ To differentiate between infection and gallstones
○ To rule out bacterial infection as the cause of persistent GI symptoms (epigastric pain, nausea, vomiting, and diarrhea)

Procedure

Preparation

○ Explain to the patient that this test determines the cause of his symptoms.
○ Instruct the patient to restrict food and fluids for 12 hours before the test.
○ Tell the patient who will perform the procedure and where it will occur.
○ Describe the insertion procedure to the patient. Assure him that although this procedure is uncomfortable, it isn't dangerous; tell him that passage of the tube may cause gagging, but that following the examiner's instructions about proper positioning, breathing, swallowing, and relaxing will minimize his discomfort.
○ Suggest that the patient empty his bladder before the procedure to increase his general comfort.

Implementation

○ After the nasoenteric tube is inserted, place the patient in a left lateral decubitus position with his feet elevated to allow peristalsis to move the tube into the duodenum.
○ Determine the pH of a small amount of aspirated fluid to ascertain the tube position. If the tube is in the stomach, pH is lower than 7; if the tube is in the duodenum, pH is higher than 7. The position of the tube can also be confirmed by fluoroscopy.
○ Aspirate duodenal contents.
○ Occasionally, a specimen for culture of duodenal contents is obtained during duodenoscopy.
○ Transfer the specimen to a sterile container and label it with the patient's name, the physician's name, the date and time of collection, and the collector's initials.
○ Wear gloves when assisting with this procedure and handling the specimen.
○ Collect the specimen for culture before antimicrobial therapy begins.
○ Send the specimen to the laboratory immediately.

Patient care

○ After duodenal tube placement or duodenoscopy, observe the patient carefully for signs of perforation, such as dysphagia, epigastric or shoulder pain, dyspnea, and fever.
○ After duodenoscopy, monitor the patient's vital signs until he's stable; keep the side rails up and enforce bed rest until he's fully alert.
○ Slowly withdraw the tube at a rate of 6″ to 8″ (15 to 20 cm) every 10 minutes until it reaches the esophagus; then clamp the tube and remove it quickly. If you can't withdraw the tube easily, report the problem; *never* force the tube.
○ Tell the patient that he may resume his usual diet.

Complications

None known

Interpretation

Normal results

○ Small amounts of polymorphonuclear leukocytes and epithelial cells with no pathogens are present; the bacterial count is usually < 100,000/ml of body fluid.

Abnormal results

○ Bacterial counts of 100,000/ml or more or the presence of pathogens in any number indicates infection. Susceptibility testing may be necessary.
○ Numerous polymorphonuclear leukocytes, copious mucus, and bile-stained epithelial cells in the bile fluid suggest inflammation of the biliary tract; many segmented neutrophils and exfoliated epithelial cells suggest pancreas, duodenum, or bile duct inflammation.
○ The presence of bile sand indicates cholelithiasis or calculi in the biliary tract. Differential diagnosis requires further testing.

Interfering factors

○ Failure to observe a 12-hour fast before the test (possible decrease)
○ Failure to use the proper collection technique

D-xylose absorption

Overview

- Evaluates the patient with symptoms of malabsorption, such as weight loss and generalized malnutrition, weakness, and diarrhea
- D-xylose is a pentose sugar that's absorbed in the small intestine without the aid of pancreatic enzymes; it passes through the liver without being metabolized and is excreted in the urine
- Because of its absorption in the small intestine without digestion, a measurement of D-xylose in the urine and blood indicates the absorptive capacity of the small intestine

Purpose

- To aid in the differential diagnosis of malabsorption
- To determine the cause of malabsorption syndrome

Procedure

Preparation

- Tell the patient that the D-xylose absorption test helps evaluate digestive function by analyzing blood samples and urine specimens after ingestion of a sugar solution.
- Explain to the patient that he must fast overnight before the test and that he'll have to fast and remain in bed during the test.
- Tell the patient that the test requires several blood samples.
- Explain who will perform the venipunctures and when.
- Explain to the patient that he may feel slight discomfort from the tourniquet and needle punctures.
- Inform the patient that all his urine will be collected for either a 5-hour or a 24-hour period.
- Tell the patient not to contaminate the urine specimens with toilet tissue or feces.
- Withhold drugs that alter test results, such as aspirin and indomethacin. Record any drugs the patient is taking on the laboratory request.

Implementation

- Perform a venipuncture to obtain a fasting blood sample, and collect the sample in a 10-ml tube without additives. Collect a first-voided morning urine specimen. Label these specimens and send them to the laboratory immediately to serve as a baseline.
- Give the patient 25 g of D-xylose dissolved in 8 ounces (240 ml) of water, followed by an additional 8 ounces of water. If the patient is a child, give 0.5 g of D-xylose per pound of body weight, up to 25 g. Record the time of D-xylose ingestion.
- For an adult, draw a blood sample 2 hours after D-xylose ingestion; for a child, 1 hour after ingestion. Collect the sample in a 10-ml tube without additives.

Occasionally, a 5-hour sample may be drawn to support the findings of the 1- or 2-hour sample.
- Collect and pool all urine during the 5 hours or 24 hours after D-xylose ingestion.
- Handle the sample gently to prevent hemolysis.
- Be sure to collect all urine and refrigerate the specimen during the collection period.

AGE AWARE Because patients age 65 and older and those with borderline or elevated creatinine levels tend to have low 5-hour urine levels but normal 24-hour levels, the physician must establish the length of the collection period.

Patient care

- Observe the patient for abdominal discomfort or mild diarrhea caused by d-xylose ingestion.
- Instruct the patient that he may resume his usual diet and medications.
- Maintain bed rest and withhold food and fluids (other than D-xylose) throughout the test period.

Complications

- Hematoma at the venipuncture site

Interpretation

Normal results

- In children, a blood concentration > 30 mg/dl in 1 hour; urine, 16% to 33% of ingested D-xylose excreted in 5 hours.
- In adults, a blood concentration 25 to 40 mg/dl in 2 hours; urine, 3.5 g excreted in 5 hours (age 65 or older, > 5 g in 24 hours).

Abnormal results

- Depressed blood and urine D-xylose levels most commonly result from malabsorption disorders that affect the proximal small intestine, such as sprue and celiac disease.
- Depressed levels may also result from regional enteritis involving the jejunum, Whipple's disease, multiple jejunal diverticula, myxedema, diabetic neuropathic diarrhea, rheumatoid arthritis, alcoholism, severe heart failure, and ascites.

Interfering factors

- Failure to observe pretest restrictions
- Aspirin (decreased D-xylose excretion by the kidneys)
- Indomethacin (decreased intestinal D-xylose absorption)
- Failure to obtain a complete urine specimen or to collect blood samples at designated times
- Intestinal overgrowth of bacteria, renal insufficiency, or renal retention of urine (possible drop in urine levels)

Echocardiography

Overview

○ Noninvasive test examines the size, shape, and motion of cardiac structures.
○ Transducer directs ultra–high-frequency sound waves toward cardiac structures, which reflect these waves; the transducer picks up the echoes, converts them to electrical impulses, and relays them to an echocardiography machine for display.
○ In M-mode (motion mode): a single, pencil-like ultrasound beam strikes the heart and produces a vertical view (useful for recording the motion and dimensions of intracardiac structures).
○ In two-dimensional echocardiography: cross-sectional view of cardiac structures used for recording lateral motion and spatial relationship between structures.

Purpose

○ To diagnose and evaluate valvular abnormalities
○ To measure and evaluate the size of the heart's chambers and valves
○ To help diagnose cardiomyopathies and atrial tumors
○ To evaluate cardiac function or wall motion after myocardial infarction
○ To detect pericardial effusion or mural thrombi

Procedure

Preparation

○ Tell the patient that he may be asked to breathe in and out slowly, to hold his breath, or to inhale a gas with a slightly sweet odor (amyl nitrite) while changes in heart function are recorded.
○ Warn about possible adverse effects of amyl nitrite (dizziness, flushing, and tachycardia), but reassure that such effects quickly subside.
○ Stress the need to remain still during the test because movement may distort results.
○ Explain that the test takes 15 to 30 minutes.

Implementation

○ The patient is placed into the supine position and conductive gel is applied to the third or fourth intercostal space to the left of the sternum. The transducer is placed directly over it.
○ The transducer is systematically angled to direct ultrasonic waves at specific parts of the patient's heart.
○ During the test, the oscilloscope screen is observed; significant findings are recorded on a strip chart recorder or on a videotape recorder.
○ For left lateral view, patient is placed on his left side.
○ Doppler echocardiography may also be used: color flow simulates red blood cell flow through the heart valves. The sound of blood flow may also be used to assess heart sounds and murmurs as they relate to cardiac hemodynamics.

Patient care

○ Remove the conductive gel from the patient's skin.

Complications

None known

Interpretation

Normal results

○ For the mitral valve, anterior and posterior mitral valve leaflets separate in early diastole and attain maximum excursion rapidly, then move toward each other during ventricular diastole; after atrial contraction, the mitral valve leaflets come together and remain together during ventricular systole.
○ For the aortic valve, aortic valve cusps move anteriorly during systole and posteriorly during diastole.
○ For the tricuspid valve, motion of the valve resembles that of the mitral valve.
○ For the pulmonic valve, movement is posterior during atrial systole and during ventricular systole. In right ventricular ejection, the cusp moves anteriorly, attaining its most anterior position during diastole.
○ For the ventricular cavities, the left ventricular cavity normally appears as an echo-free space between the interventricular septum and the posterior left ventricular wall.
○ The right ventricular cavity normally appears as an echo-free space between the anterior chest wall and the interventricular septum.

Abnormal results

○ In mitral stenosis, the valve narrows abnormally because of the leaflets' thickening and disordered motion; during diastole both mitral valve leaflets move anteriorly instead of posteriorly.
○ In mitral valve prolapse, one or both leaflets balloon into the left atrium during systole.
○ In aortic insufficiency, leaflet fluttering of the aortic valve during diastole occurs.
○ In stenosis, the aortic valve thickens and generates more echoes.
○ In bacterial endocarditis, valve motion is disrupted and fuzzy echoes usually appear on or near the valve.
○ A large chamber size may indicate cardiomyopathy, valvular disorders, or heart failure.
○ A small chamber may indicate restrictive pericarditis.
○ Hypertrophic cardiomyopathy can be identified by systolic anterior motion of the mitral valve and asymmetrical septal hypertrophy.
○ Myocardial ischemia or infarction may cause absent or paradoxical motion in ventricular walls.
○ Pericardial effusion is suggested when fluid accumulates in the pericardial space, causing an abnormal echo-free space to appear.
○ In large effusions, pressure exerted by excess fluid can restrict pericardial motion.

Interfering factors

○ Movement during test

Echocardiography, dobutamine stress

Overview

○ Two-dimensional echocardiography and dobutamine infusion detects changes in regional cardiac wall motion.
○ Dobutamine: increases myocardial contractility and stroke volume and permits study of the heart under stress conditions without exercising the patient; imaging is done during infusion of increasing amounts of dobutamine until maximum predicted heart rate is achieved.
○ Never perform without a physician and emergency resuscitation equipment immediately available.
○ Contraindicated in patients with myocardial infarction (MI) within 10 days of testing, acute myocarditis or pericarditis, ventricular or atrial arrhythmias, severe aortic or mitral stenosis.
○ Contraindicated in patients with hyperthyroidism or severe anemia, ventricular or dissecting aortic aneurysms, clinical heart failure, and acute severe infections.

Purpose

○ To identify causes of anginal symptoms
○ To measure chambers of the heart and determine functional capacity
○ To help set limits for an exercise program
○ To diagnose and evaluate valvular and wall motion abnormalities
○ To detect atrial tumors, mural thrombi, vegetative growth on valve leaflets, and pericardial effusions
○ To evaluate myocardial perfusion, coronary artery disease and obstruction, and the extent of myocardial damage following MI

Procedure

Preparation

○ Make sure the patient has signed an appropriate consent form.
○ Note and report all allergies.
○ Explain the need to refrain from eating, smoking, or drinking alcoholic or caffeine-containing beverages at least 4 hours before the test or as directed by the physician.
○ Withhold drugs the patient is currently taking before testing.
○ Warn the patient that when the dobutamine infusion begins, he may feel palpitations, some mild shortness of breath, and some fatigue.
○ Instruct the patient to report all symptoms experienced during the study.
○ Explain that the test should take 60 to 90 minutes.

Implementation

○ The patient is placed in the supine position and an echocardiogram obtained.
○ An initial electrocardiogram (ECG) is obtained.
○ ECG rhythm and blood pressure are monitored during the procedure.
○ After I.V. access is obtained, dobutamine infusion is given in increasing amounts, usually up to a maximum of 30 mcg/kg/minute.
○ The infusion continues until the patient reaches his maximum predicted heart rate or becomes symptomatic.
○ If the maximum predicted heart rate isn't reached with maximum dobutamine, I.V. atropine may be given.
○ As the maximum predicted heart rate is achieved, a second (stress) echocardiogram is obtained.
○ After the dobutamine infusion is completed, a third (recovery) echocardiogram is completed.

⚠ *ALERT Testing should be stopped for significant ECG changes, hypertension, hypotension, angina, dyspnea, syncope, or critical symptoms.*

⚠ *ALERT The procedure shouldn't be performed without a physician and emergency resuscitation equipment readily available.*

Patient care

○ If the heart rate doesn't return to baseline or the patient becomes symptomatic, give an I.V. beta blocker.
○ Remove electrodes and conductive gel from the patient's chest.
○ Monitor vital signs, ECG, heart sounds, anginal symptoms, and respiratory status.

Complications

○ Significant ECG changes, hypertension, hypotension, angina, dyspnea, syncope, or other critical symptoms

Interpretation

Normal results

○ Ventricular wall contractility increases.

Abnormal results

○ Abnormal regional wall motion may indicate cardiac ischemia or infarction.

Interfering factors

None known

Echocardiography, exercise

Overview

- Two-dimensional echocardiography and exercise detects changes in cardiac wall motion.
- Collects images before and after exercise stress testing.
- Specificity and sensitivity are an adjunct to results obtained in exercise electrocardiography.
- Also called *stress echocardiography*.
- Contraindicated in those with ventricular or dissecting aortic aneurysms, uncontrolled arrhythmias, pericarditis; myocarditis, severe anemia, uncontrolled hypertension, unstable angina, and heart failure.

Purpose

- To identify the causes of chest pain
- To determine chamber size and functional capacity of the heart
- To screen for asymptomatic cardiac disease
- To set limits for an exercise program
- To diagnose and evaluate valvular and wall motion abnormalities
- To detect atrial tumors, mural thrombi, vegetative growth on valve leaflets, pericardial effusions
- To evaluate myocardial perfusion, coronary artery disease (CAD) and obstructions, and the extent of myocardial damage after myocardial infarction (MI)

Procedure

Preparation

- Make sure the patient has signed a consent form.
- Note and report all allergies.
- The procedure shouldn't be performed without a physician and emergency resuscitation equipment readily available.
- Instruct the patient to refrain from eating, smoking, or drinking alcoholic or caffeine-containing beverages at least 3 to 4 hours before the test.
- Withhold drugs the patient is currently taking before testing.
- Warn the patient that he might feel tired, diaphoretic, and slightly short of breath. Reassure him that if symptoms become severe or if chest pain develops, the test will stop.
- Explain that the test takes about 60 minutes.

Implementation

- The patient is placed into the supine position and a baseline echocardiogram obtained.
- An initial baseline electrocardiogram (ECG) and an initial blood pressure reading are obtained.

- The patient is placed on the treadmill at slow speed until he becomes acclimated to it.
- The work rate is increased every 3 minutes as tolerated (increasing the speed of the machine slightly and increasing the degree of incline by 3% each time).
- The cardiac monitor is observed continuously for changes and blood pressure is monitored at predetermined intervals.
- The rhythm strip is checked at preset intervals for arrhythmias, premature ventricular contractions, ST-segment changes, and T-wave changes.
- The test level and the amount of time it took to reach that level are marked on each strip.
- Common responses to maximal exercise include dizziness, light-headedness, leg fatigue, dyspnea, diaphoresis, and a slightly ataxic gait. If symptoms become severe, the test is stopped.
- The test is stopped for significant ECG changes, arrhythmias, or symptoms including hypertension, hypotension, or angina.
- After the patient has reached the maximum predicted heart rate, the treadmill is slowed.
- While the patient's heart rate is still elevated, he's helped off the treadmill and placed on a litter for a second echocardiogram.

Patient care

- Remove electrodes and conductive gel.
- Monitor vital signs, ECG, and heart sounds.

Complications

- Cardiac arrhythmias
- Myocardial ischemia or MI
- Cardiac arrest
- Death

Interpretation

Normal results

- Contractility of the ventricular walls increases and results in hyperkinesis linked to sympathetic and catecholamine stimulation.
- Heart rate increases in direct proportion to the workload and metabolic oxygen demand. Systolic blood pressure also increases as the workload increases.
- The patient attains the endurance level appropriate for his age and exercise limits.

Abnormal results

- Exercise-induced myocardial ischemia suggests disease in the coronary artery supplying the involved area of myocardium.
- Hypokinesis or akinesis of the myocardium indicates significant CAD.
- Exercise-induced hypotension, ST-segment depression of 2 mm or more, or downsloping ST segments appearing within the first 3 minutes of exercise and

lasting 8 minutes after the test ends may indicate multivessel or left coronary artery disease.
- ST-segment elevation may indicate critical myocardial ischemia or injury.

Interfering factors

- Wolff-Parkinson-White syndrome, electrolyte imbalance, or the use of digoxin preparations (false-positive results)
- Conditions that cause left ventricular hypertrophy

Electrocardiography

Overview

○ Electrocardiography (ECG) graphically records the electrical current generated by the heart and measured by electrodes connected to an amplifier and strip chart recorder.
○ Measures the electrical potential from 12 different leads: the standard limb leads (I, II, III), the augmented limb leads (aV$_F$, aV$_L$, and aV$_R$), and the precordial, or chest, leads (V$_1$ through V$_6$).
○ Consists of P wave, QRS complex, and T wave.

Purpose

○ To identify conduction abnormalities, cardiac arrhythmias, myocardial ischemia or infarction (MI)
○ To monitor recovery from MI
○ To document pacemaker performance

Procedure

Preparation

○ Explain to the patient the need to lie still, relax, and breathe normally during the procedure.
○ Note current cardiac drug therapy on the test request form as well as any other pertinent clinical information, such as chest pain or pacemaker.
○ Explain that the test is painless and takes 5 to 10 minutes.

Implementation

○ Place the patient in a supine or semi-Fowler's position.
○ Expose the chest, ankles, and wrists.
○ Place electrodes on the inner aspect of the wrists, on the medial aspect of the lower legs, and on the chest.
○ After all the electrodes are in place, connect the lead wires.
○ Press the START button and input any required information.
○ Make sure that all leads are represented in the tracing. If not, determine which electrode has come loose, reattach it, and restart the tracing.
○ All recording and other nearby electrical equipment should be properly grounded.
○ Make sure that electrodes are firmly attached.

Patient care

○ Disconnect the equipment, remove the electrodes, and remove the gel with a moist cloth towel.
○ If the patient is having recurrent chest pain or if serial ECGs are ordered, leave the electrode patches in place.

Complications

○ Skin sensitivity to the electrodes

Interpretation

Normal results

○ Cardiac rate is 60 to 100 beats/minute.
○ Cardiac rhythm is normal sinus rhythm.
○ P wave precedes each QRS complex.
○ PR interval lasts 0.12 to 0.20 second.
○ QRS complex lasts 0.06 to 0.10 second.
○ ST segment is not more than 0.1 mV.
○ T wave is rounded and smooth and is positive in leads I, II, V$_3$, V$_4$, V$_5$, and V$_6$.
○ QT interval duration varies but usually lasts 0.36 to 0.44 second.

Abnormal results

○ Heart rate < 60 beats/minute is bradycardia.
○ Heart rate > 100 beats/minute is tachycardia.
○ Missing P waves may indicate atrioventricular (AV) block, atrial arrhythmia, or junctional rhythm.
○ A short PR interval may indicate a junctional arrhythmia; a prolonged PR interval may indicate an AV block.
○ A prolonged QRS complex may indicate intraventricular conduction defects; missing QRS complexes may indicate an AV block or ventricular asystole.
○ ST-segment elevation of 0.2 mV or more above the baseline may indicate myocardial injury; ST-segment depression may indicate myocardial ischemia or injury.
○ T wave inversion in leads I, II, and V$_3$ to V$_6$ may indicate myocardial ischemia; peaked T waves may indicate hyperkalemia or myocardial ischemia; variations in T wave amplitude may indicate electrolyte imbalances.
○ A prolonged QT interval may suggest life-threatening ventricular arrhythmias.

Interfering factors

○ Improper lead placement

Electrocardiography, exercise

Overview

○ Monitors patient's electrocardiogram (ECG) and blood pressure while he walks on a treadmill or pedals a stationary bicycle; response to a constant or increasing workload is observed
○ Used to evaluate the heart during physical stress
○ Commonly known as an *exercise stress test*

Purpose

○ To diagnose the cause of chest pain
○ To determine functional capacity of the heart
○ To screen for asymptomatic coronary artery disease
○ To help set limitations for an exercise program
○ To identify cardiac arrhythmias that develop during physical exercise
○ To evaluate effectiveness of antiarrhythmic or antianginal therapy
○ To evaluate myocardial perfusion

Procedure

Preparation

○ Make sure the patient has signed an appropriate consent form.
○ Note and report all allergies.
○ Check the patient's history for a recent physical examination (within 1 week) and for baseline 12-lead ECG results.
○ Instruct the patient not to eat, smoke, or drink alcoholic or caffeine-containing beverages before the test.
○ Continue drugs the patient is currently taking unless the physician directs otherwise.
○ Warn the patient that he might feel fatigued, slightly breathless, and sweaty during the test.
○ Provide reassurance that testing will stop if the patient experiences significant symptoms such as chest pain.
○ Instruct the patient to wear comfortable socks and shoes and loose, lightweight shorts or slacks during the procedure.
○ Explain that the test takes about 30 minutes.

Implementation

○ Baseline ECG and blood pressure readings are taken.
○ ECG and blood pressure readings are taken while patient walks on treadmill or pedals stationary bicycle.
○ Unless complications develop, the test continues until the patient reaches the target heart rate, determined by an established protocol (usually 85% of maximum predicted heart rate for patient's age and gender).
○ The cardiac monitor is observed continuously for changes in the heart's electrical activity.

○ The rhythm strip is checked at preset intervals for arrhythmias, premature ventricular contractions (PVCs), ST-segment changes, and T-wave changes.
○ Blood pressure is monitored at predetermined intervals (usually at the end of each test level).
○ The test stops when the patient reaches the target heart rate or if symptoms become severe.
○ The test is stopped immediately if the ECG shows significant arrhythmias or an increase in ectopy, if systolic blood pressure falls below resting level, if the heart rate falls 10 beats/minute or more below resting level, or if the patient becomes exhausted or experiences severe symptoms such as chest pain.

▶ *ALERT Stop the test if the patient has persistent ST-segment elevation, possibly indicating myocardial injury.*

▶ *ALERT Stop the test if the patient experiences a new bundle-branch block, an ST-segment depression > 1.5 mm, frequent or multifocal PVCs, blood pressure failing to rise above the resting level, systolic pressure > 220 mm Hg, or angina.*

Patient care

○ Assist the patient to a chair and continue monitoring heart rate and blood pressure for 10 to 15 minutes or until the ECG returns to the baseline.
○ Remove the electrodes and clean the application sites.
○ Have the patient resume a normal diet and activities.
○ Monitor vital signs, ECG, heart sounds, and anginal symptoms.

Complications

○ Cardiac arrhythmias
○ Myocardial ischemia or infarction

Interpretation

Normal results

○ The heart rate increases in direct proportion to the workload and metabolic oxygen demand.
○ Systolic blood pressure increases as workload increases.
○ The patient attains the endurance levels appropriate for his age and the exercise protocol.

Abnormal results

○ T-wave inversion or ST-segment depression may signify ischemia.
○ Exercise-induced hypotension, an ST-segment depression of 2 mm or more, and downsloping ST segments may indicate significant coronary artery disease.
○ ST-segment elevation may indicate myocardial injury.

Interfering factors

○ Conditions that cause left ventricular hypertrophy may interfere with testing for ischemia

Electrocardiography, signal-averaged

Overview

○ Amplifies, averages, and filters an electrocardiogram (ECG) signal recorded on the body surface
○ Detects high-frequency, low-amplitude cardiac electrical signals in the last part of the QRS complex and in the ST segment

Purpose

○ To detect destructive signals called *late potentials* that may represent delayed, disorganized activity (in patients who have survived an acute myocardial infarction)
○ To evaluate the risk of life-threatening arrhythmias

Procedure

Preparation

○ Make sure the patient has signed an appropriate consent form.
○ Note and report all allergies.
○ Record the use of antiarrhythmics on the patient's chart.
○ Tell the patient that electrodes will be attached to his arms, legs, and chest and that the procedure is painless.
○ Instruct the patient to lie still and breathe normally during the procedure.
○ Explain that there is no need to restrict food and fluids before the test.
○ Explain that the test takes about 30 minutes.

Implementation

○ The patient is placed in the supine position (or semi-Fowler position if the patient can't tolerate lying supine).
○ Electrodes are attached to the patient's chest, ankles, and wrists.
○ Multiple inputs are obtained from standard orthogonal bipolar X, Y, and Z leads over a series of ECG cycles.
○ The average is taken over a large number of beats, typically 100 or more.

Patient care

○ Wash conductive gel from the skin.

Complications

○ Skin sensitivity to the electrodes

Interpretation

Normal results

○ QRS complexes lack low potentials that would indicate disorganized activity.

Abnormal results

○ Late potentials after the QRS complex indicate a risk for ventricular arrhythmias.

Interfering factors

○ Antiarrhythmics
○ Poor tissue-electrode contact (produces an artifact)

Electroencephalography

Overview

○ Records portion of the brain's electrical activity through electrodes attached to the scalp
○ Electrical impulses transmitted, magnified, and recorded as brain waves
○ Intracranial electrodes sometimes surgically implanted to record EEG changes for localization of seizure focus

Purpose

○ To determine the presence and type of epilepsy
○ To aid in the diagnosis of intracranial lesions
○ To evaluate brain activity in metabolic disease, head injury, meningitis, encephalitis, and psychological disorders
○ To help confirm brain death

Procedure

Preparation

○ Make sure the patient has signed a consent form.
○ Note and report all allergies.
○ Wash and dry the patient's hair to remove hair sprays, creams, or oils.
○ Withhold tranquilizers, barbiturates, and other sedatives for 24 to 48 hours before the test.
○ Minimize sleep (4 to 5 hours) the night before the study.
○ If a sleep EEG is ordered, give a sedative to promote sleep during the test.
○ The patient need not restrict food and fluids before the test, but stimulants such as caffeine-containing beverages, chocolate, and tobacco aren't permitted for 8 hours before the study.
○ Reassure patient that the electrodes won't shock him.
○ If the test will involve needle electrodes, warn the patient that he might feel pricking sensations during insertion.
○ Explain that the test that takes about 1 hour.

✳ *AGE AWARE Infants and very young children may require sedation to prevent crying and restlessness, but these drugs may alter test results.*

Implementation

○ The patient is positioned and electrodes attached to the scalp.
○ During recording, the patient is carefully observed and any movements, such as blinking, swallowing, or talking are noted; these movements can cause artifacts.
○ The patient may undergo testing in various stress situations including hyperventilation and photic stimulation to elicit abnormal patterns not obvious in the resting stage.

Patient care

○ Tell the patient he may resume drug therapy.
○ Provide a safe environment.
○ Monitor the patient for seizures and maintain seizure precautions.
○ Help patient remove electrode paste from his hair.
○ If brain death is confirmed, provide emotional support for the family.

Complications

○ Adverse effects of sedation, if used
○ Possible seizure activity

Interpretation

Normal results

○ Alpha waves occur at frequencies of 8 to 13 cycles/second in a regular rhythm.
○ Alpha waves are present only in the waking state when the patient's eyes are closed but he's mentally alert and usually disappear with visual activity or mental concentration.
○ Alpha waves are decreased by apprehension or anxiety and are most prominent in the occipital leads.
○ Beta waves (13 to 30 cycles/second) indicate normal activity when the patient is alert with eyes open and are seen most readily in the frontal and central regions of the brain.
○ Theta waves (4 to 7 cycles/second) are most common in children and young adults.
○ Theta waves appear primarily in the parietal and temporal regions and indicate drowsiness or emotional stress in adults.
○ Delta waves (fewer than 4 cycles/second) are visible in deep sleep stages and in serious brain dysfunction.

Abnormal results

○ Spikes and waves at a frequency of 3 cycles/second suggest absence seizures.
○ Multiple, high-voltage, spiked waves in both hemispheres suggest generalized tonic-clonic seizures.
○ Spiked waves in the affected temporal region suggest temporal lobe epilepsy.
○ Localized, spiked discharges suggest focal seizures.
○ Slow waves (usually delta waves but possibly unilateral beta waves) suggest intracranial lesions.
○ Focal abnormalities in the injured area suggest vascular lesions.
○ Generalized, diffuse, and slow brain waves suggest metabolic or inflammatory disorders or increased intracranial pressure.
○ An absent EEG pattern or a flat tracing (except for artifacts) may indicate brain death.

Interfering factors

○ Skipping the meal before the test (can cause hypoglycemia and alter brain wave patterns)
○ Anticonvulsants, tranquilizers, barbiturates, and other sedatives

Electromyography

Overview

○ Records the electrical activity of selected skeletal muscle groups at rest and during voluntary contraction
○ Measures nerve conduction time
○ Contraindicated in patients with bleeding disorders

Purpose

○ To differentiate between primary muscle disorders such as muscular dystrophies and certain metabolic disorders
○ To identify diseases characterized by central neuronal degeneration such as amyotrophic lateral sclerosis (ALS)
○ To aid in diagnosing neuromuscular disorders such as myasthenia gravis
○ To aid in diagnosing radiculomyopathies

Procedure

Preparation

○ Make sure the patient has signed an appropriate consent form.
○ Note and report all allergies.
○ Check for and note drugs that may interfere with test results (cholinergics, anticholinergics, anticoagulants, and skeletal muscle relaxants).
○ Tell the patient he need not restrict food and fluids before the test but that it may be necessary to restrict cigarettes, coffee, tea, and cola for 2 to 3 hours beforehand.
○ Warn the patient that he might experience some discomfort as a needle is inserted into selected muscles.
○ Explain that the test takes at least 1 hour.

Implementation

○ The patient is positioned in a way that relaxes the muscle to be tested.
○ Needle electrodes are quickly inserted into the selected muscle.
○ A metal plate lies under the patient to serve as a reference electrode.
○ The resulting electrical signal is recorded during rest and contraction, amplified 1 million times, and displayed on an oscilloscope or computer screen.
○ Lead wires are usually attached to an audio-amplifier so that voltage fluctuations within the muscle are audible.

Patient care

○ Apply warm compresses and give analgesics for discomfort.
○ Resume drugs that were withheld before the test.
○ Monitor signs and symptoms of infection.
○ Monitor the patient's pain level and response to the analgesics.

Complications

○ Infection at the insertion site

Interpretation

Normal results

○ At rest, muscle exhibits minimal electrical activity.
○ During voluntary contraction, electrical activity increases markedly.
○ A sustained contraction, or one of increasing strength, produces a rapid "train" of motor unit potentials.

Abnormal results

○ Short (low-amplitude) motor unit potentials, with frequent, irregular discharges suggest possible primary muscle disease such as muscular dystrophies.
○ Isolated and irregular motor unit potentials with increased amplitude and duration suggest possible disorders such as ALS and peripheral nerve disorders.
○ Initially normal motor unit potentials that progressively diminish in amplitude with continuing contractions suggest possible myasthenia gravis.

Interfering factors

None known

Electromyography of the external sphincter

Overview

○ Measures electrical activity of the external urinary sphincter
○ Measures activity in three ways: by skin electrodes (most commonly used), by needle electrodes inserted in perineal or periurethral tissues, or by electrodes in an anal plug
○ Often used with cystometry and voiding urethrography as part of full urodynamic study

Purpose

○ To evaluate incontinence
○ To assess neuromuscular function of the external urinary sphincter
○ To assess the functional balance between bladder and sphincter muscle activity

Procedure

Preparation

○ Make sure the patient has signed a consent form.
○ Note and report all allergies.
○ If the patient is taking cholinergic or anticholinergic drugs, notify the physician and stop the drugs.
○ If the patient is to receive needle electrodes, warn him that he may feel discomfort during insertion.
○ Provide reassurance that there's no danger of electric shock.
○ If the patient is to receive an anal plug, provide reassurance that only the tip of the plug will be inserted into the rectum — the patient may feel fullness but no discomfort.
○ Explain that the test takes 30 to 60 minutes.
○ If the patient is a woman, tell her that she may notice slight bleeding with the first voiding after the procedure.

Implementation

○ The patient is placed in the lithotomy position for electrode placement; he may then lie in a supine position.
○ Electrode paste is applied to the ground plate, which is taped to the thigh and grounded. Electrodes are applied and connected to electrode adapters.
○ For a woman, skin electrodes are placed in the periurethral area; for a man, in the perineal area beneath the scrotum.
○ For a woman, needle electrodes are inserted in the periurethral area; for a man, through the perineal skin toward the apex of the prostate.
○ The electrodes are connected to adapters inserted into the preamplifier and recording begins.

○ The patient is asked alternately to relax and tighten the sphincter.
○ The patient is asked to bear down and exhale while the anal plug and needle electrodes are removed.
○ Cystometrography is sometimes done with electromyography (EMG) for a thorough evaluation of detrusor and sphincter coordination.

Patient care

○ Clean and dry the area.
○ Report hematuria after the first voiding in a woman tested with needle electrodes.
○ Report signs and symptoms of mild urethral irritation, including dysuria, hematuria, and urinary frequency.
○ Advise the patient to use warm sitz baths and increase oral fluids to 2 to 3 qt (2 to 3 L)/day, unless contraindicated.

Complications

○ Bleeding
○ Infection

Interpretation

Normal results

○ Muscle activity increases when the external urinary sphincter is tightened.
○ Muscle activity decreases when the external urinary sphincter is relaxed.
○ If EMG and cystometrography are done together, a comparison of results shows muscle activity of the sphincter that increases as the bladder fills, as the patient voids, and as the bladder contracts; and muscle activity that decreases as the sphincter relaxes.

Abnormal results

○ Failure of the sphincter to relax or increased muscle activity during voiding indicates detrusor-sphincter dyssynergia.

Interfering factors

○ Cholinergics or anticholinergics

Electronystagmography and videonystagmography

Overview

○ Electronystagmography (ENG) and videonystagmography (VNG) evaluate interactions of the vestibular system and the muscles controlling eye movement—known as the *vestibulo-ocular reflex.*
○ Nystagmus is the involuntary back-and-forth eye movements caused by this reflex, which maintains vision when the head moves.
○ Traditional ENG records nystagmus through electrodes that pick up the corneoretinal potential and chart it.
○ VNG records eye movements with an infrared camera.
○ Both tests aid in determining whether the disorder originates in the peripheral or central nervous system.

Purpose

○ To help identify the cause of dizziness and vertigo
○ To confirm the presence and location of a lesion
○ To assess neurologic disorders

Procedure

Preparation

○ Make sure the patient's ear canals are free of cerumen and that he doesn't have a tympanic membrane perforation.
○ Inform the patient that tympanometry will occur before caloric testing to ensure tympanic membrane integrity.
○ Tell the patient that his dizziness problems will be assessed by recording eye movements.
○ Reassure the patient that the test isn't painful and someone will be present to ensure that he doesn't fall, but that some portions may briefly make him dizzy. Because of this, advise him not to eat or drink for 3 to 4 hours before the test.
○ Suggest that someone accompany the patient to the evaluation, as occasionally the patient doesn't feel well enough to drive afterwards.
○ Encourage the patient to wear comfortable clothing.
○ If testing will involve traditional ENG with attachment of recording electrodes, inform the patient that make-up or facial creams shouldn't be used on the day of the test.
○ Advise the patient not to wear mascara because it can affect VNG testing.
○ Instruct the patient not to smoke or drink caffeinated beverages the day of the test, and to refrain from taking nonessential medication for 48 hours before the test.
○ Ask the patient if he has a history of back or neck problems that would be worsened by head or neck movement.
○ If the patient wears glasses, tell him to bring them to the test. The patient who wears contact lenses should bring eyeglasses to the examination, if possible.
○ Tell the patient that the audiologist will ask him to describe the dizziness, including when it began and what situations create it or make it worse. Find out about the progression of the patient's symptoms by asking him to describe the dizziness in words other than "dizzy."

Implementation

○ After the device is set up, light bars are connected to the equipment.
○ The patient is positioned a calibrated distance from the light source and asked to follow the movement of the lights using eye movement only. These movements are recorded and graphed.

Saccade testing
○ The patient watches the movement of a dot on the light bar. The accuracy and velocity of the eye tracking is measured. The traces are analyzed to determine if there's symmetrical eye movement or dysmetria. *Glissades*, a slowing of the eye movement as it approaches a target, is also ruled out.

Gaze nystagmus testing
○ The patient looks at the light on the light bar and holds the gaze steady. Gaze is directed left, right, up, and down.
○ The patient closes his eyes and retains the gaze direction in traditional ENG testing. When VNG recordings are made, goggles exclude light, and the recordings are made with the eyes open.

Smooth pursuit (sinusoidal) tracking testing
○ The patient watches the dot on the light bar as it moves back and forth at varying rates. Tracings are analyzed for left/right symmetry and smoothness of the eye's tracking of the target.

Optokinetics testing
○ The patient looks at the light bar as a series of dots moves across the screen, first in one direction and then in the other. The patient's eyes rapidly move back to center and track another dot. This creates a tracing that looks like nystagmus.
○ This test assesses the ability of the central nervous system (CNS) to control rapid eye movement and will be affected by an existing nystagmus.

Positional and positioning testing
○ The patient's eye movements are recorded as he's moved into various body positions and as he remains in them.
○ Recordings note whether nystagmus is present, and if so, which positions elicit them and have diagnostic significance.

Dix-Hallpike test
○ This test helps diagnose benign paroxysmal positional vertigo.

○ The patient is seated; then he's rapidly moved into a supine, head-hanging position, with the head deviated to the side and then returned to a sitting position.

Caloric testing

○ The patient lies supine with his head elevated 30 degrees so that the horizontal semicircular canals are perpendicular to the floor. The patient's ear is irrigated with water or air for about 60 seconds per irrigation. Four irrigations are completed.
○ Fluid in the semicircular canal or the middle ear moves when the temperature of the fluid is changed, eliciting nystagmus.
○ The patient is instructed to open his eyes during one portion of each recording. Visual fixation reduces nystagmus if the CNS is normal. The symmetry of the nystagmus elicited by irrigation of each ear is assessed. Symmetry of the left beating nystagmus and the right beating nystagmus is analyzed.
○ If the patient fails to respond to standard caloric stimulation, a small quantity of ice water or cold air is introduced into the ear canal to determine if there's residual functioning of that ear's vestibular system.

Patient care

○ After testing, the audiologist monitors the patient's status and advises him to remain in a position that reduces dizziness, if present.
○ Advise the patient not to drive until all symptoms of imbalance have subsided.

Complications

○ Dizziness

Interpretation

Normal results

○ Nystagmus accompanies a head turn.
○ In saccadic pursuit testing, square wave patterns of different amplitudes are seen along with good accuracy of eye movements.
○ In gaze testing, no nystagmus occurs with eyes open and weak nor with eyes closed.
○ In smooth pursuit, patient demonstrates volitional smooth tracking of target, accurate within age norms.
○ In optokinetic tests, eye movement follows a stimulus at speeds up to 30 degrees per second; triangular wave pattern is clear; pattern is similar for stimuli traveling in both directions.
○ In positional and positioning testing, no nystagmus occurs with eyes open, eyes closed, or with light-excluding goggles; no more than weak nystagmus occurs in one or more positions.
○ In caloric testing, with eyes closed, nystagmus occurs in all conditions; suppressed by visual fixation with cold stimuli, nystagmus beats to opposite ear; with warm stimuli, beats to same ear. Acronym COWS is used to remember *c*old, *o*pposite; *w*arm, *s*ame.

Abnormal results

○ Nystagmus after a head turn is prolonged, or nystagmus occurs when the patient isn't turning his head.
○ ENG/VNG results are reported as normal, vestibular (peripheral), CNS, or multifactorial.
○ A peripheral lesion may involve the end organ or the vestibular branch of the eighth cranial nerve and may result from conditions such as Ménière's disease, multiple sclerosis, ischemic damage to the cochlea, autoimmune disease, and vestibular ototoxicity and eighth nerve tumors.
○ A central lesion may involve the brain stem, cerebellum, cerebrum, or any of the connecting structures and may result from demyelinating diseases, tumors, or circulatory disorders.

Interfering factors

○ Drug that suppresses or stimulates CNS function
○ Poor eyesight or extraocular muscle weakness
○ Drowsiness and level of alertness
○ Poor patient compliance

Electrophysiology studies

Overview

○ Measure discrete conduction intervals
○ Record electrical conduction during the slow withdrawal of an electrode catheter from the right ventricle through the bundle of His to the sinoatrial node
○ Also known as *EPS* or *bundle of His electrography*

Purpose

○ To diagnose arrhythmias and conduction anomalies
○ To determine the need for an implanted pacemaker, internal cardioverter-defibrillator, and cardioactive drugs
○ To locate the site of a bundle-branch block, especially in asymptomatic patients with conduction disturbances
○ To determine the presence and location of accessory conducting pathways

Procedure

Preparation

○ Make sure the patient has signed an appropriate consent form.
○ Note and report all allergies.
○ Instruct the patient to restrict food and fluids for at least 6 hours before the test.
○ Provide reassurance to the patient that he will remain conscious during the test. Instruct him to report any discomfort or pain.
○ Explain that the test takes 1 to 3 hours.

Implementation

○ The patient is placed in the supine position on a special table.
○ Electrocardiography (ECG) monitoring starts.
○ The insertion site (usually the groin or antecubital fossa) is shaved and prepared.
○ A local anesthetic is injected. A catheter is inserted intravenously, using fluoroscopic guidance.
○ The catheter is advanced into the right ventricle, then slowly withdrawn.
○ Recordings of conduction intervals are taken from each pole of the catheter, either simultaneously or sequentially.
○ After recordings and measurements are complete, the catheter is removed.
○ The insertion site is cleaned and a sterile dressing applied.

▽ *ALERT Emergency resuscitation equipment should be immediately available in case of arrhythmias during the test.*

Patient care

○ Monitor the patient's vital signs.
○ Enforce bed rest.
○ Have the patient resume a usual diet.
○ Obtain a 12-lead resting ECG.
○ Monitor vital signs, the insertion site, and bleeding.
○ Monitor the patient for signs and symptoms of infection.
○ Monitor the patient for cardiac arrhythmias and anginal symptoms.
○ Watch for signs and symptoms of embolism.
○ Monitor ECG changes.
○ Emergency resuscitation equipment should be immediately available in case of arrhythmias during the test.

Complications

○ Arrhythmias
○ Pulmonary emboli and thromboemboli
○ Hemorrhage
○ Infection

Interpretation

Normal results

○ The conduction time from the bundle of His to the Purkinje fibers (HV interval) is 35 to 55 msec.
○ The conduction time from the atrioventricular node to the bundle of His (AH interval) is 45 to 150 msec.
○ The intra-atrial conduction time (PA interval) is 20 to 40 msec.

Abnormal results

○ A prolonged HV interval suggests possible acute or chronic disease.
○ AH interval delays suggest atrial pacing, chronic conduction system disease, carotid sinus pressure, recent myocardial infarction, and use of certain drugs.
○ PA interval delays suggest possible acquired, surgically induced, or congenital atrial disease and atrial pacing.

Interfering factors

None known

Endoscopic retrograde cholangio-pancreatography

Overview

- X-ray of the pancreatic ducts and hepatobiliary tree after injection of a contrast medium into the duodenal papilla
- Also known as *ERCP*

Purpose

- To evaluate obstructive jaundice
- To diagnose cancer of the duodenal papilla, pancreas, and biliary ducts
- To locate calculi and stenosis in the pancreatic ducts and hepatobiliary tree

Procedure

Preparation

- Make sure the patient has signed a consent form.
- Note and report all allergies.
- Inform the physician about the patient's hypersensitivity to iodine, seafood, or iodinated contrast media.
- Give the patient a sedative.
- Tell the patient to fast after midnight before the test.
- Explain the use of a local anesthetic spray to suppress the gag reflex and the use of a mouth guard to protect the teeth.
- Provide reassurance that oral insertion of the endoscope doesn't obstruct breathing and that the patient will remain conscious during the procedure.
- Explain that the test takes 1 to 1½ hours or longer if a procedure such as stent placement is performed.
- Explain that the patient may have a sore throat for 3 to 4 days after the examination.
- Explain that avoidance of alcohol and driving is necessary for 24 hours after the test.

Implementation

- An I.V. infusion is started.
- The patient is given a local anesthetic and I.V. sedation.
- Vital signs, cardiac rhythm, and pulse oximetry are continuously monitored.
- The patient is placed in a left lateral position.
- The endoscope is inserted into the mouth and advanced, using fluoroscopic guidance, into the stomach and duodenum.
- The patient is helped into the prone position.
- An I.V. anticholinergic or glucagon may be given to decrease GI motility.
- A cannula is passed through the biopsy channel of the endoscope, into the duodenal papilla, and into the ampulla of Vater; contrast medium is injected.
- The pancreatic duct and hepatobiliary tree become visible.
- Rapid-sequence X-rays are taken after each contrast injection.
- A tissue specimen or fluid may be aspirated for histologic and cytologic examination.
- Therapeutic measures (sphincterectomy, stent placement, stone removal, or balloon dilatation) may be performed before endoscope withdrawal, as indicated.
- After the films are reviewed, the cannula is removed.

Patient care

- Withhold food and fluids until the gag reflex returns; then have the patient resume his usual diet.
- Provide soothing lozenges and warm saline gargles for sore throat.
- Monitor vital signs, cardiac rhythm, and pulse oximetry.
- Observe the patient's level of consciousness.
- Monitor the patient for abdominal distention and bowel sounds.
- Watch for adverse drug reactions.
- Monitor for complications.
- Emergency resuscitation equipment and a benzodiazepine and opioid antagonist should be immediately available during and after the test.

Complications

- Ascending cholangitis
- Pancreatitis
- Adverse drug reactions
- Cardiac arrhythmias
- Perforation of the bowel
- Respiratory depression
- Urine retention

Interpretation

Normal results

- Duodenal papilla appears as a small red or pale erosion protruding into the lumen.
- Pancreatic and hepatobiliary ducts usually join and empty through the duodenal papilla; separate orifices are sometimes present.
- Contrast medium uniformly fills the pancreatic duct, hepatobiliary tree, and gallbladder.

Abnormal results

- Hepatobiliary tree filling defects, strictures, or irregular deviations suggest possible biliary cirrhosis, primary sclerosing cholangitis, calculi, or cancer of the bile ducts.
- Filling defects, strictures, and irregular deviations of the pancreatic duct suggest possible pancreatic cysts and pseudocysts, pancreatic tumors, chronic pancreatitis, pancreatic fibrosis, calculi, or papillary stenosis.

Interfering factors

None known

Endoscopic ultrasound

Overview

- Combines ultrasonography and endoscopy to show the GI wall and adjacent structures.
- Endoscopic ultrasound (EUS) allows ultrasound imaging with high resolution.

Purpose

- To evaluate or stage lesions of the esophagus, stomach, duodenum, pancreas, ampulla, biliary ducts, and rectum
- To evaluate submucosal tumors

Procedure

Preparation

- Make sure the patient has signed an appropriate consent form.
- Note and report all allergies.
- Tell the patient that fasting is necessary for 6 to 8 hours before the test.
- For a sigmoid EUS, inform the patient that the scope will insert through the anus. He may have to take a laxative the evening before and may feel an urge to defecate during the study.
- An I.V. sedative may be given to help the patient relax before the endoscope insertion.
- Explain that the test takes 30 to 90 minutes.

Implementation

- Vital signs are monitored throughout the procedure.
- Oxygen saturation and cardiac rhythm are monitored if the patient receives I.V. sedation.
- Follow the procedures for esophagogastroduodenoscopy or sigmoidoscopy, depending on which type of EUS is to be performed.

Patient care

- Have the patient resume his usual diet and activity.
- Monitor vital signs, level of consciousness, and cardiac rhythm.
- Monitor for bleeding and signs and symptoms of perforation.
- The patient should avoid alcohol and driving for 24 hours after the test if he received I.V. sedation.
- Esophageal stricture hinders passage of the endoscope.

Complications

- Perforation
- Bleeding

Interpretation

Normal results

- Anatomy is normal, with no evidence of tumor.

Abnormal results

- Acute or chronic ulcers
- Benign or malignant tumors
- Inflammatory disease

Interfering factors

None known

Endoscopy

Overview

○ An endoscope shows the lining of a hollow viscus.
○ A cablelike cluster of glass fibers in the endoscope transmits light into the viscus; the image then returns to the scope's optical head or video monitor.

Purpose

○ To diagnose inflammatory, ulcerative, and infectious diseases
○ To diagnose benign and malignant tumors and other lesions of the mucosa

Procedure

Preparation

○ Make sure the patient has signed a consent form.
○ Note and report all allergies.
○ Give the patient an I.V. sedative to help him relax before the endoscope insertion.
○ Explain that the study takes about 1 hour.
○ For a patient taking an anticoagulant, it may be necessary to adjust his drugs.
○ For high-risk procedures, the patient should stop taking warfarin 3 to 5 days before the procedure; an appropriate drug such as low-molecular-weight heparin should be ordered.
○ Stop aspirin or nonsteroidal anti-inflammatory drugs 3 to 7 days before the study.

Implementation

○ I.V. access is started, if indicated.
○ Vital signs, pulse oximetry, and cardiac rhythm are monitored throughout the procedure.
○ Follow the procedure for the specific endoscopy to be performed (arthroscopy, bronchoscopy, colonoscopy, colposcopy, cystourethroscopy, endoscopic retrograde cholangiopancreatography, esophagogastroduodenoscopy, hysteroscopy, laparoscopy, laryngoscopy, mediastinoscopy, proctosigmoidoscopy, sigmoidoscopy, thoracoscopy).

Patient care

○ Provide a safe environment.
○ Withhold food and fluids until the gag reflex returns.
○ Have the patient resume his usual diet.
○ Monitor vital signs.
○ Monitor respiratory status and neurologic status.
○ Monitor cardiac rhythm.

Complications

○ Adverse reaction to sedation
○ Cardiac arrhythmias
○ Respiratory depression
○ Bleeding

Interpretation

Normal results

○ See the specific endoscopy procedure.

Abnormal results

○ See the specific endoscopy procedure.

Interfering factors

○ See specific endoscopy procedure.

Enteroclysis

Overview

○ Fluoroscopic examination of the small bowel using a contrast medium
○ Also called a *small-bowel enema*

Purpose

○ To diagnose and evaluate Crohn's disease
○ To diagnose Meckel's diverticulum
○ To aid in the diagnosis of small-bowel obstruction
○ To detect tumors

Procedure

Preparation

○ Make sure the patient has signed an appropriate consent form.
○ Note and report all allergies.
○ Instruct the patient to avoid using peristalsis-inhibiting drugs (such as Demerol or Percodan) on the day of the test.
○ Instruct the patient to restrict food and fluids.
○ Give the patient a laxative the afternoon before the examination.
○ Give the patient an I.V. sedative to help him relax.
○ Inform the patient that he'll be asked to change position frequently during the procedure.
○ Explain that the test takes about 45 minutes.

Implementation

○ The patient is given a local anesthetic. A small-lumen catheter is then inserted through the nose or mouth.
○ The catheter passes through the stomach and into the distal duodenum or the jejunum.
○ A contrast medium is instilled to distend and opacify the bowel loops.
○ The patient may receive metoclopramide to facilitate peristalsis.
○ Fluoroscopy and spot films are obtained.
○ After the films are reviewed, the catheter is removed.

Patient care

○ Assist the patient to the bathroom to expel the barium.
○ Monitor vital signs, intake and output, and feces.

Complications

○ Constipation
○ Adverse reactions to sedation, if used

Interpretation

Normal results

○ Size and contours of the small intestine are unremarkable.
○ Contrast travels through the bowl at a normal rate without any sign of obstruction.
○ Bowel loops and walls are visible and free of tumors, ulcers, and constrictions.

Abnormal results

○ Anatomical abnormalities of the bowel loops, diameter, and wall thickness may indicate Crohn's disease, tumors, partial or complete bowel obstruction, Meckel's diverticula, or congenital disorders.

Interfering factors

○ Complete gastric or duodenal obstruction

Eosinophils

Overview

- Measures the number of eosinophils in the blood.
- Eosinophils are white blood cells active in allergic diseases, parasitic infections, and other disorders.

Purpose

- To detect abnormal blood differential or suspected specific diseases
- To evaluate for Hodgkin's disease

Procedure

Preparation

- Explain to the patient that this test requires a blood sample.
- Tell the patient that he need not restrict food or drink.
- Inform the patient that he may feel slight discomfort from the tourniquet and needle puncture.

Implementation

- Perform a venipuncture to collect the blood sample in a 5-ml ethylenediaminetetraacetic acid tube.

Patient care

- Apply pressure to the venipuncture site.

Complications

- Hematoma at the venipuncture site

Interpretation

Normal results

- Fewer than 350 cells per microliter (cells/µl)

Abnormal results

- Increased count is often linked to allergic diseases and parasites.
- Decreased count may indicate alcohol intoxication and excessive production of adrenocorticosteroids.

Interfering factors

- Some drugs, such as tranquilizers and certain antibiotics

Epstein-Barr virus antibodies

Overview

○ The Epstein-Barr virus (EBV) causes heterophil-positive infectious mononucleosis, Burkitt's lymphoma, and nasopharyngeal carcinoma.
○ Although the virus doesn't replicate in standard cell cultures, most EBV infections are recognizable by testing the patient's serum for heterophil antibodies (*monospot test*), which usually appear within the first 3 weeks of illness and then decline rapidly within a few weeks.
○ In about 10% of adults and a larger percentage of children, the monospot test result is negative despite primary infection with EBV.
○ EBV has been linked to lymphoproliferative processes in immunosuppressed patients; these disorders occur with reactivated, rather than primary, EBV infections and are therefore, also, monospot-negative.
○ EBV-specific antibodies, which develop to several antigens of the virus during active infection, can be measured with a high level of sensitivity and specificity by *indirect immunofluorescence*.

Purpose

○ To provide a laboratory diagnosis of heterophil- (or monospot-) negative cases of infectious mononucleosis
○ To determine the antibody status to EBV of immunosuppressed patients with lymphoproliferative processes

Procedure

Preparation

○ Explain the purpose of the test to the patient.
○ Tell the patient that the test requires a blood sample.
○ Explain who will perform the venipuncture and when.
○ Explain to the patient that he may experience slight discomfort from the tourniquet and needle puncture.

Implementation

○ Perform a venipuncture and collect 5 ml of sterile blood in a clot-activator tube.
○ Allow the blood to clot for at least 1 hour at room temperature.
○ Handle the sample gently to prevent hemolysis.
○ Transfer the serum to a sterile tube or vial and send it to the laboratory immediately.
○ If transfer can't occur immediately, store the serum at 39.2° F (4° C) for 1 to 2 days or at −4° F (−20° C) for longer periods to prevent contamination.

Patient care

○ Apply direct pressure to the venipuncture site until bleeding stops.

Complications

○ Hematoma at the venipuncture site

Interpretation

Normal results

○ Sera from patients who have never been infected with EBV have no detectable antibodies to the virus as measured by either the monospot test or the indirect immunofluorescence test.
○ The monospot test result is positive only during the acute phase of infection with EBV; the indirect immunofluorescence test detects and discriminates between acute and past infection with the virus.

Abnormal results

○ EBV infection can be ruled out if no antibodies to EBV antigens are detected in the indirect immunofluorescence test.
○ A positive monospot test result or an indirect immunofluorescence test result that's positive for immunoglobulin (Ig) M or negative for Epstein-Barr nuclear antigen (EBNA) indicates acute EBV infection.
○ A monospot-negative result doesn't necessarily rule out acute or past infection with EBV. Conversely, an IgG class antibody to viral capsid antigen and EBNA antigens (IgM-negative) indicates remote (more than 2 months) infection with EBV.
○ Most cases of monospot-negative infectious mononucleosis are caused by cytomegalovirus infections.

Interfering factors

○ Hemolysis from rough handling of the sample

Erythrocyte sedimentation rate

Overview

○ Erythrocyte sedimentation rate (ESR) measures the degree of erythrocyte settling in a blood sample during a specified period.
○ Sensitive but nonspecific test that's often the earliest indicator of disease when other chemical or physical signs are normal.
○ Usually increases significantly in widespread inflammatory disorders; prolonged elevations may exist in localized inflammation and malignant disease.

Purpose

○ To monitor inflammatory or malignant disease
○ To aid detection and diagnosis of occult disease, such as tuberculosis, tissue necrosis, or connective tissue disease

Procedure

Preparation

○ Explain to the patient that the ESR test evaluates the condition of red blood cells.
○ Tell the patient that the test requires a blood sample. Explain who will perform the venipuncture and when.
○ Explain to the patient that he may feel slight discomfort from the tourniquet and needle puncture.
○ Inform the patient that he need not restrict food and fluids.

Implementation

○ Perform a venipuncture and collect the sample in a 4.5-ml tube with ethylenediaminetetraacetic acid added or in a tube with sodium citrate added. (Check with the laboratory to determine its preference.)
○ Completely fill the collection tube and invert it gently several times to thoroughly mix the sample and the anticoagulant.
○ Because prolonged standing decreases the ESR, examine the sample for clots or clumps and send it to the laboratory immediately. It must be tested within 2 to 4 hours.
○ Handle the sample gently to prevent hemolysis.

Patient care

○ Ensure that subdermal bleeding has stopped before removing pressure.
○ For large hematoma at the venipuncture site, monitor pulses distal to the phlebotomy site.

Complications

○ Hematoma at the venipuncture site

Interpretation

Normal results

○ In men, ESR is up to 10 mm/hour (SI, 0 to 10 mm/hour); in women, up to 20 mm/hour (SI, 0 to 20 mm/hour).
○ ESR gradually increases with age.

Abnormal results

○ ESR rises in pregnancy, anemia, acute or chronic inflammation, tuberculosis, paraproteinemias (especially multiple myeloma and Waldenström's macroglobulinemia), rheumatic fever, rheumatoid arthritis, and some cancers.
○ Polycythemia, sickle cell anemia, hyperviscosity, and low plasma fibrinogen or globulin levels tend to depress the ESR.

Interfering factors

○ Failure to use the proper anticoagulant, to adequately mix the sample and the anticoagulant, or to send the sample to the laboratory immediately
○ Use of a small-gauge needle for blood aspirations
○ Hemolysis from rough handling or excessive mixing of the sample
○ Hemoconcentration from prolonged tourniquet constriction

Erythropoietin

Overview

○ Erythropoietin (EPO) test of renal hormone production measures EPO by immunoassay.
○ Evaluates anemia, polycythemia, and kidney tumors.
○ Evaluates abuse of commercially prepared EPO by athletes who believe the drug enhances performance.
○ A glycoprotein hormone, EPO is secreted by the liver in a fetus, but by the kidney in an adult.
○ The hormone acts on stem cells in the bone marrow to stimulate production of red blood cells (RBCs) and is regulated by a feedback loop involving red cell volume and oxygen saturation of the blood, especially in the brain.

Purpose

○ To aid the diagnosis of anemia and polycythemia
○ To aid the diagnosis of kidney tumors
○ To detect EPO abuse by athletes

Procedure

Preparation

○ Explain to the patient that this test determines if hormonal secretion is causing changes in his RBCs.
○ Instruct the patient to fast for 8 to 10 hours before the test.
○ Tell the patient that the test requires a blood sample. Explain who will perform the venipuncture and when.
○ Explain to the patient that he may experience slight discomfort from the tourniquet and needle puncture.
○ Keep the patient relaxed and recumbent for 30 minutes before the test.

Implementation

○ Perform a venipuncture and collect the sample in a 5-ml clot-activator tube.
○ If requested, draw a hematocrit at the same time by collecting an additional sample in a 2-ml ethylenediaminetetraacetic tube.
○ Handle the sample gently to prevent hemolysis.

Patient care

○ Apply direct pressure to the venipuncture site until bleeding stops.

Complications

○ Hematoma at the venipuncture site

Interpretation

Normal results

○ 5 to 36 mU/ml (SI, 5 to 36 IU/L)

Abnormal results

○ Low levels of EPO appear in the patient with anemia who has inadequate or absent hormone production.
○ Congenital absence of EPO can occur.
○ Severe renal disease may decrease EPO production.
○ Elevated EPO levels occur in anemias as a compensatory mechanism in the reestablishment of homeostasis.
○ Inappropriate elevations (when the hematocrit is normal to high) are present in polycythemia and EPO-secreting tumors.
○ Some athletes use EPO to enhance performance. The increased RBC volume conveys additional oxygen-carrying capacity to the blood. Adverse reactions include clotting abnormalities, headache, seizures, hypertension, nausea, vomiting, diarrhea, and rash.

Interfering factors

○ Failure to collect a sample in the fasting state
○ Hemolysis from rough handling of the sample

Esophageal acidity test

Overview

- Sensitive indicator of gastric reflux
- Indicated for patients who complain of persistent heartburn with or without regurgitation
- Measures esophageal sphincter pressure

Purpose

- To evaluate the competence of the lower esophageal sphincter
- To measure intraesophageal pH

Procedure

Preparation

- Make sure the patient has signed an appropriate consent form.
- Note and report all allergies.
- Withhold antacids, anticholinergics, cholinergics, adrenergic-receptor blockers, alcohol, corticosteroids, histamine-2 receptor antagonists, proton pump inhibitors, and reserpine for 24 hours before the test.
- Instruct the patient to fast and avoid smoking after midnight before the test.
- Warn the patient that he might experience slight discomfort and may cough or gag during passage of a tube through his mouth and into the stomach.
- Explain that the test takes about 45 minutes.

Implementation

- The patient is placed high Fowler's position.
- A catheter, with pH electrode, is inserted into the mouth and advanced to the lower esophageal sphincter.
- The patient performs a Valsalva maneuver or lifts his legs to stimulate reflux.
- The intraesophageal pH is determined.

ALERT During insertion, the catheter may enter the trachea; if respiratory distress or paroxysmal coughing occurs, clamp the catheter and remove it immediately.

Patient care

- Have the patient resume medications and his diet.
- Provide soothing lozenges for a sore throat.
- Clamp the catheter before removing it to prevent aspiration.

Complications

- Aspiration of gastric contents
- Respiratory distress

Interpretation

Normal results

- The esophagus pH is greater than 5.0.

Abnormal results

- An intra-esophageal pH of 1.5 to 2.0 indicates gastric acid reflux caused by incompetence of the lower esophageal sphincter.

Interfering factors

None known

Esophagogastro-duodenoscopy

Overview

○ Esophagogastroduodenoscopy (EGD) is the visual examination of the lining of the esophagus, stomach, and upper duodenum, using a flexible fiber-optic endoscope
○ Contraindicated in patients with Zenker's diverticulum, a large aortic aneurysm, a recent ulcer perforation, known or suspected viscus perforation, or an unstable cardiac or pulmonary condition

Purpose

○ To detect small or surface lesions missed by radiography
○ To diagnose inflammatory disease, tumors, ulcers, and structural abnormalities
○ To evaluate the stomach and duodenum postoperatively
○ To obtain specimens for laboratory evaluation
○ To allow removal of foreign bodies by suction, snare, or forceps

Procedure

Preparation

○ Note and report all allergies.
○ Instruct the patient to fast for 6 to 12 hours before the test.
○ Inform the patient that the procedure involves passing a flexible tube through the mouth.
○ Explain that a bitter-tasting local anesthetic will be sprayed into the mouth and throat to suppress the gag reflex.
○ Tell the patient that he will receive an I.V. line to allow administration of a sedative or I.V. fluids.
○ Remove the patient's dentures.
○ Insert a mouth guard to protect the patient's teeth from the endoscope.
○ Explain to the patient that he'll remain conscious during the procedure.
○ Explain that the test takes about 30 minutes.
○ Explain that belching of insufflated air after the test is normal, as is a sore throat for 3 to 4 days after the test.

Implementation

○ Vital signs, cardiac rhythm, and pulse oximetry are monitored throughout the procedure.
○ When emergent EGD is performed, the stomach contents are aspirated through a nasogastric tube.
○ Assist the patient into a left lateral position.
○ The endoscope is inserted into the mouth and advanced under direct vision to examine the esophagus and the cardiac sphincter, then advanced into the stomach.
○ After examination of the stomach, the endoscope is advanced into the duodenum.
○ The endoscope is slowly withdrawn and suspicious areas reexamined.
○ Air may be instilled to open the bowel lumen and flatten tissue folds during the test.
○ Tissue specimens are sent to the laboratory for analysis.

Patient care

○ Provide a safe environment until the patient has recovered from sedation.
○ Withhold food and fluids until the gag reflex returns.
○ Provide throat lozenges and warm saline gargles for sore throat.
○ Instruct the patient to avoid consuming alcohol, operating any machinery, and driving for 24 hours after I.V. sedation.
○ Instruct the patient to report persistent difficult swallowing, pain, fever, black feces, or bloody vomitus.

⚠ *ALERT Observe for and report evidence of aspiration of gastric contents, which could precipitate aspiration pneumonia.*

⚠ *ALERT Monitor the patient for signs and symptoms of perforation. Perforation in the cervical area of the esophagus produces pain upon swallowing and neck movement. Thoracic perforation causes substernal or epigastric pain that increases with breathing or with movement of the trunk. Diaphragmatic perforation produces shoulder pain and dyspnea. Gastric perforation causes abdominal or back pain, fever, or pleural effusion.*

○ Monitor vital signs and cardiac rhythm.
○ Monitor intake and output.
○ Observe closely for drug adverse effects and have emergency resuscitation equipment immediately available.

Complications

○ Adverse reaction to sedation
○ Aspiration of gastric contents
○ Aspiration pneumonia
○ Perforation of the esophagus, stomach, or duodenum

Interpretation

Normal results

○ The esophageal mucosa is smooth and yellow-pink with fine vascular markings.
○ The gastric mucosa is orange-red beginning at the Z line, an irregular transition line slightly above the esophagogastric junction.
○ Rugae are present in the stomach.
○ The duodenal bulb mucosa is reddish and marked by a few shallow longitudinal folds.
○ The distal duodenum has prominent circular folds, lined with villi.

Abnormal results

○ Anatomic abnormalities of the stomach and duodenum suggest acute or chronic ulcers, benign or malignant tumors, or diverticula.
○ Inflammatory changes suggest esophagitis, gastritis, and duodenitis.
○ Anatomic abnormalities of the esophagus suggest tumors, varices, Mallory-Weiss syndrome, esophageal stenoses, and esophageal hiatal hernia.

Interfering factors

○ EGD shouldn't be performed within 2 days after an upper GI series because barium can obscure visual examination

Estrogen (serum estrone, estradiol, and estriol)

Overview

○ Radioimmunoassay that measures levels of estradiol, estrone, and estriol (the only estrogens that appear in serum in measurable amounts) and can help diagnose gonadal dysfunction in women.
○ Hypothalamic pituitary function tests confirm the diagnosis.
○ Estrogens (and progesterone) are secreted by the ovaries under the influence of the pituitary gonadotropins, follicle-stimulating hormone (FSH), and luteinizing hormone (LH).
○ Estrogens — in particular, estradiol, the most potent estrogen — interact with the hypothalamic-pituitary axis through negative and positive feedback mechanisms (slowly rising or sustained high levels inhibit secretion of FSH and LH [negative feedback], but a rapid rise in estrogen just before ovulation seems to stimulate LH secretion [positive feedback]).
○ Estrogens are responsible for the development of secondary sexual characteristics in women and for normal menstruation; levels are usually undetectable in children.
○ Secreted by ovarian follicular cells during the first half of the menstrual cycle and by the corpus luteum during the luteal phase and during pregnancy.
○ In menopause, estrogen secretion drops to a constantly low level.

Purpose

○ To determine sexual maturation and fertility
○ To aid the diagnosis of gonadal dysfunction, such as precocious or delayed puberty, menstrual disorders (especially amenorrhea), and infertility
○ To determine fetal well-being
○ To aid the diagnosis of tumors known to secrete estrogen

Procedure

Preparation

○ Explain to the patient that this test helps determine whether secretion of female hormones is normal and that it may be necessary to repeat the test during the various phases of the menstrual cycle.
○ Tell the patient that she need not restrict food and fluids.
○ Tell the patient that the test requires a blood sample. Explain who will perform the venipuncture and when.
○ Explain to the patient that she may experience slight discomfort from the tourniquet and needle puncture.

○ Withhold all steroid and pituitary-based hormones. If the patient must continue them, note this on the laboratory request.

Implementation

○ Perform a venipuncture and collect the sample in a 10-ml clot-activator tube.
○ If the patient is premenopausal, indicate the phase of her menstrual cycle on the laboratory request.
○ Handle the sample gently to prevent hemolysis.
○ Send the sample to the laboratory immediately.

Patient care

○ Apply direct pressure to the venipuncture site until bleeding stops.
○ Instruct the patient that she may resume medications stopped before the test.

Complications

○ Hematoma at the venipuncture site

Interpretation

Normal results

○ For premenopausal women, 26 to 149 pg/ml (SI, 90 to 550 pmol/L)
○ For postmenopausal women, 0 to 34 pg/ml (SI, 0 to 125 pmol/L)
○ In men, 12 to 34 pg/ml (SI, 40 to 125 pmol/ L)
○ In children younger than age 6, 3 to 10 pg/ml (SI, 10 to 36 pmol/L).
○ In pregnant women, estriol level is 2 nanograms/ ml (SI, 7 nmol/L) by 30 weeks' gestation to 30 nanograms/ml (SI, 105 nmol/L) by week 40.

Abnormal results

○ Decreased levels may indicate primary hypogonadism, or ovarian failure, as in Turner's syndrome or ovarian agenesis; secondary hypogonadism, such as in hypopituitarism; or menopause.
○ Increased levels may occur with estrogen-producing tumors; in precocious puberty; in severe hepatic disease, such as cirrhosis; and in congenital adrenal hyperplasia.

Interfering factors

○ Hemolysis from rough handling of the sample
○ Pregnancy and pretest use of estrogens such as hormonal contraceptives (possible increase)
○ Clomiphene, an estrogen antagonist (possible decrease)
○ Steroids and pituitary-based hormones such as dexamethasone

Evoked potential studies

Overview

○ Measures the brain's electrical response to stimulation of the sensory organs or peripheral nerves.
○ Evaluates visual, somatosensory, and auditory nerve pathways.
○ Electrodes attached to the scalp and skin over various peripheral sensory nerves detect and record electronic impulses.
○ Computer extracts low-amplitude impulses from background brain wave activity and averages the signals from repeated stimuli.
○ The test can be used during therapeutic coma and in trauma brain-injured patients.

Purpose

○ To aid the diagnosis of nervous system lesions and abnormalities
○ To monitor spinal cord function during spinal surgery
○ To assess neurologic function
○ To evaluate neurologic function in infants
○ To monitor comatose or anesthetized patients

Procedure

Preparation

○ Make sure the patient has signed a consent form.
○ Note and report all allergies.
○ Provide reassurance to the patient that the electrodes won't hurt, but that he may feel a small shock when somatosensory evoked responses occur.
○ Encourage the patient to relax because tension can affect the test results.
○ Explain that the test takes 45 to 60 minutes.

Implementation

○ The patient is positioned in a reclining or straight-backed chair or on a bed.
○ The patient is asked to relax and remain still.
○ Depending on the specific type of evoked potential study, electrodes may be attached.
○ Visual evoked potentials, produced by exposing the eye to a rapidly reversing checkerboard pattern, help evaluate demyelinating disease (such as multiple sclerosis), traumatic injury, and puzzling visual complaints.
○ Somatosensory evoked potentials, produced by electrically stimulating a peripheral sensory nerve, help diagnose peripheral nerve disease and locate brain and spinal cord lesions.
○ Auditory brain stem evoked potentials, produced by delivering clicks to the ear, are used in locating auditory lesions and evaluating brain stem integrity and in assessing brainstem integrity when cranial nerve testing is inconclusive or cannot be performed.
○ A computer amplifies and averages the brain's response to each stimulus and plots the results as a waveform.

Patient care

○ Monitor the patient's response to testing.

Complications

None known

Interpretation

Normal results

○ In visual evoked potential testing, the most significant wave on the waveform is P100, a positive wave appearing about 100 msec after the pattern-shift stimulus is applied.
○ Normal results vary greatly among laboratories and patients.
○ In somatosensory evoked potential testing, the waveforms vary, depending on locations of the stimulating and recording electrodes.

Abnormal results

○ In visual evoked potential testing, abnormal (extended) P100 latencies confined to one eye suggest a visual pathway lesion anterior to the optic chiasm; bilateral abnormal P100 latencies suggest multiple sclerosis.
○ In somatosensory evoked potential testing, changes in the electrical waveforms may indicate damaged or degenerated nerve pathways to the brain from the eyes, ears, or limbs. Absence of activity in a pathway may mean complete loss of nerve function in that pathway.
○ Other changes may provide evidence of the type and location of nerve damage.
○ Abnormal upper-limb interwave latencies suggest possible cervical spondylosis, intracerebral lesions, or sensorimotor neuropathies.
○ Abnormalities in the lower limb suggest peripheral nerve and root lesions such as those in Guillain-Barré syndrome.

Interfering factors

○ Extremely poor visual acuity can hinder the accurate determination of visual evoked potentials

Excretory urography

Overview

○ Allows imaging of the renal parenchyma, calyces, and pelvis as well as the ureters, bladder, and sometimes the urethra after I.V. administration of a contrast medium
○ Also known as *intravenous pyelography* or *IVP*; contraindicated in patients with abnormal renal function and in children or elderly patients with actual or potential dehydration

Purpose

○ To evaluate the structure and excretory function of the kidneys, ureters, and bladder
○ To support a differential diagnosis of renovascular hypertension

Procedure

Preparation

○ Make sure the patient has signed an appropriate consent form.
○ Note and report all allergies.
○ Check the patient's history for hypersensitivity to iodine, iodine-containing foods, or iodinated contrast media.
○ Instruct the patient to fast for 8 hours before the test.
○ Give a laxative, if necessary, the night before the test.
○ Obtain and report any abnormal results of renal function testing, such as blood urea nitrogen and creatinine.
○ Warn the patient that he might experience a transient burning sensation and metallic taste with injection of the contrast agent.
○ Explain that the test takes about 30 to 45 minutes.

Implementation

○ The patient is assisted into a supine position.
○ A kidney-ureter-bladder X-ray is performed.
○ I.V. contrast medium is injected.
○ X-rays are obtained at regular intervals.
○ Ureteral compression is performed after the 5-minute film to facilitate retention of the contrast medium by the upper urinary tract.
○ After the 10-minute film, ureteral compression is released.
○ Another film is taken of the lower halves of both ureters and bladder.
○ The patient voids and final films are taken immediately to show residual bladder contents or mucosal abnormalities of the bladder or urethra.

Patient care

○ Observe the patient for delayed reactions to the contrast medium.
○ Continue I.V. fluids or provide oral fluids to promote hydration.
○ If the patient has pyelonephritis, he may have to take antibiotics.

Complications

○ Adverse reaction to the contrast media
○ Dehydration
○ Impaired renal function.

Interpretation

Normal results

○ Kidneys, ureters, and bladder show no gross evidence of soft- or hard-tissue lesions.
○ Visualization of the contrast medium in the kidneys occurs promptly.
○ Bilateral renal parenchyma and pelvicaliceal systems have normal conformity.
○ No postvoiding mucosal abnormality and little residual urine.

Abnormal results

○ Anatomic abnormalities may suggest renal and ureteral calculi, supernumerary or absent kidney, polycystic kidney disease, redundant pelvis or ureter, space-occupying lesions or tumors, renal, bladder, or ureteral hematoma, laceration, or trauma, or hydronephrosis.

Interfering factors

○ Fecal matter, gas, or retained barium in the colon from a previous diagnostic study

Exophthalmometry

Overview

○ Determines the relative forward protrusion of the eye from its orbit, or the anteroposterior position of the globe in the orbit.
○ An exophthalmometer is a horizontal calibrated bar with movable carriers holding mirrors inclined at a 45-degree angle; it measures the distance from the apex of the cornea to the lateral orbital margin.

Purpose

○ To measure the amount of forward protrusion of the eye
○ To evaluate progression or regression of exophthalmos
○ To provide information about conditions that displace the eye in the orbit, such as thyroid disease, tumors of the eye, cavernous sinus thrombosis, and orbital filtration from leukemia

Procedure

Preparation

○ Make sure the patient has signed an appropriate consent form.
○ Note and report all allergies.
○ Explain that the study takes 5 to 10 minutes.

Implementation

○ The patient sits upright facing the examiner with his eyes on the same level.
○ The horizontal bar of the exophthalmometer is held in front of the patient's eyes, parallel to the floor.
○ The two small concave mirrors of the device are moved against the lateral orbital margins at the deepest angle.
○ The calibrated bar reading is recorded for a baseline reading.
○ The patient fixates his right eye on the examiner's left eye.
○ Using the inclined mirrors, the apex of the right cornea is superimposed on the millimeter scale.
○ Left eye, right eye, and biocular readings are obtained, representing the eye's relative forward displacement from its orbit.
○ The patient fixates his left eye on the examiner's right eye, and the procedure is repeated.
○ For follow-up examinations, the calibrated bar is set at the baseline reading.

Patient care

○ Refer the patient to an appropriate specialist as needed.
○ Inform the patient that exophthalmos resulting from a systemic disorder, such as thyroid disease as well as xanthomatosis or a blood dyscrasia, will require a complete medical examination.

Complications

None known

Interpretation

Normal results

○ Average readings are 15 to 17 mm for adults, with a range of 12 to 22 mm.
○ Measurements for each eye are similar, usually differing by 1.5 mm or less and rarely by more than 3 mm.
○ Repeated readings shouldn't vary more than 1 mm.

Abnormal results

○ A difference between the eyes of > 2 mm suggests exophthalmos or enophthalmos.
○ A single reading > 20 mm may indicate exophthalmos.
○ A reading < 12 mm may indicate enophthalmos.
○ Bilateral exophthalmos suggests a possible systemic disorder such as thyroid disease as well as xanthomatosis or a blood dyscrasia.

Interfering factors

None known

External fetal monitoring

Overview

○ Electronic transducer and a cardiotachometer amplify and record fetal heart rate (FHR) while a pressure-sensitive transducer (tocodynamometer) records uterine contractions. (See *Understanding fetal monitoring terminology*.)
○ Records the baseline FHR (average FHR over two contraction cycles or 10 minutes), periodic fluctuations in the baseline FHR, and beat to beat heart rate variability.
○ Also used during other tests of fetal health, notably the nonstress test and the contraction stress test (CST).

Purpose

○ To measure FHR and the frequency of uterine contractions
○ To evaluate antepartum and intrapartum fetal health during stress and nonstress situations
○ To detect fetal distress
○ To determine the necessity for internal fetal monitoring

Procedure

Preparation

○ Explain to the patient that external fetal monitoring assesses fetal health.
○ Explain the procedure to the patient and answer all her questions. Assure her that external fetal monitoring is painless and won't hurt the fetus or interfere with normal labor.
○ If monitoring will occur antepartum, instruct the patient to eat a meal just before the test to increase fetal activity, which decreases the test time.
○ If the patient is still smoking, advise her to abstain for 2 hours before testing because smoking decreases fetal activity.
○ Explain to the patient that she may have to restrict movement during baseline readings but that she may change position between the readings.

Implementation

○ Place the patient in the semi-Fowler or left lateral position with her abdomen exposed. Cover the ultrasound transducer receiver crystal with ultrasound transmission jelly.
○ Palpate the patient's abdomen to identify the fetal chest area and locate the most distinct fetal heart sounds; secure the ultrasound transducer over the area with the elastic band, stockinette, or abdominal strap.

○ Check the recording equipment to ensure an adequate printout and verify the alarm boundaries of the fetal monitor.
○ During monitoring, check the elastic band, stockinette, or abdominal strap to ensure that the fit is comfortable yet tight enough to produce a good tracing.
○ As labor progresses, reposition the pressure transducer as necessary so that it remains on the fundal portion of the uterus.
○ Reposition the ultrasound transducer whenever fetal or maternal position changes.

For antepartum monitoring with nonstress tests
○ Tell the patient to hold the pressure transducer in her hand and to push it each time she feels the fetus move.
○ Within a 20-minute period, monitor baseline FHR until you record two fetal movements that last longer than 15 seconds each and cause heart rate accelerations of more than 15 beats/minute from the baseline. If you can't obtain two FHR accelerations within 30 minutes, gently shake the patient's abdomen to stimulate the fetus and repeat the test.

For antepartum monitoring with a CST
○ Induce contractions by oxytocin infusion or nipple stimulation (endogenous oxytocin).
○ When giving oxytocin, infuse a dilute solution at a rate of 1 mU/minute, increasing the oxytocin rate until the patient experiences three contractions within 10 minutes, each lasting longer than 45 seconds.
○ When using nipple stimulation, tell the patient to stimulate one nipple by hand until contractions begin. If a second contraction doesn't occur in 2 minutes, have her stimulate the nipple again. Stimulate both nipples if contractions don't occur in 15 minutes. Continue the test until contractions occur in 10 minutes.
○ If no decelerations occur during three contractions, the patient may be discharged. Late decelerations during any of the contractions require notification of the physician and further tests.
○ Intrapartum monitoring: Secure the pressure transducer with an elastic band, a stockinette, or an abdominal strap over the area of greatest uterine electrical activity during contractions (usually the fundus).
○ Adjust the machine to record 0 to 10 mm Hg of pressure between palpable contractions.
○ Reposition the ultrasound and pressure transducers as necessary to ensure continuous accurate readings. Review the tracings frequently for baseline abnormalities, periodic changes, variability of changes, and uterine contraction abnormalities.
○ Record maternal movement, administration of drugs, and procedures performed directly on the tracing to assist in the evaluation of changes in the tracing.
○ Report abnormalities immediately.
○ Repeat antepartum monitoring weekly as long as indications, such as pregnancy over 42 weeks' gestation or fetal growth retardation, persist.

Patient care

○ Answer the patient's questions about the test.

Complications

○ Fetal distress with oxytocin infusion or nipple stimulation

Interpretation

Normal results

○ FHR ranges from 120 to 160 beats/minute, with a variability of 5 to 25 beats/minute.
○ *Antepartum nonstress test:* The fetus is considered healthy and should remain so for another week if two fetal movements causing a heart rate acceleration of more than 15 beats/minute from baseline FHR occur in a 20-minute period.
○ *Nonstress test:* A normal, healthy fetus usually has three rises in FHR within 10 to 15 minutes, but fetuses may sleep up to 45 minutes at a time. If there's no change in FHR in a 10-minute period, consider shaking the patient's abdomen gently, clapping loudly, or having the patient drink ice water or apple juice. If the FHR remains unchanged, a contraction stress test or biophysical profile test should be ordered. The fetus is assessed by watching fetal movements, muscle tone, fetal breathing, and the amniotic fluid index.
○ *CST:* The fetus is assumed to be healthy and should remain so for another week if three contractions occur during a 10-minute period, with no late decelerations.

Abnormal results

○ Bradycardia (FHR ≤ 120 beats/minute) may indicate fetal heart block, malposition, or hypoxia. Fetal bradycardia may also be drug-induced.
○ Tachycardia (FHR > 160 beats/minute) may result from maternal fever, tachycardia, hyperthyroidism, or use of vagolytic drugs or opioids; early fetal hypoxia; or fetal infection or arrhythmia.
○ Decreased variability (a fluctuation of < 5 beats/minute in the FHR) may indicate fetal arrhythmia or heart block; fetal hypoxia, central nervous system malformation, or infections; or vagolytic drugs.
○ FHR accelerations may result from early hypoxia. They may precede or follow variable decelerations and may indicate that the fetus is in a breech position.
○ Antepartum nonstress test: A positive result (fewer than two accelerations of FHR that last longer than 15 seconds each, with a heart rate acceleration of over 15 beats/minute) indicates an increased risk of perinatal morbidity and mortality and usually requires a CST.
○ CST: Persistent late decelerations during two or more contractions may indicate an increased risk of fetal morbidity or mortality.
○ Hyperstimulation (long or frequent uterine contractions) or suspicious results require biophysical profile assessment.

Understanding fetal monitoring terminology

- Baseline fetal heart rate (FHR): Average FHR over two contraction cycles or 10 minutes
- Baseline changes: Fluctuations in FHR unrelated to uterine contractions
- Periodic changes: Fluctuations in FHR related to uterine contractions
- Amplitude: Difference in beats per minute between baseline readings and fluctuation in FHR
- Recovery time: Difference between the end of the contraction and the return to the baseline FHR
- Acceleration: Transient rise in FHR lasting longer than 15 seconds and related to a uterine contraction
- Deceleration: Transient fall in FHR related to a uterine contraction
- Lag time: Difference between the peak of the contraction and the lowest point of deceleration

○ If findings are unsatisfactory, cesarean delivery may be indicated.

Interfering factors

○ Maternal position, particularly if supine (may cause artifactual fetal distress)
○ Drugs that affect the sympathetic and parasympathetic nervous systems (possible low FHR)
○ Excessive maternal or fetal activity (possible difficulty in recording uterine contractions or FHR)
○ Maternal obesity (possible difficulty caused by density of abdominal wall)
○ Loose or dirty leads or transducer connections (possible production of artifacts)

Extractable nuclear antigen antibodies

Overview

○ Extractable nuclear antigen (ENA) is a complex of at least four antigens.
○ Ribonucleoprotein (RNP) is susceptible to degradation by ribonuclease.
○ Smith (Sm) antigen is an acidic nuclear protein that resists ribonuclease degradation.
○ The third and fourth antigens that are sometimes included in this group — Sjögren's syndrome A (SS-A) antigen and Sjögren's syndrome B (SS-B) antigen — form a precipitate when an antibody is present.
○ The RNP antibody test detects RNP autoantibodies, which are associated with systemic lupus erythematosus (SLE), progressive systemic sclerosis, and other rheumatic disorders; it aids in the differential diagnosis of systemic rheumatic disease and is a useful follow-up test for collagen vascular autoimmune disease.
○ The anti-Sm antibody test detects Sm autoantibodies, which are a specific marker for SLE; thus, positive results strongly suggest a diagnosis of SLE; also helps monitor collagen vascular autoimmune disease.
○ The Sjögren's antibody test detects the SS-B autoantibodies produced by Sjögren's syndrome (an immunologic abnormality sometimes associated with rheumatic arthritis and SLE) but doesn't confirm a diagnosis of Sjögren's syndrome.

Purpose

○ To aid in the differential diagnosis of autoimmune disease
○ To distinguish between anti-RNP and anti-Sm antibodies
○ To screen for anti-RNP antibodies (common in mixed connective tissue disease)
○ To screen for anti-Sm antibodies (common in SLE)
○ To support the diagnosis of collagen vascular autoimmune diseases
○ To monitor the patient's response to therapy

Procedure

Preparation

○ Explain to the patient that this test detects certain antibodies and that test results help determine diagnosis and treatment.
○ Explain that the test assess the effectiveness of treatment, when appropriate.
○ Inform the patient that he need not restrict food and fluids.
○ Tell the patient that the test requires a blood sample. Explain who will perform the venipuncture and when.

○ Explain to the patient that he may experience slight discomfort from the tourniquet and needle puncture.

Implementation

○ Perform a venipuncture and collect the sample in a 7-ml tube without additives.

Patient care

○ Because a patient with an autoimmune disease has a compromised immune system, check the venipuncture site for infection, and report changes promptly.
○ Keep a clean, dry bandage over the site for at least 24 hours.
○ Apply direct pressure to the venipuncture site until bleeding stops.

Complications

○ Hematoma at the venipuncture site

Interpretation

Normal results

○ Serum is negative for anti-RNP, anti-Sm, and SS-B antibodies.

Abnormal results

○ Anti-RNP antibodies are elevated in SLE (35% to 40% of cases) and in mixed connective tissue disease.
○ Anti-Sm antibodies are specific for SLE.
○ Anti–SS-A and anti–SS-B antibodies are elevated in Sjögren's syndrome (40% to 45% of cases).
○ Anti–SS-B antibodies are also elevated in SLE.

Interfering factors

○ Failure to send the sample to the laboratory immediately

Fasting plasma glucose

Overview

○ Measures plasma glucose levels after a 12- to 14-hour fast.
○ In patients with diabetes mellitus, absence or deficiency of insulin allows persistently high glucose levels.

Purpose

○ To screen for diabetes mellitus
○ To monitor drug or diet therapy in patients with diabetes mellitus

Procedure

Preparation

○ Explain to the patient that this test detects disorders of glucose metabolism and aids in the diagnosis of diabetes.
○ Tell the patient that the test requires a blood sample. Explain who will perform the venipuncture and when.
○ Explain to the patient that he may experience slight discomfort from the tourniquet and needle puncture.
○ Instruct the patient to fast for 12 to 14 hours before the test.
○ Notify the laboratory and physician of medications the patient is taking that may affect test results; it may be necessary to restrict them.
○ Alert the patient to the symptoms of hypoglycemia (weakness, restlessness, nervousness, hunger, and sweating) and tell him to report such symptoms immediately.

Implementation

○ Perform a venipuncture and collect the sample in a 5-ml clot-activator tube.
○ Send the sample to the laboratory immediately.
○ Note on the laboratory request when the patient last ate, when the sample was collected, and when the patient received the last pretest dose of insulin or oral antidiabetic drug (if applicable).

Patient care

○ Apply direct pressure to the venipuncture site until bleeding stops.
○ Provide a balanced meal or a snack.
○ Instruct the patient that he may resume his usual medications that were stopped before the test.

Complications

○ Hematoma at the venipuncture site

Interpretation

Normal results

○ Results vary according to the laboratory procedure.
○ After at least an 8-hour fast, 70 to 100 mg of true glucose per deciliter of blood (SI, 3.9 to 5.6 mmol/L).

Abnormal results

○ Levels of 126 mg/dl (SI, 7 mmol/L) or more, obtained on two or more occasions, confirm diabetes mellitus.
○ Borderline or transient increased levels require a 2-hour after-meal plasma glucose test or oral glucose tolerance test to confirm the diagnosis of diabetes.
○ Increased levels may indicate pancreatitis, recent acute illness (such as myocardial infarction), Cushing's syndrome, acromegaly, and pheochromocytoma.
○ Increased fasting plasma glucose levels may also stem from hyperlipoproteinemia (especially types III, IV, or V), chronic hepatic disease, nephrotic syndrome, brain tumor, sepsis, or gastrectomy with dumping syndrome and is typical in eclampsia, anoxia, and seizure disorders.
○ Low levels may result from hyperinsulinism, insulinoma, von Gierke's disease, functional and reactive hypoglycemia, myxedema, adrenal insufficiency, congenital adrenal hyperplasia, hypopituitarism, malabsorption syndrome, and hepatic insufficiency.

Interfering factors

○ Failure to observe pretest restrictions (possible increase)
○ Recent illness, infection, or pregnancy (possible increase)
○ Glycolysis because of failure to refrigerate the sample or send it to the laboratory immediately (possible false-negative)
○ Acetaminophen, if using the glucose oxidase or hexokinase method (possible false-positive)
○ Chlorthalidone, thiazide diuretics, furosemide, triamterene, hormonal contraceptives, benzodiazepines, phenytoin, phenothiazines, lithium, epinephrine, arginine, phenolphthalein, dextrothyroxine, diazoxide, large doses of nicotinic acid, corticosteroids, and recent I.V. glucose infusions (increase)
○ Ethacrynic acid (may cause hyperglycemia); large doses in patients with uremia (can cause hypoglycemia)
○ Beta blockers, ethanol, clofibrate, insulin, oral antidiabetic agents, and monoamine oxidase inhibitors (decrease)
○ Strenuous exercise (decrease)

Febrile agglutination

Overview

○ Provides important diagnostic information in patients with a fever of undetermined origin, with infection, and with other conditions in which microorganisms are difficult to isolate from blood or excreta
○ Includes Weil-Felix test for rickettsial disease, Widal's test for *Salmonella,* and tests for brucellosis and tularemia
Weil-Felix test
○ Establishes rickettsial antibody titers, using three forms of *Proteus* antigens (OX-19, OX-2, and OX-K) that cross-react with the various strains of rickettsiae.
○ Antibodies to certain rickettsial strains react with more than one *Proteus* antigen; antibodies to other strains don't react with any *Proteus* antigens.
Widal's test
○ Establishes titers for flagellar (H) and somatic (O) antigens, which may indicate *Salmonella* gastroenteritis and extraintestinal focal infections, caused by *S. enteritidis,* or enteric (typhoid) fever, caused by *S. typhosa.*
○ A third (Vi or envelope) antigen, which may indicate typhoid carrier status, commonly tests negative for H and O antigens.
Slide agglutination and tube dilution tests
○ Uses killed suspensions of the disease organisms as antigens.
○ Establishes titers for the gram-negative coccobacilli *Brucella* and *Francisella tularensis,* which cause brucellosis and tularemia, respectively.

Purpose

○ To support clinical findings in diagnosis of disorders caused by *Rickettsia, Salmonella, Brucella,* and *F. tularensis* organisms
○ To identify the cause of a fever of undetermined origin

Procedure

Preparation

○ Explain to the patient that this test detects and quantifies microorganisms that may cause fever and other symptoms.
○ Inform the patient that he need not restrict food and fluids.
○ Tell the patient that the test requires a blood sample. Explain who will perform the venipuncture and when.
○ Explain to the patient that he may experience slight discomfort from the tourniquet and needle puncture.

○ Explain to the patient that this test requires a series of blood samples to detect a pattern of titers characteristic of the suspected disorder, if appropriate. Reassure him that a positive result only suggests a disorder.
○ Note on the laboratory request when antimicrobial therapy began, if appropriate.

Implementation

○ Perform a venipuncture and collect the sample in a 7-ml clot-activator tube.

Patient care

○ Apply pressure to the venipuncture site until bleeding stops.
○ In a fever of undetermined origin and suspected infection, contact the facility's infection control department. Isolation may be necessary.

Complications

○ Hematoma at the venipuncture site

Interpretation

Normal results

○ Dilutions for rickettsial antibody are < 1:40, Salmonella antibody, < 1:80, brucellosis antibody, < 1:80, tularemia antibody, < 1:40.

Abnormal results

○ Observing the rise and fall of titers is crucial for detecting active infection. If this isn't possible, certain titer levels can suggest the disorder.
○ For all febrile agglutinins, a fourfold increase in titers is strong evidence of infection.
○ The Weil-Felix test result is positive for rickettsiae with antibodies to *Proteus* occurring 6 to 12 days after infection; titers peak in 1 month and usually drop to negative in 5 to 6 months. This test can't diagnose rickettsialpox or Q fever because the antibodies of these diseases don't cross-react with *Proteus* antigens; the test shows positive titers in *Proteus* infections and, in such cases, is nonspecific for rickettsiae.
○ In *Salmonella* infection, H and O agglutinins usually appear in serum after 1 week, and titers rise for 3 to 6 weeks. O agglutinins usually fall to insignificant levels in 6 to 12 months. Agglutinin titers may remain increased for years.
○ Although the absence of *Brucella* agglutinins doesn't rule out brucellosis, titers usually rise after 2 to 3 weeks and peak between 4 and 8 weeks.
○ In tularemia, titers usually become positive during the second week of infection, exceed 1:320 by the third week, peak within 4 to 7 weeks, and usually decline gradually 1 year after recovery.

Interfering factors

○ Failure to send the sample to the laboratory immediately

○ Vaccination or continuous exposure to bacterial or rickettsial infection, resulting in immunity (high titers)

○ Antibody cross-reaction with bacteria causing other infectious diseases, such as tularemia antibodies cross-reacting with *Brucella* antigens

○ Immunodeficiency (negative titers even during symptomatic infection because of inability to form antibodies)

○ Antibiotics (low titers early in the course of infection)

○ Hepatic disease or excessive drug use (high *Salmonella* titers)

○ Skin tests with *Brucella* antigen (possible high *Brucella* titers); *Proteus* infections (possible positive Weil-Felix titers for rickettsial disease)

Fecal lipids

Overview

- Lipids excreted in feces include monoglycerides, diglycerides, triglycerides, phospholipids, glycolipids, soaps (fatty acids and fatty acid salts), sterols, and cholesterol esters.
- Excessive excretion of fecal lipids (steatorrhea) occurs in several malabsorption syndromes.
- Qualitative and quantitative tests detect excessive excretion of lipids in patients exhibiting signs of malabsorption, such as weight loss, abdominal distention, and scaly skin.
- Qualitative test involves staining a specimen of feces with Sudan III dye and then examining it microscopically for evidence of malabsorption, such as undigested muscle fibers and various fats.
- The quantitative test involves drying and weighing a 72-hour specimen and then using a solvent to extract the lipids, which are subsequently evaporated and weighed.
- Only the quantitative test confirms steatorrhea.

Purpose

- To confirm steatorrhea

Procedure

Preparation

- Explain to the patient that the fecal lipid test evaluates fat digestion.
- Instruct the patient to abstain from alcohol and to maintain a high-fat diet (100 g/day) for 3 days before the test and during the collection period.
- Tell the patient that the test requires a 72-hour fecal collection.
- Notify the laboratory and physician of drugs the patient is taking that may affect test results; it may be necessary to restrict them.
- Explain to the patient how to collect a timed fecal specimen and provide him with the necessary equipment.
- Inform the patient that the laboratory requires 1 or 2 days to complete the analysis.

Implementation

- Collect a 72-hour fecal specimen.
- Don't use a waxed collection container because the wax may become incorporated in the feces and interfere with accurate testing.
- Tell the patient to avoid contaminating the fecal specimen with toilet tissue or urine.
- Refrigerate the collection container and keep it tightly covered.

Patient care

- Answer the patient's questions about the test.
- Instruct the patient that he may resume his usual diet and medications after the test.

Complications

None known

Interpretation

Normal results

- Less than 20% of excreted solids, with excretion more than 7 g/24 hours

Abnormal results

- Digestive disorders may affect the production and release of pancreatic lipase or bile; absorptive disorders may affect the intestine's integrity, causing steatorrhea.
- In pancreatic insufficiency, impaired lipid digestion may result from insufficient lipase production.
- Pancreatic resection, cystic fibrosis, chronic pancreatitis, or ductal obstruction by stone or tumor may prevent the normal release or action of lipase.
- In impaired hepatic function, faulty lipid digestion may result from inadequate bile salt production.
- Biliary obstruction may prevent the normal release of bile salts into the duodenum.
- Extensive small-bowel resection or bypass may also interrupt normal enterohepatic bile salt circulation.
- Diseases of the intestinal mucosa affect the normal absorption of lipids.
- Regional ileitis and atrophy caused by malnutrition cause gross structural changes in the intestinal wall; celiac disease and tropical sprue produce mucosal abnormalities.
- Scleroderma, radiation enteritis, fistulas, intestinal tuberculosis, small intestine diverticula, and altered intestinal flora may also cause steatorrhea.
- Whipple's disease and lymphomas cause lymphatic obstruction that may inhibit fat absorption.

Interfering factors

- Failure to observe pretest restrictions or the use of a waxed collection container
- Contaminated or incomplete specimen (total weight < 300 g)
- Alcohol, aluminum hydroxide, azathioprine, bisacodyl, calcium carbonate, colchicines, cholestyramine, kanamycin, neomycin, mineral oil, and potassium chloride (possible increase or decrease caused by inhibited absorption or altered chemical digestion)

Fecal occult blood

Overview

- Detectable by microscopic analysis or by chemical tests for hemoglobin, such as the guaiac test.
- Normally, feces contain small amounts of blood (2 to 2.5 ml/day); therefore, tests for occult blood detect quantities larger than this.
- Indicated when clinical symptoms and preliminary blood studies suggest GI bleeding.
- Additional tests are necessary to pinpoint the origin of the bleeding.

Purpose

- To detect GI bleeding
- To aid in the early diagnosis of colorectal cancer

Procedure

Preparation

- Explain to the patient that this test detects abnormal GI bleeding.
- Instruct the patient to maintain a high-fiber diet and to refrain from eating red meats, turnips, and horseradish for 48 to 72 hours before the test as well as throughout the collection period.
- Tell the patient that the test usually requires three fecal specimens but that sometimes only one sample is needed.
- Instruct the patient to avoid contaminating the fecal specimen with toilet tissue or urine.
- Notify the laboratory and physician of drugs the patient is taking that may affect test results; it may be necessary to restrict them. If the patient must continue using these drugs, note this on the laboratory request.

Implementation

- Collect three fecal specimens or a random fecal specimen.
- Obtain specimens from two different areas of each fecal specimen.

Hematest

- Use a wooden applicator to smear a bit of the fecal specimen on the filter paper supplied with the kit. Or, after performing a digital rectal examination, wipe the finger you used for the examination on a square of the filter paper. Place the filter paper with the fecal smear on a glass plate.
- Remove a reagent tablet from the bottle and immediately replace the cap tightly. Place the tablet in the center of the fecal smear on the filter paper. Add 1 drop of water to the tablet, and allow it to soak in for 5 to 10 seconds. Add a second drop, letting it run from the tablet onto the specimen and filter paper.
- After 2 minutes, the filter paper will turn blue if the test result is positive. Don't read the color that appears on the tablet itself or develops on the filter paper after the 2-minute period. Note the results and discard the filter paper. Remove and discard your gloves and wash your hands thoroughly.

Hemoccult test

- Open the flap on the slide pack and use a wooden applicator to apply a thin smear of the fecal specimen to the guaiac-impregnated filter paper exposed in box A. Apply a second smear from another part of the specimen to the filter paper exposed in box B.
- Let the specimen dry for 3 to 5 minutes. Open the flap at the rear of the slide package and place 2 drops of Hemoccult developing solution on the paper over each smear. A positive result yields a blue reaction in 30 to 60 seconds. Record the results and discard the slide package. Remove and discard your gloves and wash your hands thoroughly.

Instant-View fecal occult blood test

- Add a fecal sample to the collection tube. Shake it to mix the sample with the extraction buffer, and then dispense 4 drops into the sample well of the cassette.
- Results will appear on the test region and the control region of the cassette in 5 to 10 minutes, indicating whether the hemoglobin level is > 0.05 μg/ml of feces.

Patient care

- Answer the patient's questions about the test.
- After testing is complete, inform the patient that he may resume his normal diet and drug therapy.

Complications

None known

Interpretation

Normal results

- Less than 2.5 ml of blood in feces, resulting in a green reaction

Abnormal results

- GI bleeding, which may result from many disorders, such as varices, a peptic ulcer, carcinoma, ulcerative colitis, dysentery, or hemorrhagic disease

Interfering factors

- Failure to observe pretest restrictions
- Failure to test the specimen immediately or to send it to the laboratory immediately after collection
- Bromides, colchicines, indomethacin, iron preparations, phenylbutazone, rauwolfia derivatives, and steroids (possible increase from GI blood loss)
- Ascorbic acid (false-negative, even with significant bleeding)
- Ingestion of 2 to 5 ml of blood (for example, from bleeding gums)
- Active bleeding from hemorrhoids (possible false-positive results)

Ferritin

Overview

- Protein that stores iron in the body.
- This test provides information about the body's ability to store iron for later use.
- Usually performed with iron testing and total iron-binding capacity.

Purpose

- To measure a patient's iron level to determine whether there is too much or too little iron in the blood

Procedure

Preparation

- Inform the patient that he need not restrict food or beverages.
- Explain that the test will require a blood sample.
- Inform the patient that he may feel discomfort from the tourniquet and needle puncture.

Implementation

- Perform a venipuncture and collect the sample.

Patient care

- Apply direct pressure to the venipuncture site until bleeding stops.

Complications

- Hematoma at the venipuncture site

Interpretation

Normal results

- In men, 20 to 300 nanograms/ml (SI, 20 to 300 mcg/L)
- In women, 20 to 120 nanograms/ml (SI, 20 to 120 mcg/L)

Abnormal results

- Low levels may indicate iron deficiency, chronic GI bleeding, or heavy menstrual bleeding.
- High levels may indicate alcoholic liver disease, hemochromatosis, hemolytic anemia, Hodgkin's lymphoma, and megaloblastic anemia.

Interfering factors

None known

Fetal hemoglobin

Overview

○ Fetal hemoglobin (HbF) is a normal hemoglobin produced in the red blood cells of a fetus and in smaller amounts in infants.
○ Constitutes 50% to 90% of the hemoglobin level in a neonate; the remaining hemoglobin level consists of HbA_1 and HbA_2 (the hemoglobin level in adults).
○ Normally, the body stops making HbF during the first years of life and begins to make HbA.
○ If changeover doesn't occur and HbF continues to constitute more than 5% of the hemoglobin level after age 6 months, an abnormality may be present, particularly thalassemia.

Purpose

○ To diagnose thalassemia

Procedure

Preparation

○ Explain to the patient that the test detects thalassemia disease.
○ Tell the patient that the test requires a blood sample. Explain who will perform the venipuncture and when.
○ Reassure the patient that drawing the sample will take less than 3 minutes.
○ Explain to the patient that he may feel slight discomfort from the tourniquet and needle puncture.
○ If the patient is a child, explain to his parents that a small amount of blood will be taken from his finger or earlobe.
○ Inform the patient or his parents that he need not restrict food and fluids.

Implementation

○ Perform a venipuncture and collect the sample of blood in a 4.5-ml ethylenediaminetetraacetic acid tube.

 AGE AWARE For a young child, collect capillary blood in a microcollection device.

○ Completely fill the collection tube and invert it gently several times to mix the sample and the anticoagulant thoroughly.
○ Handle the sample gently to prevent hemolysis.

Patient care

○ Apply direct pressure to the venipuncture site until bleeding stops.
○ Ensure that subdermal bleeding has stopped before removing pressure.
○ If hematoma at the venipuncture site is large, monitor pulses distal to the site.

Complications

○ Hematoma at the venipuncture site

Interpretation

Normal results

○ In neonates up to age 1 month: 60% to 90% (SI, 0.60 to 0.90)
○ In children ages 1 to 23 months: 2% (SI, 0.02)
○ From age 24 months to adult: 0% to 2% (SI, 0 to 0.02)

Abnormal results

○ HbF level may be 30% or more of the total hemoglobin level in those with beta-thalassemia major.
○ HbF level may be slightly increased in unrelated hematologic disorders, such as aplastic anemia, homozygous sickle cell disease, and myeloproliferative disorders.
○ HbF level commonly increases to as much as 5% during normal pregnancy.

Interfering factors

○ Hemolysis from rough handling of the sample
○ Delay in analyzing the specimen for more than 2 to 3 hours (possible false-high)

Fetal-maternal erythrocyte distribution

Overview

- Measures the number of fetal red blood cells (RBCs) in the maternal circulation.
- Some transfer of RBCs from the fetal to the maternal circulation occurs during most spontaneous or elective abortions and most normal deliveries.
- Usually, the amount of blood transferred is minimal and has no clinical significance.
- Transfer of significant amounts of blood from an Rh-positive fetus to an Rh-negative mother can result in maternal immunization to the D antigen and the development of anti-D antibodies in the maternal circulation
- During a subsequent pregnancy, the maternal immunization subjects an Rh-positive fetus to potentially fatal hemolysis and erythroblastosis

Purpose

- To detect and measure fetal-maternal blood transfer
- To determine the amount of $Rh_0(D)$ immune globulin needed to prevent maternal immunization to the D antigen

Procedure

Preparation

- Explain to the patient that this test determines the amount of fetal blood transferred to the maternal circulation and helps determine the appropriate treatment, if necessary.
- Inform the patient that she need not restrict food and fluids.
- Tell the patient that the test requires a blood sample. Explain who will perform the venipuncture and when.
- Explain to the patient that she may experience slight discomfort from the tourniquet and needle puncture.
- Check the patient's history for recent administration of dextran, I.V. contrast media, or drugs that may alter results.

Implementation

- Perform a venipuncture and collect the sample in a 7-ml EDTA tube.
- Label the sample with the patient's name, the hospital or blood bank number, the date, and the phlebotomist's initials.
- Send the sample to the laboratory immediately with a properly completed laboratory request.

Patient care

- Apply direct pressure to the venipuncture site until bleeding stops.

Complications

- Hematoma at the venipuncture site

Interpretation

Normal results

- Maternal whole blood contains no fetal RBCs.

Abnormal results

- Increased fetal RBC volume in the maternal circulation requires more than one dose of $Rh_0(D)$ immune globulin.
- To determine the number of vials needed, divide the calculated milliliters of fetal-maternal hemorrhage by 30. (A single vial of $Rh_0(D)$ immune globulin protects against a 30-ml fetal-maternal hemorrhage.)
- To prevent complications in later pregnancies in an unsensitized Rh-negative mother, give her $Rh_0(D)$ immune globulin as soon as possible (no later than 72 hours) after the birth of an Rh-positive infant or after a spontaneous or elective abortion. Most physicians are now giving $Rh_0(D)$ immune globulin prophylactically at 28 weeks' gestation to women who are Rh-negative but have no detectable Rh antibodies.
- The following patients should be screened for Rh isoimmunization or irregular antibodies: all Rh-negative mothers during their first prenatal visit and at 28 weeks' gestation, and all Rh-positive mothers with histories of transfusion, a jaundiced infant, stillbirth, cesarean delivery, or induced or spontaneous abortion.

Interfering factors

- Delay of testing for more than 72 hours after sample collection

Fibrin split products

Overview

○ After a fibrin clot forms in response to vascular injury, the clot is eventually degraded by plasmin, a fibrin-dissolving enzyme.
○ Resulting fragments are known as fibrin split products (FSP), or *fibrinogen degradation products*.
○ Test detects FSP in the diluted serum that's left in a blood sample after clotting.

Purpose

○ To detect FSP in the circulation
○ To help determine the presence and severity of a hyperfibrinolytic state (such as disseminated intravascular coagulation [DIC]) that may result in primary fibrinogenolysis or hypercoagulability (See *Causes of disseminated intravascular coagulation.*)

Procedure

Preparation

○ Explain to the patient that the FSP test determines whether blood clots normally.
○ Tell the patient that the test requires a blood sample. Explain who will perform the venipuncture and when.
○ Explain to the patient that he may feel slight discomfort from the tourniquet and needle puncture.
○ Notify the laboratory and physician of drugs the patient is taking that may affect test results; it may be necessary to restrict them.

Causes of disseminated intravascular coagulation

Obstetric	Amniotic fluid embolism, eclampsia, retained dead fetus, retained placenta, abruptio placentae, and toxemia
Neoplastic	Sarcoma, metastatic carcinoma, acute leukemia, prostate cancer, and giant hemangioma
Infectious	Acute bacteremia, septicemia, and rickettsemia; viral, fungal, or protozoal infection
Necrotic	Trauma, destruction of brain tissue, extensive burns, heatstroke, rejection of transplant, and hepatic necrosis
Cardiovascular	Fat embolism, acute venous thrombosis, cardiopulmonary bypass surgery, hypovolemic shock, cardiac arrest, and hypotension
Other	Snakebite, cirrhosis, transfusion of incompatible blood, purpura, and glomerulonephritis

○ Inform the patient that he need not restrict food and fluids.

Implementation

○ Perform a venipuncture and draw 2 ml of blood into a plastic syringe.
○ Draw the sample before giving heparin to avoid false-positive test results.
○ Transfer the sample to the tube provided by the laboratory, which contains a soybean trypsin inhibitor and bovine thrombin.
○ Gently invert the collection tube several times to mix the contents thoroughly.
○ The blood clots within 2 seconds; after clotting, the sample must be sent immediately to the laboratory for incubation at 98.6° F (37° C) for 30 minutes before testing proceeds.

Patient care

○ Ensure that subdermal bleeding has stopped before removing pressure.
○ If hematoma at the venipuncture site is large, monitor pulses distal to the site.
○ Instruct the patient that he may resume any medications stopped before the test.

Complications

○ Hematoma at the venipuncture site

Interpretation

Normal results

○ Serum contains < 10 µg/ml (SI, , 10 mg/L) of FSP. A quantitative assay shows levels of < 3 µg/ml (SI, < 3 mg/L).

Abnormal results

○ FSP levels increase in primary fibrinolytic states because of increased levels of circulating profibrinolysin; in secondary states because of DIC and subsequent fibrinolysis; and in alcoholic cirrhosis, preeclampsia, abruptio placentae, congenital heart disease, sunstroke, burns, intrauterine death, pulmonary embolus, deep vein thrombosis (transient increase), and myocardial infarction (after 1 or 2 days).
○ FSP levels usually exceed 100 µg/ml (SI, >100 mg/L) in active renal disease or renal transplant rejection.

Interfering factors

○ Pretest administration of heparin (false-high)
○ Failure to fill the collection tube completely, to adequately mix the sample and additive, or to send the sample to the laboratory immediately
○ Hemolysis from rough handling of the sample
○ Fibrinolytic drugs, such as urokinase, streptokinase, and tissue plasminogen activator, and large doses of barbiturates (increase)

Fluorescein angiography

Overview

- Rapid-sequence blue-colored flash photographs of the fundus taken with a special camera after I.V. injection of a vegetable-based dye, sodium fluorescein
- Enhanced visibility of microvascular structures of the retina and choroids from fluorescein dye and sophisticated photographic equipment
- Permits evaluation of the entire retinal vascular bed, including retinal circulation
- May be used in conjunction with a photographic technique called indocyanine green (ICG) angiography in certain diseases to obtain further information

Purpose

- To document retinal circulation and the layers beneath the retina
- To aid in evaluating intraocular abnormalities

Procedure

Preparation

- Make sure the patient has signed an appropriate consent form.
- Note and report all allergies.
- Check the patient's history for glaucoma.
- Don't give miotic eyedrops on the day of the test.
- Warn the patient that he may experience a strobe-light effect during the test.
- Explain that the test takes about 30 minutes.
- Explain that the study is fairly painless and adverse effects are uncommon but may include nausea and mild urticaria.
- Inform the patient that skin and urine may appear yellow for 24 to 48 hours.

Implementation

- The patient is given mydriatic eyedrops.
- The patient is positioned in an examination chair facing the camera with his chin on the chin rest and his forehead against the bar.
- He is asked to open his eyes as widely as possible and stare straight ahead.
- The contrast medium is injected rapidly into the antecubital vein. Photographs — 25 to 30 — are taken in rapid sequence (1 second apart). Photographs may be taken up to 1 hour after the injection.

Patient care

- Encourage oral fluid intake to help excrete the dye.
- Caution the patient that his near vision will be blurred for up to 12 hours.
- Instruct the patient to avoid direct sunlight and driving during the period of blurred vision.
- Instruct the patient that his skin and urine will be slightly discolored for 24 to 48 hours after the test.

Complications

- Serious adverse effects (laryngeal edema, bronchospasm, and respiratory arrest) are possible. Have emergency resuscitation equipment at hand.
- Extravasation of the dye is painful and toxic to the tissues.

Interpretation

Normal results

- After rapid injection, sodium fluorescein reaches the retina in 12 to 15 seconds (filling phase).
- The retinal background appears evenly mottled (choroidal flush) during choroidal vessel and choriocapillary filling.
- The contrast fills the arteries (arterial phase).
- No leakage of contrast from retinal vessels is visible.

Abnormal results

- Abnormalities in the early filling phase suggest possible microaneurysms, arteriovenous shunts, and neovascularization.
- Delayed or absent flow of the dye through the arteries may indicate arterial stenosis or occlusion.
- Dilation of the vessels and fluorescein leakage may suggest venous occlusion.
- Recanalization and collateral circulation suggest chronic obstruction.
- Increased vascular tortuosity suggests hypertensive retinopathy.
- Leaking of fluorescence, surrounded by hard, yellow exudate, suggests possible aneurysms and capillary hemangiomas.
- Vascular leakage in the disk area suggests papilledema.

Interfering factors

None known

Fluorescent treponemal antibody absorption

Overview

○ The fluorescent treponemal antibody absorption (FTA-ABS or FTA) test uses indirect immunofluorescence to detect antibodies to the spirochete *Treponema pallidum* in serum.
○ Spirochete causes syphilis.
○ Prepared *T. pallidum* is fixed on a slide, and the patient's serum is added after the addition of an absorbed preparation of Reiter treponema.
○ This addition to the test serum prevents interference by antibodies from nonsyphilitic treponemas; Reiter treponema combines with most nonsyphilitic antibodies, making the FTA-ABS test specific for *T. pallidum.*
○ If syphilitic antibodies are present in the test serum, they will coat the treponemal organisms.
○ Slide is then stained with fluorescein-labeled antiglobulin; this antiglobulin attaches to the coated spirochetes, which fluoresce when viewed under an ultraviolet microscope.
○ Although the FTA-ABS test is generally performed on a serum sample to detect primary or secondary syphilis, a cerebrospinal fluid (CSF) specimen is required to detect tertiary syphilis.
○ Because antibody levels remain constant for long periods, the FTA-ABS test isn't recommended for monitoring the patient's response to therapy.

Purpose

○ To confirm primary and secondary syphilis
○ To screen for suspected false-positive results of the Venereal Disease Research Laboratory tests

Procedure

Preparation

○ Explain to the patient that this test can confirm or rule out syphilis.
○ Inform the patient that he need not restrict food and fluids.
○ Tell the patient that the test requires a blood sample. Explain who will perform the venipuncture and when.
○ Explain to the patient that he may experience slight discomfort from the tourniquet and needle puncture.

Implementation

○ Perform a venipuncture and collect the sample in a 7-ml clot-activator tube.
○ Handle the sample gently to prevent hemolysis.

Patient care

○ Apply direct pressure to the venipuncture site until bleeding stops.
○ If the test is reactive, explain the nature of syphilis and stress the importance of proper treatment and the need to find and treat the patient's sexual contacts.
○ Provide the patient with additional information about syphilis and how it's spread; emphasize the need for antibiotic therapy, if appropriate. Report positive results to state public health authorities and prepare the patient for mandatory inquiries.
○ If the test is nonreactive or findings are borderline but syphilis hasn't been ruled out, instruct the patient to return for follow-up testing; explain that inconclusive results don't necessarily indicate that he's free from the disease.

Complications

○ Hematoma at the venipuncture site

Interpretation

Normal results

○ Nonreactive result

Abnormal results

○ The presence of treponemal antibodies in the serum — a reactive test result — doesn't indicate the stage or severity of infection. (The presence of these antibodies in CSF is strong evidence of tertiary neurosyphilis.)
○ Increased antibody levels appear in most patients with primary syphilis and in almost all patients with secondary syphilis.
○ Increased antibody levels persist for several years, with or without treatment.
○ The absence of treponemal antibodies, a nonreactive test result, doesn't necessarily rule out syphilis. *T. pallidum* causes no detectable immunologic changes in the blood for 14 to 21 days after initial infection.
○ Organisms may be detected earlier by examining suspicious lesions with a darkfield microscope.
○ Low antibody levels and other nonspecific factors produce borderline findings. In such cases, repeated testing and a thorough review of the patient's history may be productive.
○ Although the FTA-ABS test is specific, some patients with nonsyphilitic conditions, such as systemic lupus erythematosus, genital herpes, and increased or abnormal globulins, or those who are pregnant may show minimally reactive levels.
○ The FTA-ABS test doesn't always distinguish between *T. pallidum* and certain other treponemas, such as those that cause pinta, yaws, and bejel.

Interfering factors

○ Hemolysis from rough handling of the sample

Fluoroscopy, thoracic

Overview

○ Provides visualization of physiologic or pathologic structural motion of thoracic contents
○ Dynamic shadows of the heart, lungs, and diaphragm on a fluorescent screen created by a continuous stream of X-rays passing through the patient

Purpose

○ To assess lung expansion and contraction
○ To assess movement of the diaphragm and chest wall
○ To assist with placement of tubes or catheters such as a pulmonary artery catheter

Procedure

Preparation

○ Make sure the patient has signed an appropriate consent form.
○ Note and report all allergies.
○ Advise the patient that he will be asked to breathe deeply and cough during imaging.
○ Explain the need to remove all metallic objects (including jewelry) in the X-ray field.
○ Explain the need to wear a lead apron to protect the gonads.
○ Explain that the test usually takes 5 minutes.

Implementation

○ The patient is placed in the supine position on the fluoroscopy table or upright to best visualize diaphragmatic motion.
○ Equipment may be used to intensify the images or a videotape recording may be made for later study.
○ Check that no tubes have been dislodged during positioning.

Patient care

○ Monitor the patient's response to testing.

Complications

○ Inadvertent dislodgment of the patient lines or tubes

Interpretation

Normal results

○ Diaphragmatic movement is synchronous and symmetrical.
○ Diaphragmatic excursion ranges from 5 to 6 cm.

Abnormal results

○ Diminished diaphragmatic movement may indicate pulmonary disease or phrenic nerve injury.
○ Increased lung translucency may indicate loss of elasticity or bronchiolar obstruction.
○ Diminished or paradoxical diaphragmatic movement may indicate phrenic paralysis.

Interfering factors

None known

Folic acid

Overview

- Quantitative analysis of serum folic acid (also called *pteroylglutamic acid, folacin,* or *folate*) levels by radioisotope assay of competitive binding.
- Usually combined with measurement of serum vitamin B_{12} levels (like vitamin B_{12}, folic acid is a water-soluble vitamin that influences hematopoiesis, deoxyribonucleic acid synthesis, and overall body growth).
- Normally, food supplies folic acid in organ meats, such as liver or kidneys, yeast, fruits, leafy vegetables, fortified breads and cereals, eggs, and milk.
- Inadequate dietary intake may cause a deficiency, especially during pregnancy.
- Because of folic acid's vital role in hematopoiesis, the usual indication for this test is a suspected hematologic abnormality.

Purpose

- To aid in the differential diagnosis of megaloblastic anemia, which may result from folic acid or vitamin B_{12} deficiency
- To assess folate stores in pregnancy

Procedure

Preparation

- Explain to the patient that this test determines the folic acid level in the blood.
- Instruct the patient to fast overnight before the test.
- Tell the patient that the test requires a blood sample. Explain who will perform the venipuncture and when.
- Explain to the patient that he may experience slight discomfort from the tourniquet and needle puncture.
- Check the patient's history for drugs that may affect test results, such as phenytoin or pyrimethamine.

Implementation

- Perform a venipuncture and collect the sample in a 4.5-ml tube without additives.
- Handle the sample gently to prevent hemolysis.
- Protect the sample from light.
- Send the sample to the laboratory immediately.

Patient care

- Apply direct pressure to the venipuncture site until bleeding stops.
- Instruct the patient that he may resume his usual diet.

Complications

- Hematoma at the venipuncture site

Interpretation

Normal results

- 1.8 to 20 nanograms/ml (SI, 4 to 45.3 nmol/L)

Abnormal results

- Low serum levels may indicate hematologic abnormalities, such as anemia (especially megaloblastic anemia), leukopenia, and thrombocytopenia.
- The Schilling test is usually performed to rule out vitamin B_{12} deficiency, which also causes megaloblastic anemia.
- Decreased folic acid levels can also result from hypermetabolic states (such as hyperthyroidism), inadequate dietary intake, small-bowel malabsorption syndrome, hepatic or renal diseases, chronic alcoholism, or pregnancy.
- Serum levels greater than normal may indicate excessive dietary intake of folic acid or folic acid supplements. Even when taken in large doses, this vitamin is nontoxic.

Interfering factors

- Hemolysis from rough handling of the sample
- Alcohol, anticonvulsants (such as primidone), antimalarials, antineoplastics, hormonal contraceptives, phenytoin, and pyrimethamine (possible decrease)

Follicle-stimulating hormone, serum

Overview

○ The follicle-stimulating hormone (FSH) test of go-nadal function, performed more commonly on women than on men, measures FSH levels and is vital in infertility studies.
○ A glycoprotein secreted by the anterior pituitary gland, FSH stimulates gonadal activity in both sexes.
○ In women, it spurs development of primary ovarian follicles into graafian follicles for ovulation (secretion varies diurnally and fluctuates during the menstrual cycle, peaking at ovulation).
○ In men, continuous secretion of FSH (and testosterone) stimulates and maintains spermatogenesis.
○ Plasma levels fluctuate widely in women; to obtain a true baseline level, daily testing may be necessary (for 3 to 5 days), or multiple samples may be drawn on the same day.

Purpose

○ To aid in the diagnosis and treatment of infertility and disorders of menstruation such as amenorrhea
○ To aid in the diagnosis of precocious puberty in girls (before age 9) and in boys (before age 10)
○ To aid in the differential diagnosis of hypogonadism

Procedure

Preparation

○ Explain to the patient, or her parents if she's a minor, that this test helps determine if her hormonal secretion is normal.
○ Tell the patient that the test requires a blood sample.
○ Explain to the patient that she may experience slight discomfort from the tourniquet and needle puncture.
○ Withhold drugs that may interfere with accurate determination of test results for 48 hours before the test. If the patient must continue them (for example, for infertility treatment), note this on the laboratory request.
○ Make sure the patient is relaxed and recumbent for 30 minutes before the test.

Implementation

○ Perform a venipuncture, preferably between 6 a.m. and 8 a.m., and collect the sample in a 7-ml clot-activator tube. Send the sample to the laboratory immediately.
○ Handle the sample gently to prevent hemolysis.
○ If the patient is a woman, indicate the phase of her menstrual cycle on the laboratory request. If she's menopausal, note this on the laboratory request.

Patient care

○ Apply direct pressure to the venipuncture site until bleeding stops.
○ Instruct the patient that he may resume medications stopped before the test.

Complications

○ Hematoma at the venipuncture site

Interpretation

Normal results

○ Reference values vary greatly, depending on the patient's age, stage of sexual development, and—for a woman—phase of her menstrual cycle.
○ For the menstruating woman, FSH values are follicular phase 5 to 20 mIU/ml (SI, 5 to 20 IU/L), ovulatory phase 15 to 30 mIU/ml (SI, 15 to 30 IU/L), luteal phase 5 to 15 mIU/ml (SI, 5 to 15 IU/L).
○ FSH values for menopausal women range from 50 to 100 mIU/ ml (SI, 50 to 100 IU/L).
○ FSH values for men range from 5 to 20 mIU/ml (SI, 5 to 20 IU/L).

Abnormal results

○ Low FSH levels may cause aspermatogenesis in men and anovulation in women.
○ Low FSH levels may indicate secondary hypogo-nadotropic states, which can result from anorexia nervosa, panhypopituitarism, or hypothalamic lesions.
○ High FSH levels in women may indicate ovarian failure from Turner's syndrome (primary hypogo-nadism) or Stein-Leventhal syndrome (polycystic ovary syndrome).
○ High FSH levels may occur in patients with precocious puberty (idiopathic or with central nervous system lesions) and in postmenopausal women.
○ High FSH levels in men may indicate destruction of the testes (from mumps orchitis or X-ray exposure), testicular failure, seminoma, or male climacteric.
○ Congenital absence of the gonads and early-stage acromegaly may cause FSH levels to rise in both sexes.

Interfering factors

○ Failure to observe pretest restrictions
○ Hemolysis from rough handling of the sample
○ Ovarian steroid hormones, such as estrogen and progesterone, related compounds, and phenothiazines such as chlorpromazine (possible decrease through negative feedback by inhibiting FSH flow from the hypothalamus and pituitary gland)
○ Radioactive scan performed within 1 week before the test

Fractionated erythrocyte porphyrins

Overview

○ Measures erythrocyte porphyrins (also called *erythropoietic porphyrins*): coproporphyrin, protoporphyrin, and uroporphyrin.
○ Porphyrins are present in all protoplasm and are significant in energy storage and use; they're produced during heme biosynthesis and usually appear in small amounts in the blood, urine, and feces.
○ Production and excretion of porphyrins or their precursors increase in porphyria.

Purpose

○ To aid in the diagnosis of congenital and acquired erythropoietic porphyrias
○ To help confirm the diagnosis of disorders affecting red blood cell (RBC) activity

Procedure

Preparation

○ Explain to the patient that the fractionated erythrocyte porphyrin test detects RBC disorders.
○ Tell the patient that the test requires a blood sample. Explain who will perform the venipuncture and when.
○ Explain to the patient that he may experience slight discomfort from the tourniquet and needle puncture.

Implementation

○ Perform a venipuncture and collect the sample in a 5-ml or larger heparinized tube.
○ Handle the sample gently to prevent hemolysis.
○ Label the sample, place it on ice, and send it to the laboratory immediately.

Patient care

○ Apply direct pressure to the venipuncture site until bleeding stops.

Complications

○ Hematoma at the venipuncture site

Interpretation

Normal results

○ Total porphyrin levels range from 16 to 60 µg/dl (SI, 0.25 to 1.062 µmol/L) of packed RBCs.
○ Protoporphyrin levels range from 16 to 60 µg/dl.
○ Coproporphyrin and uroporphyrin levels are normally less than 2 µg/dl (SI, < 0.035 µmol/L).

Abnormal results

○ Increased total porphyrin levels suggest the need for further enzyme testing to identify the specific porphyria.
○ Increased protoporphyrin levels may indicate erythropoietic protoporphyria, infection, increased erythropoiesis, thalassemia, sideroblastic anemia, iron deficiency anemia, or lead poisoning.
○ Increased coproporphyrin levels may indicate congenital erythropoietic porphyria, erythropoietic protoporphyria or coproporphyria, or sideroblastic anemia.
○ Increased uroporphyrin levels may indicate congenital erythropoietic porphyria or erythropoietic protoporphyria.

Interfering factors

○ Hemolysis from rough handling of the sample
○ Exposure of the sample to direct sunlight or ultraviolet light

Free cortisol, urine

Overview

- A screen for adrenocortical hyperfunction, the free cortisol test measures urine levels of the portion of cortisol not bound to the corticosteroid-binding globulin transcortin (one of the best diagnostic tools for detecting Cushing's syndrome).
- Unlike a single measurement of plasma cortisol, radioimmunoassay determinations of free cortisol levels in a 24-hour urine specimen reflect overall secretion levels instead of diurnal variations.
- Concurrent measurements of plasma cortisol and corticotropin, with urine 17-hydroxycorticosteroids and the dexamethasone suppression test, may confirm the diagnosis.

Purpose

- To aid in the diagnosis of Cushing's syndrome
- To evaluate adrenocortical function

Procedure

Preparation

- Explain to the patient that the urine free cortisol test helps evaluate adrenal gland function.
- Inform the patient that he need not restrict food and fluids but should avoid stressful situations and excessive physical exercise during the collection period.
- Tell the patient that the test requires collection of urine over a 24-hour period.
- Teach the patient the proper collection technique for a 24-hour urine specimen.
- Notify the laboratory and physician of drugs the patient is taking that may affect test results; it may be necessary to restrict them.

Implementation

- Collect the urine over a 24-hour period, discarding the first specimen and retaining the last specimen. Use a bottle containing a preservative to keep the specimen at a pH of 4.0 to 4.5.
- Refrigerate the specimen or place it on ice during the collection period.
- Instruct the patient that he may resume his usual activities and medications.

Patient care

- Answer the patient's questions about the test.

Complications

None known

Interpretation

Normal results

- Less than 50 µg/24 hours (SI, <138 mmol/24 hours)

Abnormal results

- High free cortisol levels may indicate Cushing's syndrome resulting from adrenal hyperplasia, adrenal or pituitary tumor, or ectopic corticotropin production.
- High plasma cortisol levels but normal urine levels of free cortisol may result from hepatic disease or obesity.
- Low cortisol levels have little significance and don't necessarily indicate adrenocortical hypofunction.

Interfering factors

- Failure to collect all urine during the test period or to properly store the specimen
- Pregnancy (possible increase)
- Amphetamines, danazol, hormonal contraceptives, morphine, phenothiazines, prolonged steroid therapy, reserpine, and spironolactone (possible increase)
- Dexamethasone, ethacrynic acid, ketoconazole, and thiazides (decrease)

Free thyroxine and free triiodothyronine

Overview

○ The free thyroxine (FT_4) and free triiodothyronine (FT_3) tests measure serum levels of FT_4 and FT_3, the minute portions of T_4 and T_3 not bound to thyroxine-binding globulin (TBG) and other serum proteins.
○ Because of disagreement as to whether FT_4 or FT_3 is the better indicator, laboratories usually measure both.
○ These unbound hormones are responsible for the thyroid's effects on cellular metabolism.
○ Measurement of free hormone levels is best indicator of thyroid function.
○ Disadvantages: a cumbersome and difficult laboratory method, inaccessibility, and cost.
○ May be useful in the 5% of patients in whom the standard T_3 or T_4 test fails to produce diagnostic results.

Purpose

○ To measure the metabolically active form of the thyroid hormones
○ To aid diagnosis of hyperthyroidism and hypothyroidism when TBG levels are abnormal

Procedure

Preparation

○ Explain to the patient that this special test helps evaluate thyroid function.
○ Tell the patient that the test requires a blood sample. Explain who will perform the venipuncture and when.
○ Explain to the patient that he may experience slight discomfort from the tourniquet and needle puncture.

Implementation

○ Perform a venipuncture and collect the sample in a 7-ml clot-activator tube.
○ Handle the sample gently to prevent hemolysis.

Patient care

○ Apply direct pressure to the venipuncture site until bleeding stops.

Complications

○ Hematoma at the venipuncture site

Interpretation

Normal results

○ Normal range for FT_4 is 0.9 to 2.3 nanograms/dl (SI, 10 to 30 nmol/L); for FT_3, 0.2 to 0.6 nanogram/dl (SI, 0.003 to 0.009 nmol/L).

○ Values vary, depending on the laboratory.

Abnormal results

○ High FT_4 and FT_3 levels indicate hyperthyroidism, unless the patient has peripheral resistance to thyroid hormone.
○ High FT_3 levels with normal or low FT_4 levels indicate T_3 toxicosis, a distinct form of hyperthyroidism.
○ Low FT_4 levels usually indicate hypothyroidism, except in patients receiving replacement therapy with T_3.
○ FT_4 and FT_3 levels may vary in patients receiving thyroid therapy, depending on the preparation used and the time of sample collection.

Interfering factors

○ Hemolysis from rough handling of the sample
○ Thyroid therapy, depending on dosage (possible increase)

Fungal serology

Overview

- Most fungal organisms enter the body as spores inhaled into the lungs or infiltrated through wounds in the skin or mucosa.
- Body's defenses can't destroy the organisms initially, the fungi multiply to form lesions; blood and lymph vessels may then spread the mycosis throughout the body.
- Most healthy people easily overcome initial mycotic infection, but elderly people and others with a deficient immune system are more susceptible to acute or chronic mycotic infection and to disorders secondary to such infection.
- Mycosis may be deep-seated (usually in the lungs) or superficial (in the skin or mucosal linings).
- Serologic tests occasionally provide the sole evidence for mycosis.
- Such serologic tests use immunodiffusion, complement fixation, precipitin, latex agglutination, or agglutination methods to demonstrate the presence of specific mycotic antibodies.

Purpose

- To rapidly detect the presence of antifungal antibodies, aiding in the diagnosis of a mycosis
- To monitor the effectiveness of therapy for a mycosis

Procedure

Preparation

- Explain that this test aids in the diagnosis of certain fungal infections. If appropriate, tell the patient that this test monitors his response to antimycotic therapy and that it may be necessary to repeat the test.
- Instruct the patient to restrict food and fluids for 12 to 24 hours before the test. Tell him that the test requires a blood sample.
- Explain to the patient that he may experience slight discomfort from the tourniquet and needle puncture.

Implementation

- Perform a venipuncture and collect the sample in a 10-ml sterile clot-activator tube.
- Send the sample to the laboratory immediately.
- If transport to the laboratory is delayed, store the sample at 39.2° F (4° C).

Patient care

- Apply direct pressure to the venipuncture site until bleeding stops.

Complications

- Hematoma at the venipuncture site

Interpretation

Normal results

- Depending on the test method, a negative result or normal titer

Abnormal results

- Aspergillosis
- Blastomycosis
- Coccidiomycosis
- Cryptococcosis.
- Histoplasmosis
- Sporotrichosis

Interfering factors

- Failure to observe dietary restrictions
- Failure to send a sterile sample to the laboratory immediately or to properly store the sample in case of delay in transportation
- Cross-reaction of antibodies with other antigens, such as blastomycosis and histoplasmosis antigens (possible false-positive or high titers)
- Recent skin testing with fungal antigens (possible high titers)
- Mycosis-caused immunosuppression (low titers or false-negative)

Galactose-1-phosphate uridyltransferase

Overview

- Helps convert galactose to glucose during lactose metabolism.
- Deficiency may cause galactosemia, a hereditary disorder that can impair eye, brain, and liver development and cause irreversible cataracts, mental retardation, and cirrhosis, unless discovered and treated immediately.
- Qualitative test screens for the deficiency; some facilities require it for all neonates.
- Quantitative test is performed after a positive qualitative test result, measures the amount of a fluorescent substance generated during a coupled enzyme reaction, and identifies adults who are galactosemia carriers.
- Prenatal testing of amniotic fluid can also detect deficiency; rarely performed because neonatal screening can detect the deficiency in time to prevent irreversible damage.

Purpose

- To screen the infant for galactosemia
- To detect a heterozygous carrier of galactosemia

Procedure

Preparation

- When testing a neonate, explain to the parents that the test screens for galactosemia, a potentially dangerous enzyme deficiency.
- If a blood sample wasn't taken from the umbilical cord at birth, tell the parents that a small amount of blood will be drawn from the infant's heel. Explain that the procedure is safe and quick.
- When testing an adult, explain that this test identifies carriers of galactosemia, a genetic disorder that may be transmitted to offspring.
- Tell the patient that the test requires a blood sample. Explain who will perform the venipuncture and when.
- Explain to the patient that he may experience slight discomfort from the tourniquet and the needle puncture.
- Inform the patient that he need not restrict food and fluids.

Implementation

- For a qualitative (screening) test, collect cord blood or blood from a heelstick on special filter paper, saturating all three circles.
- A follow-up quantitative test should occur as soon as possible after a positive qualitative test result.

- For a quantitative test, perform a venipuncture and collect a 4-ml sample in a heparinized or ethylenediaminetetraacetic acid tube, depending on the laboratory method used.
- Indicate the patient's age on the laboratory request.
- Check the patient's history for a recent exchange transfusion.
- Note this on the laboratory request or postpone the test.
- Handle the sample gently to prevent hemolysis.
- Send the sample to the laboratory on wet ice.

Patient care

- Apply direct pressure to the venipuncture site until bleeding stops.
- If test results indicate galactosemia, refer the parents for nutrition counseling and provide a galactose- and lactose-free diet for their infant.
- Inform parents that a soybean- or meat-based formula can substitute for formulas based on cow's milk.

Complications

- Hematoma at the venipuncture site

Interpretation

Normal results

- Negative qualitative test result
- Quantitative test result of 18.5 to 28.5 units/g of hemoglobin (Hb) (Confirm the normal range with the particular laboratory in case a different method is used.)

Abnormal results

- A positive qualitative test result may indicate a transferase deficiency.
- Quantitative test result of < 5 units/g of Hb indicates galactosemia.
- Quantitative test result of 5 to 18.5 units/g of Hb may indicate that the patient is a carrier.

Interfering factors

- Hemolysis from rough handling of the sample
- Failure to use the proper collection tube or to send the sample to the laboratory on wet ice (possible false-positive because heat inactivates transferase)
- Total exchange transfusion (transient false-negative because normal blood contains enzyme)

Gallium scanning

Overview

- Total body scan performed 24 to 72 hours after I.V. injection of radioactive gallium (GA 67) citrate
- Contraindicated in children and in pregnant or breast-feeding women, unless the benefit outweighs the risks

Purpose

- To detect primary or metastatic neoplasms
- To detect inflammatory lesions
- To evaluate malignant lymphoma
- To identify recurrent tumors
- To clarify focal defects in the liver when scanning and ultrasonography are inconclusive
- To evaluate bronchogenic carcinoma
- To screen for the cause of a fever of unknown origin

Procedure

Preparation

- Make sure the patient has signed an appropriate consent form.
- Note and report all allergies.
- Inform the patient that he need not restrict food or fluids.
- Give the patient a laxative or cleansing enema (or both).
- Explain that the test takes 30 to 60 minutes.
- Reassure the patient that radiation exposure is minimal.

Implementation

- Various patient positions may be necessary, depending on the condition.
- Scans or scintigrams are taken from various views 24, 48, and 72 hours after the injection of gallium.
- If bowel disease is suggested and additional scans are necessary, give the patient a cleansing enema.

Patient care

- Inform the patient that he may resume previous activity.

Complications

- Infection at the injection site

Interpretation

Normal results

- Gallium activity is demonstrated in the liver, spleen, bones, and large bowel.

Abnormal results

- Abnormally high activity suggests inflammatory bowel disease and colon cancer.
- Abnormal activity in one or more lymph nodes or in extranodal locations suggests possible Hodgkin's disease and non-Hodgkin's lymphoma.
- Localization of gallium suggests possible hepatoma, abscess, or tumor.

Interfering factors

- Hepatic and splenic uptake (may obscure the detection of abnormal para-aortic nodes in Hodgkin's disease, causing false-negative scans)
- Barium studies within 1 week before this scan
- Other isotope studies may be postponed for up to 7 days after a gallium scan because of the slow elimination of gallium
- Previous treatment with antibiotics or high doses of steroids (may decrease the inflammatory response and result in false negative gallium imaging)

Gamma globulin

Overview

○ A form of protein electrophoresis that examines globulin proteins

Purpose

○ To examine the amount of globulin proteins in the blood

Procedure

Preparation

○ Inform the patient that this test requires a blood sample.
○ Instruct the patient to fast for 4 hours before the test.
○ Ask the patient what drugs he's taking; it may be necessary to restrict them.

Implementation

○ Perform the venipuncture and collect the sample in a 7-ml clot-activator tube.

Patient care

○ Apply direct pressure to the venipuncture site.

Complications

○ Hematoma at the venipuncture site

Interpretation

Normal results

○ Serum globulin count is 2.0 to 3.5 g/dl.
○ Immunoglobulin (Ig) M component is 75 to 300 mg/dl.
○ IgG component is 650 to 1,850 mg/dl.
○ IgA component is 90 to 350 mg/dl.

Abnormal results

○ Increased gamma globulin proteins may indicate multiple myeloma, chronic inflammatory disease (for example, rheumatoid arthritis and systemic lupus erythematosus), hyperimmunization, acute infection, or Waldenström's macroglobulinemia.

Interfering factors

○ Chlorpromazine, corticosteroids, isoniazid, neomycin, phenacemide, salicylates, sulfonamides, and tolbutamide

Gamma-glutamyltransferase

Overview

○ Measures serum gamma-glutamyltransferase (GGT) level.
○ GGT helps transfer amino acids across cellular membranes and may aid in glutathione metabolism.
○ Highest GGT levels in kidney; also present in the liver, biliary tract, epithelium, pancreas, lymphocytes, brain, and testes.
○ More sensitive indicator of hepatic necrosis than the aspartate aminotransferase assay and at least as sensitive as the alkaline phosphatase (ALP) assay because GGT isn't elevated in bone growth or pregnancy.
○ Test is nonspecific, providing little data about the type of hepatic disease, because increased levels also occur in renal, cardiac, and prostatic disease and with the use of certain drugs.
○ GGT is particularly sensitive to the effects of alcohol on the liver (therefore, levels may be elevated after moderate alcohol intake and in chronic alcoholism, even without clinical evidence of hepatic injury).

Purpose

○ To provide information about hepatobiliary diseases, to assess liver function, and to detect alcohol ingestion
○ To distinguish between skeletal and hepatic disease when the serum ALP level is elevated (a normal GGT level suggests that such elevation stems from skeletal disease)

Procedure

Preparation

○ Explain to the patient that this test evaluates liver function.
○ Tell the patient that the test requires a blood sample. Explain who will perform the venipuncture and when.
○ Explain to the patient that he may experience slight discomfort from the tourniquet and the needle puncture.
○ Inform the patient that he need not restrict food and fluids.

Implementation

○ Perform a venipuncture and collect the sample in a 4-ml tube without additives.
○ Handle the sample gently to prevent hemolysis.
○ GGT activity is stable in serum at room temperature for 2 days.

Patient care

○ Apply direct pressure to the venipuncture site until bleeding stops.

Complications

○ Hematoma at the venipuncture site

Interpretation

Normal results

○ In children, 3 to 30 units/L (SI, 0.05 to 0.51 μkat/L)
○ In men age 16 and older, 6 to 38 units/L (SI, 0.10 to 0.63 μkat/L)
○ In women ages 16 to 45, 4 to 27 units/L (SI, 0.08 to 0.46 μKat/L); age 45 and older, 6 to 37 units/L (SI, 0.10 to 0.63 μkat/L)

Abnormal results

○ Serum GGT levels rise in acute hepatic disease.
○ Moderate increases occur in acute pancreatitis, renal disease, and prostatic metastases; postoperatively; and in some patients with epilepsy or brain tumors.
○ Levels also increase after alcohol ingestion because of enzyme induction. The sharpest elevations occur in patients with obstructive jaundice and hepatic metastatic infiltrations.
○ Levels may also increase 5 to 10 days after acute myocardial infarction, either as a result of tissue granulation and healing or as an indication of the effects of cardiac insufficiency on the liver.

Interfering factors

○ Hemolysis from rough handling of the sample
○ Clofibrate and hormonal contraceptives (decrease)
○ Aminoglycosides, barbiturates, phenytoin glutethimide, and methaqualone (increase)
○ Moderate alcohol intake (increase for at least 60 hours)

Gastric acid stimulation

Overview

- Measures secretion of gastric acid for 1 hour after subcutaneous injection of pentagastrin or a similar drug that stimulates gastric acid output
- Usually performed immediately after a basal secretion test suggests abnormal gastric secretion

Purpose

- To aid in the diagnosis of duodenal ulcer, Zollinger-Ellison syndrome, pernicious anemia, and gastric carcinoma

Procedure

Preparation

- Make sure the patient has signed an appropriate consent form.
- Note and report all allergies.
- Check the patient's history for hypersensitivity to pentagastrin.
- Withhold antacids, anticholinergics, adrenergic-receptor blockers, histamine-2 receptor antagonists, corticosteroids, proton pump inhibitors, and reserpine before the test.
- Instruct the patient to refrain from eating, drinking, and smoking after midnight before the test.
- Tell the patient to immediately report to the physician adverse effects (abdominal pain, nausea, vomiting, flushing, transitory dizziness, faintness, and numbness of the extremities).
- Explain that the test takes 1 hour.

Implementation

- A nasogastric (NG) tube is inserted.
- Basal gastric secretions are collected using the NG tube.
- Pentagastrin is injected.

> ⚠ ALERT *Watch for the adverse effects of pentagastrin, such as rash, hives, nausea, vomiting, abdominal pain, blurred vision, diaphoresis, and shortness of breath.*

- Prevent contamination of specimens with saliva.
- After 15 minutes, a specimen is collected every 15 minutes for 1 hour.
- The color, odor, and presence of food, mucus, bile, or blood in specimens are noted and recorded.
- All specimens are labeled "stimulated contents," and numbered 1 through 4.
- Specimens are sent to the laboratory immediately.

Patient care

- If the NG tube is to remain in place, clamp it or attach it to low intermittent suction.
- Watch for and report nausea, vomiting, abdominal distention, or pain after removal of the NG tube.
- For a sore throat, provide soothing lozenges.
- Tell the patient he may resume his diet and drugs.

Complications

- Adverse effects of pentagastrin

Interpretation

Normal results

- For men, 8 to 28 mEq/hour
- For women, 11 to 21 mEq/hour

Abnormal results

- Elevated gastric secretion may indicate duodenal ulcer.
- Markedly elevated secretion suggests Zollinger-Ellison syndrome.
- Depressed secretion may indicate gastric carcinoma.
- Achlorhydria may indicate pernicious anemia.

Interfering factors

None known

Gastric culture

Overview

- Requires aspiration of gastric contents and cultivation of any microbes present.
- Accompanies a chest X-ray and a purified protein derivative skin test; it's especially useful when a sputum specimen isn't obtainable by expectoration or nebulization.
- Also provides specimen for rapid presumptive identification of bacteria (by Gram's stain) in neonatal septicemia.

Purpose

- To aid in the diagnosis of mycobacterial infections
- To identify the infectious bacteria in neonatal septicemia

Procedure

Preparation

- Explain to the patient (or parents, if the patient is a child) that gastric culture helps diagnose tuberculosis.
- Instruct the patient to fast for 8 hours before the test.
- Tell the patient who will perform the test. Explain that it may be necessary to repeat the procedure on three consecutive mornings.
- Instruct the patient to remain in bed each morning until the specimen collection is complete to prevent premature emptying of stomach contents.
- Tell him that the nasogastric (NG) tube may make him gag but that it passes more easily if he relaxes and follows instructions about breathing and swallowing.
- Just before the procedure, obtain baseline oxygen saturation and heart rate and rhythm. Assist the patient into high Fowler's position.
- Inform the patient (or his parents) that it may take a while to get test results because acid-fast bacteria are slow growing.
- Check the patient's history for recent antimicrobial therapy and inform the physician of your findings; it may be necessary to stop drugs before the test.

Implementation

- As soon as the patient awakens in the morning, put on gloves, perform the NG insertion, confirming the position, and obtain gastric washings.
- Clamp the tube before quickly removing it from the patient.
- Note recent antimicrobial therapy on the laboratory request, along with the site and time of collection.
- Label the specimen container with the patient's name, the physician's name, and the facility number.
- If possible, obtain the specimens before the start of antimicrobial therapy.

- Never inject water into an NG tube unless you're sure the tube is correctly placed in the patient's stomach. During lavage, use sterile distilled water to decrease the risk of contamination with saprophytic mycobacteria.
- Check the patient's pulse rate for irregularities during this procedure to detect arrhythmias and monitor for signs of hypoxia.
- Wear gloves when performing the procedure and when handling specimens and the NG tube.
- Put the specimen in a tightly capped container, wipe the outside of the container with disinfectant, and place it upright in a plastic bag.

Patient care

- Tell the patient that he may resume his usual diet and medications.
- Instruct the patient not to blow his nose for 4 hours to prevent bleeding.

Complications

- Tube enters the trachea: coughing, cyanosis, decreasing oxygen saturation readings, and gasping result.

Interpretation

Normal results

- The culture specimen tests negative for pathogenic mycobacteria.

Abnormal results

- Isolation and identification of the organism *Mycobacterium tuberculosis* indicates the presence of active tuberculosis; other species, such as *M. bovis*, *M. kansasii*, and *M. avium-intracellulare*, may cause pulmonary disease that's clinically indistinguishable from tuberculosis.
- These mycobacterial infections may be difficult to treat and commonly require susceptibility studies to determine the most effective antimicrobial therapy.
- Pathogenic bacteria causing neonatal septicemia may also be identified through culture.

Interfering factors

- Failure to observe an 8-hour fast before the test
- Tetracycline and aminoglycosides (possible false-negative)
- Presence of saprophytic mycobacteria in gastric contents because these mycobacteria can't be microscopically distinguished from pathogenic mycobacteria (possible false-positive acid-fast smears)

Gastrin

Overview

○ A polypeptide hormone produced and stored in the antrum of the stomach and in the islets of Langerhans
○ Facilitates food digestion by triggering gastric acid secretion
○ Stimulates release of pancreatic enzymes and the gastric enzyme pepsin, increases gastric and intestinal motility, and stimulates bile flow from the liver
○ Radioimmunoassay of gastrin levels is especially useful in patients suspected of having gastrinomas (Zollinger-Ellison syndrome)

Purpose

○ To confirm a diagnosis of gastrinoma, the gastrin-secreting tumor in Zollinger-Ellison syndrome
○ To aid in the differential diagnosis of gastric and duodenal ulcers and pernicious anemia; gastrin estimation has limited value in the patient with a duodenal ulcer

Procedure

Preparation

○ Explain to the patient that this test helps determine the cause of GI symptoms.
○ Instruct the patient to abstain from alcohol for at least 24 hours before the test and to fast and avoid caffeinated drinks for 12 hours before the test, although he may drink water.
○ Tell the patient that the test requires a blood sample. Explain who will perform the venipuncture and when.
○ Explain to the patient that he may experience slight discomfort from the tourniquet and the needle puncture.
○ Withhold all drugs that may interfere with test results, especially insulin and anticholinergics, such as atropine and belladonna, as ordered. If the patient must continue them, note this on the laboratory request.
○ Tell the patient to lie down and relax for at least 30 minutes before the test.

Implementation

○ Perform a venipuncture and collect the sample in a 10- to 15-ml clot-activator tube.
○ Handle the sample gently to avoid hemolysis.
○ To prevent destruction of serum gastrin by proteolytic enzymes, immediately send the sample to the laboratory to have the serum separated and frozen.

Patient care

○ Apply direct pressure to the venipuncture site until bleeding stops.
○ Instruct the patient that he may resume his usual diet and medications stopped before the test.

Complications

○ Hematoma at the venipuncture site

Interpretation

Normal results

○ 50 to 150 pg/ml (SI, 50 to 150 ng/L)

Abnormal results

○ Strikingly high serum gastrin levels (> 1,000 pg/ml [SI, > 1,000 nanograms/L]) confirm Zollinger-Ellison syndrome.
○ Levels as high as 450,000 pg/ml (SI, 450,000 ng/L) have been reported.
○ Increased serum levels of gastrin may occur in a few patients with duodenal ulceration (<1 %) and in patients with achlorhydria (with or without pernicious anemia) or extensive stomach carcinoma (because of hyposecretion of gastric juices and hydrochloric acid).

Interfering factors

○ Failure to observe pretest restrictions
○ Hemolysis from rough handling of the sample
○ Amino acids (especially glycine), calcium carbonate, acetylcholine, calcium chloride, and ethanol (increase)
○ Anticholinergics, such as atropine, as well as hydrochloric acid and secretin, a strongly basic polypeptide (decrease)
○ Insulin-induced hypoglycemia (increase)

Given diagnostic imaging system (camera pill)

Overview

○ Tiny video camera with light source and transmitter inside a capsule records images along its path.
○ Capsule measures 11 mm × 30 mm; propelled along the digestive tract by peristalsis.
○ Clear end of the capsule records images of the stomach walls and small intestine (where other diagnostic techniques may not reach or make visible); transmits them to data recorder on a belt around the patient's waist.
○ Contraindicated in patients with a suspected obstruction, fistula, or stricture and in infants, young children, and others unable to swallow capsules.
○ Battery is short lived, so images of the large intestine aren't obtainable.
○ Capsule can't stop bleeding, take tissue samples, remove growths, or repair other detected problems (it may be necessary to use other invasive studies).

Purpose

○ To detect polyps or cancer
○ To detect the causes of bleeding and anemia

Procedure

Preparation

○ Explain to the patient that this test shows the stomach and small intestine, helping to detect disorders.
○ Tell the patient who will perform the test and where it will take place.
○ Inform the patient that he may need to fast for 12 hours before the test but may have fluids for up to 2 hours before the test.
○ Usually no bowel preparation is involved, but some patients may benefit from it.
○ Explain to the patient that he'll need to swallow the camera pill and that it will send information to a receiver he'll wear on his belt.
○ Tell the patient that the procedure is painless and that after swallowing the pill he can go home or go to work.
○ Explain to the patient that walking helps facilitate movement of the pill.
○ Tell the patient that he'll need to return to the facility in 24 hours (or as directed) so the recorder can be removed from his belt.
○ Tell the patient that he will excrete the pill normally in his feces in 8 to 72 hours.

Implementation

○ The patient ingests the camera pill, and a receiver is attached to his belt.
○ The pill records images for up to 6 hours along its path through the stomach, small intestine, and mouth of the large intestine, transmitting the information to the receiver.
○ The patient returns to the facility, as instructed, so the images can be transmitted to the computer, where they're displayed on the screen.

Patient care

○ Tell the patient that he may resume his usual diet after the images are obtained.
○ Explain that he will excrete the pill normally in feces.

Complications

None known

Interpretation

Normal results

○ Normal anatomy of the stomach and small intestine

Abnormal results

○ Bleeding sites or abnormalities of the stomach and small bowel, such as erosions, Crohn's disease, celiac disease, benign and malignant tumors of the small intestine, vascular disorders, medication-related small-bowel injuries, and pediatric small-bowel disorders

Interfering factors

○ Narrowing or obstruction of the intestine, causing the pill to become lodged

Glucose oxidase

Overview

○ Uses commercial, plastic-coated reagent strips (Clinistix, Diastix) or glucose enzymatic test strips
○ A specific, qualitative test for glycosuria
○ Primarily for monitoring urine glucose in patients with diabetes
○ Can be performed at home because of its simplicity and convenience

Purpose

○ To detect glycosuria and determine the renal threshold for glucose
○ To monitor urine glucose levels during insulin therapy

Procedure

Preparation

○ Explain to the patient that the glucose oxidase test determines urine glucose concentration.
○ If the patient is newly diagnosed with diabetes, teach him how to perform a reagent strip test.
○ If the patient is taking ascorbic acid, hypochlorites, levodopa, peroxides, phenazopyridine, or salicylates use Clinitest tablets instead.

Implementation

○ Have the patient void; then give him a drink of water.
○ Collect a second-voided specimen after 30 to 45 minutes.

Clinistix test
○ Dip the test area of the reagent strip in the specimen for 2 seconds.
○ Remove excess urine by tapping the strip against a clean surface or the side of the container and begin timing.
○ Hold the Clinistix strip in the air and "read" the color *exactly 10 seconds* after taking the strip out of the urine by comparing it with the reference color blocks on the label of the container.
○ Record the results; ignore color changes that develop after 10 seconds.

Diastix test
○ Dip the reagent strip in the specimen for 2 seconds.
○ Remove excess urine by tapping the strip against the container and begin timing.
○ Hold the Diastix strip in the air and compare the color to the color chart *exactly 30 seconds* after taking the strip out of the urine.
○ Record the results; ignore color changes that develop after 30 seconds.

Glucose enzymatic test strip
○ Withdraw about 1″ (2.5 cm) of the reagent tape from the dispenser; dip ¼″ (0.6 cm) in the specimen for 2 seconds.

○ Remove excess urine by tapping the strip against the side of the container and begin timing.
○ Hold the glucose enzymatic test strip in the air and compare the color of the darkest part of the tape to the color chart *exactly 60 seconds* after taking the strip out of the urine.
○ If the tape indicates 0.5% or higher, wait an additional 60 seconds to make the final color comparison.
○ Record the results.

Patient care

○ Instruct the patient not to contaminate the urine specimen with toilet tissue or feces.
○ Keep the test strip container tightly closed to prevent deterioration of the strips by exposure to light or moisture.
○ Store the container under 86° F (30° C) to avoid heat degradation.
○ Don't use discolored or darkened Clinistix or Diastix, or dark yellow or yellow-brown glucose enzymatic test strips.

Complications

None known

Interpretation

Normal results

○ No glucose in the urine

Abnormal results

○ Glycosuria occurs in diabetes mellitus, adrenal and thyroid disorders, hepatic and central nervous system diseases, conditions involving low renal threshold (such as Fanconi's syndrome), toxic renal tubular disease, heavy metal poisoning, glomerulonephritis, and nephrosis; in pregnant women; and in those receiving total parenteral nutrition.
○ Glycosuria occurs with prolonged use of phenothiazines and with ingestion of large amounts of glucose and of certain drugs, such as ammonium chloride, asparaginase, carbamazepine, corticosteroids, dextrothyroxine, lithium carbonate, nicotinic acid, and thiazide diuretics.

Interfering factors

○ Dilute, stale urine or contamination of the specimen by toilet tissue, feces, or bacteria
○ Use of reagent strips after the expiration date, failure to keep the reagent strip container tightly closed, or failure to record the reagent strip method used
○ Presence of reducing substances, such as levodopa, ascorbic acid, phenazopyridine, methyldopa, and salicylates (possible false-negative)
○ Tetracyclines (false-negative)

Glucose-6-phosphate dehydrogenase

Overview

○ Glucose-6-phosphate dehydrogenase (G6PD), an enzyme found in most body cells, helps metabolize glucose.
○ Test detects G6PD deficiency — a hereditary, sex-linked condition that impairs stability of the red cell membrane and allows strong oxidizing agents to destroy red blood cells (RBCs).
○ RBC enzyme levels normally decrease as cells age, but G6PD deficiency accelerates this process, making older red cells more prone to destruction than younger ones.
○ In mild deficiency, young RBCs retain enough G6PD to survive; in severe deficiency, all RBCs are destroyed.
○ About 10% of Black males in the United States inherit a mild G6PD deficiency; some people of Mediterranean descent inherit a severe deficiency.
○ In some Whites, fava beans may produce hemolytic episodes.
○ Although a deficiency of G6PD provides partial immunity to falciparum malaria, it precipitates an adverse reaction to antimalarials.

Purpose

○ To detect hemolytic anemia caused by G6PD deficiency
○ To aid differential diagnosis of hemolytic anemia

Procedure

Preparation

○ Explain to the patient that this test detects an inherited enzyme deficiency that may affect red blood cells.
○ Tell the patient that the test requires a blood sample. Explain who will perform the venipuncture and when.
○ Explain to the patient that he may experience slight discomfort from the tourniquet and the needle puncture.
○ Inform the patient that he need not restrict food and fluids.
○ Check the patient's history and report recent blood transfusion or ingestion of aspirin, sulfonamides, phenacetin, nitrofurantoin, vitamin K derivatives, antimalarials, or fava beans, which cause hemolysis in someone who's G6PD-deficient.

Implementation

○ Perform a venipuncture and collect the sample in a 4-ml ethylenediaminetetraacetic acid tube.

○ Completely fill the collection tube and invert it gently several times to mix the sample and the anticoagulant.
○ Handle the sample gently to prevent hemolysis.
○ Refrigerate the sample if you can't send it to the laboratory immediately.

Patient care

○ Apply direct pressure to the venipuncture site until bleeding stops.

Complications

○ Hematoma at the venipuncture site

Interpretation

Normal results

○ Values vary with the measurement method but usually range from 4.3 to 11.8 units/g (SI, 0.28 to 0.76 mU/mmol) of hemoglobin.

Abnormal results

○ Fluorescent spot testing or staining for Heinz bodies or erythrocytes can test for G6PD deficiency.
○ If results are positive, the kinetic quantitative assay for G6PD may be necessary.
○ Electrophoretic techniques assess genetic variants of deficiencies (which may cause lifelong, mild, or asymptomatic anemia).
○ Some variants are symptomatic only when the patient experiences stress or illness or has been exposed to drugs or agents that elicit hemolytic episodes.

Interfering factors

○ Performing the test after a hemolytic episode or a blood transfusion (possible false-negative)
○ Failure to use the proper anticoagulant or to adequately mix the sample and the anticoagulant
○ Hemolysis from rough handling of the sample
○ Aspirin, fava beans, nitrofurantoin, primaquine, sulfonamides, and vitamin K derivatives (decreased G6PD enzyme activity, precipitating a hemolytic episode)

Glycosylated hemoglobin

Overview

- Also called *total fasting hemoglobin (Hb)*, monitors diabetes therapy by measuring glycosylated Hb levels, provides information about the average blood glucose level during the preceding 2 to 3 months.
- Requires only one venipuncture every 6 to 8 weeks; can be used to evaluate the long-term effectiveness of diabetes therapy.
- Values are reported as a percentage of the total Hb in an erythrocyte.

Purpose

- To assess control of diabetes mellitus

Procedure

Preparation

- Explain to the patient that the glycosylated Hb test evaluates diabetes therapy.
- Tell the patient that the test requires a blood sample. Explain who will perform the venipuncture and when.
- Explain to the patient that he may experience slight discomfort from the tourniquet and the needle puncture.
- Inform the patient that he need not restrict food and fluids, and instruct him to maintain his prescribed medication and diet regimens.

Implementation

- Perform a venipuncture and collect the sample in a 5-ml ethylenediaminetetraacetic acid tube.
- Completely fill the collection tube.
- Invert the sample gently several times to mix the sample and the anticoagulant adequately.

Patient care

- Apply direct pressure to the venipuncture site until bleeding stops.
- Schedule the patient for an appointment in 6 to 8 weeks for appropriate follow-up testing.

Complications

- Hematoma at the venipuncture site

Interpretation

Normal results

- 4% to 7%

Abnormal results

- In diabetes, the patient has good control of blood glucose levels when the glycosylated Hb value is less than 8%.
- A glycosylated Hb value greater than 10% indicates poor control.

Interfering factors

- Failure to adequately mix the sample and the anticoagulant
- Hemolytic anemia (decreased)
- Hyperglycemia, thalassemia, chronic renal failure, the patient receiving dialysis, the patient that has a splenectomy, and the patient with elevated triglycerides or Hb F levels (increased)

Growth hormone suppression

Overview

- Also called *glucose loading,* evaluates excessive baseline levels of human growth hormone (hGH) from the anterior pituitary gland.
- Normally, hGH raises plasma glucose and fatty acid concentrations; in response, insulin secretion increases to counteract these effects (consequently, a glucose load should suppress hGH secretions).
- In a patient with excessive hGH levels, failure of suppression indicates anterior pituitary dysfunction and confirms a diagnosis of acromegaly or gigantism

Purpose

- To assess elevated baseline levels of hGH
- To confirm a diagnosis of gigantism in children and acromegaly in adults and adolescents

Procedure

Preparation

- Explain to the patient, or his parents if the patient is a child, that this test helps determine the cause of his abnormal growth.
- Instruct the patient to fast and limit physical activity for 10 to 12 hours before the test.
- Tell him that the test will require two blood samples. Warn him that he may experience nausea after drinking the glucose solution and some discomfort from the needle punctures and the tourniquet.
- Withhold all steroids and other pituitary-based hormones. If the patient must continue these or other drugs, note this on the laboratory request.
- Tell the patient to lie down and relax for 30 minutes before the test.

Implementation

- Perform a venipuncture and collect 6 ml of blood (basal sample) in a 7-ml clot-activator tube between 6 a.m. and 8 a.m.
- Give the patient 100 g of glucose solution by mouth. To prevent nausea, advise the patient to drink the glucose slowly.
- About 1 hour later, draw venous blood into a 7-ml clot-activator tube. Label the tubes appropriately and send them to the laboratory immediately.
- Handle the samples gently to prevent hemolysis.
- Send each sample to the laboratory immediately because hGH has a half-life of only 20 to 25 minutes.

Patient care

- Apply direct pressure to the venipuncture site until bleeding stops.

- Instruct the patient that he may resume his usual diet, activities, and medications stopped before the test.

Complications

Hematoma at the venipuncture site

Interpretation

Normal results

- Glucose suppresses hGH to levels ranging from undetectable to 3 nanograms/ml (SI, 3 µg/L) in 30 minutes to 2 hours.
- In children, rebound stimulation may occur after 2 to 5 hours.

Abnormal results

- In a patient with active acromegaly, elevated baseline hGH levels (5 nanograms/ml [SI, 5 µg/L]) aren't suppressed to less than 5 nanograms/ml during the test.
- Unchanged or rising hGH levels in response to glucose loading indicate hGH hypersecretion and may confirm suspected acromegaly and gigantism. This response may be verified by repeating the test after a 1-day rest.

Interfering factors

- Failure to observe pretest restrictions
- Hemolysis from rough handling of the sample
- Corticosteroids and phenothiazines such as chlorpromazine (possible decrease in hGH secretion)
- Amphetamines, arginine, estrogens, glucagon, levodopa, and niacin (possible increase in hGH secretion)
- Radioactive scan performed within 1 week before the test
- Delay in sending the specimen to the laboratory

Ham test

Overview

○ Ham test, *or acidified serum lysis test,* determines the cause of hemolytic anemia, hemoglobinuria, and bone marrow aplasia and the stability of the red blood cell (RBC) membrane.
○ Helps establish a diagnosis of paroxysmal nocturnal hemoglobinuria (PNH), a rare hematologic disease.
○ Relies on the susceptibility of RBCs to lyse — RBCs from patients with PNH are unusually susceptible to lysis by complement.
○ Washed RBCs are mixed with ABO-compatible normal serum and acid; after incubation at 98.6° F (37° C), the cells are examined for hemolysis.
○ In the presence of acidified human serum, a substantial portion of PNH cells are lysed, whereas normal RBCs show no hemolysis.

Purpose

○ To aid in the diagnosis of PNH

Procedure

Preparation

○ Explain to the patient that this test helps determine the cause of his anemia or other signs.
○ Inform the patient that he need not restrict food and fluids.
○ Tell the patient that the test requires a blood sample. Explain who will perform the venipuncture and when.
○ Explain to the patient that he may experience slight discomfort from the tourniquet and the needle puncture.

Implementation

○ Because the blood sample must be defibrinated immediately, laboratory personnel perform the venipuncture and collect the sample.

Patient care

○ Apply direct pressure to the venipuncture site until bleeding stops.

Complications

○ Hematoma at the venipuncture site

Interpretation

Normal results

○ RBCs don't undergo hemolysis.
○ Test results should be negative.

Abnormal results

Hemolysis of RBCs indicates PNH.

Interfering factors

○ Blood containing large numbers of spherocytes (possible false-positive)
○ Blood from patients with congenital dyserythropoietic anemia (false-positive)

Haptoglobin

Overview

○ Measures serum levels of haptoglobin, a glycoprotein produced in the liver.
○ In acute intravascular hemolysis, the haptoglobin concentration decreases rapidly and may remain low for 5 to 7 days, until the liver synthesizes more glyco-protein.

Purpose

○ To serve as an index of hemolysis
○ To distinguish between hemoglobin and myoglobin in plasma because haptoglobin doesn't bind with myo-globin
○ To investigate hemolytic transfusion reactions
○ To establish proof of paternity using genetic (pheno-typic) variations in haptoglobin structure.

Procedure

Preparation

○ Explain to the patient that this test determines the condition of red blood cells.
○ Tell the patient that the test requires a blood sample. Explain who will perform the venipuncture and when.
○ Explain to the patient that he may experience slight discomfort from the tourniquet and the needle punc-ture.
○ Inform the patient that he need not restrict food and fluids.
○ Notify the laboratory and physician of drugs the pa-tient is taking that may affect test results; it may be necessary to restrict them.

Implementation

○ Perform a venipuncture and collect the sample in a 7-ml clot-activator tube.
○ Handle the sample gently to prevent hemolysis.

Patient care

○ Apply direct pressure to the venipuncture site until bleeding stops.
○ Inform the patient that he may resume his usual medications.
○ If serum haptoglobin values are very low, watch for symptoms of hemolysis: chills, fever, back pain, flushing, distended jugular veins, tachycardia, tachypnea, and hypotension.

Complications

○ Hematoma at the venipuncture site

Interpretation

Normal results

○ Serum haptoglobin concentrations, measured in terms of the protein's hemoglobin-binding capacity, range from 40 to 180 mg/dl (SI, 0.4 to 1.8 g/L).
○ Nephelometric procedures yield lower results.
○ Haptoglobin is absent in 90% of neonates, but in most cases, levels gradually increase to normal by age 4 months.

Abnormal results

○ Markedly decreased serum haptoglobin levels are characteristic in acute and chronic hemolysis, severe hepatocellular disease, infectious mononucleosis, and transfusion reactions.
○ Hepatocellular disease inhibits haptoglobin synthesis.
○ In hemolytic transfusion reactions, haptoglobin levels begin decreasing after 6 to 8 hours and drop to 40% of pretransfusion levels after 24 hours.
○ In about 1% of the population, including 4% of blacks, haptoglobin is permanently absent; this dis-order is known as congenital ahaptoglobinemia.
○ Strikingly elevated serum haptoglobin levels occur in diseases marked by chronic inflammatory reactions or tissue destruction, such as rheumatoid arthritis and malignant neoplasms.

Interfering factors

○ Hemolysis from rough handling of the sample
○ Corticosteroids and androgens (possible increase in levels; may mask hemolysis in patients with inflam-matory disease)

Heinz bodies

Overview

○ Particles of decomposed hemoglobin (Hb) that precipitate from the cytoplasm of red blood cells (RBCs) and accumulate on RBC membranes.
○ Form as a result of drug injury to RBCs, the presence of unstable Hb, unbalanced globin chain synthesis caused by thalassemia, or a red cell enzyme deficiency (such as glucose-6-phosphate dehydrogenase deficiency).
○ Although removed from RBCs by the spleen, they're a major cause of hemolytic anemias. (See *Identifying Heinz bodies*.)
○ Detectable in a whole blood sample using phase microscopy or supravital stains; when they don't form spontaneously, various oxidant drugs added to the sample induce their formation.

Purpose

○ To help detect causes of hemolytic anemia

Procedure

Preparation

○ Explain that this test determines the cause of anemia.
○ Tell the patient that the test requires a blood sample.
○ Explain that he may feel slight discomfort from the tourniquet and the needle puncture.
○ Notify the laboratory and physician of drugs the patient is taking that may affect test results; it may be necessary to restrict them.
○ Inform the patient that he need not restrict food and fluids.

Identifying Heinz bodies

After supravital staining, Heinz bodies (particles of denatured hemoglobin that are usually attached to the cell membrane) appear as small, purple inclusions at cell margins. Heinz bodies are present in certain hemolytic anemias.

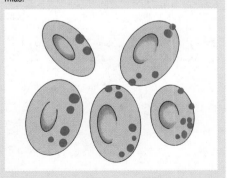

Implementation

○ Perform a venipuncture and collect the sample in a 3- or 4.5-ml ethylenediaminetetraacetic acid tube.
○ Fill the sample collection tube completely.
○ Invert the tube gently several times to mix the sample and the anticoagulant.

Patient care

○ Apply direct pressure to the venipuncture site until bleeding stops.
○ Instruct the patient that he may resume medications stopped before the test.
○ If large hematoma develops at venipuncture site, monitor pulses distal to the site.

Complications

○ Hematoma at the venipuncture site

Interpretation

Normal results

○ A negative test result indicates an absence of Heinz bodies.

Abnormal results

○ The presence of Heinz bodies may indicate an inherited RBC enzyme deficiency, the presence of unstable Hb, thalassemia, or drug-induced RBC injury.
○ Heinz bodies may also be present after splenectomy.

Interfering factors

○ Failure to fill the collection tube completely, to use the appropriate anticoagulant, to adequately mix the sample and the anticoagulant, or to send the sample to the laboratory immediately
○ Antimalarials, furazolidone (in infants), nitrofurantoin, phenacetin, procarbazine, and sulfonamides (possible false-positive)
○ Recent blood transfusion

Helicobacter pylori antibodies

Overview

○ Spiral, gram-negative bacterium linked to chronic gastritis and idiopathic chronic duodenal ulceration.
○ Although a gastric specimen can be obtained by endoscopy and cultured for *H. pylori*, the *H. pylori* antibody blood test is a more useful noninvasive screening procedure; may be performed using the enzyme-linked immunosorbent assay. (See *Other tests for* Helicobacter pylori.)

Purpose

○ To help diagnose *H. pylori* infection in patients with GI symptoms (used only for patients with GI symptoms, as a large number of healthy people have *H. pylori* antibodies)

Procedure

Preparation

○ Inform the patient that this test diagnoses the infection that may cause ulcers.

Other tests for *Helicobacter pylori*

H. pylori is detectable through blood, breath, feces, and tissue tests. Blood, breath, and feces tests are usually done before a tissue test because they are less invasive. Blood tests aren't used to detect *H. pylori* after treatment because a patient's blood can test positive even after *H. pylori* has been eliminated.

Blood test
The most common method, this test detects antibodies to *H. pylori* bacteria.

Urea breath test
Effective as a diagnostic tool for H. pylori, this test can also monitor whether treatment has been effective. In the physician's office, the patient drinks a urea solution that contains a special carbon atom. If H. pylori is present, it breaks down the urea, releasing the carbon. Blood carries the carbon to the lungs, and the patient exhales it. The breath test is 96% to 98% accurate.

Feces test
The *H. pylori* stool antigen (HpSA) test is another accurate way to detect *H. pylori* infection. It is a noninvasive test.

Tissue test
Normally, this test uses a biopsy sample taken with an endoscope, using one of three types:
● The rapid urease test detects the enzyme disease caused by *H. pylori*.
● A histology test allows the physician to find and examine the actual bacteria.
● A culture test grows *H. pylori* in the tissue sample.

○ Inform the patient that he need not restrict food and fluids.
○ Tell the patient that the test requires a blood sample.
○ Explain to the patient that he may experience slight discomfort from the tourniquet and the needle puncture.

Implementation

○ Perform a venipuncture and collect the sample in a 7-ml clot-activator tube.
○ Send the sample to the laboratory immediately.

Patient care

○ Apply direct pressure to the venipuncture site until bleeding stops.

Complications

○ Hematoma at the venipuncture site

Interpretation

Normal results

○ No antibodies to *H. pylori*
○ Test results reported as negative or positive

Abnormal results

○ A positive *H. pylori* test result indicates that the patient has antibodies to the bacterium.
○ The serologic results should be interpreted in light of the clinical findings.

Interfering factors

None known

Hematocrit

Overview

- A hematocrit (HCT) test is performed separately or as part of a complete blood count.
- Measures percentage by volume of packed red blood cells (RBCs) in a whole blood sample; for example, an HCT of 40% indicates that a 100-ml sample of blood contains 40 ml of packed RBCs.
- Packing is achieved by centrifuging anticoagulated whole blood in a capillary tube so that RBCs pack tightly without hemolysis.
- Test results may be used to calculate two RBC indices: mean corpuscular volume and mean corpuscular hemoglobin concentration.

Purpose

- To aid diagnosis of polycythemia, anemia, or abnormal states of hydration
- To aid in the calculation of erythrocyte indices.

Procedure

Preparation

- Explain to the patient that the HCT test detects anemia and other abnormal blood conditions.
- Tell the patient that the test requires a blood sample.
- Explain to the patient that he may feel slight discomfort from the tourniquet and the needle puncture.
- Inform the patient that he need not restrict food and fluids.
- If the patient is a child, explain to him (if he's old enough) and his parents that a small amount of blood will be taken from his finger or earlobe.

Implementation

- Perform a fingerstick using a heparinized capillary tube with a red band on the anticoagulant end. Fill the tube from the red-banded end to about two-thirds capacity; seal this end with clay.
- Or, perform a venipuncture and fill a 3- or 4.5-ml ethylenediaminetetraacetic acid tube.
- Invert the tube gently several times to mix the sample.
- Send the sample to the laboratory immediately.
- After you complete the testing, place the tube in the centrifuge with the red end pointing outward.

Patient care

- Ensure subdermal bleeding has stopped before removing pressure.
- If large hematoma develops at the venipuncture site, monitor pulses distal to the site.

Complications

- Hematoma at the venipuncture site

Interpretation

Normal results

- HCT is usually measured electronically; electronic results are 3% lower than manual measurements, which trap plasma in the column of packed RBCs.
- In men, 42% to 52% (SI, 0.42 to 0.52).
- In women, 36% to 48% (SI, 0.36 to 0.48).
- In neonates younger than age 1 week: 55% to 68% (SI, 0.55 to 0.68).
- Neonates age 1 week, 47% to 65% (SI, 0.47 to 0.65).
- Infants age 1 month, 37% to 49% (SI, 0.37 to 0.49).
- Infants age 3 months, 30% to 36% (SI, 0.3 to 0.36).
- Age 1 year, 29% to 41% (SI, 0.29 to 0.41).
- Age 10 years, 36% to 40% (SI, 0.36 to 0.4).

Abnormal results

- Low HCT suggests anemia, hemodilution, or massive blood loss.
- High HCT indicates polycythemia or hemoconcentration caused by blood loss and dehydration.

Interfering factors

- Failure to fill the tube properly, to use the proper anticoagulant, or to adequately mix the sample and the anticoagulant
- Hemolysis from rough handling of the sample or drawing the blood through a small-gauge needle for venipuncture
- Hemoconcentration caused by tourniquet constriction for longer than 1 minute (increase, typically 2.5% to 5%)
- Hemodilution from drawing the blood from the arm above an I.V. infusion

Hemoglobin

Overview

○ Total hemoglobin (Hb) measures the amount of Hb present in a deciliter (dl, or 100 ml) of whole blood.
○ Hb level correlates closely with the red blood cell (RBC) count and affects the Hb-to-RBC ratio (mean corpuscular hemoglobin [MCH] and mean corpuscular hemoglobin concentration [MCHC]).

Purpose

○ To measure the severity of anemia or polycythemia and to monitor the patient's response to therapy
○ To obtain data for calculating the MCH and MCHC

Procedure

Preparation

○ Explain to the patient that the Hb test detects anemia or polycythemia, or assesses his response to treatment.
○ Tell the patient that the test requires a blood sample. Explain who will perform the venipuncture and when.
○ Explain to the patient that he may feel slight discomfort from the tourniquet and the needle puncture.
○ If the patient is an infant or child, explain to the parents that a small amount of blood will be taken from his finger or earlobe.
○ Inform the patient that he need not restrict food and fluids.

Implementation

○ For adults and older children, perform a venipuncture and collect the sample in a 3- or 4.5-ml ethylenediaminetetraacetic acid (EDTA) tube.
○ For younger children and infants, collect the sample by fingerstick or heelstick in a microcollection device with EDTA.
○ Completely fill the collection tube and invert it gently several times to thoroughly mix the sample and the anticoagulant.
○ Handle the sample gently to prevent hemolysis.

Patient care

○ Apply direct pressure to the venipuncture site until bleeding stops.
○ If large hematoma develops at the venipuncture site, monitor pulses distal to the site.

Complications

○ Hematoma at the venipuncture site

Interpretation

Normal results

○ In men before middle age, 14 to 17.4 g/dl (SI, 140 to 174 g/L).
○ In men after middle age, 12.4 to 14.9 g/dl (SI, 124 to 149 g/L).
○ In women, 12 to 16 g/dl (SI, 120 to 160 g/L).
○ In women after middle age, 11.7 to 13.8 g/dl (SI, 117 to 138 g/L).
○ In neonates, 17 to 22 g/dl (SI, 170 to 220 g/L).
○ In neonates age 1 week, 15 to 20 g/dl (SI, 150 to 200 g/L).
○ In infants age 1 month, 11 to 15 g/dl (SI, 110 to 150 g/L).
○ In children, 11 to 13 g/dl (SI, 110 to 130 g/L).
○ Those who are more active or who live at high altitudes may have higher normal values.

Abnormal results

○ Low Hb level may indicate anemia, recent hemorrhage, or fluid retention, causing hemodilution.
○ High Hb level suggests hemoconcentration from polycythemia or dehydration.

Interfering factors

○ Failure to use the proper anticoagulant or to adequately mix the sample and the anticoagulant
○ Hemolysis from rough handling of the sample
○ Hemoconcentration from prolonged tourniquet constriction
○ Very high white blood cell counts, lipemia, or RBCs that are resistant to lysis (false-high)

Hemoglobin electrophoresis

Overview

- Probably the most useful laboratory method for separating and measuring normal and abnormal hemoglobin (Hb).
- Through electrophoresis, different types of Hb are separated to form a series of distinctly pigmented bands in a medium.
- Results compared with those of a normal sample

Purpose

- To measure the amount of HbA and to detect abnormal Hb
- To aid in the diagnosis of thalassemia

Procedure

Preparation

- Explain that Hb electrophoresis evaluates Hb.
- Tell the patient that the test requires a blood sample.
- If the patient is an infant or child, explain to the parents that a small amount of blood will be taken from his finger.
- Inform the patient that he need not restrict food and fluids.

Implementation

- Ask the patient if he has received a blood transfusion within the past 4 months.
- Perform a venipuncture and collect the sample in a 3- or 4.5-ml ethylenediaminetetraacetic acid tube.
- For young children, collect capillary blood in a microcollection device.
- Completely fill the collection tube and invert it gently several times; don't shake the tube vigorously.

Patient care

- Apply pressure to the venipuncture site until bleeding stops.

Complications

- Hematoma at the venipuncture site

Interpretation

Normal results

- In adults, HbA accounts for 95% (SI, 0.95) of all Hb; HbA$_2$, 1.5% to 3% (SI, 0.015 to 0.030); and HbF, < 2% (SI, < 0.02).
- In neonates, HbF normally accounts for half the total. HbS and HbC are normally absent.

Abnormal results

- Hb electrophoresis allows the identification of various types of Hb: Certain types may indicate a hemolytic disease. (See *Common variations of hemoglobin type and distribution.*)

Interfering factors

- Failure to fill the tube completely, to use the proper anticoagulant, or to adequately mix the sample and the anticoagulant
- Hemolysis from rough handling of the sample
- Blood transfusion within the past 4 months

Common variations of hemoglobin type and distribution

Hemoglobin (Hb)	Percentage of total hemoglobin	Clinical implications
HbA$_2$	4% to 5.8% (SI, 0.04 to 0.058)	Beta-thalassemia minor
	Less than 1.5% (SI, < 0.015)	Hb H disease
HbF	2% to 5% (SI, 0.02 to 0.05)	Beta-thalassemia minor
	10% to 90% (SI, 0.1 to 0.9)	Beta-thalassemia major
	5% to 15% (SI, 0.05 to 0.15)	Beta-δ-thalassemia minor
Homozygous HbS	70% to 98% (SI, 0.7 to 0.98)	Sickle cell disease

Hemoglobin, urine

Overview

○ Free hemoglobin (Hb) in the urine may occur in hemolytic anemias, infection, strenuous exercise, or severe intravascular hemolysis from a transfusion reaction.
○ Contained in red blood cells (RBCs), Hb consists of an iron-protoporphyrin complex (heme) and a polypeptide (globin).
○ Usually, RBCs are destroyed in the reticuloendothelial system, but when they're destroyed in the circulation, free Hb enters the plasma and binds with haptoglobin.
○ If the plasma level of Hb exceeds that of haptoglobin, the excess free Hb is excreted in the urine (hemoglobinuria).
○ Heme proteins act like enzymes that catalyze oxidation of organic substances.
○ This reaction produces a blue coloration; the intensity of color depends on the amount of Hb present.
○ Microscopic examination is necessary to identify intact RBCs in urine (hematuria), which can occur in the presence of free Hb.

Purpose

○ To aid in the diagnosis of hemolytic anemias, infection, or severe intravascular hemolysis from a transfusion reaction

Procedure

Preparation

○ If a woman is menstruating, reschedule the test, as menstrual blood can interfere with the result.
○ Explain to the patient that the urine hemoglobin test detects excessive RBC destruction.
○ Inform the patient that he need not restrict food and fluids.
○ Tell the patient that the test requires a random urine specimen, and teach him the proper collection technique.
○ Notify the laboratory and physician of drugs the patient is taking that may affect test results; it may be necessary to restrict them.

Implementation

○ Collect a random urine specimen.
Dipstik, Multistix, or Chemstrip method
○ Dip stick into the specimen and withdraw it.
○ After 30 seconds, read results using the chart provided by the manufacturer.
Occult tablet test
○ Put one drop of urine on filter paper, place tablet on urine, and apply 2 drops of water to the tablet.
○ After 2 minutes, inspect the filter paper.
○ Blue indicates a positive test.

Occult solution
○ Place a drop of urine on filter paper, close the package, and turn it over.
○ Apply 2 drops of solution to the site indicated. Read test after 30 seconds.
○ Blue indicates a positive reaction.

Patient care

○ Instruct the patient that he may resume his usual medications.

Complications

○ None known

Interpretation

Normal results

○ The urine contains no Hb.

Abnormal results

○ Hemoglobinuria may result from severe intravascular hemolysis caused by a blood transfusion reaction, burns, or a crush injury.
○ It may result from acquired hemolytic anemias caused by chemical or drug intoxication or malaria; congenital hemolytic anemias, such as hemoglobinopathies or enzyme defects; or paroxysmal nocturnal hemoglobinuria (another type of hemolytic anemia).
○ It may signal cystitis, ureteral calculi, or urethritis.
○ Hemoglobinuria and hematuria occur in renal epithelial damage (which may result from acute glomerulonephritis or pyelonephritis), renal tumor, and tuberculosis.

Interfering factors

○ Nephrotoxic drugs and anticoagulants (positive results)
○ Large doses of vitamin C or drugs that contain vitamin C as a preservative (false-negative)
○ Lysis of RBCs in stale or alkaline urine and contamination of the specimen by menstrual blood
○ Bacterial peroxidases in highly infected specimens (false-positive)

Hepatitis A antibodies

Overview

○ This test identifies hepatitis A antibodies that appear in the serum or body fluid of patients with hepatitis A virus (HAV).
○ Hepatitis A antibodies are present in blood and feces only briefly before symptoms appear.

Purpose

○ To aid in the differential diagnosis of viral hepatitis

Procedure

Preparation

○ Check the patient's history for administration of hepatitis vaccine.
○ Explain to the patient that this test helps identify a type of viral hepatitis.
○ Inform the patient that he need not restrict food or fluids before the test.
○ Tell the patient that the test requires a blood sample.
○ Explain to the patient that he may experience discomfort from the tourniquet and the needle puncture.

Implementation

○ Perform a venipuncture and collect the sample in two 3- or 4.5-ml ethylenediaminetetraacetic acid tubes.

Patient care

○ Apply direct pressure to the venipuncture site until bleeding stops.
○ Tell the patient that confirmed viral hepatitis is reported to public health authorities in most states.

Complications

○ Hematoma at the venipuncture site

Interpretation

Normal results

○ Serum is negative for hepatitis A antibodies.

Abnormal results

○ A single positive test result may indicate previous exposure to the virus, but because these antibodies persist so long in the bloodstream, only evidence of rising anti-HAV titers confirms HAV as the cause of current or very recent infection.

Interfering factors

○ Hepatitis vaccine (possible positive)

Hepatitis B core antibodies

Overview

○ This test identifies past or present hepatitis B virus (HBV) infection.
○ HBV core antibodies are produced during or after an acute HBV infection.
○ The core antigen is part of HBV, and the antibodies to the core antigen are usually present in chronic carriers.
○ HBV is identified by the presence of hepatitis B antibodies, protein molecules (immunoglobulins) in serum or body fluid that either neutralize antigens or tag them for attack by other cells or chemicals.

Purpose

○ To screen blood donors for hepatitis B
○ To screen people at high risk for contracting hepatitis B, such as hemodialysis nurses
○ To aid in the differential diagnosis of viral hepatitis

Procedure

Preparation

○ Explain to the patient that this test helps identify a type of viral hepatitis.
○ Inform the patient that he need not restrict food or fluids before the test.
○ Tell the patient that the test requires a blood sample.
○ Explain to the patient that he may experience discomfort from the tourniquet and the needle puncture.
○ Check the patient's history for administration of hepatitis vaccine.

Implementation

○ Perform a venipuncture and collect the sample in two 3- or 4.5-ml ethylenediaminetetraacetic acid tubes.

Patient care

○ Apply direct pressure to the venipuncture site until bleeding stops.
○ Tell the patient that confirmed viral hepatitis is reported to public health authorities in most states.

Complications

○ Hematoma at the venipuncture site

Interpretation

Normal results

○ Serum is negative for hepatitis B core antibodies.

Abnormal results

○ Positive findings may indicate that the patient is recovering from an acute HBV infection.

Interfering factors

○ Hepatitis vaccine (possible positive)
○ Undetectable level of hepatitis B surface antigens (false-negative)

Hepatitis B surface antibodies

Overview

- The hepatitis B virus is identified by the presence of hepatitis B antibodies, protein molecules (immunoglobulins) in serum or body fluid that either neutralize antigens or tag them for attack by other cells or chemicals.
- The presence of hepatitis B surface antigens indicates that a patient who has been exposed to the hepatitis B virus (HBV) is no longer contagious.
- These antigens protect the body from future HBV infection.

Purpose

- To screen blood donors
- To screen people at high risk for contracting hepatitis B, such as hemodialysis nurses
- To aid in the differential diagnosis of viral hepatitis

Procedure

Preparation

- Explain to the patient that this test helps identify a type of viral hepatitis.
- Inform the patient that he need not restrict food or fluids before the test.
- Tell the patient that the test requires a blood sample.
- Explain to the patient that he may experience discomfort from the needle and the tourniquet.
- Check the patient's history for administration of hepatitis vaccine.

Implementation

- Perform a venipuncture and collect the sample in two 3- or 4.5-ml ethylenediaminetetraacetic acid tubes.

Patient care

- Apply direct pressure to the venipuncture site until bleeding stops.
- Tell the patient that confirmed viral hepatitis is reported to public health authorities in most states.

Complications

- Hematoma at the venipuncture site

Interpretation

Normal results

- Serum is negative for hepatitis B core surface antigens.

Abnormal results

- Positive findings indicate that the patient is immune to HBV infection.

Interfering factors

- Hepatitis vaccine (possible positive)

Hepatitis B surface antigen

Overview

- Hepatitis B surface antigen (HBsAg), also called *hepatitis-associated antigen* or *Australia antigen,* appears in the serum of the patient with hepatitis B virus.
- HBsAg is detectable by radioimmunoassay or, less commonly, reverse passive hemagglutination during the extended incubation period and usually during the first 3 weeks of acute infection or when the patient is a carrier.
- Because hepatitis transmission is one of the gravest complications associated with blood transfusion; all donors must undergo screening for hepatitis B before their blood is stored.
- This screening, required by the Food and Drug Administration's Bureau of Biologics, has helped reduce the incidence of hepatitis.
- This test doesn't screen for hepatitis A virus (infectious hepatitis).

Purpose

- To screen blood donors for hepatitis B
- To screen people at high risk for contracting hepatitis B such as hemodialysis nurses
- To aid in the differential diagnosis of viral hepatitis

Procedure

Preparation

- Explain to the patient that this test helps identify a type of viral hepatitis.
- Inform the patient that he need not restrict food and fluids.
- Tell the patient that the test requires a blood sample. Explain who will perform the venipuncture and when.
- Explain to the patient that he may experience slight discomfort from the tourniquet and the needle puncture.
- Check the patient's history for administration of hepatitis B vaccine.
- If the patient is giving blood, explain the donation procedure to him.

Implementation

- Perform a venipuncture and collect the sample in a 10-ml clot-activator tube.
- Wash your hands carefully after the procedure.
- Remember to wear gloves when drawing blood and dispose of the needle properly.

Patient care

- Apply direct pressure to the venipuncture site until bleeding stops.
- Tell the patient that confirmed viral hepatitis is reported to public health authorities in most states.

Complications

- Hematoma at the venipuncture site

Interpretation

Normal results

- Normal serum is negative for HBsAg.

Abnormal results

- The presence of HBsAg in patients with hepatitis confirms hepatitis B.
- In chronic carriers and in people with chronic active hepatitis, HBsAg may be present in the serum several months after the onset of acute infection.
- It may also occur in more than 5% of patients with certain diseases other than hepatitis, such as hemophilia, Hodgkin's disease, and leukemia.
- If HBsAg is found in donor blood, that blood must be discarded because it carries a risk of transmitting hepatitis.
- Blood samples that test positive should be retested because inaccurate results do occur.

Interfering factors

- Hepatitis B vaccine (possible positive)

Hepatitis C virus antibodies

Overview

○ Detects hepatitis C virus (HCV) by checking for antibodies in the blood.
○ Patients with risk factors for the disease and those who exhibit symptoms may be tested.
○ Antibodies may indicate an infection or past infection.

Purpose

○ To test for the presence of HCV antibodies

Procedure

Preparation

○ Explain to the patient that the test can't distinguish between an acute or chronic infection.
○ Explain that the test doesn't indicate whether the HCV infection has been cured.
○ Explain that the test requires a blood sample.
○ Inform the patient that he may feel discomfort from the tourniquet and the needle puncture.

Implementation

○ Perform the venipuncture and collect the sample in two 3- or 4.5-ml ethylenediaminetetraacetic acid tubes.

Patient care

○ Apply direct pressure to the venipuncture site.
○ Offer appropriate referrals after testing.
○ Tell the patient that confirmed viral hepatitis is reported to public health authorities in most states.

Complications

○ Hematoma at the venipuncture site

Interpretation

Normal results

○ Absence of HCV antibodies in the blood.

Abnormal results

○ The absence of antibodies doesn't always mean the patient is free of Hepatitis C; antibodies can take a few weeks to develop.
○ Most people develop antibodies within three months of becoming infected.
○ A positive sample for antibodies cannot determine whether the infection is current or from the past. Further testing is required.
○ False-positive results are possible; repeat the test to confirm.

Interfering factors

○ Patients with weakened immune systems, such as those having HIV, end stage kidney disease, and organ transplants, may not be able to produce HCV antibodies even though they are infected

Hepatitis D antibodies

Overview

- Hepatitis D occurs primarily in patients with acute or chronic episodes of hepatitis B.
- Infection requires the presence of the hepatitis B surface antigen, while the hepatitis D virus (HDV) depends on the double-shelled type B virus to replicate.
- Type D infection can't outlast a type B infection.

Purpose

- To aid in the differential diagnosis of viral hepatitis

Procedure

Preparation

- Explain to the patient that the test can't distinguish between an acute and a chronic infection.
- Explain that the test doesn't indicate whether the HCV infection is cured.
- Explain that the test requires a blood sample.
- Inform the patient that he may feel discomfort from the tourniquet and the needle puncture.

Implementation

- Perform the venipuncture and collect the sample in two 3- or 4.5-ml ethylenediaminetetraacetic acid tubes.

Patient care

- Apply direct pressure to the venipuncture site.
- Tell the patient that confirmed viral hepatitis is reported to public health authorities in most states.

Complications

- Hematoma at the venipuncture site

Interpretation

Normal results

- Serum is negative for HDV antibodies.

Abnormal results

- Detection of intrahepatic delta antigens or immunoglobulin (Ig) M anti-delta antigens in acute disease (or IgM and IgG in chronic disease) confirm HDV.

Interfering factors

- Lipemia (possible false-positive)
- High titer rheumatoid factor (possible false-positive)

Herpes simplex antibodies

Overview

- The herpes simplex virus (HSV), a member of the herpes virus group, causes various clinically severe manifestations, including genital lesions, keratitis or conjunctivitis, generalized dermal lesions, and pneumonia.
- Severe involvement is associated with intrauterine or neonatal infections and encephalitis; such infections are most severe in immunosuppressed patients.
- Of the two closely related antigenic types, type 1 usually causes infections above the waistline; type 2 infections predominantly involve the external genitalia.
- Primary contact with this virus occurs in early childhood as acute stomatitis or, more commonly, as an inapparent infection.
- More than 50% of adults have antibodies to HSV.
- Sensitive assays, such as indirect immunofluorescence and enzyme immunoassay, demonstrate immunoglobulin (Ig) M class antibodies to HSV or detect a fourfold or greater increase in IgG class antibodies between acute- and convalescent-phase sera.

Purpose

- To confirm infections caused by HSV
- To detect recent or past HSV infection

Procedure

Preparation

- Explain the purpose of the test to the patient.
- Tell the patient that the test requires a blood sample.
- Explain to the patient that he may experience slight discomfort from the tourniquet and the needle puncture.

Implementation

- Perform a venipuncture and collect the sample in a 7-ml clot-activator tube.
- Allow the blood to clot for at least 1 hour at room temperature.
- Handle the sample gently to prevent hemolysis.
- Transfer the serum to a sterile tube or vial and send it to the laboratory promptly.
- If transfer cannot occur immediately, store the serum at 39.2° F (4° C) for 1 to 2 days or at −4° F (−20° C) for longer periods to avoid contamination.

Patient care

- Apply direct pressure to the venipuncture site until bleeding stops.
- If the patient's immune system is compromised, check the venipuncture site for changes and report them immediately.

Complications

- Hematoma at the venipuncture site

Interpretation

Normal results

- Sera from patients who have never been infected with HSV have no detectable antibodies (less than 1:5).

Abnormal results

- HSV infection can be ruled out in a patient whose serum shows no detectable antibodies to the virus.
- The presence of IgM or a fourfold or greater increase in IgG antibodies indicates active HSV infection.

Interfering factors

- Hemolysis from rough handling of the sample

Heterophil antibodies

Overview

○ Detects and identifies two immunoglobulin (Ig) M antibodies in human serum that react against foreign red blood cells (RBCs): Epstein-Barr virus (EBV) antibodies and Forssman antibodies.
○ In the Paul-Bunnell test — also called the presumptive test — EBV antibodies, found in the sera of patients with infectious mononucleosis, agglutinate with sheep RBCs in a test tube.
○ Forssman antibodies, present in the sera of some normal persons as well as in the sera of patients with such conditions as serum sickness, also agglutinate with sheep RBCs, thus rendering test results inconclusive for infectious mononucleosis.
○ If the Paul-Bunnell test establishes a presumptive titer, the Davidsohn differential absorption test can then distinguish between EBV and Forssman antibodies.

Purpose

○ To aid in the differential diagnosis of infectious mononucleosis

Procedure

Preparation

○ Explain to the patient that this test helps detect infectious mononucleosis.
○ Tell the patient that the test requires a blood sample.
○ Explain to the patient that he may experience slight discomfort from the tourniquet and the needle puncture.

Implementation

○ Perform a venipuncture and collect the sample in a 7-ml clot-activator tube.

Patient care

○ Apply direct pressure to the venipuncture site until bleeding stops.
○ If the titer is positive and infectious mononucleosis is confirmed, explain the treatment plan to the patient.
○ If the titer is positive but infectious mononucleosis isn't confirmed, or if the titer is negative but symptoms persist, explain that additional testing will be necessary in a few days or weeks to confirm the diagnosis and plan effective treatment.

Complications

○ Hematoma at the venipuncture site

Interpretation

Normal results

○ The titer is less than 1:56. It may be higher in elderly people.
○ Some laboratories refer to a normal titer as "negative" or as having "no reaction."

Abnormal results

○ Although heterophil antibodies are present in the sera of about 80% of patients with infectious mononucleosis 1 month after its onset, a positive finding — a titer higher than 1:56 — doesn't confirm this disorder.
○ A high titer can also result from systemic lupus erythematosus, syphilis, cryoglobulinemia, or the presence of antibodies to nonsyphilitic treponemata (yaws, pinta, bejel).
○ A gradual increase in the titer during week 3 or 4 followed by a gradual decrease during weeks 4 to 8 proves most conclusive for infectious mononucleosis.
○ A negative titer doesn't always rule out this disorder; occasionally, the titer becomes reactive 2 weeks later. If symptoms persist, repeat the test in 2 weeks.
○ Confirming infectious mononucleosis depends on heterophil agglutination and hematologic tests that show absolute lymphocytosis with 10% or more atypical lymphocytes.

Interfering factors

○ Hemolysis from rough handling of the sample
○ Hepatitis, leukemia, lymphomas, opioid use, and phenytoin therapy (false-positive)

Hexosaminidase A and B, serum

Overview

○ This fluorometric test measures the hexosaminidase A and B content of serum samples drawn by venipuncture or collected from a neonate's umbilical cord or of amniotic fluid obtained by amniocentesis.
○ Testing cultured skin fibroblasts can also identify a hexosaminidase deficiency; however, this procedure is costly and technically complex.
○ A reference center for congenital disease can recommend the preferred screening method and specimen.
○ Hexosaminidase refers to a group of enzymes that are necessary for metabolism of gangliosides, water-soluble glycolipids found primarily in brain tissue.
○ The hexosaminidase A and B test measures the hexosaminidase A and B content of serum and amniotic fluid.
○ Deficiency of hexosaminidase A indicates Tay-Sachs disease, which affects people of eastern European Jewish ancestry about 100 times more often than the general population.
○ Both parents must carry the defective gene to transmit Tay-Sachs disease to their children.
○ Sandhoff disease, which results from a deficiency of hexosaminidase A and B, is uncommon and not prevalent in any ethnic group.

Purpose

○ To confirm or rule out Tay-Sachs disease in the neonate
○ To screen for a Tay-Sachs carrier
○ To establish prenatal diagnosis of hexosaminidase A deficiency

Procedure

Preparation

○ Explain to the patient that this test identifies carriers of Tay-Sachs disease.
○ Tell the patient that the test requires a blood sample. Explain who will perform the venipuncture and when.
○ Explain to the patient that he may experience slight discomfort from the tourniquet and the needle puncture.
○ Inform the patient that he need not restrict food and fluids.
○ When testing a neonate, explain to the parents that this test detects Tay-Sachs disease.
○ Tell them that blood will be drawn from the neonate's arm, neck, or umbilical cord; that the procedure is safe and quickly performed; and that the neonate will have a small bandage on the venipuncture site.

○ Inform the parents that no pretest restrictions of food or fluid are needed.
○ If the test is prenatal, advise the patient of preparations for amniocentesis.

Implementation

○ Perform a venipuncture, collect cord blood, or assist with amniocentesis, as appropriate.
○ Collect the sample in a 7-ml clot-activator tube.
○ Handle the sample gently to prevent hemolysis.
○ The serum of a pregnant woman can't be tested, but her leukocytes or amniotic fluid can be, if necessary; if the father's blood test result is negative, the child will not inherit Tay-Sachs disease.
○ If the test can't occur immediately, freeze the sample.

Patient care

○ Apply direct pressure to the venipuncture site until bleeding stops.

Complications

○ Hematoma at the venipuncture site

Interpretation

Normal results

○ Total serum levels of hexosaminidase range from 5 to 12.9 U/L; hexosaminidase A accounts for 55% to 76% of the total.

Abnormal results

○ Absence of hexosaminidase A indicates Tay-Sachs disease (total hexosaminidase levels can be normal).
○ Absence of hexosaminidase A and B indicates Sandhoff disease, an uncommon, virulent variant of Tay-Sachs disease in which deterioration occurs more rapidly.

Interfering factors

○ Hemolysis from rough handling of the sample
○ Hormonal contraceptives (false-high)
○ Rifampin and isoniazid (increase in levels)

Holter monitoring

Overview

- Continuous recording of heart activity as the patient follows his normal routine, usually for 24 hours
- Patient-activated monitor: worn for 5 to 7 days, allows patient to manually initiate recording of heart activity when he experiences symptoms
- Also known as *ambulatory electrocardiography (ECG)* or *dynamic monitoring*

Purpose

- To detect cardiac arrhythmias
- To evaluate chest pain
- To evaluate the effectiveness of antiarrhythmic drug therapy
- To monitor pacemaker function
- To correlate symptoms and palpitations with actual cardiac events and patient activities
- To detect sporadic arrhythmias missed by an exercise or resting ECG

Procedure

Preparation

- Make sure the patient has signed an appropriate consent form.
- Note and report all allergies.
- Provide bathing instructions because some equipment must not get wet.
- Instruct the patient to avoid magnets, metal detectors, high-voltage areas, and electric blankets.
- Explain the importance of logging activities, as well as emotional upsets, physical symptoms, and ingestion of medication, in a diary.
- Explain how to mark the tape at the onset of symptoms, if applicable.
- Explain how to check the recorder to make sure it's working properly.

Implementation

- Electrodes are applied to the chest wall and securely attached to the lead wires and monitor.
- Placing electrodes over large muscles masses, such as the pectorals, is avoided to limit artifact.
- A new or fully charged battery is inserted in the recorder.
- A tape is inserted and the recorder turned on.
- The electrode attachment circuit is tested by connecting the recorder to a standard ECG machine, noting artifact during normal patient movement.

Patient care

- Remove all chest electrodes.
- Clean the electrode sites.

Complications

- Skin sensitivity to the electrodes

Interpretation

Normal results

- The ECG shows no significant arrhythmias or ST-segment changes.
- Changes in heart rate occur during various activities.

Abnormal results

- Abnormalities in cardiac rate or rhythm suggest possible serious arrhythmias, which may be symptomatic or asymptomatic.
- ST-T wave changes may coincide with patient symptoms or increased patient activity and may suggest possible myocardial ischemia.

Interfering factors

None known

Homocysteine, total, plasma

Overview

○ Homocysteine (tHcy), a sulfur-containing amino acid, is a transmethylation product of methionine.
○ tHcy is an intermediate in the synthesis of cysteine, which is produced by the enzymatic or acid hydrolysis of proteins.
○ This test is useful for the biochemical diagnosis of inborn errors of methionine, folate, and vitamins B_6 and B_{12} metabolism.

Purpose

○ To make a biochemical diagnosis of inborn errors of methionine, folate, and vitamins B_6 and B_{12} metabolism
○ To indicate acquired folate or cobalamin deficiency
○ To evaluate the risk factors for atherosclerotic vascular disease
○ To evaluate as a contributing factor in the pathogenesis of neural tube defects
○ To evaluate the cause of recurrent spontaneous abortions
○ To evaluate delayed child development or failure to thrive in infants

Procedure

Preparation

○ Inform the patient that this test detects homocysteine levels in plasma.
○ Advise him to fast for 12 to 14 hours before the test.
○ Tell the patient that this test requires a blood sample.
○ Tell him who will perform the venipuncture and when.
○ Inform him that he may experience slight discomfort from the tourniquet and the needle puncture.

Implementation

○ Perform a venipuncture and collect the sample in a 5-ml tube with ethylenediaminetetraacetic acid added.
○ Handle the sample gently to prevent hemolysis.
○ Immediately put the sample on ice and send it to the laboratory.

Patient care

○ Apply direct pressure to the venipuncture site until bleeding stops.

Complications

○ Hematoma at the venipuncture site

Interpretation

Normal results

○ 4 to 17 µmol/L

Abnormal results

○ Low homocysteine levels indicate inborn or acquired folate or cobalamine deficiency and inborn B_6 or B_{12} deficiency.
○ Elevated homocysteine levels indicate a higher incidence of atherosclerotic vascular disease.
○ In patients with type 2 diabetes mellitus, studies show that tHcy levels increase with even a modest deterioration in renal function.

Interfering factors

○ Failure to adhere to dietary restrictions
○ Failure to immediately freeze the specimen
○ Penicillamine (reduces the plasma levels of tHcy)
○ Azauridine, nitrous oxide, and a methotrexate deficiency (will cause increased plasma levels of tHcy)

Human chorionic gonadotropin

Overview

○ Human chorionic gonadotropin (hCG) is a glycoprotein hormone produced in the placenta.
○ If conception occurs, a specific assay for hCG — commonly called the beta-subunit assay — may detect this hormone in the blood 9 days after ovulation.
○ This interval coincides with the implantation of the fertilized ovum into the uterine wall.
○ Although the precise function of hCG is still unclear, it appears that hCG, with progesterone, maintains the corpus luteum during early pregnancy.
○ Production of hCG increases steadily during the first trimester, peaking around 10 weeks' gestation.
○ Levels then fall to less than 10% of first-trimester peak levels during the remainder of the pregnancy.
○ About 2 weeks after delivery, the hormone may no longer be detectable.
○ This serum immunoassay, a quantitative analysis of hCG beta-subunit level, is more sensitive (and costlier) than the routine pregnancy test using a urine sample.

Purpose

○ To detect early pregnancy
○ To determine adequacy of hormonal production in high-risk pregnancies (for example, habitual abortion)
○ To aid in the diagnosis of trophoblastic tumors, such as hydatidiform mole and choriocarcinoma, and tumors that ectopically secrete hCG
○ To monitor treatment for induction of ovulation and conception

Procedure

Preparation

○ Explain to the patient that this test determines if she's pregnant.
○ If detection of pregnancy isn't the diagnostic objective, offer the appropriate explanation.
○ Inform the patient that she need not restrict food and fluids.
○ Tell the patient that the test requires a blood sample. Explain who will perform the venipuncture and when.
○ Explain to the patient that she may experience slight discomfort from the tourniquet and the needle puncture.

Implementation

○ Perform a venipuncture and collect the sample in a 7-ml clot-activator tube.
○ Handle the sample gently to prevent hemolysis.

○ Send the sample to the laboratory immediately.

Patient care

○ Apply direct pressure to the venipuncture site until bleeding stops.

Complications

○ Hematoma at the venipuncture site

Interpretation

Normal results

○ Less than 4 IU/L
○ During pregnancy, hCG levels vary widely, depending partly on the number of days after the last normal menstrual period

Abnormal results

○ Elevated hCG beta-subunit levels indicate pregnancy; significantly higher concentrations are present in a multiple pregnancy.
○ Increased levels may also suggest hydatidiform mole, trophoblastic neoplasms of the placenta, and nontrophoblastic carcinomas that secrete hCG (including gastric, pancreatic, and ovarian adenocarcinomas).
○ Low hCG beta-subunit levels can occur in an ectopic pregnancy or a pregnancy of less than 9 days.
○ Beta-subunit levels can't differentiate between pregnancy and tumor recurrence because they're high in both conditions.

Interfering factors

○ Hemolysis from rough handling of the sample
○ Heparin anticoagulants and ethylenediaminetetraacetic acid (decrease; ask the laboratory whether the test will occur on plasma or serum)

Human chorionic gonadotropin, urine

Overview

○ Qualitative analysis of urine levels of human chorionic gonadotropin (hCG) detects pregnancy as early as 14 days after ovulation.
○ Production of hCG, a glycoprotein that prevents degeneration of the corpus luteum at the end of a normal menstrual cycle, begins after conception.
○ During the first trimester, hCG levels rise steadily and rapidly, peaking around 10 weeks' gestation, subsequently tapering off to less than 10% of peak levels.
○ Most common method of evaluating hCG in urine is hemagglutination inhibition.
○ Provides qualitative and quantitative information.
○ Qualitative urine test is easier and less expensive than the serum hCG test (*beta-subunit assay*); therefore, it's a more common test for detecting pregnancy.

Purpose

○ To detect and confirm pregnancy
○ To aid in the diagnosis of hydatidiform mole or hCG-secreting tumors, threatened abortion, or dead fetus

Procedure

Preparation

○ If appropriate, explain to the patient that the urine hCG test determines whether she's pregnant or determines the status of her pregnancy.
○ Alternatively, explain how the test functions as a screen for some types of cancer.
○ Tell the patient that she need not restrict food but should restrict fluids for 8 hours before the test.
○ Inform the patient that the test requires a first-voided morning specimen or urine collection over a 24-hour period, depending on whether the test is qualitative or quantitative.
○ Notify the laboratory and physician of drugs the patient is taking that may affect test results; it may be necessary to restrict them.

Implementation

○ For verification of pregnancy (qualitative analysis), collect a first-voided morning specimen. If this isn't possible, collect a random specimen.
○ For quantitative analysis of hCG, collect the patient's urine over a 24-hour period in the appropriate container, discarding the first specimen and retaining the last.
○ Specify the date of the patient's last menstrual period on the laboratory request.
○ Refrigerate the 24-hour specimen or keep it on ice during the collection period.

○ Be sure the test occurs at least 5 days after a missed period to avoid a false-negative result.

Patient care

○ Instruct the patient that she may resume her usual diet and medications.

Complications

None known

Interpretation

Normal results

○ In a qualitative immunoassay analysis, results are negative (nonpregnant) or positive (pregnant) for hCG.
○ In a quantitative analysis, urine hCG levels in the first trimester of a normal pregnancy may be as high as 500,000 IU/24 hours; in the second trimester, from 10,000 to 25,000 IU/24 hours; and in the third trimester, from 5,000 to 15,000 IU/24 hours.
○ Measurable hCG levels don't normally appear in the urine of men or nonpregnant women.

Abnormal results

○ During pregnancy, elevated urine hCG levels may indicate multiple pregnancy or erythroblastosis fetalis; depressed urine hCG levels may indicate threatened abortion or ectopic pregnancy.
○ Measurable levels of hCG in men and nonpregnant women may indicate choriocarcinoma, ovarian or testicular tumors, melanoma, multiple myeloma, or gastric, hepatic, pancreatic, or breast cancer.

Interfering factors

○ Gross proteinuria (> 1 g/24 hours), hematuria, or an elevated erythrocyte sedimentation rate (possible false-positive, depending on the laboratory method)
○ Early pregnancy, ectopic pregnancy, or threatened abortion (possible false-negative)
○ Phenothiazine (possible false-negative or false-positive)

Human growth hormone, serum

Overview

○ Human growth hormone (hGH), protein secreted by pituitary gland; primary regulator of human growth
○ Has no easily defined feedback mechanism or single target gland; affects many body tissues
○ Like insulin, promotes protein synthesis and stimulates amino acid uptake by cells; raises plasma glucose levels by inhibiting glucose uptake and utilization by cells, and increases free fatty acid levels by enhancing lipolysis
○ Secretion regulated by the hypothalamus through a growth hormone–releasing factor and a growth hormone release–inhibiting factor (somatostatin)
○ Secretion diurnal; varies with exercise, sleep, stress, and nutritional status
○ Hyposecretion or hypersecretion may induce pathologic states (such as dwarfism or gigantism); altered levels are common in pituitary dysfunction
○ Quantitative analysis of plasma hGH levels, part of an anterior pituitary stimulation or suppression test
○ Such testing crucial because clinical manifestations of an hGH deficiency are rarely reversible by therapy
○ Also called *somatotropin*

Purpose

○ To differentiate between pituitary or thyroid hypofunction in diagnosis of dwarfism
○ To confirm the diagnosis of acromegaly and gigantism in the adult
○ To help diagnose pituitary and hypothalamic tumors
○ To help evaluate hGH therapy

Procedure

Preparation

○ Explain to the patient, or his parents if the patient is a child, that this test measures hormone levels and helps determine the cause of abnormal growth.
○ Instruct the patient to fast and limit activity for 10 to 12 hours before the test.
○ Tell the patient that the test requires a blood sample.
○ Inform him that another sample may be necessary the next day for comparison.
○ Tell the patient he may have slight discomfort from the tourniquet and the needle puncture.
○ Withhold all drugs that affect hGH levels such as pituitary-based steroids. If the patient must continue them, note this on the laboratory request.
○ Make sure the patient is relaxed and recumbent for 30 minutes before the test; stress and activity elevate hGH levels.

Implementation

○ Between 6 a.m. and 8 a.m. on 2 consecutive days, perform a venipuncture and collect at least 7 ml of blood in a clot-activator tube.
○ Handle the sample gently to prevent hemolysis.
○ Send it to the laboratory immediately because hGH has a half-life of only 20 to 25 minutes.

Patient care

○ Apply direct pressure to the venipuncture site until bleeding stops.
○ Tell the patient that he may resume his usual diet, activities, and medications stopped before the test.

Complications

○ Hematoma at the venipuncture site

Interpretation

Normal results

○ Normal hGH levels for men range from undetectable to 5 nanograms/ml (SI, 5 µg/L); for women, from undetectable to 10 nanograms/ml (SI, 10 µg/L).
○ Children's values may range from undetectable to 16 nanograms/ml (SI, 16 µg/L) and are usually higher.

Abnormal results

○ Increased hGH levels may indicate a pituitary or hypothalamic tumor, frequently an adenoma, which causes gigantism in children and acromegaly in adults and adolescents.
○ Some patients with diabetes mellitus have elevated hGH levels without acromegaly.
○ Suppression testing is necessary to confirm diagnosis.
○ Pituitary infarction, metastatic disease, and tumors may decrease hGH levels.
○ Dwarfism may result from low hGH levels, although only 15% of all cases of growth failure relate to endocrine dysfunction.
○ Confirming the diagnosis requires stimulation testing with arginine or insulin.

Interfering factors

○ Failure to observe pretest restrictions
○ Hemolysis from rough handling of the sample
○ Arginine, beta blockers such as propranolol, and estrogens (increase)
○ Amphetamines, bromocriptine, levodopa, dopamine, pituitary-based steroids, methyldopa, and histamine (increase)
○ Insulin (induced hypoglycemia), glucagon, and nicotinic acid (increase)
○ Phenothiazines (such as chlorpromazine) and corticosteroids (decrease)
○ Radioactive scan performed within 1 week before the test

Human immunodeficiency virus antibodies

Overview

○ Detects antibodies to human immunodeficiency virus (HIV) in serum.
○ HIV is the virus that causes acquired immunodeficiency syndrome (AIDS); transmission occurs by direct exposure of a person's blood to body fluids containing the virus.
○ Virus may be transmitted from one person to another through exchange of contaminated blood and blood products, during sexual intercourse with an infected partner, when I.V. drugs are shared, and from an infected mother to her child during pregnancy or breast-feeding.
○ Initial identification of HIV usually occurs through enzyme-linked immunosorbent assay.
○ Western blot test and immunofluorescence confirm positive finding; other tests available, which may detect antibodies.

Purpose

○ To screen for HIV in a high-risk patient
○ To screen donated blood for HIV

Procedure

Preparation

○ Explain to the patient that this test detects HIV infection.
○ Provide adequate counseling about the reasons for performing the test; usually, a patient's physician requests it.
○ If the patient has questions about his condition, be sure to provide full and accurate information.
○ Tell the patient that the test requires a blood sample. Explain who will perform the venipuncture and when.
○ Explain to the patient that he may experience slight discomfort from the tourniquet and the needle puncture.

Implementation

○ Perform a venipuncture and collect the sample in a 10-ml barrier tube.
○ Barrier tubes help prevent contamination when pouring the serum in the laboratory.
○ Observe standard precautions when drawing a blood sample.
○ Use gloves, properly dispose of needles, and use blood-fluid precaution labels on tubes, as necessary.

Patient care

○ Apply direct pressure to the venipuncture site until bleeding stops.
○ Keep the venipuncture site clean and dry, as the patient may have a compromised immune system.
○ Keep test results confidential.
○ When the patient receives the results, give him another opportunity to ask questions.
○ Encourage the patient with positive screening tests to seek medical follow-up care, even if he's asymptomatic.
○ Tell the patient to report early signs of AIDS, such as fever, weight loss, axillary or inguinal lymphadenopathy, rash, and persistent cough or diarrhea. Women should also report gynecologic symptoms.
○ Tell the patient to assume that he can transmit HIV to others until conclusively proved otherwise.
○ To prevent possible virus transmission, advise him about safer sex practices.
○ Instruct the patient not to share razors, toothbrushes, or utensils (which may be contaminated with blood) and to clean such items with household bleach diluted 1:10 in water.
○ Advise the patient against donating blood, tissues, or an organ.
○ Warn the patient to inform his physician and dentist about his condition so that they can take proper precautions.

Complications

○ Hematoma at the venipuncture site
○ Infection

Interpretation

Normal results

○ Test results are normally negative.

Abnormal results

○ The test detects previous exposure to HIV — it does not identify a patient who has been exposed to the virus but hasn't yet made antibodies.
○ In most cases, the patient with AIDS has antibodies to HIV.
○ A positive test for the HIV antibody can't determine whether a patient harbors actively replicating virus or when the patient will manifest signs and symptoms of AIDS.
○ Many apparently healthy people have been exposed to HIV and have circulating antibodies. The test results for such people aren't false-positives.
○ Patients in the later stages of AIDS may exhibit no detectable antibody in their sera because they can no longer mount an antibody response.

Interfering factors

None known

Human leukocyte antigens

Overview

○ Identifies a group of antigens present on the surface of all nucleated cells but most easily detected on lymphocytes.
○ The four types of human leukocyte antigen (HLA) are HLA-A, HLA-B, HLA-C, and HLA-D.
○ Essential to immunity and determine the degree of histocompatibility between transplant recipients and donors.
○ Numerous antigenic determinants (more than 60, for instance, at the HLA-B locus) are present for each site; one set of each antigen is inherited from each parent.
○ High incidence of specific HLA types linked to specific diseases, such as rheumatoid arthritis and multiple sclerosis, but these findings have little diagnostic significance.

Purpose

○ To provide histocompatibility typing of transplant recipients and donors
○ To aid in genetic counseling
○ To aid in paternity testing

Procedure

Preparation

○ Explain that this test detects antigens on white blood cells.
○ Inform the patient that he need not restrict food and fluids.
○ Tell the patient that the test requires a blood sample.
○ Tell him who will perform the venipuncture and when.
○ Explain to the patient that he may experience slight discomfort from the tourniquet and the needle puncture.
○ Check the patient's history for recent blood transfusions. It may be necessary to postpone HLA testing if he has recently undergone a transfusion.

Implementation

○ Perform a venipuncture and collect the sample in a tube containing anticoagulant acid citrate dextrose solution.
○ Handle the sample gently to prevent hemolysis.

Patient care

○ Apply direct pressure to the venipuncture site until bleeding stops.
○ Refer the patient and family to appropriate counseling services.

Complications

○ Hematoma at the venipuncture site

Interpretation

Normal results

○ No reaction of lymphocytes in HLA-A, -B, and -C testing
○ No reaction of leukocytes in HLA-D testing

Abnormal results

○ In HLA-A, HLA-B, and HLA-C testing, lymphocytes that react with the test antiserum undergo lysis; they're detectable by phase microscopy.
○ In HLA-D testing, leukocyte incompatibility is marked by blast formation, deoxyribonucleic acid synthesis, and proliferation.
○ Incompatible HLA-A, HLA-B, HLA-C, and HLA-D groups may cause unsuccessful tissue transplantation.
○ Many diseases have a strong association with certain types of HLAs. For example, HLA-DR5 is associated with Hashimoto's thyroiditis.
○ B8 and Dw3 are associated with Graves' disease, whereas B8 alone is associated with chronic autoimmune hepatitis, celiac disease, and myasthenia gravis.
○ Dw3 alone is associated with Addison's disease, Sjögren's syndrome, dermatitis herpetiformis, and systemic lupus erythematosus.
○ In paternity testing, a putative father who presents a phenotype (two haplotypes: one from the father and one from the mother) with no haplotype or antigen pair identical to one of the child's is excluded as the father.
○ A putative father with one haplotype identical to one of the child's may be the father; the probability varies with the incidence of the haplotype in the population.

Interfering factors

○ Hemolysis from rough handling of the sample
○ HLA from blood transfusion within 72 hours before sample collection

Human placental lactogen

Overview

○ A polypeptide hormone, human placental lactogen (hPL) — also known as *human chorionic somato-mammotropin* — displays lactogenic and somato-tropic (growth hormone) properties in a pregnant woman.
○ In combination with prolactin, hPL prepares the breasts for lactation.
○ Indirectly provides energy for maternal metabolism and fetal nutrition
○ Facilitates protein synthesis and mobilization essential to fetal growth.
○ Secretion is autonomous, beginning at about 5 weeks' gestation and declining rapidly after delivery.
○ This radioimmunoassay measures plasma hPL levels, which are roughly proportional to placental mass.
○ Assays may be necessary in high-risk pregnancies and suspected placental tissue dysfunction.
○ Because values vary widely during the latter half of pregnancy, serial determinations over several days provide the most reliable test results.
○ Combined with the measurement of estriol levels, is a reliable indicator of placental function and fetal well-being.
○ Also useful as a tumor marker in certain malignant states such as ectopic tumors that secrete hPL.

Purpose

○ To assess placental function and fetal well-being
○ To aid diagnosis of hydatidiform mole and choriocarcinoma
○ To aid in the diagnosis and monitor treatment of nontrophoblastic tumors that ectopically secrete hPL

Procedure

Preparation

○ Explain to the patient that this test helps assess placental function and fetal well-being.
○ If assessing fetal well-being isn't the diagnostic objective, offer an appropriate explanation.
○ Explain to the patient that she may experience slight discomfort from the tourniquet and the needle puncture.
○ Inform the pregnant patient that it may be necessary to repeat this test during her pregnancy.

Implementation

○ Perform a venipuncture and collect the sample in a 7-ml clot-activator tube.
○ Handle the sample gently to prevent hemolysis.

Patient care

○ Apply direct pressure to the venipuncture site until bleeding stops.

Complications

○ Hematoma at the venipuncture site

Interpretation

Normal results

○ For pregnant women, normal hPL levels vary with the gestational phase and slowly increase throughout pregnancy, reaching 8.6 µg/ml at term is normal.
○ 5 to 27 weeks: < 4.6 µg/ml.
○ 28 to 31 weeks: 2.4 to 6.1 µg/ml.
○ 32 to 35 weeks: 3.7 to 7.7 µg/ml.
○ 36 weeks to term: 5.0 to 8.6 µg/ml.
○ At term, patients with diabetes may have mean levels of 9 to 11 µg/ml.
○ Normal levels for men and nonpregnant women are less than 0.5 µg/ml.

Abnormal results

○ For reliable interpretation, correlate hPL levels with gestational age; for example, after 30 weeks' gestation, levels below 4 µg/ml may indicate placental dysfunction.
○ Low hPL concentrations are also characteristically associated with postmaturity syndrome, intrauterine growth retardation, preeclampsia, and eclampsia.
○ Declining concentrations may help differentiate incomplete abortion from threatened abortion.
○ Be aware that low hPL concentrations don't confirm fetal distress.
○ Concentrations over 4 µg/ml after 30 weeks' gestation don't guarantee fetal well-being because elevated levels have been reported after fetal death.
○ An hPL value above 6 µg/ml after 30 weeks' gestation may suggest an unusually large placenta, commonly occurring in a patient with diabetes mellitus, multiple pregnancy, or Rh isoimmunization.
○ The test's usefulness in predicting fetal death in a patient with diabetes mellitus and in managing Rh isoimmunization during pregnancy is limited.
○ Below-normal concentrations of hPL may indicate trophoblastic neoplastic disease, such as hydatidiform mole and choriocarcinoma.
○ Abnormal concentrations of hPL have occurred in the sera of patients with other neoplastic disorders, including bronchogenic carcinoma, hepatoma, lymphoma, and pheochromocytoma. In these patients, hPL levels are used as tumor markers for evaluating chemotherapy, monitoring tumor growth and recurrence, and detecting residual tissue after excision.

Interfering factors

○ Hemolysis from rough handling of the sample

Hypotonic duodenography

Overview

- Fluoroscopic examination of the duodenum after instillation of barium sulfate and air through an intestinal catheter.
- Used in patients with symptoms of duodenal or pancreatic pathology such as persistent upper abdominal pain.
- Patients with upper GI tract strictures, particularly with ulcerations or large masses, shouldn't undergo this procedure.
- After the catheter is passed through the patient's nose into the duodenum, I.V. infusion of glucagon or I.M. injection of propantheline bromide (or another anticholinergic) induces duodenal atony.
- Instillation of barium and air distends the relaxed duodenum, flattening its deep circular folds; spot films then record the precise delineation of the duodenal anatomy.
- Although these films readily demonstrate small duodenal lesions and tumors of the head of the pancreas that impinge on the duodenal wall, differential diagnosis requires further studies.

Purpose

- To detect small, postbulbar duodenal lesions, tumors of the head of the pancreas, and tumors of the ampulla of Vater
- To aid in the diagnosis of chronic pancreatitis

Procedure

Preparation

- Explain to the patient that hypotonic duodenography permits examination of the duodenum and pancreas after the instillation of barium and air.
- Instruct the patient to fast after midnight the night before the test.
- Describe the test, including who will perform it and where it will take place.
- Inform the patient that a tube will be passed through his nose into the duodenum to serve as a channel for the barium and air.
- Tell the patient that he may experience a cramping pain as air is introduced into the duodenum. Instruct him to breathe deeply and slowly through his mouth if he experiences this pain to help relax the abdominal muscles.
- If the patient is to receive glucagon or an anticholinergic during the procedure, describe the possible adverse effects of glucagon (nausea, vomiting, hives, and flushing) or of anticholinergics (dry mouth, thirst, tachycardia, urine retention, and blurred vi-

sion). If an anticholinergic is given to an outpatient, advise him to have someone accompany him home.
- Just before the test, tell the patient to remove dentures, glasses, necklaces, hairpins, combs, and constricting undergarments; also ask him to void.

Implementation

- While the patient is sitting, a catheter is passed through his nose and into the stomach.
- The patient is then placed into a supine position on an X-ray table; the catheter is advanced into the duodenum under fluoroscopic guidance.
- The patient is given I.V. glucagon, which quickly induces duodenal atony for about 20 minutes; or an I.M. anticholinergic is injected.
- Barium is instilled through the catheter; spot films are taken of the duodenum.
- Some of the barium is then withdrawn, air is instilled, and additional spot films are taken.
- When the required films have been obtained, the catheter is removed.
- Throughout the procedure, the patient is observed for adverse reactions. Be aware that such reactions may follow administration of glucagon or an anticholinergic.

Patient care

- If the patient received an anticholinergic, make sure he voids within a few hours after the test.
- Advise the outpatient to rest in a waiting area until his vision clears (about 2 hours) unless someone can take him home.
- Give a cathartic.
- Tell the patient that he may burp instilled air or pass flatus and that the barium colors the feces chalky white for 24 to 72 hours.
- After the procedure, encourage the patient to drink extra fluids, unless contraindicated, to help eliminate the barium.
- Record a description of feces the patient passed in the hospital and notify the physician if the patient hasn't expelled the barium after 2 to 3 days.

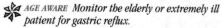 *AGE AWARE Monitor the elderly or extremely ill patient for gastric reflux.*

Complications

- Adverse reaction to the drugs

Interpretation

Normal results

- When barium and air distend the atonic duodenum, the mucosa normally appears smooth and even.
- The regular contour of the pancreas head also appears on the duodenal wall.

Abnormal results

○ Irregular nodules or masses on the duodenal wall could mean duodenal lesions, tumors of the ampulla of Vater, tumors of the pancreas head, or chronic pancreatitis.
○ A differential diagnosis requires further tests, such as endoscopic retrograde cholangiopancreatography, serum and urine amylase tests, ultrasonography of the pancreas, and computed tomography of the pancreas.

Interfering factors

○ Failure to fast

Hysterosalpingography

Overview

- Radiologic examination that shows the uterine cavity, fallopian tubes, and peritubal area.
- Fluoroscopic X-rays obtained as contrast medium flows through the uterus and the fallopian tubes.
- Performed as part of an infertility study.

Purpose

- To confirm tubal abnormalities such as adhesions
- To confirm uterine abnormalities such as congenital malformations
- To confirm the presence of fistulas or peritubal adhesions
- To evaluate the cause of repeated miscarriage

Procedure

Preparation

- Make sure the patient has signed an appropriate consent form.
- Note and report all allergies, including iodinated contrast media.
- Check the patient's history for recent pelvic infection.
- A test for pelvic infections may be necessary before the study.
- Antibiotics may be prescribed before the test.
- Explain that the procedure should take place 2 to 5 days after menstruation ends.
- Warn the patient that she might experience moderate cramping.
- Explain that she may receive a mild sedative or a nonprescription prostaglandin inhibitor 30 minutes before the procedure.
- Explain that the test takes about 15 minutes.
- Explain that a small amount of vaginal bleeding and pelvic cramping is normal for a few days after the study.

Implementation

- The patient is assisted into the lithotomy position; a scout film is taken.
- A bimanual examination determines uterine size and position.
- A speculum is inserted in the vagina, and the vagina and cervix are cleaned.
- A cannula is inserted into the cervix and anchored to a tenaculum.
- Contrast medium is injected through the cannula.
- The uterus and fallopian tubes are viewed fluoroscopically and X-rays are taken.
- For oblique views, the table is tilted or the patient is asked to change position.
- Films may be taken later to evaluate the spillage of contrast medium into the peritoneal cavity.

Patient care

- Instruct the patient to return to normal activities gradually.
- Tell the patient that additional tests and studies may be necessary to establish a precise diagnosis.
- Monitor the patient's vital signs.
- Monitor for signs and symptoms of infection and uterine perforation.
- Monitor for bleeding.
- Watch for an adverse reaction to the contrast medium.

Complications

- Uterine perforation
- Infection
- Bleeding
- Adverse reaction to the contrast medium

Interpretation

Normal results

- The uterine cavity is symmetrical.
- The fallopian tubes are a normal caliber.
- Contrast medium spills freely into the peritoneal cavity.
- Contrast medium doesn't leak from the uterus.

Abnormal results

- The uterus is asymmetrical, suggesting intrauterine adhesions or masses.
- contrast medium flow through the fallopian tubes is impaired, suggesting partial or complete blockage.
- Contrast medium leaks through the uterine wall, suggesting fistulas.

Interfering factors

None known

Hysteroscopy

Overview

- Small-diameter endoscope shows the interior of the uterus.
- Usually performed in the physician's office after giving patient a local anesthetic or mild sedative, within the first week after the end of a patient's menstrual cycle.

Purpose

- To investigate abnormal uterine bleeding
- To remove polyps
- To evaluate infertile patients
- To direct the removal of intrauterine devices
- To aid in the diagnosis and treatment of intrauterine adhesions
- To diagnose uterine fibroids

Procedure

Preparation

- Make sure the patient has signed an appropriate consent form.
- Note and report all allergies.
- Check the patient's history for hypersensitivity to the anesthetic.
- Obtain the results of the patient's last Pap test.
- Food and fluids may be restricted before the test.
- The doctor will perform a complete pelvic examination.
- Cultures of the vagina and cervix may be taken.
- Instruct the patient to empty her bladder before the test.
- Warn the patient that the doctor may inflate her uterus with carbon dioxide (CO_2); tell her that her body will absorb it but that it may cause upper abdominal or shoulder pain lasting 24 to 36 hours after the test.
- Explain that some vaginal bleeding and mild abdominal cramping may occur after the test.
- Recommend that patient have a friend or relative drive her home after the procedure.

Implementation

- The patient is assisted into a modified dorsal lithotomy position with her legs in stirrups.
- A local anesthetic is given.
- The vagina is cleaned and the hysteroscope inserted.
- Visualization begins at the level of the internal os.
- In contact hysteroscopy, the uterus isn't distended; only the area in direct contact with the hysteroscope is visible.
- In panoramic hysteroscopy, an external illumination source and media (such as CO_2) for distention are used; this makes the tissue visible from a distance.

Patient care

- Provide the patient with a sanitary pad if needed.
- Provide analgesics as needed.
- Monitor vital signs.
- Monitor for bleeding
- Watch for adverse reaction to analgesics.
- Watch for signs and symptoms of infection, such as fever and pain.

Complications

- Severe cramps, dyspnea, upper abdominal and right shoulder pain can develop if CO_2 passes into the peritoneal cavity
- Adverse reaction to drugs
- Infection

Interpretation

Normal results

- The interior of the uterus is normal in size and shape and free from adhesions and lesions.

Abnormal results

- The interior of the uterus is abnormally shaped, suggesting polyps, uterine wall tumors, or adhesions.

Interfering factors

- Heavy bleeding or a distended bladder may interfere with visualization

Immune complex assays

Overview

○ Immune complex diseases, such as postinfectious syndromes, serum sickness, drug sensitivity, rheumatoid arthritis, and systemic lupus erythematosus (SLE) may occur when immune complexes develop faster than the lymphoreticular system can clear them.
○ Immune complexes can develop when a certain ratio of antigen reacts with antibody of isotypes immunoglobulin (Ig) G 1, 2, 3, or IgM in tissues.
○ Immune complexes are usually detected by histologic examination of biopsy tissue and use of fluorescence or peroxidase staining with antibodies specific for immunologic types.
○ Tissue biopsies can't evaluate complexes still in circulation, but serum assays detect circulating immune complexes indirectly. More than one test may be necessary to achieve accurate results.
○ Appropriate serum test methods are those using C1, rheumatoid factor (RF), or cellular substrates, such as Raji cells, as reagents.

Purpose

○ To demonstrate circulating immune complexes in serum
○ To monitor the patient's response to therapy
○ To estimate disease severity

Procedure

Preparation

○ Explain to the patient that these tests help evaluate his immune system.
○ Inform the patient that the test will be repeated to monitor his response to therapy, if appropriate.
○ Inform the patient that he need not restrict food and fluids.
○ Tell the patient that the test requires a blood sample. Explain who will perform the venipuncture and when.
○ Explain to the patient that he may experience slight discomfort from the needle puncture and the tourniquet.
○ If the patient is scheduled for C1q assay (a component of C1), check his history for recent heparin therapy and report such therapy to the laboratory.

Implementation

○ Perform a venipuncture and collect the sample in a 7-ml clot-activator tube.
○ Send the sample to the laboratory immediately to prevent deterioration of immune complexes.

Patient care

○ Because many patients with immune complexes have a compromised immune system, keep the venipuncture site clean and dry.
○ Apply direct pressure to the venipuncture site until bleeding stops.

Complications

○ Hematoma at the venipuncture site

Interpretation

Normal results

○ Immune complexes are not detectable in serum.

Abnormal results

○ The presence of detectable immune complexes in serum has etiologic importance in many autoimmune diseases, such as SLE and rheumatoid arthritis.
○ For definitive diagnosis, the presence of these complexes must be considered with the results of other studies. For example, in SLE, immune complexes are associated with high titers of antinuclear antibodies and circulating antinative deoxyribonucleic acid antibodies.
○ Because of their filtering function, renal glomeruli seem vulnerable to immune complex deposition, although blood vessel walls and choroid plexuses (vascular folds in the ventricles of the brain) can be affected.
○ Renal biopsy to detect immune complexes can provide conclusive evidence for immune complex (type III) glomerulonephritis, differentiating it from other types of glomerulonephritis.

Interfering factors

○ Failure to send the sample to the laboratory immediately
○ Presence of cryoglobulins in the serum
○ Inability to standardize RF inhibition tests and platelet aggregation assays

Impedance plethysmography

Overview

○ Reliable, widely used, noninvasive test that measures venous flow in the limbs
○ Plethysmograph electrodes applied to the patient's leg record changes in electrical resistance (impedance) from blood volume variations that may result from respiration or venous occlusion
○ Also called *occlusive impedance phlebography*

Purpose

○ To detect deep vein thrombosis (DVT) in the proximal deep veins of the leg
○ To screen the patient at high risk for thrombophlebitis
○ To evaluate the patient with suspected pulmonary embolism (because most pulmonary emboli are complications of DVT in the leg)

Procedure

Preparation

○ Explain to the patient that impedance plethysmography helps detect DVT.
○ Inform the patient that he need not restrict food, fluids, and medications.
○ Explain that both legs will receive the test and that three to five tracings may be made for each leg.
○ Assure the patient that the test is painless and safe.
○ Emphasize that accurate testing requires that leg muscles be relaxed and breathing be normal.
○ Reassure the patient that, if he experiences pain that interferes with leg relaxation, he may receive a mild analgesic.
○ Urge the patient to lie quietly and relax as much as possible.
○ Keep the room temperature as warm as possible to help prevent the patient's extremities from becoming cold.
○ Just before the test, instruct the patient to void and to put on a hospital gown.

Implementation

○ Assist the patient into the supine position, elevating the leg to be tested 30 to 35 degrees. To promote venous drainage, place the calf above the patient's heart level.
○ Ask the patient to flex his knee slightly and to rotate his hips by shifting his weight to the same side as the leg being tested.
○ After the electrodes (connected to the plethysmograph) have been loosely attached to the calf about 3″ to 4″ (7.5 to 10 cm) apart, the pressure cuff (connected to the air pressure system) is wrapped snugly around the thigh about 2″ (5 cm) above the knee.
○ The pressure cuff is inflated to 45 to 60 cm H$_2$O, allowing full venous distention without interfering with arterial blood flow.
○ Pressure is maintained for 45 seconds or until the tracing stabilizes.
○ In a patient with reduced arterial blood flow, pressure is maintained for 2 minutes or longer, after which the pressure cuff is rapidly deflated.
○ The strip chart tracing, which records the increase in venous volume after cuff inflation and the decrease in venous volume 3 seconds after deflation, is checked.
○ The test is repeated for the other leg.
○ If necessary, three to five tracings for each leg are obtained to confirm full venous filling and outflow; the tracing showing the greatest rise and fall in venous volume is used as the test result.
○ If the result is ambiguous, the position of the patient's leg and placement of the cuff and electrode are checked.

Patient care

○ Be sure to remove the conductive gel from the patient's skin after the test.

Complications

None known

Interpretation

Normal results

○ Temporary venous occlusion normally produces a sharp rise in venous volume; release of the occlusion produces rapid venous outflow.

Abnormal results

○ When clots in a major deep vein obstruct venous outflow, calf vein pressure rises; these veins become distended and can't expand further when more pressure is applied with an occlusive thigh cuff.
○ Blockage of major deep veins also decreases the rate at which blood flows from the leg.
○ If significant thrombi are present in a major deep vein of the lower leg (popliteal, femoral, or iliac), calf vein filling and venous outflow rates are reduced. In such cases, the physician will evaluate the need for further treatment, such as anticoagulant therapy, taking the patient's overall condition into consideration.

Interfering factors

○ Decreased peripheral arterial blood flow caused by shock, increased vasoconstriction, low cardiac output, or arterial occlusive disease
○ Extrinsic venous compression, as from pelvic tumors, large hematomas, constricting clothing, or bandages
○ The patient's failure to breathe normally or to completely relax his leg muscles because of pain
○ Cold extremities from cold room temperature

Insulin, serum

Overview

○ This radioimmunoassay is a quantitative analysis of serum insulin levels.
○ Insulin is usually measured along with glucose levels because glucose is the primary stimulus for insulin release from pancreatic islet cells.
○ Insulin regulates the metabolism and transport or mobilization of carbohydrates, amino acids, proteins, and lipids.
○ Stimulated by increased plasma levels of glucose, insulin secretion peaks after meals, when metabolism and food storage are greatest.

Purpose

○ To aid in the diagnosis of hyperinsulinemia as well as hypoglycemia resulting from a tumor or hyperplasia of pancreatic islet cells, glucocorticoid deficiency, or severe hepatic disease
○ To aid in the diagnosis of diabetes mellitus and insulin-resistant states

Procedure

Preparation

○ Explain to the patient that this test helps determine if the pancreas is functioning normally.
○ Instruct the patient to fast for 10 to 12 hours before the test.
○ Tell the patient that the test requires a blood sample.
○ Explain to the patient that he may experience slight discomfort from the needle puncture and the tourniquet.
○ Explain that questionable results may require a repeat test or a simultaneous glucose tolerance test, which requires that the patient drink a glucose solution.
○ Withhold corticotropin, corticosteroids (including hormonal contraceptives), thyroid supplements, epinephrine, and other drugs that may interfere with test results. If the patient must continue them, note this on the laboratory request.
○ Make sure the patient is relaxed and recumbent for 30 minutes before the test.

▽ ALERT *In the patient with an insulinoma, fasting for this test may precipitate dangerously severe hypoglycemia — keep an ampule of dextrose 50% available to counteract possible hypoglycemia.*

Implementation

○ Perform a venipuncture and collect one sample for insulin level in a 7-ml EDTA tube.
○ Collect a sample for glucose level in a tube with sodium fluoride and potassium oxalate.

○ Pack the insulin sample in ice and send it, along with the glucose sample, to the laboratory immediately.
○ Handle the samples gently to prevent hemolysis.

Patient care

○ Apply direct pressure to the venipuncture site until bleeding stops.
○ Instruct the patient that he may resume his usual activities, diet, and medications stopped before the test.

Complications

○ Hematoma at the venipuncture site

Interpretation

Normal results

○ 0 to 35 µU/ml (SI, 144 to 243 pmol/L)

Abnormal results

○ Insulin levels are interpreted in light of the prevailing glucose level.
○ A normal insulin level may be inappropriate for the glucose results.
○ High insulin and low glucose levels after a significant fast suggest the presence of an insulinoma.
○ Prolonged fasting or stimulation testing may be necessary to confirm the diagnosis.
○ In insulin-resistant diabetes mellitus, insulin levels are elevated; in non-insulin-resistant diabetes, they're low.

Interfering factors

○ Failure to observe pretest restrictions
○ Agitation and stress
○ Hemolysis from rough handling of the sample
○ Failure to pack the insulin sample in ice and send it to the laboratory promptly
○ Corticotropin, corticosteroids (including hormonal contraceptives), thyroid hormones, and epinephrine (possible increase)
○ Use of insulin by the patient with type 2 diabetes mellitus (possible increase)
○ High levels of insulin antibodies in the patient with type 1 diabetes mellitus

Insulin tolerance test

Overview

○ Measures serum levels of human growth hormone (hGH) and corticotropin after a patient receives a loading dose of insulin (more reliable than direct measurement of hGH and corticotropin because many healthy people have undetectable fasting levels of these hormones).

○ Insulin-induced hypoglycemia stimulates hGH and corticotropin secretion in persons with an intact hypothalamic-pituitary-adrenal axis.

○ Failure of stimulation indicates anterior pituitary or adrenal hypofunction and helps confirm an hGH or a corticotropin deficiency.

○ Because the insulin tolerance test stimulates an adrenergic response, it isn't recommended for patients with cardiovascular or cerebrovascular disorders, epilepsy, or low basal plasma cortisol levels.

Purpose

○ To aid in the diagnosis of hGH and corticotropin deficiency
○ To identify pituitary dysfunction
○ To aid differential diagnosis of primary and secondary adrenal hypofunction

Procedure

Preparation

○ Explain to the patient, or his parents if the patient is a child, that his test evaluates hormonal secretion.

○ Instruct the patient to fast and restrict physical activity for 10 to 12 hours before the test.

○ Explain that the test involves I.V. infusion of insulin and the collection of multiple blood samples.

○ Warn the patient that he may experience an increased heart rate, diaphoresis, hunger, and anxiety after administration of insulin.

○ Reassure him that these symptoms are transient, and that if they become severe, the test will be stopped.

○ Tell the patient to lie down and relax for 90 minutes before the test.

Implementation

○ Between 6 a.m. and 8 a.m., perform a venipuncture and collect three 5-ml samples of blood for basal levels: one in a gray-top tube (for blood glucose) and two in green-top tubes (for hGH and corticotropin).

○ Give an I.V. bolus of U-100 regular insulin (0.15 units/kg) over 1 to 2 minutes.

○ Use an indwelling venous catheter to avoid repeated venipunctures.

○ Collect additional blood samples 15, 30, 45, 60, 90, and 120 minutes after giving the insulin.

○ At each interval, collect three samples: one in a tube with sodium fluoride and potassium oxidate and two in heparinized tubes.

○ Label the tubes appropriately and send them to the laboratory immediately.

○ Handle the samples gently to prevent hemolysis.

▼ ALERT *Be sure to have concentrated glucose solution readily available in case the patient has severe hypoglycemic reaction to insulin.*

Patient care

○ Apply direct pressure to the venipuncture site until bleeding stops.

○ Instruct the patient that he may resume his usual diet, activities, and medications stopped before the test.

Complications

○ Hematoma at the I.V. or venipuncture site

Interpretation

Normal results

○ Blood glucose falls to 50% of the fasting level 20 to 30 minutes after the patient receives insulin.

○ This stimulates a 10- to 20-nanogram/dl (SI, 10 to 20 µg/L) increase in baseline values for hGH and corticotropin, with peak levels occurring 60 to 90 minutes after the patient receives insulin.

Abnormal results

○ Failure of stimulation or a blunted response suggests dysfunction of the hypothalamic-pituitary-adrenal axis.

○ An hGH increase of less than 10 nanograms/dl (SI, < 10 µg/L) above baseline suggests hGH deficiency.

○ A definitive diagnosis of hGH deficiency requires a supplementary stimulation test such as the arginine test.

○ Additional testing is necessary to determine the site of the abnormality.

○ An increase in corticotropin levels of less than 10 nanograms/dl above baseline suggests adrenal insufficiency.

○ The metyrapone or corticotropin stimulation test then confirms the diagnosis and determines whether the insufficiency is primary or secondary.

Interfering factors

○ Failure to observe pretest restrictions
○ Hemolysis from rough handling of the sample
○ Corticosteroids and pituitary-based drugs (increase in hGH)
○ Glucocorticoids and beta blockers (decrease in hGH)
○ Glucocorticoids, estrogens, calcium gluconate, amphetamines, methamphetamines, spironolactone, and ethanol (decrease in corticotropin)

Internal fetal monitoring

Overview

○ Invasive procedure that involves attaching an electrode to the fetal scalp to directly monitor fetal heart rate (FHR).
○ A catheter introduced into the uterine cavity measures the frequency and pressure of uterine contractions.
○ Performed only during labor, after the membranes have ruptured and the cervix has dilated 3 cm, with the fetal head lower than the −2 station and only if external monitoring provides inadequate data.
○ Provides more accurate information about fetal health than external monitoring and is especially useful in determining whether cesarean delivery is necessary.
○ Carries minimal risks to the patient (perforated uterus and intrauterine infection) and fetus (scalp abscess and hematoma).

Purpose

○ To monitor FHR, especially beat-to-beat variability (short-term variability)
○ To measure the frequency and pressure of uterine contractions to assess the progress of labor
○ To evaluate intrapartum fetal health
○ To supplement or replace external fetal monitoring

Procedure

Preparation

○ Explain to the patient that internal fetal monitoring accurately assesses fetal health and uterine activity and that it doesn't necessarily mean there's a problem.
○ Warn the patient that she may feel mild discomfort when the uterine catheter and scalp electrode are inserted.
○ Make sure the patient or a responsible family member has signed an informed consent form.

Implementation

○ The steps vary depending on whether the procedure is being used to measure FHR or uterine contractions.
To measure fetal heart rate
○ Assist the patient into the dorsal lithotomy position and prepare her perineal area for a vaginal examination, explaining each step of the procedure as it's performed by a physician or certified nurse-midwife.
○ As the procedure begins, ask the patient to breathe through her mouth and relax her abdominal muscles.

○ After the vaginal examination, the fetal scalp is palpated and an appropriate site is identified.
○ A plastic tube carrying the small electrode is introduced into the cervix, pressed firmly against the fetal scalp, and rotated clockwise to attach the electrode to the scalp.
○ The electrode wire is tugged gently to ensure proper attachment and the tube is withdrawn, leaving the electrode in place.
○ Apply a conduction medium to a leg plate and strap it to the patient's thigh. Attach electrode wires to the leg plate and plug a cable from the leg plate into the fetal monitor.
○ To check proper placement of the scalp electrode, turn on the monitor and press the electrocardiogram button; an FHR signal indicates proper electrode attachment.
To measure uterine contractions
○ Before the uterine catheter is inserted, fill it with sterile normal saline solution to prevent air emboli. Explain each step of the procedure to the patient.
○ Ask the patient to breathe deeply through her mouth and to relax her abdominal muscles.
○ After the vagina has been examined and the presenting part of the fetus palpated, the catheter and guide are inserted ⅜″ to ¾″ (1 to 2 cm) into the cervix, usually between the fetal head and the posterior cervix.
○ The catheter is then gently advanced into the uterus until the black mark on the catheter is flush with the vulva. (The catheter guide should *never* be passed deeply into the uterus.)
○ The guide is removed and the catheter is connected to a transducer that converts the intrauterine pressure, as measured by the fluid in the catheter, to an electrical signal. (See *Understanding internal fetal monitoring*.)

Patient care

○ After removing the fetal scalp electrode, apply antiseptic or antibiotic solution to the attachment site.
○ If FHR patterns indicate distress, fetal oxygenation commonly can be improved by loading maternal fluids to increase placental perfusion, turning the mother on her side (preferably left) to alleviate supine hypotension, and giving oxygen to the mother. If these measures return FHR patterns to normal, labor may continue. If abnormal patterns persist, cesarean birth may be necessary.
○ Make sure to remove the fetal scalp electrode and the uterine catheter before cesarean delivery.

Complications

○ Fetal scalp abscess or maternal intrauterine infection

Internal fetal monitoring uses an electrode attached to the fetal scalp. The resultant fetal electrocardiograms (FECGs) are transmitted to an amplifier. Then, a cardiotachometer measures the interval between FECGs and plots a continuous fetal heart rate (FHR) graph, which is displayed on a two-channel oscilloscope screen. Intrauterine catheters attached to a transducer in a leg plate measure the frequency and pressure of uterine contractions, which are plotted below the FHR graph.

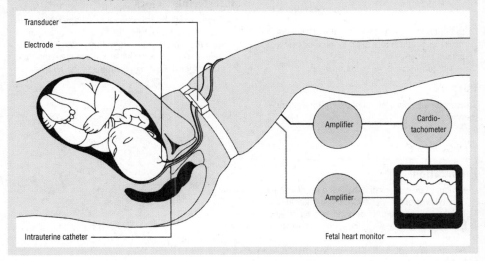

Interpretation

Normal results

○ 120 to 160 beats/minute, with a variability of 5 to 25 beats/minute

Abnormal results

○ Bradycardia (FHR < 120 beats/minute) may indicate fetal heart block, malposition, or hypoxia.
○ Fetal bradycardia may also result from maternal ingestion of certain drugs, such as propranolol and opioid analgesics.
○ Tachycardia (FHR > 160 beats/minute) may result from early fetal hypoxia, fetal infection or arrhythmia, prematurity, or maternal fever, tachycardia, hyperthyroidism, or use of vagolytics.
○ Decreased variability (fluctuation of < 5 beats/minute from baseline) may result from fetal arrhythmia or heart block, hypoxia, central nervous system malformation, or infections, or from maternal use of opioids or vagolytics.
○ Early decelerations (slowing of FHR at the onset of a contraction with recovery to baseline within no more than 15 seconds after the contraction ends) are related to fetal head compression and usually ensure fetal health.
○ Late decelerations (slowing of FHR after a contraction begins, a lag time of more than 20 seconds, and a recovery time of more than 15 seconds) may be related to uteroplacental insufficiency, fetal hypoxia, or acidosis.

○ Recurrent and persistently late decelerations with decreased variability usually indicate serious fetal distress, possibly resulting from conduction (spinal, caudal, or epidural) anesthesia or fetal hypoxia.
○ Variable decelerations (sudden precipitous drops in FHR unrelated to uterine contractions) are often related to cord compression.
○ A severe drop in FHR (to < 70 beats/minute for more than 60 seconds) with a decrease in variability indicates fetal distress and may result in a compromised neonate.
○ Poor beat-to-beat variability without periodic patterns may indicate fetal distress, requiring further evaluation such as analysis of fetal blood gas levels.
○ Low intrauterine pressure during labor that isn't progressing normally may indicate a need for oxytocin stimulation.
○ High intrauterine pressure may indicate abruptio placentae or overstimulation from oxytocin, possibly resulting in fetal distress caused by decreased placental perfusion.

Interfering factors

○ Drugs that affect the parasympathetic and sympathetic nervous systems
○ Clogged pressure transducer and catheter obstruction (prevent artifactual pressure readings by flushing the transducer with normal saline solution; relieve a catheter obstruction — by vernix caseosa, for example — by injecting a small amount of sterile normal saline solution into the catheter while the transducer is isolated from the system)

International normalized ratio

Overview

- The International Normalized Ratio (INR) system measures prothrombin time, to monitor oral anticoagulant therapy.
- Isn't used to screen for coagulopathies.

Purpose

To evaluate the effectiveness of oral anticoagulant therapy

Procedure

Preparation

- Explain to the patient that the INR test determines the effectiveness of his oral anticoagulant therapy.
- Tell the patient that the test requires a blood sample. Explain who will perform the venipuncture and when.
- Explain to the patient that he may feel slight discomfort from the needle puncture and the tourniquet.

Implementation

- Perform a venipuncture and collect the sample in a 4.5-ml tube with sodium citrate added.
- Completely fill the collection tube; otherwise, an excess of citrate appears in the sample.
- Gently invert the tube several times to thoroughly mix the sample and the anticoagulant.
- To prevent hemolysis, avoid excessive probing during venipuncture and handle the sample gently.
- Put the sample on ice and send it to the laboratory immediately.

Patient care

- Apply direct pressure to the venipuncture site until bleedings stops.

Complications

- Hematoma at the venipuncture site; if large, monitor pulses distal to the venipuncture site

Interpretation

Normal results

- For those receiving warfarin therapy, 2.0 to 3.0 (SI, 2.0 to 3.0)
- For those with mechanical prosthetic heart valves, 2.5 to 3.5 (SI, 2.5 to 3.5)

Abnormal results

- Increased INR values may indicate disseminated intravascular coagulation, cirrhosis, hepatitis, vitamin K deficiency, salicylate intoxication, uncontrolled oral anticoagulation, or massive blood transfusion.

Interfering factors

- Failure to fill the collection tube completely, to adequately mix the sample and the anticoagulant, or to send the sample to the laboratory immediately
- Hemolysis from excessive probing at the venipuncture site or from rough handling of the sample

Iron, serum

Overview

- A person's blood contains about 70% of the total iron in his body.
- Iron is carried in the hemoglobin of red blood cells.
- A patient suspected of having anemia may receive this test.

Purpose

- To determine the serum iron level in the blood

Procedure

Preparation

- Explain to the patient that this test requires a blood test.
- Inform the patient that he may feel slight discomfort from the tourniquet and needle puncture.
- Tell the patient to refrain from eating for 12 hours before the test. He need not restrict water.

Implementation

- Perform a venipuncture to collect the blood sample.

Patient care

- Apply direct pressure to the venipuncture site until bleeding stops.

Complications

- Hematoma at the venipuncture site

Interpretation

Normal results

- In men, 65 to 176 µg/dl (SI, 11.6 to 31.3 µmol/L)
- In women, 50 to 170 µg/dl (SI, 9 to 30.4 µmol/L)
- In children, 50 to 120 µg/dl (SI, 9 to 21.6 µmol/L)
- In neonates, 100 to 250 µg/dl (SI, 18 to 45 µmol/L)

Abnormal results

- High levels may indicate hemolytic anemia, hemosiderosis, hemochromatosis, or iron poisoning.
- Low levels may be a sign of chronic blood loss, such as in GI bleeding, of dietary iron insufficiency.

Interfering factors

- Failure to fast before test

Ketones, urine

Overview

- Routine, semi-quantitative screening test; commercially prepared product measures the urine level of ketone bodies.
- Ketones are by-products of fat metabolism; they include acetoacetic acid, acetone, and beta-hydroxybutyric acid.
- Commercially available tests include the Acetest tablet, Ketostix, or Keto-Diastix.
- Each product measures a specific ketone body.

Purpose

- To screen for ketonuria
- To identify diabetic ketoacidosis (DKA) and carbohydrate deprivation
- To distinguish between a diabetic and a nondiabetic coma
- To check for a metabolic complication of total parenteral nutrition.
- To monitor control of diabetes mellitus, ketogenic weight reduction, and treatment of DKA

Procedure

Preparation

- Explain to the patient that the ketone test evaluates fat metabolism.
- If the patient is newly diagnosed with diabetes, tell him how to perform the test.

▼ *ALERT If the patient is taking levodopa or phenazopyridine or has recently received sulfobromophthalein, use Acetest tablets because reagent strips may produce inaccurate results.*

Implementation

- Instruct the patient to void; then give him a drink of water.
- Collect a second-voided midstream specimen about 30 minutes later.

Acetest
- Lay the tablet on a piece of white paper, and place 1 drop of urine on the tablet.
- Compare the tablet color (white, lavender, or purple) with the color chart after 30 seconds.

Ketostix
- Dip the reagent stick into the specimen and remove it immediately.
- Compare the stick color (buff or purple) with the color chart after 15 seconds. Record the results as negative, small, moderate, or large amounts of ketones.

Keto-Diastix
- Dip the reagent strip into the specimen and remove it immediately. Tap the edge of the strip against the container or a clean, dry surface to remove excess urine.
- Hold the Keto-Diastix strip horizontally to prevent mixing the chemicals from the two areas. Interpret each area of the strip separately. Compare the color of the ketone section (buff or purple) with the appropriate color chart after exactly 15 seconds; compare the color of the glucose section after 30 seconds.

All tests
- Ignore color changes that occur after the specified waiting periods. Record the results as negative or positive for small, moderate, or large amounts of ketones.
- Test the specimen within 1 hour after it's obtained, or refrigerate it until ready to test.
- Let refrigerated specimens return to room temperature before testing.
- Don't use tablets or strips that have become discolored or darkened.

Patient care

- Answer the patient's questions about the test.

Complications

None known

Interpretation

Normal results

- No ketones present

Abnormal results

- Ketones are present in urine, indicating carbohydrate dehydration, which may suggest DKA, starvation, or a metabolic complication of total parenteral nutrition.

Interfering factors

- Failure to keep the reagent container tightly closed to prevent absorption of light or moisture, or bacterial contamination of the specimen (false-negative)
- Failure to test the specimen within 1 hour or to refrigerate it
- Levodopa, phenazopyridine, and sulfobromophthalein (false-positive results when Ketostix or Keto-Diastix is used instead of Acetest)

Kidney-ureter-bladder radiography

Overview

○ Surveys the abdomen even if renal function isn't intact
○ Also known as a *flat plate of the abdomen*

Purpose

○ To evaluate the size, structure, and position of the kidneys and bladder
○ To screen for abnormalities, such as calcifications, in the area of the kidneys, ureters, and bladder

Procedure

Preparation

○ Make sure the patient has signed an appropriate consent form.
○ Note and report all allergies.
○ Tell the patient that he need not restrict food or fluids.
○ Explain that the test takes only a few minutes.

Implementation

○ The patient is assisted into a supine position with his arms extended over his head on an X-ray table.
○ Symmetrical positioning of the iliac crests is noted.
○ A single X-ray is taken.

▼ *ALERT During the X-ray, a man's gonads should be shielded; however, a woman's ovaries can't be shielded because they're too close to the kidneys, ureters, and bladder.*

Patient care

○ Answer the patient's questions about the test.

Complications

None known

Interpretation

Normal results

○ Kidney shadows appear bilaterally, the right slightly lower than the left.
○ Both kidneys are about the same size, with the superior poles tilted slightly toward the vertebral column, paralleling the shadows of the psoas muscles.
○ The bladder shadow isn't as clearly visible as the kidney shadows.

Abnormal results

○ Bilateral renal enlargement suggests possible polycystic kidney disease, multiple myeloma, lymphoma, amyloidosis, hydronephrosis, or compensatory renal hypertrophy.
○ Unilateral renal enlargement suggests a possible tumor, cyst, or hydronephrosis.
○ Abnormally small kidneys suggest possible end-stage glomerulonephritis or bilateral atrophic pyelonephritis.
○ An apparent decrease in the size of one kidney suggests possible congenital hypoplasia, atrophic pyelonephritis, or ischemia.
○ Renal displacement may be the result of a retroperitoneal tumor.
○ Obliteration or bulging of a portion of the psoas muscle stripe suggests possible tumor, abscess, or hematoma.
○ Abnormal location or absence of a kidney suggests possible congenital anomalies.
○ A lobulated edge or border suggests possible polycystic kidney disease or patchy atrophic pyelonephritis.
○ Opaque bodies suggest possible calculi, vascular calcification, cystic tumors, fecaliths, foreign bodies, soft tissue mass, or abnormal fluid or gas collection.

Interfering factors

○ Recent instillation of barium

Lactate dehydrogenase

Overview

○ Lactate dehydrogenase (LD) catalyzes the reversible conversion of muscle lactic acid into pyruvic acid, which ultimately produces cellular energy.
○ Because LD is present in almost all body tissues, cellular damage increases total serum LD, limiting its diagnostic usefulness.
○ Immunochemical separation and quantification or electrophoresis can identify and measure five tissue-specific isoenzymes.
○ Two of these isoenzymes, LD_1 and LD_2, appear primarily in the heart, red blood cells (RBCs), and kidneys; LD_3, primarily in the lungs; and LD_4 and LD_5, in the liver and the skeletal muscles.
○ The specificity of LD isoenzymes and their distribution pattern are useful in diagnosing hepatic, pulmonary, and erythrocyte damage.
○ Their widest clinical application is in aiding the diagnosis of acute myocardial infarction (MI).
○ An LD isoenzyme assay is useful when creatine kinase (CK) hasn't been measured within 24 hours of an acute MI.
○ The myocardial LD level rises later than CK (12 to 48 hours after infarction begins), peaks in 2 to 5 days, and drops to normal in 7 to 10 days if tissue necrosis doesn't persist.

Purpose

○ To aid in the differential diagnosis of an MI, pulmonary infarction, anemias, hepatic disease, granulocytic leukemia, lymphomas, and platelet disorders
○ To support CK isoenzyme test results in diagnosing an MI or to provide diagnosis when CK-MB samples are drawn too late to display an increase
○ To monitor patient's response to chemotherapy

Procedure

Preparation

○ Explain to the patient that this test primarily detects tissue alterations.
○ Tell the patient that the test requires a blood sample. Explain who will perform the venipuncture and when.
○ Explain to the patient that he may experience slight discomfort from the tourniquet and the needle puncture.
○ Inform the patient that he need not restrict food and fluids.
○ If an MI is suspected, tell the patient that the test will be repeated on the next two mornings to monitor progressive changes.

Implementation

○ Perform a venipuncture and collect the sample in a 4-ml clot-activator tube.
○ Draw the samples on schedule to avoid missing peak levels, and mark the collection time on the laboratory request.
○ Handle the sample gently to prevent artifact blood sample hemolysis because RBCs contain LD_1.
○ Send the sample to the laboratory immediately or, if transport is delayed, keep the sample at room temperature. Changes in temperature inactivate LD_5, thus altering isoenzyme patterns.

Patient care

○ Apply direct pressure to the venipuncture site until bleeding stops.

Complications

○ Hematoma at the venipuncture site

Interpretation

Normal results

○ Total LD levels, 71 to 207 units/L (SI, 1.2 to 3.52 μkat/L)
○ LD_1, 14% to 26% (SI, 0.14 to 0.26) of total
○ LD_2, 29% to 39% (SI, 0.29 to 0.39) of total
○ LD_3, 20% to 26% (SI, 0.20 to 0.26) of total
○ LD_4, 8% to 16% (SI, 0.08 to 0.16) of total
○ LD_5, 6% to 16% (SI, 0.06 to 0.16) of total

Abnormal results

○ Because many common diseases increase total LD levels, isoenzyme electrophoresis is usually necessary for diagnosis.
○ In some disorders, total LD may be within normal limits, but abnormal proportions of each enzyme indicate specific organ tissue damage.
○ In an acute MI, the level of LD_1 is greater than that of LD_2 within 12 to 48 hours after the onset of symptoms; therefore, the LD_1-to-LD_2 ratio is greater than 1. This reversal of the normal isoenzyme pattern is typical of myocardial damage and is known as *flipped LD*.
○ Increased midzone fractions (LD_2, LD_3, LD_4) can indicate granulocytic leukemia, lymphomas, and platelet disorders.

Interfering factors

○ Hemolysis from rough handling of the sample
○ Failure to draw the sample on schedule, for diagnosis of an acute MI
○ Failure to send the sample to the laboratory immediately (may obscure LD isoenzyme patterns)
○ Failure to centrifuge the sample and separate the cells from the serum
○ Recent surgery or pregnancy (possible increase)
○ Prosthetic heart valve (possible increase caused by chronic hemolysis)
○ Anabolic steroids, anesthetics, alcohol, opioids, and procainamide (increase)

Lactic acid and pyruvic acid

Overview

○ Lactic acid, present in blood as lactate ions, is derived primarily from muscle cells and erythrocytes.
○ An intermediate product of carbohydrate metabolism; usually metabolized by the liver.
○ Blood lactate level depends on the rates of production and metabolism; levels may increase significantly during exercise.
○ Lactate and pyruvate together form a reversible reaction that's regulated by the oxygen supply
○ When oxygen levels are deficient, pyruvate converts to lactate; when oxygen levels are adequate, lactate converts to pyruvate.
○ When the hepatic system fails to metabolize lactose sufficiently or when excess pyruvate converts to lactate, lactic acidosis may result.
○ Measurement of blood lactate levels is recommended for all patients with symptoms of lactic acidosis such as Kussmaul's respiration.
○ Comparison of pyruvate and lactate levels provides reliable information about tissue oxidation, but measurement of pyruvate is technically difficult and occurs infrequently.

Purpose

○ To assess tissue oxidation
○ To help determine the cause of lactic acidosis

Procedure

Preparation

○ Explain to the patient that this blood test evaluates the oxygen level in tissues.
○ Tell the patient that the test requires a blood sample. Explain who will perform the venipuncture and when.
○ Explain to the patient that he may experience slight discomfort from the tourniquet and the needle puncture.
○ Withhold food overnight and make sure the patient rests for at least 1 hour before the test.

Implementation

▷ *ALERT Because venostasis may raise blood lactate levels, tell the patient that he must not clench his fist during the venipuncture.*

○ Avoid using a tourniquet; however, if it is necessary to use one, release it at least 2 minutes before collecting the sample so blood can circulate.
○ Perform a venipuncture and collect the sample in a 5-ml tube with sodium fluoride and potassium oxalate added.

○ Because lactate and pyruvate are extremely unstable, place the sample container in an ice-filled cup and send it to the laboratory immediately.

Patient care

○ Apply direct pressure to the venipuncture site until bleeding stops.
○ Instruct the patient that he may resume his usual diet and activity stopped before the test.

Complications

○ Hematoma at the venipuncture site

Interpretation

Normal results

○ Blood lactate values range from 0.93 to 1.65 mEq/L (SI, 0.93 to 1.65 mmol/L); pyruvate levels, from 0.08 to 0.16 mEq/L (SI, 0.08 to 0.16 mmol/L).
○ The lactate-pyruvate ratio is less than 10:1.

Abnormal results

○ Elevated blood lactate levels associated with hypoxia may result from strenuous muscle exercise, shock, hemorrhage, septicemia, myocardial infarction, pulmonary embolism, and cardiac arrest.
○ When no reason for diminished tissue perfusion is apparent, increased lactate levels may result from systemic disorders, such as diabetes mellitus, leukemias and lymphomas, hepatic disease, and renal failure, or from enzymatic defects, such as von Gierke's disease (glycogen storage disease) and fructose-1,6-diphosphatase deficiency.
○ Lactic acidosis can follow ingestion of large doses of acetaminophen and ethanol, as well as I.V. infusion of epinephrine, glucagon, fructose, or sorbitol.

Interfering factors

○ Failure to observe pretest restrictions
○ Failure to pack the sample in ice and transport it to the laboratory immediately (possible increase)

Laparoscopy of peritoneal cavity

Overview

○ Makes peritoneal cavity visible through a small fiber-optic telescope (*laparoscope*) inserted through the anterior abdominal wall
○ Requires only a small incision, resulting in lower cost and faster recovery
○ Allows many types of abdominal surgery, such as tubal ligation and cholecystectomy, to be performed simultaneously

Purpose

○ To identify the cause of pelvic pain
○ To detect endometriosis, ectopic pregnancy, or pelvic inflammatory disease (PID)
○ To evaluate pelvic masses
○ To evaluate infertility
○ To stage a carcinoma

Procedure

Preparation

○ Make sure the patient has signed an appropriate consent form.
○ Note and report all allergies.
○ Check the patient's history for hypersensitivity to the anesthetic.
○ Inform the physician if the patient takes aspirin, nonsteroidal anti-inflammatory drugs, or other drugs that affect clotting.
○ Tell the patient to fast after midnight before the test or for at least 8 hours before surgery.
○ Explain the use of a local or general anesthetic.
○ Warn the patient that she may experience pain at the puncture site and in the shoulder.
○ Instruct the patient to empty her bladder just before the test.
○ Explain that the test takes 15 to 30 minutes.

Implementation

○ The patient is anesthetized and helped into the lithotomy position.
○ The bladder is catheterized.
○ A bimanual examination of the pelvic area may be performed to detect abnormalities.
○ An incision is made at the inferior rim of the umbilicus.
○ The peritoneal cavity is insufflated with carbon dioxide or nitrous oxide.
○ A laparoscope is inserted to examine the pelvis and abdomen.
○ A second incision may be made just above the pubic hair line for some procedures.

○ After the examination, minor surgical procedures, such as ovarian biopsy, may be performed.

Patient care

○ Instruct the patient to resume her usual diet.
○ Instruct the patient to restrict activity for 2 to 7 days.
○ Explain that abdominal and shoulder pain should disappear within 24 to 36 hours.
○ Provide analgesics.
○ Monitor vital signs.
○ Monitor the patient for adverse reactions to anesthetic.
○ Monitor intake and output.
○ Watch for bleeding and signs and symptoms of infection.

Complications

○ Punctured visceral organ
○ Peritonitis

Interpretation

Normal results

○ The uterus and fallopian tubes are a normal size and shape, free from adhesions, and mobile.
○ The ovaries are a normal size and shape.
○ No cysts and no endometriosis are found.

Abnormal results

○ A bubble on the surface of the ovary suggests a possible ovarian cyst.
○ Sheets or strands of tissue suggest possible adhesions.
○ Small, blue powder burns on the peritoneum or serosa suggest endometriosis.
○ Growths on the uterus suggests fibroids.
○ An enlarged fallopian tube suggests possible hydrosalpinx.
○ An enlarged or ruptured fallopian tube suggests a possible ectopic pregnancy.
○ Infection or abscess suggests possible PID.

Interfering factors

None known

Laryngoscopy, direct

Overview

○ Makes the larynx visible using a fiber-optic endoscope, or laryngoscope, passed through the mouth or nose and pharynx to the larynx
○ Usually follows indirect laryngoscopy

Purpose

○ To detect lesions, strictures, or foreign bodies in the larynx
○ To aid the diagnosis of laryngeal cancer or vocal cord impairment
○ To remove benign lesions or foreign bodies from the larynx
○ To examine the larynx when the view provided by indirect laryngoscopy is inadequate
○ To evaluate symptoms of pharyngeal or laryngeal disease (stridor or hemoptysis)

Procedure

Preparation

○ Make sure the patient has signed an appropriate consent form.
○ Note and report all allergies.
○ Check the patient's history for hypersensitivity to the anesthetic.
○ Instruct the patient to fast for 6 to 8 hours before the test.
○ Give the patient a sedative to help him relax and a drug to reduce secretions.
○ Give a general or local anesthetic to numb the gag reflex.
○ Explain that the study takes about 30 minutes; it takes longer if minor surgery is performed as part of the procedure.

Implementation

○ The patient is assisted into the supine position.
○ A general anesthetic is given, or the mouth or nose and throat are sprayed with local anesthetic
○ The laryngoscope is inserted through the mouth.
○ The larynx is examined for abnormalities.
○ Specimens may be collected for further study.
○ Minor surgery (polyp removal) may occur at this time.

Patient care

○ Assist the patient onto his side with his head slightly elevated to prevent aspiration.
○ Restrict food and fluids until the gag reflex returns (usually 2 hours).
○ Reassure that voice loss, hoarseness, and sore throat are most likely temporary.
○ Provide throat lozenges or a soothing liquid gargle after the gag reflex returns.

○ Monitor patient and immediately report to the physician any adverse reaction to the anesthetic or sedative.
○ Apply an ice collar to prevent or minimize laryngeal edema.
○ Observe sputum for blood and notify the physician immediately if excessive bleeding or respiratory compromise occurs.
○ After a biopsy, instruct the patient to refrain from clearing his throat and coughing, and to avoid smoking.
○ Monitor vital signs, respiratory status, sputum, and voice quality.

▼ *ALERT Immediately report signs of respiratory difficulty, such as laryngeal stridor or dyspnea. Keep emergency resuscitation equipment and a tracheotomy tray readily available for 24 hours.*

○ Watch for edema, bleeding, and subcutaneous emphysema.

Complications

○ Subcutaneous crepitus around the patient's face and neck — a sign of tracheal perforation
○ Airway obstruction (in the patient with epiglottiditis)
○ Adverse reaction to anesthetic
○ Bleeding

Interpretation

Normal results

○ No inflammation, lesions, strictures, or foreign bodies are found.

Abnormal results

○ Combined with the results of a biopsy, abnormal lesions suggest possible laryngeal cancer or benign lesions.
○ Narrowing suggests stricture.
○ Inflammation suggests possible laryngeal edema secondary to radiation or tumor.
○ Asynchronous vocal cords suggest possible vocal cord dysfunction.

Interfering factors

None known

Leucine aminopeptidase

Overview

○ Measures serum levels of leucine aminopeptidase (LAP), an isoenzyme of alkaline phosphatase (ALP) widely distributed in body tissues.
○ Greatest LAP levels appear in the hepatobiliary tissues, pancreas, and small intestine.
○ Serum LAP levels parallel serum ALP levels in hepatic disease.

Purpose
○ To provide information about suspected liver, pancreatic, and biliary diseases
○ To differentiate skeletal disease from hepatobiliary or pancreatic disease
○ To evaluate neonatal jaundice

Procedure

Preparation
○ Explain to the patient that this test evaluates liver and pancreatic function.
○ Tell the patient that the test requires a blood sample. Explain who will perform the venipuncture and when.
○ Explain to the patient that he may experience slight discomfort from the tourniquet and the needle puncture.
○ Tell the patient to fast for at least 8 hours before the test.
○ Notify the laboratory and physician of drugs the patient is taking that may affect test results; it may be necessary to restrict them.

Implementation
○ Perform a venipuncture and collect the sample in a 4-ml clot-activator tube.
○ Handle the sample gently to prevent hemolysis.
○ Transport the sample to the laboratory immediately.

Patient care
○ Apply direct pressure to the venipuncture site until bleeding stops.
○ Instruct the patient to resume his usual diet and medications stopped before the test.

Complications
○ Hematoma at the venipuncture site

Interpretation

Normal results
○ In men, 80 to 200 units/ml (SI, 80 to 200 kU/L)
○ In women, 75 to 185 units/ml (SI, 75 to 185 kU/L)

Abnormal results
○ Elevated levels can occur in biliary obstruction, tumors, strictures, and atresia; advanced pregnancy; and therapy with drugs containing estrogen or progesterone.

Interfering factors
○ Advanced pregnancy (false-high)
○ Estrogen or progesterone (false-high)

Leukoagglutinins

Overview

○ Detects leukoagglutinins (also known as *white blood cell [WBC] antibodies or human leukocyte antigen [HLA] antibodies*) — antibodies that react with WBCs and may cause a transfusion reaction.
○ Antibodies usually develop after exposure to foreign WBCs through transfusions, pregnancies, and allografts.
○ If a blood recipient has these antibodies, a febrile nonhemolytic reaction may occur 1 to 4 hours after the start of whole blood, red blood cell, platelet, or granulocyte transfusion (this kind of reaction must be distinguished from a true hemolytic reaction before further transfusion can proceed).
○ Technique for detecting leukoagglutinins is the microlymphocytotoxicity test: The recipient serum is tested against donor lymphocytes or against a panel of lymphocytes of known HLA phenotype.
○ Antibodies in the recipient serum bind to the corresponding antigen present in the lymphocytes and cause cell membrane injury when the complement is added to the test system.
○ Cell injury is detectable by examining the lymphocytes under a microscope.

Purpose

○ To detect leukoagglutinins in blood recipients who develop transfusion reactions, thus differentiating between hemolytic and febrile nonhemolytic transfusion reactions
○ To detect leukoagglutinins in blood donors after transfusion of donor blood causes a reaction

Procedure

Preparation

○ Explain to the patient that this test helps determine the cause of his transfusion reaction.
○ Tell the patient that the test requires a blood sample. Explain who will perform the venipuncture and when.
○ Explain to the patient that he may experience slight discomfort from the tourniquet and the needle puncture.
○ Check the patient's history for recent administration of blood, dextran, or I.V. contrast media and note this on the laboratory request.

Implementation

○ Perform a venipuncture and collect a sample in a 10-ml clot-activator tube. The laboratory requires 3 to 4 ml of serum for testing.
○ Label the sample with the patient's name, the hospital or blood bank number, the date, and the phlebotomist's initials.

○ Be sure to include on the laboratory request the patient's suspected diagnosis and history of blood transfusions, pregnancies, and drug therapy.

Patient care

○ Apply direct pressure to the venipuncture site until bleeding stops.
○ If a transfusion recipient has a positive leukoagglutinin test, know that continued transfusions require premedication with acetaminophen 1 to 2 hours before the transfusion, specially prepared leukocyte-poor blood, or use of leukocyte-removal blood filters to prevent further reactions.
○ Note that tests for these antibodies aren't useful in deciding which patient should receive leukocyte-poor blood components; the decision must be based on clinical experience.

Complications

○ Hematoma at the venipuncture site

Interpretation

Normal results

○ If the lymphocytes don't absorb the added dye, the test result is negative.
○ Agglutination doesn't occur because the serum contains no antibodies.

Abnormal results

○ If the lymphocytes show dye uptake, the test result is positive.
○ A positive result in a transfusion recipient indicates the presence of leukoagglutinins in his blood, identifying his transfusion reaction as a febrile nonhemolytic reaction to these antibodies.
○ Recipients who test positive for HLA antibodies may need HLA-matched platelets to control bleeding episodes caused by thrombocytopenia.

Interfering factors

None known

Lipase

Overview

- Originates in the pancreas and is secreted into the duodenum, where it converts triglycerides and other fats into fatty acids and glycerol.
- Destruction of pancreatic cells, which occurs in acute pancreatitis, causes large amounts of lipase to release into the blood.
- Test measures serum lipase levels; it's most useful when performed with a serum or urine amylase test.

Purpose
- To aid in the diagnosis of acute pancreatitis

Procedure

Preparation
- Explain to the patient that this test evaluates pancreatic function.
- Tell the patient that the test requires a blood sample. Explain who will perform the venipuncture and when.
- Inform the patient that he may experience slight discomfort from the tourniquet and the needle puncture.
- Instruct the patient to fast overnight before the test.
- Notify the laboratory of drugs the patient is taking that may affect test results; it may be necessary to restrict them.

Implementation
- Perform a venipuncture and collect the sample in a 4-ml clot-activator tube.
- Handle the sample gently to prevent hemolysis.

Patient care
- Apply direct pressure to the venipuncture site until bleeding stops.
- Instruct the patient that he may resume his usual diet and medications stopped before the test.

Complications
- Hematoma at the venipuncture site

Interpretation

Normal results
- Less than 160 units/L (SI, < 2.72 µkat/L)

Abnormal results
- Increased levels suggest acute pancreatitis or pancreatic duct obstruction. After an acute attack, levels remain elevated for up to 14 days.
- Increased levels may occur in other pancreatic injuries, such as perforated peptic ulcer with chemical pancreatitis caused by gastric juices, and in a patient with high intestinal obstruction, pancreatic cancer, or renal disease with impaired excretion.

Interfering factors
- Hemolysis from rough handling of the sample
- Cholinergics, codeine, meperidine, and morphine (false-high caused by spasm of the sphincter of Oddi)

Lipoprotein-cholesterol fractionation

Overview

○ Isolates and measures the types of cholesterol in serum: low-density lipoproteins (LDLs) and high-density lipoproteins (HDLs).
○ The HDL level is inversely related to the risk of coronary artery disease (CAD); the higher the HDL level, the lower the incidence of CAD (conversely, the higher the LDL level, the higher the incidence of CAD).

Purpose

○ To assess the risk of CAD
○ To assess the efficacy of lipid-lowering drug therapy

Procedure

Preparation

○ Tell the patient that this test determines his risk for CAD.
○ Tell the patient that the test requires a blood sample. Explain who will perform the venipuncture and when.
○ Explain to the patient that he may experience slight discomfort from the tourniquet and the needle puncture.
○ Instruct the patient to maintain his normal diet for 2 weeks before the test, to abstain from alcohol for 24 hours before the test, and to fast and avoid exercise for 12 to 14 hours before the test.
○ Notify the laboratory and physician of drugs the patient is taking that may affect test results; it may be necessary to restrict them.

Implementation

○ Perform a venipuncture and collect the sample in a 7-ml ethylenediaminetetraacetic acid tube.
○ Send the sample to the laboratory immediately to avoid spontaneous redistribution among the lipoproteins.
○ If the sample can't be transported immediately, refrigerate it but don't freeze it.

Patient care

○ Apply direct pressure to the venipuncture site until bleeding stops.
○ Instruct the patient to resume his usual diet and medications stopped before the test.

Complications

○ Hematoma at the venipuncture site

Interpretation

Normal results

○ Normal lipoprotein values vary by age, sex, geographic area, and ethnic group; check the laboratory for reference values.
○ Desirable HDL levels are greater than 60 mg/dl (SI, > 1.55 mmol/L)
○ Optimal LDL levels are less than 100 mg/dl (SI, < 2.59 mmol/L); above optimal levels range from 100 to 129 mg/dl (SI, 2.59 to 3.34 mmol/L).

Abnormal results

○ Undesirable HDL levels are below 40 mg/dl (SI, < 1.03 mmol/L).
○ Borderline high LDL levels range from 130 to 159 mg/dl (SI, 3.36 to 4.12 mmol/L); high levels range from 160 to 189 mg/dl (SI, 4.14 to 4.90 mmol/L). Levels above 190 mg/dl (SI, > 4.92 mmol/L) are considered very high.

Interfering factors

○ Concurrent illness, especially if accompanied by fever, recent surgery, or myocardial infarction
○ Collecting the sample in a heparinized tube (possible false-high from activation of the enzyme lipase, which causes the release of fatty acids from triglycerides)
○ Failure to send the sample to the laboratory immediately
○ Antilipemic drugs, such as clofibrate, cholestyramine, colestipol, dextrothyroxine, niacin, probucol, and gemfibrozil (decrease)
○ Hormonal contraceptives, disulfiram, alcohol, miconazole, and high doses of phenothiazines (possible increase)
○ Estrogens (possible increase or decrease)
○ Presence of bilirubin, hemoglobin, salicylates, iodine, and vitamins A and D

Lipoprotein phenotyping

Overview

- Test determines levels of the four major lipoproteins: chylomicrons, very-low-density (pre-beta) lipoproteins, low-density (beta) lipoproteins, and high-density (alpha) lipoproteins.
- Familial lipoprotein disorders are either hyperlipoproteinemias or hypolipoproteinemias; detecting altered lipoprotein patterns is essential in identifying hyperlipoproteinemia and hypolipoproteinemia.
- Types of hyperlipoproteinemias and hypolipoproteinemias are characterized by electrophoretic patterns.
- Six types of hyperlipoproteinemias: I, IIa, IIb, III, IV, and V (types IIa, IIb, and IV are relatively common).
- All hypolipoproteinemias are rare, including hypobetalipoproteinemia, betalipoproteinemia, and alpha-lipoprotein deficiency.

Purpose

- To determine the classification of hyperlipoproteinemia and hypolipoproteinemia

Procedure

Preparation

- Explain to the patient that lipoprotein typing determines how the body metabolizes fats.
- Tell the patient that the test requires a blood sample.
- Explain to the patient that he may experience slight discomfort from the tourniquet and the needle puncture.
- Instruct the patient to abstain from alcohol for 24 hours before the test and to fast after midnight before the test. Provide a low-fat meal the night before the test.
- Check the patient's drug history for heparin use. Withhold antilipemics such as cholestyramine about 2 weeks before the test.
- Notify the laboratory if the patient is receiving treatment for another condition that might significantly alter lipoprotein metabolism, such as diabetes mellitus, nephrosis, or hypothyroidism.

Implementation

- Perform a venipuncture and collect the sample in a 4-ml ethylenediaminetetraacetic acid tube.
- When you draw multiple samples, collect the sample for lipoprotein phenotyping first because venous obstruction for 2 minutes can affect test results.
- Fill the collection tube completely and invert it gently several times to mix the sample and the anticoagulant thoroughly.
- Handle the sample gently to prevent hemolysis.

Patient care

- Apply direct pressure to venipuncture site until bleeding stops.

Complications

- Hematoma at the venipuncture site

Interpretation

Normal results

- No altered lipoprotein patterns detected

Abnormal results

- Altered lipoprotein patterns

Interfering factors

- Recent use of antilipemics (decrease)
- Failure to observe pretest restrictions
- Hemolysis from rough handling of the sample
- Administration of heparin (which activates the enzyme lipase, producing fatty acids from triglycerides) or collection of the sample in a heparinized tube (possible false-high)

Liver biopsy, percutaneous

Overview

○ Needle aspiration of a core of liver tissue for histologic analysis
○ Usually performed under local anesthesia with image-guidance

Purpose

○ To diagnose hepatic parenchymal disease
○ To diagnose malignant tumors and granulomatous infections

Procedure

Preparation

○ Make sure the patient has signed an appropriate consent form.
○ Note and report all allergies.
○ Check the patient's history for hypersensitivity to the local anesthetic.
○ Report any abnormal coagulation study results to the physician.
○ Ensure that all aspirin products and nonsteroidal anti-inflammatory drugs were stopped at least 5 days before the study.
○ Instruct the patient to restrict food and fluids for 4 to 8 hours before the test.
○ Warn the patient that he might experience right shoulder pain.
○ Explain that the test takes about 10 to 15 minutes.

Implementation

○ The patient is placed in the supine position with his right hand under his head.
○ After the biopsy site is selected, a local anesthetic is injected.
○ The patient takes a deep breath, exhales, then holds his breath at the end of expiration.
○ The biopsy needle is quickly inserted into the liver and withdrawn in 1 second while the patient is holding his breath.
○ After the needle is withdrawn, the patient resumes normal breathing.
○ The tissue specimen is placed in a properly labeled specimen cup.

Patient care

○ Apply direct pressure to the biopsy site to stop bleeding.
○ Maintain bed rest.
○ Give the patient an analgesic.
○ Instruct the patient to resume his normal diet.
○ Monitor vital signs.

○ Monitor the patient for bleeding and respiratory distress.
○ Watch for and immediately report to the physician bleeding or signs and symptoms of bile peritonitis (tenderness and rigidity around the biopsy site).
○ Watch for signs and symptoms of pneumothorax (tachypnea, decreased breath sounds, dyspnea, persistent shoulder pain, pleuritic chest pain).

Complications

▽ *ALERT Abdominal pain or dyspnea after the biopsy may indicate perforation of an abdominal organ or pneumothorax*

○ Peritonitis
○ Bleeding
○ Infection

Interpretation

Normal results

○ The normal liver consists of sheets of hepatocytes supported by a reticulum framework.

Abnormal results

○ Examination of hepatic tissue may indicate diffuse hepatic disease, such as cirrhosis and hepatitis; granulomatous infections such as tuberculosis.
○ Primary malignant tumors suggest possible hepatocellular carcinoma, cholangiocellular carcinoma, and angiosarcoma.

Interfering factors

None known

Liver-spleen scanning

Overview

- Liver-spleen scanning involves the distribution of radioactivity within the liver and spleen, recorded by a gamma camera after I.V. injection of a radioactive colloid, technetium 99m (^{99m}Tc).
- Test demonstrates focal disease nonspecifically as a cold spot (a defect that fails to take up the colloid).
- In conjunction with flow studies, liver-spleen scanning may help to distinguish among metastases, tumors, cysts, and abscesses.
- Scanning may not show focal lesions smaller than 2 cm in diameter.
- Scanning may not show early hepatocellular disease.
- More than one radionuclide scan shouldn't occur in the same day.

Purpose

- To screen for hepatic metastases and hepatocellular disease
- To detect focal disease (tumors, cysts, abscesses)
- To demonstrate hepatomegaly, splenomegaly, and splenic infarcts
- To assess the condition of the liver and spleen after abdominal trauma

Procedure

Preparation

- Make sure the patient has signed an appropriate consent form.
- Note and report all allergies.
- Tell the patient that he need not restrict food or fluids before the test.
- Stress the importance of lying still during the study.
- Explain that the test takes about 1 hour.
- Reassure the patient that the procedure involves only trace amounts of radioactivity and that adverse reactions are rare.

Implementation

- ^{99m}Tc is injected I.V.
- After 10 to 15 minutes the abdomen is scanned using various views.
- Scintigraphs are reviewed for clarity.
- Additional views are obtained as needed.

Patient care

▼ ALERT *Watch for anaphylactoid reactions (shortness of breath, chest tightness, itching, headache) or pyrogenic (fever-producing) reactions that may result from a stabilizer, such as dextran or gelatin, added to ^{99m}Tc.*

- Encourage oral fluid intake (unless contraindicated) to assist elimination of the radioactive material.
- Instruct the patient to flush the toilet immediately after urinating to reduce exposure to radiation in the urine.
- Monitor vital signs and respiratory status.
- Monitor intake and output.

Complications

- Anaphylactoid reactions
- Pyrogenic reactions

Interpretation

Normal results

- The liver and spleen appear equally bright on images.
- The distribution of radioactive colloid is usually more homogeneous in the spleen than in the liver.

Abnormal results

- A uniformly decreased or patchy appearance suggests hepatocellular disease.
- Uniformly decreased distribution of the colloid suggests hepatitis.
- Failure to take up the radioactive colloid and the appearance of solitary or multiple focal defects suggest cysts, abscesses, and tumors.
- Focal defects suggest intrahepatic hematoma.
- Lentiform defects on the periphery of the liver suggest subcapsular hematoma.
- Linear defects suggest hepatic laceration.
- Focal defects in or next to the spleen, which may transect it, suggest splenic hematoma.

Interfering factors

None known

Lumbar puncture

Overview

○ Permits sampling of cerebral spinal fluid (CSF) for qualitative analysis
○ More common than cisternal or ventricular puncture
○ Also known as a *spinal tap*

Purpose

○ To measure CSF pressure
○ To aid in the diagnoses of viral or bacterial meningitis; subarachnoid or intracranial hemorrhage; tumors and brain abscesses; neurosyphilis and chronic central nervous system infections

Procedure

Preparation

○ Make sure the patient has signed a consent form.
○ Note and report all allergies.
○ Inform the patient that he need not restrict food and fluids.
○ Explain that the test takes at least 15 minutes.
○ Explain that headache is the most common adverse effect.

Implementation

○ Position the patient on his side at the edge of the bed with his knees drawn up to his abdomen and his chin tucked against his chest (the fetal position); or position the patient sitting while leaning over a bedside table.
○ If the patient is in a supine position, provide pillows to support the spine on a horizontal plane.
○ The skin site is prepared and draped.
○ A local anesthetic is injected.
○ The spinal needle is inserted in the midline between the spinous processes of the vertebrae (usually between the third and fourth lumbar vertebrae or between the fourth and fifth).
○ The stylet is removed from the needle; CSF will drip out of the needle if properly positioned.
○ A stopcock and manometer are attached to the needle to measure the initial (opening) CSF pressure.
○ Specimens are collected and placed in the appropriate containers.
○ The needle is removed and a small sterile dressing applied.

▼ *ALERT During the procedure, observe closely for signs of an adverse reaction (elevated pulse rate, pallor, or clammy skin).*

Patient care

○ Keep the patient lying flat for 4 to 6 hours.
○ Inform him that he can turn from side to side.
○ Encourage the patient to drink fluids and assist him as needed.
○ Give analgesics.
○ Monitor the patient's vital signs, neurologic status, and intake and output.
○ Monitor the puncture site for redness, swelling, and drainage.

Complications

○ Adverse reaction to the anesthetic
○ Infection
○ Meningitis
○ Bleeding into the spinal canal
○ Leakage of CSF
○ Cerebellar herniation
○ Medullary compression

Interpretation

Normal results

○ Pressure is 50 to 180 mm H_2O.
○ Appearance is clear, colorless.
○ Protein is 15 to 45 mg/dl.
○ Gamma globulin is 3% to 12% of total protein.
○ Glucose is 50 to 80 mg/dl.
○ Cell count, 0 to 5 white blood cells; no red blood cells (RBCs).
○ Venereal Disease Research Laboratories (VDRL) test is nonreactive.
○ Chloride is 118 to 130 mEq/L.
○ Gram stain shows no organisms.

Abnormal results

○ Increased intracranial pressure (ICP), indicating tumor, hemorrhage, or edema caused by trauma
○ Decreased ICP, indicating spinal subarachnoid obstruction
○ Cloudy appearance, suggesting infection
○ Yellow or bloody appearance, suggesting intracranial hemorrhage or spinal cord obstruction
○ Brown or orange appearance, indicating increased protein levels or RBC breakdown
○ Increased protein, suggesting tumor, trauma, diabetes mellitus, or blood in CSF
○ Decreased protein, indicating rapid CSF production
○ Increased gamma globulin, associated with demyelinating disease or Guillain-Barré syndrome
○ Increased glucose, suggesting hyperglycemia
○ Decreased glucose, which could result from hypoglycemia, infection, or meningitis
○ Increased cell count, indicating meningitis, tumor, abscess, demyelinating disease
○ The presence of RBCs from hemorrhage
○ A positive VDRL test result, indicating neurosyphilis
○ Decreased chloride, pointing to infected meninges
○ Gram-positive or gram-negative organisms, indicating bacterial meningitis

Interfering factors

○ Inability of patient to remain in proper position.

Lung biopsy

Overview

- Obtains a pulmonary tissue specimen for histologic examination (three types).
- *Needle biopsy* is performed when the lesion is readily accessible, when it originates in the lung parenchyma, or when it's affixed to the chest wall.
- *Transbronchial biopsy* is removal of multiple tissue specimens through a fiber-optic bronchoscope; used for diffuse infiltrative pulmonary disease, tumors, or severe debilitation that contraindicates open biopsy.
- *Open biopsy* is appropriate for a well-circumscribed lesion that may require resection.

Purpose

- To confirm the diagnosis of diffuse parenchymal pulmonary disease
- To confirm the diagnosis of pulmonary lesions

Procedure

Preparation

- Make sure the patient has signed an appropriate consent form.
- Note and report all allergies.
- Obtain results of pre-study tests; report abnormal results to the physician.
- Check the patient's history for hypersensitivity to local anesthetic.
- Instruct the patient to fast after midnight before the procedure.
- The patient will receive chest X-ray and blood studies before the biopsy.
- Give the patient a mild sedative 30 minutes before the biopsy.
- Explain that the test takes 30 to 60 minutes.

Implementation

- The procedure depends on the type of approach: needle, transbronchial, or open biopsy.
- Tissue specimens are obtained for histologic examination.
- Specimens are placed in appropriate and properly labeled containers.
- Repeat the chest X-ray immediately after the biopsy is complete.

Patient care

- Instruct the patient to resume his normal diet.
- Monitor vital signs, intake and output, respiratory status, pulse oximetry, and breath sounds.
- Watch for bleeding and infection.
- Coughing or movement during the biopsy can cause pneumothorax.

Complications

- Bleeding
- Infection
- Pneumothorax

Interpretation

Normal results

- Pulmonary tissue exhibits uniform texture of the alveolar ducts, alveolar walls, bronchioles, and small vessels.

Abnormal results

- Histologic examination of a pulmonary tissue specimen reveals possible squamous cell or oat cell carcinoma and adenocarcinoma.

Interfering factors

- Failure to obtain a representative tissue specimen

Lung perfusion scan

Overview

○ Produces a visual image of pulmonary blood flow after I.V. injection of a radiopharmaceutical
○ Human serum albumin microspheres (particles) or macroaggregated albumin, bonded to technetium, possibly used

Purpose

○ To assess arterial perfusion of the lungs
○ To detect pulmonary emboli
○ To evaluate pulmonary function

Procedure

Preparation

○ Make sure the patient has signed an appropriate consent form.
○ Note and report all allergies.
○ Tell the patient that he need not restrict food and fluids before the test.
○ Stress the importance of lying still during imaging.
○ Explain that the test takes about 30 minutes
○ Explain that the amount of radioactivity is minimal.

Implementation

○ The patient is assisted into the supine position on a nuclear medicine table.
○ The radiopharmaceutical is injected I.V.
○ A gamma camera takes a series of images in various views.
○ Images projected on an oscilloscope screen show the distribution of radioactive particles.

Patient care

○ Monitor the injection site for hematoma and apply warm soaks if one develops.

Complications

○ Hematoma at the injection site
○ Sensitivity to the radiopharmaceutical

Interpretation

Normal results

○ Hot spots (areas of high uptake) indicate normal blood perfusion.
○ The uptake pattern is uniform.

Abnormal results

○ Cold spots (areas of low uptake) indicate poor perfusion, suggesting an embolism.
○ Decreased regional blood flow, without vessel obstruction, suggests possible pneumonitis.

Interfering factors

○ Failure to obtain a representative tissue specimen may affect test results

Lung ventilation scan

Overview

○ Nuclear scan after inhalation of air mixed with radioactive gas
○ Differentiates areas of ventilated lung from areas of underventilated lung

Purpose

○ To diagnose pulmonary emboli when used in combination with a lung perfusion scan
○ To identify areas of the lung that are capable of ventilation
○ To evaluate regional respiratory function
○ To locate regional hypoventilation

Procedure

Preparation

○ Make sure the patient has signed an appropriate consent form.
○ Note and report all allergies.
○ Tell the patient that he need not restrict food or fluids.
○ Stress the importance of lying still during imaging.
○ Tell the patient that he will wear a tight-fitting mask during the study.
○ Explain that the test takes 15 to 30 minutes.

Implementation

○ The patient is assisted into the supine position on a nuclear medicine table.
○ A tight-fitting mask is applied covering the patient's nose and mouth.
○ The patient inhales air mixed with a small amount of radioactive gas through the tightly fitted mask.
○ Distribution of the gas in the lungs is monitored on a nuclear scanner.
○ The patient's chest is scanned as the gas is exhaled.

Patient care

○ Reinstate oxygen therapy as appropriate.
○ Monitor the patient's vital signs and respiratory status.

Complications

○ Panic attacks from wearing the tight-fitting mask

Interpretation

Normal results

○ Gas is equally distributed in both lungs.

Abnormal results

○ Gas distributed unequally in both lungs suggests poor ventilation or airway obstruction in areas with low radioactivity.
○ When performed with a lung perfusion scan, vascular obstruction with normal ventilation suggests decreased perfusion as in pulmonary embolism.
○ Both ventilation and perfusion abnormalities suggest possible parenchymal disease.

Interfering factors

None known

Lupus erythematosus cell preparation

Overview

- In vitro procedure used in diagnosing systemic lupus erythematosus (SLE).
- Although less sensitive and reliable than either the antinuclear antibody (ANA) or the anti-deoxyribonucleic acid (DNA) antibody test, it's commonly used because it requires minimal equipment and reagents.
- Blood sample is mixed with laboratory-treated nucleoprotein (the antigen).
- If sample contains ANAs, they react with the nucleoprotein, causing swelling and rupture.
- Phagocytes from the serum then engulf the extruded nuclei, forming LE cells, which are then detected by microscopic examination of the sample.

Purpose

- To aid in the diagnosis of SLE
- To monitor treatment of SLE (about 60% of successfully treated patients fail to show LE cells after 4 to 6 weeks of therapy)

Procedure

Preparation

- Explain to the patient that this test helps detect antibodies to his own tissue.
- If appropriate, inform the patient that the test will be repeated to monitor his response to therapy.
- Inform the patient that he need not restrict food and fluids.
- Tell the patient that the test requires a blood sample. Explain who will perform the venipuncture and when.
- Explain to the patient that he may experience slight discomfort from the tourniquet and the needle puncture.
- Check the patient's medication history for drugs that may affect test results, such as isoniazid, hydralazine, and procainamide. If the patient must continue such drugs, be sure to note this on the laboratory request.

Implementation

- Perform a venipuncture and collect the sample in a 7-ml red-top tube.
- Handle the sample gently to prevent hemolysis.

Patient care

- Because the patient with SLE may have a compromised immune system, keep a clean, dry bandage over the venipuncture site for at least 24 hours and check for infection.
- Apply direct pressure to the venipuncture site until bleeding stops.

- If test results indicate SLE, tell the patient further tests may be necessary to monitor treatment.

Complications

- Hematoma at the venipuncture site

Interpretation

Normal results

- No LE cells present in serum

Abnormal results

- The presence of at least two LE cells may indicate SLE. Although these cells occur primarily in SLE, they may also appear in chronic active hepatitis, rheumatoid arthritis, scleroderma, and certain drug reactions.
- Up to 25% of patients with SLE demonstrate no LE cells.
- Apart from supportive clinical signs, a definitive diagnosis of SLE may require a confirming ANA or anti-DNA test.
- The ANA test detects autoantibodies in the serum of many patients with SLE who have negative LE cell tests.
- Anti-DNA antibodies appear in two-thirds of all patients with SLE but are rare in other conditions; thus, the presence of these antibodies is strong evidence of SLE.

Interfering factors

- Hemolysis from rough handling of the sample
- Isoniazid, hydralazine, and procainamide (may produce a syndrome resembling SLE)
- Chlorpromazine, clofibrate, ethosuximide, gold salts, griseofulvin, hormonal contraceptives, mephenytoin, methyldopa, methysergide, para-aminosalicylic acid, penicillin, phenytoin, phenylbutazone, primidone, propylthiouracil, quinidine, reserpine, streptomycin, sulfonamides, tetracyclines, and trimethadione

Lyme disease serology

Overview

- Multisystem disorder characterized by dermatologic, neurologic, cardiac, and rheumatic manifestations in various stages.
- Epidemiologic and serologic studies implicate a common tickborne spirochete, *Borrelia burgdorferi,* as the causative agent.
- Serologic tests for Lyme disease, both indirect immunofluorescent and enzyme-linked immunosorbent assays, measure antibody response to this spirochete and indicate current infection or past exposure.
- Serologic tests can identify 50% of patients with early-stage Lyme disease and all patients with later complications of carditis, neuritis, and arthritis, or patients in remission.
- In an indirect immunofluorescent assay, *B. burgdorferi* is grown in culture, fixed to a microscope slide, and then incubated with a human serum sample.
- A fluorescein-labeled antiglobulin is then introduced into the antigen-antibody complex.
- Any human antibody that binds to the spirochete is detected by viewing (under an ultraviolet microscope) the fluorescent antiglobulin that attaches to it.

Purpose

- To confirm a diagnosis of Lyme disease

Procedure

Preparation

- Explain to the patient that this test helps determine whether his symptoms are caused by Lyme disease.
- Instruct the patient to fast for 12 hours before the sample is drawn, but to drink fluids as usual.
- Tell the patient that the test requires a blood sample. Explain who will perform the venipuncture and when.
- Explain to the patient that he may experience slight discomfort from the tourniquet and the needle puncture.

Implementation

- Perform a venipuncture and collect the sample in a 7-ml clot-activator tube.
- Handle the specimen carefully to prevent hemolysis.
- Send the specimen to the laboratory immediately.

Patient care

- Apply direct pressure to the venipuncture site until bleeding stops.

Complications

- Hematoma at the venipuncture site

Interpretation

Normal results

- Normal serum values are nonreactive.

Abnormal results

- A positive result can help confirm the diagnosis, but it isn't definitive.
- Other treponemal diseases and high rheumatoid factor titers can cause false-positive results.
- More than 15% of patients with Lyme disease fail to develop antibodies.

Interfering factors

- High serum lipid levels (possible inaccurate results, requiring a repeat test after a period of restricted fat intake)
- Samples contaminated with other bacteria (possible false-positive)
- Hemolysis from rough handling of the sample

Lymph node biopsy

Overview

○ Surgical excision of an active lymph node or the needle aspiration of a nodal specimen for histologic examination

Purpose

○ To determine the cause of lymph node enlargement
○ To distinguish between benign and malignant lymph node tumors
○ To stage metastatic cancer

Procedure

Preparation

○ Make sure the patient has signed an appropriate consent form.
○ Note and report all allergies.
○ Check the patient's history for hypersensitivity to anesthetic.
○ For excisional biopsy, instruct the patient to restrict food from midnight and to drink clear liquids only.
○ If the patient will receive a general anesthetic, tell him to restrict fluids.
○ For a needle biopsy, no restriction of food or fluids is necessary.
○ Explain that the test takes 15 to 30 minutes.

Implementation

Excisional biopsy
○ The skin over the biopsy site is prepared and draped.
○ An anesthetic is given; an incision is made and an entire node removed.
○ The specimen is placed in an appropriate, properly labeled container.
○ After the wound is sutured, a sterile dressing is applied.

Needle biopsy
○ The biopsy site is prepared and draped.
○ A local anesthetic is given.
○ The biopsy needle is directed into the node and a small core specimen obtained.
○ The specimen is placed in a properly labeled container.
○ Pressure is applied to the biopsy site to control bleeding.
○ A dressing is applied after bleeding stops.

Patient care

○ Tell the patient to resume his usual diet and activity.
○ Monitor vital signs.
○ Watch for bleeding and infection.
○ Observe the biopsy site.

Complications

○ Bleeding
○ Infection

Interpretation

Normal results

○ The lymph node is encapsulated by collagenous connective tissue.
○ The lymph node is divided into smaller lobes by tissue strands called trabeculae.
○ The outer cortex is composed of lymphoid cells and nodules or follicles containing lymphocytes.
○ The inner medulla is composed of reticular phagocytic cells.

Abnormal results

○ Histologic examination may be necessary to distinguish between malignant and nonmalignant causes of lymph node enlargement.
○ A lymphoma affecting the entire lymph system suggests possible Hodgkin's disease.
○ Lymph node malignancy suggests possible metastatic cancer.

Interfering factors

None known

Lymphangiography

Overview

○ Radiographic examination of the lymphatic system after the injection of an oil-based contrast medium.
○ X-rays taken immediately after injection show the lymphatic system; those taken 24 hours later show the lymph nodes.
○ Contrast medium remains in the nodes for up to 2 years.
○ Subsequent X-rays assess disease progression and monitor treatment effectiveness.
○ Staging of lymphoma is determined by the number of nodes affected; unilateral or bilateral node involvement; extent of extranodal involvement.
○ Also known as *lymphography*.

Purpose

○ To detect and stage lymphomas
○ To identify metastatic involvement of the lymph nodes
○ To distinguish primary from secondary lymphedema
○ To evaluate effectiveness of chemotherapy or radiation therapy
○ To investigate enlarged lymph nodes

Procedure

Preparation

○ Make sure the patient has signed an appropriate consent form.
○ Note and report all allergies.
○ Check the patient's history for hypersensitivity to iodine, seafood, or iodinated contrast media.
○ Tell the patient that he need not restrict food or fluids before the test.
○ Advise the patient that he will receive a local anesthetic.
○ Explain that the test takes about 3 hours.
○ Explain that additional X-rays will be taken the next day (taking less than 30 minutes).
○ Explain that the contrast medium discolors urine, feces, and skin, and that vision will have a bluish tinge for 48 hours.
○ Explain that the incision site may be sore for several days.

Implementation

○ A preliminary chest X-ray is taken.
○ The skin is cleaned over the dorsum of each foot.
○ Blue contrast medium is injected intradermally into the area between the toes of each foot (usually into the first and fourth toe webs) and makes the lymphatic vessels appear as small blue lines on the upper surface of each instep.
○ A local anesthetic is injected into the dorsum of each foot.
○ A 1″ (2.5 cm) transverse incision is made to expose the lymphatic vessels.
○ Each vessel is catheterized, and contrast injected.
○ Fluoroscopy may be used to monitor filling of the lymphatic system.
○ Needles are removed, incisions sutured, and sterile dressings applied.
○ X-rays of the legs, pelvis, abdomen, and chest are taken.
○ Injection into the foot allows visualization of the lymphatics of the leg, inguinal and iliac regions, and the retroperitoneum up to the thoracic duct.
○ Injection into the hand allows visualization of the axillary and supraclavicular nodes.

Patient care

○ Instruct the patient to maintain bed rest for 24 hours, with feet elevated.
○ Apply ice packs to the incision sites.
○ Give analgesics.
○ Prepare the patient for follow-up X-rays as needed.
○ Monitor vital signs and respiratory status.

> ◢ *ALERT Watch for signs and symptoms of pulmonary complications caused by embolization of contrast medium, such as shortness of breath, pleuritic pain, hypotension, low-grade fever, and cyanosis*

○ Watch for bleeding and infection.
○ Observe incision sites.

Complications

○ Bleeding
○ Infection

Interpretation

Normal results

○ Homogeneous and complete filling with contrast medium is evident on the initial X-rays.
○ On 24-hour X-rays, the lymph nodes are fully opacified and well circumscribed; lymph nodes should be of normal size and architecture.
○ Lymphatic channels empty a few hours after injection.

Abnormal results

○ Enlarged, foamy-looking nodes suggest lymphoma.
○ Filling defects or lack of opacification suggests metastatic involvement.
○ Shortened or decreased lymphatic vessels suggest primary lymphedema.
○ Abruptly terminating lymphatic vessels suggest secondary lymphedema.

Interfering factors

None known

Lymphocyte transformation

Overview

- Evaluates lymphocyte competency without injection of antigens into the patient's skin.
- These in vitro tests eliminate the risk of adverse effects but can still accurately assess the ability of lymphocytes to proliferate and to recognize and respond to antigens.
- Mitogen assay evaluates the mitotic response of T and B lymphocytes to a foreign antigen.
- Antigen assay uses specific substances, such as purified protein derivative, *Candida*, mumps, tetanus toxoid, and streptokinase, to stimulate lymphocyte transformation.
- Mixed lymphocyte culture (MLC) assay is useful in matching transplant recipients and donors and in testing immunocompetence.
- Ability of neutrophils to engulf and destroy bacteria and foreign particles can also be determined.

Purpose

- To assess and monitor genetic and acquired immunodeficiency states
- To provide histocompatibility typing of tissue transplant recipients and donors
- To detect whether a patient has been exposed to various pathogens, such as those that cause malaria, hepatitis, and mycoplasmal pneumonia

Procedure

Preparation

- Explain to the patient that this test evaluates lymphocyte function, which is crucial to the immune system.
- Inform the patient that the test monitors his response to therapy, if appropriate.
- For histocompatibility typing, explain that this test helps determine the best match for a transplant.
- Inform the patient that he need not restrict food and fluids.
- Tell the patient that the test requires a blood sample. Explain who will perform the venipuncture and when.
- Explain to the patient that he may experience slight discomfort from the tourniquet and the needle puncture.
- If the patient is to receive a radioisotope scan, make sure to draw the serum sample for this test first.

Implementation

- Perform a venipuncture.
- If the patient is an adult, collect the sample in a 7-ml heparinized tube; for a child, use a 5-ml heparinized tube.
- Completely fill the collection tube and invert it gently several times to mix the sample and the anticoagulant.
- Send the sample to the laboratory immediately.
- Don't refrigerate or freeze the sample.

Patient care

- Because the patient may have a compromised immune system, take special care to keep the venipuncture site clean and dry.
- Apply direct pressure to the venipuncture site until bleeding stops.

Complications

- Hematoma at the venipuncture site

Interpretation

Normal results

- Results depend on the mitogens used. Reference ranges accompany test results.
- A positive test is normal; a negative test indicates a deficiency.

Abnormal results

- In the mitogen and antigen assays, a low stimulation index or unresponsiveness indicates a depressed or defective immune system.
- Serial testing can monitor the effectiveness of therapy in a patient with an immunodeficiency disease.
- In the MLC test, the stimulation index is a measure of compatibility. A high index indicates poor compatibility.
- A low stimulation index indicates good compatibility.
- A high stimulation index, in response to the relevant pathogen, can also demonstrate exposure to malaria, hepatitis, mycoplasmal pneumonia, periodontal disease, and certain viral infections in a patient who no longer has detectable serum antibodies.

Interfering factors

- Pregnancy or use of hormonal contraceptives, depressing lymphocyte response to phytohemagglutinin (low stimulation index)
- Chemotherapy (unless pretherapy baseline values are available for comparison)
- Radioisotope scan within 1 week before the test
- Failure to send the sample to the laboratory immediately

Lymphocytes

Overview

- Class of leukocytes
- Two main types: T lymphocytes and B lymphocytes

Purpose

- To determine lymphocyte blood count

Procedure

Preparation

- Explain to the patient that this test requires a blood sample.
- Inform the patient that he may feel discomfort from the tourniquet and the needle puncture.

Implementation

- Perform the venipuncture and collect the sample in a 5-ml ethylenediaminetetraacetic acid tube.

Patient care

- Apply direct pressure to venipuncture site until bleeding stops.

Complications

- Hematoma at the venipuncture site

Interpretation

Normal results

- Total lymphocytes, 800 to 2,600/mm^3

Abnormal results

- Increased absolute lymphocyte count is (> 4,500/mm^3).
- Increased counts can occur in conditions such as influenza and mononucleosis.
- Decreased counts occur in conditions, such as acquired immunodeficiency syndrome, aplastic anemia, and bone marrow suppression.

Interfering factors

None known

Lysozyme

Overview

- Lysozyme, also known as *muramidase*, is a low–molecular-weight enzyme that's present in mucus, saliva, tears, skin secretions, and various internal body cells and fluids.
- Enzyme splits, or *lyses*, the cell walls of gram-positive bacteria and, with complement and other blood factors, acts to destroy them.
- Lysozyme seems to be synthesized in granulocytes and monocytes, first appearing in serum after the destruction of such cells.
- When the serum lysozyme level exceeds three times the normal level, the enzyme appears in the urine — however, renal tissue also contains lysozyme, and renal injury alone can cause measurable excretion of this enzyme.
- Test measures urine lysozyme levels with a turbidimeter; serum lysozyme determinations, using the same method, confirm the results of urine testing.

Purpose

- To aid in the diagnosis of acute monocytic or granulocytic leukemia and to monitor the progression of these diseases
- To evaluate proximal tubular function and to diagnose renal impairment
- To detect rejection or infarction of kidney transplantation

Procedure

Preparation

- Explain to the patient that this test evaluates renal function and the immune system.
- Advise the patient that he need not restrict food and fluids.
- Tell the patient that the test requires collection of urine over a 24-hour period, and teach him how to collect the specimen correctly.

Implementation

- Collect the patient's urine over a 24-hour period, discarding the first specimen and retaining the last specimen in the appropriate container.
- Cover and refrigerate the specimen throughout the collection period.
- Keep the collection bag on ice if the patient has an indwelling urinary catheter in place.
- Send the specimen to the laboratory as soon as the test is complete.

Patient care

- If a woman is menstruating, anticipate possible test rescheduling.

- Tell the patient to avoid contaminating the urine specimen with toilet tissue or feces.

Complications

None known

Interpretation

Normal results

- Urine lysozyme values are 0 to 3 mg/24 hours.

Abnormal results

- Elevated urine lysozyme levels are characteristic of impaired renal proximal tubular reabsorption, acute pyelonephritis, nephrotic syndrome, tuberculosis of the kidney, severe extrarenal infection, rejection or infarction of kidney transplantation (levels normally increase during the first few days after transplantation), and polycythemia vera.
- Urine levels rise markedly after the acute onset or relapse of monocytic or myelomonocytic leukemia and rise moderately after acute onset or relapse of granulocytic (myeloid) leukemia.
- Urine lysozyme levels remain normal or decrease in lymphocytic leukemia and remain normal in myeloblastic and myelocytic leukemias.

Interfering factors

- Failure to collect all urine
- Bacteriuria (decrease)
- Blood or saliva in the specimen (increase)

Magnesium, serum

Overview

○ Measures serum levels of magnesium, an electrolyte vital to neuromuscular function that aids intracellular metabolism, activates many essential enzymes, affects the metabolism of nucleic acids and proteins, helps transport sodium and potassium across cell membranes, and influences intracellular calcium levels.
○ Most found in bone and intracellular fluid; small amount found in extracellular fluid.
○ Absorbed by the small intestine and excreted in urine and stool.

Purpose

○ To evaluate electrolyte status
○ To assess neuromuscular and renal function

Procedure

Preparation

○ Explain to the patient that the serum magnesium test determines the magnesium content of the blood.
○ Tell the patient that the test requires a blood sample.
○ Instruct the patient not to use magnesium salts (such as milk of magnesia or Epsom salt) for at least 3 days before the test, but tell him that he need not restrict food and fluids.
○ Explain to the patient that he may experience slight discomfort from the tourniquet (if one becomes necessary) and the needle puncture.

Implementation

○ Perform a venipuncture without a tourniquet, if possible, and collect the sample in a 3- or 4-ml clot-activator tube.
○ Handle the sample gently to prevent hemolysis.

Patient care

○ Apply pressure to the venipuncture site until bleeding stops.
○ In hypermagnesemia, watch for lethargy; flushing; diaphoresis; decreased blood pressure; slow, weak pulse; muscle weakness; diminished deep tendon reflexes; slow, shallow respiration; and electrocardiogram (ECG) changes (prolonged PR interval, wide QRS complex, elevated T waves, atrioventricular block, premature ventricular contractions [PVCs]).
○ In hypomagnesemia, watch for leg and foot cramps, hyperactive deep tendon reflexes, arrhythmias, muscle weakness, seizures, twitching, tetany, tremors, PVCs, and ventricular fibrillation.

Complications

○ Hematoma at the venipuncture site

Interpretation

Normal results

○ 1.3 to 2.1 mg/dl (SI, 0.65 to 1.05 mmol/L)

Abnormal results

○ Hypermagnesemia is most common in renal failure, when the kidneys excrete inadequate amounts of magnesium, in magnesium administration or ingestion, and in adrenal insufficiency (Addison's disease).
○ Hypomagnesemia is most common in chronic alcoholism; also in malabsorption syndrome, diarrhea, faulty absorption after bowel resection, prolonged bowel or gastric aspiration, acute pancreatitis, primary aldosteronism, severe burns, hypercalcemic conditions (including hyperparathyroidism), malnutrition, and certain diuretic therapy.

Interfering factors

○ Venous stasis from tourniquet use
○ Obtaining a sample above an I.V. site that's receiving a solution containing magnesium
○ Excessive use of antacids or cathartics or excessive infusion of magnesium sulfate (increase)
○ Prolonged I.V. infusions without magnesium; excessive use of diuretics (decrease)
○ I.V. administration of calcium gluconate (possible false-low if measured using the Titan yellow method)
○ Hemolysis of the sample (false-high)

Magnesium, urine

Overview

- Magnesium is found primarily in bones and intracellular fluid, with small amount in extracellular fluid.
- Activates enzyme systems, helps transport sodium and potassium across cell membranes, affects nucleic acid and protein metabolism, and influences intracellular calcium levels by affecting parathyroid hormone secretion.
- Deficiency detectable in urine before serum.
- Rules out magnesium deficiency as the cause of neurologic symptoms and helps evaluate glomerular function in renal disease.

Purpose

- To rule out magnesium deficiency in the patient with symptoms of central nervous system irritation
- To detect excessive urinary excretion of magnesium
- To help evaluate glomerular function in renal disease

Procedure

Preparation

- Explain to the patient that the urine magnesium test determines urine magnesium levels.
- Tell the patient that this test requires urine collection over a 24-hour period.
- Notify the laboratory and physician of drugs the patient is taking that may affect test results; it may be necessary to restrict them.

Implementation

- Tell the patient not to use a metal bedpan for collection.
- Instruct the patient not to contaminate the urine specimen with toilet tissue or feces.
- Collect the patient's urine over a 24-hour period, discarding the first specimen and retaining the last.

Patient care

- Inform the patient that he may resume his usual medications.

Complications

None known

Interpretation

Normal results

- 6 to 10 mEq/24 hours (SI, 3 to 5 mmol/d)

Abnormal results

- Low urine magnesium levels possibly result from decreased dietary intake of magnesium, malabsorption, acute or chronic diarrhea, diabetic ketoacidosis, de-

hydration, pancreatitis, advanced renal failure, and primary aldosteronism.
- Elevated urine magnesium levels possibly result from early chronic renal disease, adrenocortical insufficiency (Addison's disease), chronic alcoholism, or chronic ingestion of magnesium-containing antacids.

Interfering factors

- Failure to collect all urine during the test period
- Spirolactone (decrease)
- Increased calcium intake (decrease)
- Magnesium-containing antacids, ethacrynic acid, thiazide diuretics, and aldosterone (possible increase)

Magnetic resonance imaging

Overview

- Uses a powerful magnetic field and radiofrequency waves to produce computerized images of internal organs and tissues
- Eliminates the risks associated with exposure to X-ray beams and causes no harm to cells
- Also known as *MRI*

Purpose

- To obtain images of internal organs and tissues not readily visible on standard X-rays

Procedure

Preparation

- Patients requiring life support equipment, including ventilators, require special preparation; contact MRI staff ahead of time.
- Tell the patient that he need not restrict food or fluids.
- Make sure the patient has signed an appropriate consent form.
- Note and report all allergies.
- A claustrophobic patient may require sedation or an open MRI to reduce anxiety.
- Instruct the patient to remove any metal objects he's wearing or carrying.
- Advise the patient that he'll be asked to remain still during the procedure.
- Warn the patient that the machine makes loud clacking sounds.
- Explain that the test takes about 30 to 90 minutes.

Implementation

- If the patient is to receive a contrast medium, an I.V. line is started and the medium is administered before the procedure.
- The patient is checked for metal objects at the scanner room door.
- The patient is placed in the supine position on a padded scanning table.
- The table is positioned in the opening of the scanning gantry.
- A call bell or intercom is used to maintain verbal contact.
- The patient may wear earplugs if needed.
- Varying radiofrequency waves are directed at the area being scanned.
- A computer reconstructs information as images on a television screen.

Patient care

- Tell the patient to resume his normal diet and activities unless otherwise indicated.
- Monitor vital signs.
- Watch for orthostatic hypotension.

Complications

- Orthostatic hypotension
- Anxiety
- Claustrophobia

Interpretation

Normal results

- Refer to the specific type of MRI.

Abnormal results

- Refer to the specific type of MRI.

Interfering factors

- Metal objects, such as I.V. pumps, ventilators, other metallic equipment, or computer-based equipment, in the MRI area

Magnetic resonance imaging of bone and soft tissue

Overview

○ Produces clear and sensitive tomographic images of bone and soft tissue using a noninvasive technique
○ Provides superior contrast of body tissues and allows imaging of multiple planes, including direct sagittal and coronal views
○ Eliminates the risks associated with exposure to radiation from X-rays and causes no known harm to cells

Purpose

○ To evaluate bony and soft-tissue tumors
○ To identify changes in the bone marrow cavity
○ To identify spinal disorders

Procedure

Preparation

○ Make sure the patient has signed an appropriate consent form.
○ Note and report all allergies.
○ Make sure the scanner can accommodate the patient's weight and abdominal girth.
○ Screen for surgically implanted joints, pins, clips, valves, pumps, or pacemakers containing metal.
○ Stress the importance of removing all metallic objects, such as jewelry, hairpins, and wrist watch.
○ Stop I.V. infusion pumps, feeding tubes with metal tips, pulmonary artery catheters, and similar devices before the test.
○ Explain that the patient will hear the scanner clicking, whirring, and thumping, and that he may use earplugs.
○ Provide reassurance to the patient that he'll be able to communicate with the technician at all times.
○ For certain types of magnetic resonance imaging (MRI), start an I.V. for injection of a contrast medium.
○ Explain that the test takes 30 to 90 minutes.
○ Explain that MRI is painless and involves no exposure to radiation.
○ A claustrophobic patient may require sedation or an open MRI to reduce anxiety.
○ An anesthesiologist may need to be present to monitor a heavily sedated patient.
○ If the patient is unstable, make sure an I.V. line without metal components is in place and that all equipment is compatible with MRI imaging; monitor oxygen saturation, cardiac rhythm, and respiratory status during the test.

Implementation

○ The patient is checked for metal objects at the scanner room door.
○ The patient is placed on a narrow, padded, nonmetallic table that moves into the scanner tunnel.
○ A call bell or intercom is used to maintain verbal contact.
○ The patient is instructed to remain still during the procedure.
○ The patient is monitored for claustrophobia and anxiety.
○ The area to be studied is stimulated with radiofrequency waves.
○ A computer measures resulting energy changes at these body sections and uses them to generate images.

Patient care

○ Provide the patient with comfort measures as needed.
○ Tell the patient he may resume his normal activities.
○ Monitor vital signs.
○ Monitor the patient for orthostatic hypotension.

Complications

○ Orthostatic hypotension
○ Anxiety
○ Claustrophobia

Interpretation

Normal results

○ No evidence of pathology in bone, muscles, and joints

Abnormal results

○ Structural abnormalities suggest possible primary and metastatic tumors and various disorders of the bone, muscles, and joints.

Interfering factors

○ Metal objects, such as I.V. pumps, ventilators, other metallic equipment, or computer-based equipment, in the MRI area

Magnetic resonance imaging of the ear

Overview

- Assesses cranial nerves and bone using a noninvasive technique
- Provides high-quality, cross-sectional images of the body without X-rays or other radiation
- Fast spin echo (FSE) magnetic resonance imaging (MRI): for otologic assessment, especially with suspected retrocochlear lesion

Purpose

- To assess the cause of sudden unilateral sensorineural hearing loss
- To show early nonossified soft-tissue scarring in the membranous labyrinth
- To investigate lesions of the petrous apex
- To diagnose vestibular schwannomas as small as 2 mm
- To make visible cranial nerves VII and VIII, especially when anticipating excision of an auditory neuroma

Procedure

Preparation

- Make sure the patient has signed an appropriate consent form.
- Note and report all allergies.
- Inform the physician of a patient's pacemaker or other implant.
- Warn the patient that the MRI machine emits a loud, banging noise when operating, and that he may wear foam hearing protectors.
- Have the patient remove all jewelry and metal objects.
- Explain the need to remain still during the procedure.
- Explain that without I.V. contrast, the test takes about 15 minutes. FSE MRI is faster.
- A claustrophobic patient may require sedation or an open MRI to reduce anxiety.

Implementation

- Each MRI protocol depends on the purpose of the test.
- The patient is prepared and placed on the MRI table.
- The patient's head is moved into a large, hollow, cylindrical magnet.
- The scan is performed and images obtained.

Patient care

- Monitor vital signs.
- Monitor for orthostatic hypotension.

Complications

- Orthostatic hypotension
- Anxiety
- Claustrophobia

Interpretation

Normal results

- Cranial nerves and auditory bones appear normal.

Abnormal results

- Structural abnormalities suggest possible disorders, such as viral labyrinthitis, increased intracranial pressure, or paragangliomas.

Interfering factors

- Metal objects, such as I.V. pumps, ventilators, other metallic equipment, or computer-based equipment, in the MRI area

Magnetic resonance imaging of the neurologic system

Overview

○ Produces cross-sectional images of the brain and spine in multiple planes
○ Enables ability to "see through" bone and to delineate fluid-filled soft tissue

Purpose

○ To aid in the diagnosis of intracranial and spinal lesions
○ To aid in the diagnosis of soft-tissue abnormalities
○ To detect small tumors and hemorrhages and cerebral infarction earlier than possible with computed tomography scanning

Procedure

Preparation

○ Make sure the patient has signed an appropriate consent form.
○ Note and report all allergies.
○ Screen for surgically implanted joints, pins, clips, valves, pumps, or pacemakers containing metal.
○ Remove all metallic objects from the patient.
○ Because of powerful magnetic fields, magnetic resonance imaging (MRI) is contraindicated in patients with pacemakers, intracranial clips, ferrous metal implants, or gunshot wounds to the head.
○ Metallic or computer-based equipment (for example, ventilators and I.V. pumps) must not enter the MRI area.
○ Explain that MRI is painless and involves no exposure to radiation.
○ Explain the need to remain still for the entire procedure.
○ A claustrophobic patient may require sedation or an open MRI to reduce anxiety.
○ Warn the patient that he will hear clicking, whirring, and thumping sounds during the procedure, and that he may wear earplugs.
○ Provide reassurance to the patient that he'll be able to communicate with the technician at all times.
○ Explain that the test takes up to 90 minutes.

Implementation

○ The patient is placed in the supine position on a narrow table.
○ The table is moved to the desired position inside the scanner.
○ Radiofrequency energy is directed at the head or spine.
○ Resulting images are displayed on a monitor.
○ Images are recorded on film or magnetic tape.

Patient care

○ Instruct the patient to resume his normal activity.
○ Monitor vital signs.
○ Monitor the patient for orthostatic hypotension.

Complications

○ Orthostatic hypotension
○ Anxiety
○ Claustrophobia

Interpretation

Normal results

○ The appearance of brain and spinal cord structures is defined and distinct.

Abnormal results

○ Structural changes that increase tissue water content suggest possible cerebral edema, demyelinating disease, and pontine and cerebellar tumors.
○ Areas of demyelination (curdlike gray or gray-white areas) around the edges of ventricles suggest multiple sclerosis lesions.
○ Changes in normal anatomy suggest possible tumors.

Interfering factors

○ Metal objects, such as I.V. pumps, ventilators, other metallic equipment, or computer-based equipment, in the MRI area

Magnetic resonance imaging of the urinary tract

Overview

- Uses radiofrequency waves and magnetic fields to show specific structures (kidney or prostate), which are then converted to computer-generated images
- Can reveal blood vessel size and anatomy when imaging the soft-tissue structures of the kidneys, but not useful for detecting calculi or calcified tumors

Purpose

- To diagnose urinary tract disorders
- To evaluate genitourinary tumors and abdominal or pelvic masses
- To detect prostate calculi and cysts
- To detect cancer invasion into seminal vesicles and pelvic lymph nodes

Procedure

Preparation

- Make sure that the patient or family member has signed an appropriate consent form.
- Explain to the patient that magnetic resonance imaging (MRI) of the urinary tract helps evaluate abnormalities in the urinary system.
- Tell the patient who will perform the test, where it will take place, and how long it will last — about 30 to 90 minutes.
- Advise the patient to avoid alcohol, caffeine-containing beverages, and smoking for at least 2 hours before the test, and food for at least 1 hour beforehand.
- Explain to the patient that he can continue taking medications, except for iron, which interferes with the imaging.
- Before the test, tell the patient that he'll need to remove all clothing, jewelry, and metallic objects and wear a special hospital gown without snaps or closures.
- Inform the patient that he won't feel pain but may feel claustrophobic while lying supine in the tubular MRI chamber. Tell him the physician may order an anxiolytic.
- Tell the patient that he'll hear loud, crushing noises throughout the test but may receive a music headset to decrease this noise.
- If the patient will receive a contrast medium, obtain a history of allergies or hypersensitivity to these drugs. Mark sensitivities on the chart and notify the physician.
- Ask the patient if he or she has any implanted metal devices or prostheses, such as vascular clips, shrapnel, pacemakers, joint implants, filters, and intrauterine devices. If so, the patient may not be able to have the test.
- Just before the procedure, have the patient void.

Implementation

- The patient is placed in the supine position on a narrow, flat table.
- If the patient is to receive a contrast medium, start an I.V. line so that the medium is infused before the procedure.
- The table is moved to the enclosed cylindrical scanner.
- The patient is told to lie very still in the scanner while the images are being produced.
- Varying radiofrequency waves are directed at the area being scanned.
- Although the patient's face remains uncovered to allow him to see out, the patient is advised to keep his eyes closed to promote relaxation and prevent a closed-in feeling.
- If the patient feels nauseated because of claustrophobia, he's encouraged to take deep breaths.

Patient care

- If the patient received sedatives, monitor his vital signs until he's awake and responsive.
- Advise the patient that he may resume his usual diet, fluids, and medications.
- Monitor the patient for adverse reactions to the contrast medium (flushing, nausea, urticaria, and sneezing).

Complications

- Anxiety
- Adverse reactions to contrast medium

Interpretation

Normal results

- Visualization of the soft tissue structures of the kidneys
- Visualization of blood vessels

Abnormal results

- The discovery of tumors, strictures, stenosis, thrombosis, malformations, abscess, inflammation, edema, fluid collection, bleeding, hemorrhage, or organ atrophy

Interfering factors

- Uncooperative behavior, unstable medical conditions (confusion, combativeness), or inability to remain still during the procedure
- Metal objects in the MRI area

Mammography

Overview

- Detects breast cysts or tumors, especially those not palpable on physical examination.
- Questionable findings may warrant a follow-up ultrasound.
- Follow American Cancer Society guidelines.
- Never substitute for biopsy; mammography may not reveal all cancers.
- Many false-positive results.

Purpose

- To screen for malignant breast tumors
- To investigate breast masses, breast pain, or nipple discharge
- To differentiate between benign breast disease and malignant tumors
- To monitor patients with breast cancer who are treated with breast-conserving surgery and radiation

Procedure

Preparation

- Instruct the patient to avoid using underarm deodorant or powder the day of the exam.
- Explain that the test takes about 15 minutes.
- Explain to the patient that she may be asked to wait while the films are checked.
- When scheduling the test, inform the staff if patient has breast implants.
- Make sure the patient has signed an appropriate consent form.
- Note and report all allergies.

Implementation

- The patient rests one breast on a table above the X-ray cassette.
- The compressor is placed on the breast.
- The patient holds her breath until the X-ray is taken and she's told to breathe again.
- An X-ray of the craniocaudal view is taken.
- The machine is rotated, and the breast is compressed again.
- An X-ray of the lateral view is taken.
- The procedure is repeated for the other breast.
- The film is developed and checked for quality.

Patient care

- Answer the patient's questions about the test.

Complications

- Vasovagal reaction during compression

Interpretation

Normal results

- The test reveals normal ducts, glandular tissue, and fat architecture.
- No abnormal masses or calcifications are present.

Abnormal results

- Irregular, poorly outlined, opaque areas suggest malignant tumor, especially if solitary and unilateral.
- Well-outlined, regular, clear spots may be benign, especially if bilateral.

Interfering factors

- Improper positioning for testing

Manganese

Overview

- Analysis by atomic absorption spectroscopy, to measure serum levels of manganese, a trace element that activates several enzymes — including cholinesterase and arginase — which are essential to metabolism.
- Dietary sources are unrefined cereals, green leafy vegetables, and nuts.
- Toxicity may result from inhaling manganese dust or fumes — a hazard in the steel and dry-cell battery industries — or drinking contaminated water.

Purpose
- To detect manganese toxicity

Procedure

Preparation
- Explain to the patient that this test determines the level of manganese in the blood.
- Check the patient's history for drugs that may influence serum manganese levels, such as estrogens and glucocorticoids.
- Inform the patient that he need not restrict food and fluids.
- Tell the patient that the test requires a blood sample.
- Explain to the patient that he may experience slight discomfort from the tourniquet and the needle puncture.

Implementation
- Perform a venipuncture and collect the sample in a metal-free collection tube. Laboratories supply a special kit for this test on request.
- Handle the sample gently to prevent hemolysis.
- Send the sample to the laboratory immediately.

Patient care
- Apply direct pressure to the venipuncture site until bleeding stops.

Complications
- Hematoma at the venipuncture site

Interpretation

Normal results
- 0.4 to 1.4 µg/ml

Abnormal results

> ⚠ *ALERT Significantly elevated serum levels indicate manganese toxicity, which requires prompt medical attention to prevent central nervous system deterioration.*

- Low serum manganese levels may indicate deficient dietary intake, although not necessarily disease.

Interfering factors
- Failure to use a metal-free collection tube
- Hemolysis from rough handling of the sample
- High dietary intake of calcium and phosphorus (possible decrease caused by interference with intestinal absorption of manganese)
- Estrogen (increase)
- Glucocorticoids (increase or decrease caused by altered distribution of manganese in the body)

Mean corpuscular hemoglobin

Overview

- Gives the hemoglobin to red blood cell (RBC) ratio (Hb-MCH)
- Gives the weight of Hb in an average red cell

Purpose

- To measure the Hb-MCH
- To help determine anemia

Procedure

Preparation

- Explain to the patient that this test requires a venipuncture.
- Tell him that he may feel discomfort from the tourniquet and the needle puncture.

Implementation

- Perform a venipuncture, and collect the sample in a 3- or 4.5-ml ethylenediaminetetraacetic acid tube.

Patient care

- Apply direct pressure to the venipuncture site until bleeding stops.

Complications

- Hematoma at the venipuncture site

Interpretation

Normal results

- 26 to 32 pg/cell

Abnormal results

- A level of 5 to 25 pg/cell results in iron deficiency anemia.
- A level of 33 to 53 pg/cell results in pernicious anemia. (See *Comparative red cell indices in anemias.*)

Interfering factors

- Failure to use proper anticoagulant or to adequately mix the sample and the anticoagulant
- Hemolysis from rough handling of the sample
- Hemoconcentration from prolonged tourniquet constriction
- Diseases that cause RBCs to agglutinate or form *rouleaux* (false-low RBC count)

Comparative red cell indices in anemias

	Normal values (normocytic, normochromic)	Iron deficiency anemia (microcytic, hypochromic)	Pernicious anemia (macrocytic, normochromic)
MCV	84 to 99 µm³	60 to 80 µm³	96 to 150 µm³
MCH	26 to 32 pg/cell	5 to 25 pg/cell	33 to 53 pg/cell
MCHC	30 to 36 g/dl	20 to 30 g/dl	33 to 38 g/dl

Key:
MCV = Mean corpuscular volume
MCH = Mean corpuscular hemoglobin
MCHC = Mean corpuscular hemoglobin concentration

Mean corpuscular hemoglobin concentration

Overview

- Measures the ratio of hemoglobin (Hb) weight to hematocrit
- Defines the level of Hb in 100 ml of packed red blood cells (RBCs)
- Helps distinguish normochromic RBCs from hypochromic RBCs

Purpose

- To measure the ratio of Hb weight to hematocrit

Procedure

Preparation

- Explain to the patient that this test requires a venipuncture.
- Tell the patient that he may feel discomfort from the tourniquet and the needle puncture.

Implementation

- Perform a venipuncture, and collect the sample in a 3- or 4.5-ml ethylenediaminetetraacetic acid tube.

Patient care

- Apply direct pressure to the site until bleeding stops.

Complications

- Hematoma at the venipuncture site

Interpretation

Normal results

- 30 to 36 g/dl

Abnormal results

- A level of 20 to 30 g/dl results in iron deficiency anemia.
- A level of 33 to 38 g/dl results in pernicious anemia.

Interfering factors

- Failure to use proper anticoagulant or to adequately mix the sample and the anticoagulant
- Hemolysis from rough handling of sample
- Hemoconcentration from prolonged tourniquet constriction
- Diseases that cause RBCs to agglutinate or form *rouleaux* (false-low RBC count)

Mean corpuscular volume

Overview

- Measures the ratio of hematocrit to red blood cell (RBC) count
- Expresses the average size of erythrocytes and indicates whether they are microcytic, macrocytic, or normocytic
- Also known as *MCV*

Purpose

- To measure the ratio of hematocrit (packed cell volume) to RBC count

Procedure

Preparation

- Explain to the patient that this test requires a venipuncture.
- Tell the patient that he may feel discomfort from the tourniquet and the needle puncture.

Implementation

- Perform a venipuncture and collect the sample in a 3- or 4.5-ml ethylenediaminetetraacetic acid tube.

Patient care

- Apply direct pressure to the site until bleeding stops.

Complications

- Hematoma at the venipuncture site

Interpretation

Normal results

- 84 to 99 mm^3

Abnormal results

- 60 to 80 mm^3 indicates iron deficiency anemia.
- A high MCV suggests macrocytic anemias caused by megaloblastic anemias, folic acid or vitamin B$_{12}$ deficiency, inherited disorders of deoxyribonucleic acid synthesis or reticulocytosis.
- 96 to 150 mm^3 indicates pernicious anemia.

Interfering factors

- Failure to use proper anticoagulant or to adequately mix the sample and the anticoagulant
- Hemolysis from rough handling of sample
- Hemoconcentration from prolonged tourniquet constriction
- Diseases that cause RBCs to agglutinate or form *rouleaux* (false-low RBC count)

Mediastinoscopy

Overview

○ Operative procedure that shows mediastinal structures through a mediastinoscope with a built-in light source
○ Used when sputum cytology, lung scans, radiography, and bronchoscopic biopsy fail to confirm a diagnosis

Purpose

○ To detect bronchogenic carcinoma, lymphoma, and sarcoidosis
○ To stage lung cancer
○ To permit biopsy of paratracheal and carinal lymph nodes

Procedure

Preparation

○ Instruct the patient to fast after midnight before the test.
○ Make sure the patient has signed an appropriate consent form.
○ Note and report all allergies.
○ Check the patient's history for hypersensitivity to the anesthetic.
○ Inform the patient that he will receive a general anesthetic.
○ Warn the patient that he may have temporary chest pain, tenderness at the incision site, and a sore throat (from intubation).
○ Explain that he'll have an incision above the suprasternal notch.
○ Explain that the test takes about 1 hour.

Implementation

○ The patient is intubated and anesthetized.
○ A small transverse suprasternal incision is made.
○ A channel is formed using finger dissection, and lymph nodes are palpated.
○ The mediastinoscope is inserted.
○ Tissue specimens are collected and sent to the laboratory for frozen section examination.
○ If analysis confirms malignancy of a resectable tumor, thoracotomy and pneumonectomy may follow immediately.

Patient care

○ Give the prescribed analgesic.
○ Have the patient resume his diet and activity.
○ Monitor vital signs and intake and output.
○ Watch the patient for bleeding and signs of infection.
○ Observe the incision and dressings.
○ Monitor the patient's respiratory and neurologic status.

○ Observe the patient for signs and symptoms of complications: fever (mediastinitis); crepitus (subcutaneous emphysema); dyspnea, cyanosis, and diminished breath sounds (pneumothorax); tachycardia and hypotension (hemorrhage or cardiac tamponade); or loss of voice and obstruction of breathing (laryngeal nerve damage).

Complications

○ Pneumothorax
○ Perforated esophagus
○ Mediastinitis
○ Infection
○ Hemorrhage
○ Left recurrent laryngeal nerve damage
○ Cardiac tamponade

Interpretation

Normal results

○ The lymph nodes appear as small, smooth, flat oval bodies of lymphoid tissue.

Abnormal results

○ Anatomical abnormalities suggest various disorders including lung or esophageal cancer, and lymphomas such as Hodgkin's disease.

Interfering factors

○ Previous mediastinoscopy with scarring (makes dissection of nodes difficult or impossible)

Methemoglobin

Overview

○ Methemoglobin (MetHb) is a structural hemoglobin (Hb) variant, formed when the heme portion of deoxygenated Hb is oxidized to a ferric state.
○ This oxidization prevents the heme from combining with oxygen and transporting it to the tissues, and the patient becomes cyanotic.

Purpose

○ To detect methemoglobinemia acquired from excessive radiation or the toxic effects of chemicals or drugs
○ To detect congenital methemoglobinemia

Procedure

Preparation

○ If possible, obtain a history of the patient's hematologic status and Hb disorder, conditions that produce nitrite, and exposure to sources of nitrites in drugs.
○ Notify the laboratory and physician of drugs the patient is taking that may affect test results; it may be necessary to restrict them.
○ Explain to the patient that this test detects abnormal Hb in the blood.
○ Tell the patient that the test requires a blood sample.
○ Explain to the patient that he may feel slight discomfort from the tourniquet and the needle puncture.

Implementation

○ Perform a venipuncture and collect the sample in a 4.5-ml heparinized tube.
○ Fill the collection tube completely and invert it gently several times.
○ To avoid hemolysis, don't shake the tube vigorously.
○ Place the collection tube on ice and send it to the laboratory immediately.

Patient care

○ Apply direct pressure until bleeding stops.
○ Ensure subdermal bleeding has stopped before removing pressure.
○ If a large hematoma develops at the venipuncture site, monitor pulses distal to the site.

Complications

○ Hematoma at the venipuncture site

Interpretation

Normal results

○ 0% to 1.5% (SI, 0 to 0.015) of total Hb

Abnormal results

○ Increased MetHb levels may indicate acquired or hereditary methemoglobinemia, carbon monoxide poisoning, ingestion of certain drugs, or being exposed to certain substances.
○ Decreased MetHb levels may occur in pancreatitis.

Interfering factors

○ Aniline dyes, nitroglycerin, benzocaine, chlorates, lidocaine, nitrates, nitrites, phenacetin, sulfonamides, radiation, primaquine, and resorcinol (possible increase)
○ Nitrite toxicity in breast-feeding infants (increase caused by conversion of inorganic nitrate to nitrite ion)

Monocytes

Overview

- Mononuclear cells
- A type of white blood cell
- Phagocytic; develop into macrophages
- Help protect the body against infection

Purpose

- To help diagnose an illness such as infection or inflammatory disease

Procedure

Preparation

- Explain to the patient that this test requires a blood sample.
- Inform the patient that he may feel discomfort from the tourniquet and the needle puncture.

Implementation

- Perform a venipuncture and collect the blood sample.
- Send specimen to the laboratory promptly.

Patient care

- Apply direct pressure to the venipuncture site until bleeding stops.

Complications

- Hematoma at the venipuncture site

Interpretation

Normal results

- 0.21 to 0.92 $\times$ 10^9/L

Abnormal results

- Increased counts indicate carcinomas, monocytic leukemia, or lymphomas, collagen vascular disease such as systemic lupus erythematosus and rheumatoid arthritis infections, subacute bacterial endocarditis, tuberculosis, hepatitis, and malaria.

Interfering factors

None known

Multiple-gated acquisition imaging: rest and stress

Overview

○ Shows moving image of the beating heart and important features that reveal health of cardiac ventricles
○ Useful, noninvasive tool for assessing heart function
○ Often given at rest and then repeated with exercise or after patient receives certain drugs

Purpose

○ To assess the function of the heart
○ To detect certain heart conditions

Procedure

Preparation

○ Describe the test to the patient, including who will perform it, where it will take place, and how long it will last.
○ Tell the patient that he need not restrict food and fluids.
○ Make sure the patient or a responsible family member has signed an informed consent form.
○ Explain to the patient that he'll receive an I.V. injection of a radioactive tracer and that a detector positioned above his chest will record the circulation of this tracer through the heart.
○ Inform the patient that he may experience slight discomfort from the needle puncture, but that the imaging itself is painless.
○ Reassure the patient that the tracer poses no radiation hazard and rarely produces adverse effects.
○ Instruct the patient to remain silent and motionless during imaging, unless otherwise instructed.

Implementation

○ A radioactive isotope is injected into the patient's vein.
○ Radioactive isotopes attach to red blood cells and pass through the heart in the circulation.
○ The isotopes are traced through the heart by a scintillation camera.
○ For the next minute, the scintillation camera records the first pass of the isotope through the heart so that the aortic and mitral valves can be located.
○ Using an electrocardiogram, the camera is gated for selected 60-msec intervals, representing end-systole and end-diastole, and 500 to 1,000 cardiac cycles are recorded on X-ray or Polaroid film.

Patient care

○ Answer the patient's questions about the test.

Complications

None known

Interpretation

Normal results

○ The left ventricle contracts symmetrically, and the isotope appears evenly distributed in the scans.

Abnormal results

○ The patient with coronary artery disease usually has asymmetrical blood distribution to the myocardium, which produces segmental abnormalities of ventricular wall motion; such abnormalities may also result from preexisting conditions such as myocarditis.
○ The patient with a cardiomyopathy shows globally reduced ejection fractions. In the patient with a left-to-right shunt, the recirculating radioisotope prolongs the downslope of the curve of scintigraphic data; early arrival of activity in the left ventricle or aorta signifies a right-to-left shunt.

Interfering factors

None known

Myelography

Overview

○ Combines fluoroscopy and radiography to evaluate the spinal subarachnoid space after injection of a contrast medium.
○ Fluoroscopy shows flow of contrast medium and outlines the subarachnoid space.

Purpose

○ To demonstrate lesions partially or totally blocking cerebrospinal fluid (CSF) flow in the subarachnoid space (tumors and herniated intervertebral disks)
○ To detect arachnoiditis, spinal nerve root injury, or tumors in the posterior fossa of the skull

Procedure

Preparation

○ Instruct the patient to restrict food and fluids for 8 hours before the test.
○ Make sure the patient has signed a consent form.
○ Check the patient's history for hypersensitivity to iodine and iodine-containing substances (such as shellfish) and contrast media.
○ Notify the radiologist if the patient has a history of epilepsy or of antidepressant or phenothiazine use; phenothiazines given with metrizamide during myelography increases the risk of toxicity.
○ A patient undergoing lumbar puncture may need an enema.
○ Give the patient a sedative and an anticholinergic.
○ Warn the patient that he may feel transient burning, flushing, warmth, headache, salty taste, or nausea and vomiting when the contrast medium is injected.

Implementation

○ The patient is positioned on his side at the edge of the table with his knees drawn up to his abdomen and his chin on his chest.
○ Patient may receive a cisternal puncture if lumbar deformity or infection at the puncture site is present.
○ A lumbar puncture is performed.
○ Fluoroscopy verifies proper needle position in the subarachnoid space.
○ Some CSF may be removed for routine laboratory analysis.
○ The patient is placed in the prone position.
○ The contrast medium is injected.
○ If a subarachnoid space obstruction blocks the upward flow of the contrast medium, a cisternal puncture may be performed.
○ The flow of the contrast medium is studied with fluoroscopy; X-rays are taken.
○ The contrast medium is withdrawn, if oil-based, and the needle is removed.

○ The puncture site is cleaned and a small dressing applied.
○ If a spinal tumor is confirmed, the patient may go directly to the operating room.

Patient care

○ If the patient received an oil-based contrast medium, keep him flat in bed for 8 to 12 hours.
○ If he received a water-based contrast medium, elevate the head of the bed for 6 to 8 hours.
○ If test involved a water-based contrast, make sure that the large dye load doesn't reach the surface of the brain; to prevent this, keep the patient's head elevated for 30 to 45 degrees after the procedure.
○ Encourage the patient to drink fluids to assist the kidneys in eliminating the contrast medium.
○ Notify physician if patient fails to void within 8 hours.
○ Instruct the patient to resume his usual diet and activities the day after the test.
○ Monitor vital signs and intake and output.
○ Monitor the patient's neurological status.
○ Observe the puncture site.
○ Watch for bleeding and infection.
○ Monitor the patient for seizure activity.
○ If radicular pain, fever, back pain, or signs and symptoms of meningeal irritation (headache, irritability, or neck stiffness) develop, inform the physician immediately. Keep the room quiet and dark, and provide an analgesic or an antipyretic.

Complications

○ Bleeding
○ Infection
○ Meningeal irritation
○ Seizures
○ Dehydration

Interpretation

Normal results

○ The contrast medium flows freely through the subarachnoid space.
○ No obstruction or structural abnormality found.

Abnormal results

○ Extradural lesions suggest possible herniated intervertebral disks, or metastatic tumors.
○ Lesions within the subarachnoid space suggest possible neurofibromas or meningiomas.
○ Lesions within the spinal cord suggest possible ependymomas or astrocytomas.
○ Fluid-filled cavities in the spinal cord and widening of the cord itself suggest possible syringomyelia.

Interfering factors

○ Improper positioning after test may affect recovery

Myocardial perfusion imaging, radiopharmaceutical

Overview

○ An alternative way to assess coronary arteries in patients who can't tolerate exercise stress tests.
○ Adenosine, dobutamine, or dipyridamole used to chemically stress patient, simulating effects of exercise by increasing blood flow in coronary arteries or by increasing heart rate and contractility.
○ A radiopharmaceutical is injected; resting and stress images are obtained and compared to evaluate coronary perfusion.
○ Also known as *chemical stress test imaging.*

Purpose

○ To assess the presence and degree of coronary artery disease
○ To evaluate a patient's response after therapeutic procedures (such as bypass surgery and coronary angioplasty)

Procedure

Preparation

○ Confirm that the patient isn't pregnant.
○ For dobutamine administration, withhold beta blockers for 48 hours before the test. Give drugs such as antihypertensives.
○ Withhold theophylline for 24 to 36 hours and nitrates 6 hours before the examination.
○ Instruct the patient to avoid caffeine for 12 hours before testing.
○ Tell the patient that he must fast — but may drink water — for 3 to 4 hours before the test.
○ Make sure the patient has signed an appropriate consent form.
○ Note and report all allergies to the physician.
○ Screen for bronchospastic lung disease or asthma (adenosine and dipyridamole are contraindicated).
○ Screen for the presence of a pacemaker; dobutamine may be contraindicated.
○ Weigh the patient to determine the appropriate drug dosage.
○ A cardiologist, nurse, electrocardiogram (ECG) technician, and nuclear medicine technologist are usually present during the test.
○ Provide reassurance that emergency equipment is available if needed.
○ Warn the patient that he may experience flushing, shortness of breath, dizziness, headache, chest pain, increased heart rate, or palpitations during the infusion, depending on the drug in use.
○ Explain that signs and symptoms generally stop as soon as the infusion ends.
○ Explain that the study takes 1 to 2 hours but may take longer, depending on the type of nuclear medicine equipment.
○ Give adenosine or dipyridamole.

Implementation

○ The patient is placed in the supine position on the examination table.
○ I.V. access is obtained.
○ Baseline ECG and vital signs are obtained.
○ The chemical stress medication is infused.
○ During the infusion, vital signs and cardiac rhythm are monitored continuously.
○ At the appropriate time, the radiopharmaceutical is injected.
○ Rest imaging may be done before stress imaging or 3 to 4 hours after stress imaging, depending on the radiopharmaceutical used.
○ After the images are completed, the I.V. access is removed.

Patient care

○ Tell the patient to resume his regular diet and activity.
○ Monitor vital signs, ECG, and cardiac rhythm.
○ Monitor the patient's respiratory status.
○ Monitor anginal symptoms and heart sounds.
○ Monitor breath sounds.
○ Reversal drugs that should be readily available include I.V. aminophylline for adenosine and dipyridamole, and I.V. beta blocker for dobutamine.

Complications

○ Serious arrhythmias
○ Myocardial ischemia or infarction

Interpretation

Normal results

○ No perfusion defects are found on imaging.
○ No ischemic changes are found on ECG.

Abnormal results

○ Cold spots, indicating areas of decreased uptake, may suggest coronary artery disease (most common), myocardial fibrosis, attenuation caused by soft tissue (breast and diaphragm), or coronary spasm.

Interfering factors

None known

Myoglobin

Overview

○ This oxygen-binding muscle protein is usually found in skeletal and cardiac muscle.
○ Ischemia, trauma, and inflammation of muscle cause myoglobin to release into the bloodstream.
○ Release of myoglobin into the bloodstream is especially important when determining damaged cardiac muscle.
○ Creatine kinase and its isoform CK-MB are released more slowly than myoglobin during a myocardial infarction (MI).
○ Myoglobin, which is detectable as soon as 2 hours after the onset of chest pain and peaks in 4 hours, can be an early indicator of MI.

Purpose

○ To estimate damage to skeletal or cardiac muscle tissue (nonspecific test)
○ To determine if an MI has occurred (specific test)
○ To predict flare-ups of polymyositis

Procedure

Preparation

○ Explain the purpose of the test to the patient.
○ Obtain a patient history, including disorders that may be associated with increased myoglobin levels.
○ Tell the patient that the test requires a blood sample. Explain who will perform the venipuncture and when.
○ Tell the patient that he may experience slight discomfort from the tourniquet and the needle puncture.
○ Inform the patient that the results need to be correlated with other tests for a definitive diagnosis.

Implementation

○ Perform a venipuncture and collect the sample in a 4-ml tube with no additives.
○ Expect to collect blood samples 4 to 8 hours after the onset of an acute MI.
○ Handle the sample gently to prevent hemolysis.
○ Send the sample to the laboratory immediately.

Patient care

○ Apply direct pressure to the venipuncture site until bleeding stops.

Complications

○ Hematoma at the venipuncture site

Interpretation

Normal results

○ Normal myoglobin values are 0 to 0.09 µg/ml (SI, 5 to 70 µ/L).

Abnormal results

○ Besides MI, increased myoglobin levels may occur in acute alcohol intoxication, dermatomyositis, hypothermia (with prolonged shivering), muscular dystrophy, polymyositis, rhabdomyolysis, severe burns, trauma, severe renal failure, and systemic lupus erythematosus.

Interfering factors

○ Hemolysis or radioactive scans performed within 1 week of the test
○ Recent angina, cardioversion, or improper timing of the test (possible increase)
○ I.M. injection (possible false-positive)

Myoglobin, urine

Overview

○ Detects presence of myoglobin — a red pigment found in the cytoplasm of cardiac and skeletal muscle cells — in urine.
○ When muscle cells are extensively damaged, as by disease or severe crushing trauma, myoglobin is released into the blood, quickly cleared by renal glomerular filtration, and eliminated in the urine (*myoglobinuria*).
○ Appears in urine within 24 hours after a myocardial infarction (MI).
○ Must be differentiated from urine hemoglobin because of marked structural similarities.
○ Most commonly used test method is differential precipitation test.
○ Hemoglobin — bound to haptoglobin — precipitates when urine is mixed with ammonium sulfate; myoglobin, however, remains soluble and can be measured.

Purpose

○ To aid in the diagnosis of muscular disease or rhabdomyolysis
○ To detect extensive infarction of muscle tissue
○ To assess the extent of muscular damage from crushing trauma

Procedure

Preparation

○ Explain to the patient that the urine myoglobin test detects a red pigment found in muscle cells and helps evaluate muscle injury or disease.
○ Inform the patient that he need not restrict food and fluids.
○ Tell the patient that this test requires a random urine specimen, and teach him the proper collection technique.

Implementation

○ Collect a random urine specimen.
○ Send the specimen to the laboratory immediately.

Patient care

○ Answer the patient's questions about the test.

Complications

None known

Interpretation

Normal results

○ Myoglobin doesn't appear in urine.

Abnormal results

○ Myoglobinuria occurs in acute or chronic muscular disease, alcoholic polymyopathy, familial myoglobinuria, extensive MI, and in severe trauma to the skeletal muscles (which may result from a crush injury, extreme hyperthermia, or severe burns).
○ It also occurs in strenuous or prolonged exercise but disappears after rest.

Interfering factors

○ Extremely dilute urine (reduces sensitivity)
○ Contamination with iodine during surgery (positive results)
○ Recent ingestion of large amounts of vitamin C (inhibits reaction if testing is performed with Chemstrip or other reagent strips)
○ Failure to send the specimen to the laboratory immediately after collection

Nasopharyngeal culture

Overview

○ Makes preliminary identification of organisms to guide clinical management and determine the need for additional testing
○ Requires subsequent susceptibility testing to determine appropriate antimicrobial therapy

Purpose

○ To identify pathogens causing upper respiratory tract symptoms
○ To identify *B. pertussis* and *N. meningitidis,* especially in very young, elderly, or debilitated patients and asymptomatic carriers
○ To isolate viruses, especially in carriers of influenza viruses A and B

Procedure

Preparation

○ Explain to the patient that this test isolates the cause of nasopharyngeal infection.
○ Tell the patient who will collect the specimen and how it's done; tell him that secretions will be obtained from the back of his nose and throat, using a cotton-tipped swab.
○ Warn the patient that he may experience slight discomfort and gagging. Reassure him that obtaining the specimen takes less than 15 seconds.

Implementation

○ Wear gloves when performing the procedure and handling the specimen.
○ Moisten the swab with sterile water or saline solution.
○ Ask the patient to cough before you begin collecting the specimen.
○ Position the patient with his head tilted back.
○ Using a penlight and a tongue blade, inspect the nasopharyngeal area.
○ Gently pass the swab through the nostril and into the nasopharynx, keeping the swab near the septum and floor of the nose. Rotate the swab quickly and remove it.
○ Or, place a glass tube in the patient's nostril and carefully pass the swab through the tube into the nasopharynx. Rotate the swab for 5 seconds and then place it in the culture tube with transport medium. Remove the glass tube.
○ Label the specimen with the patient's name, the physician's name, the date and time of collection, the origin of the material, and the suspected organism.
○ Ideally, fresh culture medium should be inoculated with specimens for *B. pertussis* at the patient's bed-

side because of the organism's susceptibility to environmental changes.
○ If the purpose of specimen collection is to isolate a virus, follow the laboratory's recommended collection technique.
○ To prevent specimen contamination, don't let the swab touch the sides of the patient's nostril or his tongue.
○ Note antimicrobial therapy or chemotherapy on the laboratory request.
○ Keep the container upright.
○ Tell the laboratory if the suspected organism is *Corynebacterium diphtheriae* or *B. pertussis* because these need special growth media.
○ Refrigerate a viral specimen according to your laboratory's procedure.
○ If *B. pertussis* is suspected, use Dacron or calcium alginate mini-tipped swabs for collection.
○ When specimens can't be directly placed onto growth media, the best media-based transport is one supplemented with antibiotics to reduce the growth of normal flora.

Patient care

○ Answer the patient's questions about the test.

Complications

⚠ *ALERT Laryngospasm after the culture is obtained if the patient has epiglottiditis or diphtheria (keep resuscitation equipment nearby)*

Interpretation

Normal results

○ Nonhemolytic streptococci, alpha-hemolytic streptococci, *Neisseria* species (except *N. meningitidis* and *N. gonorrhoeae*), coagulase-negative staphylococci such as *Staphylococcus epidermidis,* and occasionally coagulase-positive *S. aureus* are present.

Abnormal results

○ Group A beta-hemolytic streptococci; occasionally groups B, C, and G beta-hemolytic streptococci; *B. pertussis, C. diphtheriae,* and *S. aureus;* large numbers of pneumococci; *Haemophilus influenzae;* myxovirus influenzae; paramyxoviruses; *Candida albicans;* mycoplasma species; and *Mycobacterium tuberculosis* are present.

Interfering factors

○ Recent antimicrobial therapy (decrease in bacterial growth)
○ Failure to use the proper collection technique
○ Failure to place the specimen in transport medium
○ Failure to keep a viral specimen cold
○ Failure to send the specimen to the laboratory immediately

Nephrotomography

Overview

- Presents images as "slices" or linear layers of the kidneys; structures in front of and behind the selected planes appear blurry.
- Produces film images of the renal arterial network and parenchyma before and after opacification with contrast medium.
- A separate procedure or adjunct to excretory urography.

Purpose

- To differentiate between a simple renal cyst and a solid neoplasm
- To assess renal lacerations
- To assess post-traumatic nonperfused areas of the kidneys
- To localize adrenal tumors
- To show space-occupying lesions

Procedure

Preparation

- Instruct the patient to fast for 8 hours before the test.
- Make sure the patient has signed an appropriate consent form.
- Note and report all allergies.
- Check the patient's history for hypersensitivity to iodine or iodine-containing foods (such as shellfish) or to iodinated contrast media.
- If the patient has a history of I.V. contrast hypersensitivity, inform the physician so that a prophylaxis (such as diphenhydramine) or a low osmolar contrast medium can be used.
- Check the serum creatinine level and inform the physician if it's greater than 1.5 mg/dl. (I.V. fluids may be ordered.)
- Nephrotomography is performed with extreme caution in patients with impaired renal function (serum creatinine levels greater than 1.5 mg/dl), especially in elderly and dehydrated patients.
- Warn the patient that he may experience transient adverse effects from the injection of the contrast medium (burning, stinging at the injection site, flushing, and a metallic taste).
- Tell the patient that he may hear loud, clacking sounds as the films are exposed.
- Explain that the test takes less than 1 hour.

Implementation

- A plain film of the kidneys is obtained.
- Preliminary tomograms are obtained and reviewed.
- A contrast medium is administered I.V., using either a bolus or infusion method.
- Serial tomograms are obtained.

Patient care

- Ensure adequate hydration.
- Tell the patient to resume his normal diet and activity.
- Monitor vital signs and intake and output.
- Monitor the patient's serum creatinine levels.
- Observe the patient for signs and symptoms of a post-test allergic reaction to the contrast medium (flushing, nausea, urticaria, and sneezing) or an anaphylactic reaction.

Complications

- Adverse reaction to the contrast medium
- Impaired renal function

Interpretation

Normal results

- The size, shape, and position of the kidneys are normal.
- No space-occupying lesions or other abnormalities.

Abnormal results

- Various structural abnormalities, such as simple cysts and solid tumors

Interfering factors

- Residual barium from a recently performed barium study obscuring the kidneys

Neutrophils

Overview

○ One of five types of white blood cells (WBCs).
○ Help protect the body against infection and aid immune system.
○ More than half the white cells in the peripheral circulation are neutrophils.
○ Because they quickly phagocytize significant quantities of microorganisms, neutrophils are the body's first line of defense against infection.
○ Each mature neutrophil can inactivate 5 to 20 bacteria.

Purpose

○ To reveal whether neutrophils are present in normal proportion to one another, if one cell type is increased or decreased, or if immature cells are present
○ To help diagnose specific types of illnesses that affect the immune system

Procedure

Preparation

○ Explain to the patient that this test requires a blood sample.
○ Inform the patient that he may feel discomfort from the needle puncture and the tourniquet.

Implementation

○ Perform the venipuncture.

Patient care

○ Apply direct pressure to the site until bleeding stops.

Complications

○ Hematoma at the venipuncture site

Interpretation

Normal results

○ A small number of slightly immature neutrophils, known as *band cells*, are present in peripheral blood.

Abnormal results

○ The presence of many band cells and their precursors, known as a *shift to the left,* indicate infection.
○ The presence of mature, hypersegmented neutrophils that have more nuclear segments than normal, known as a *shift to the right*, indicate pernicious anemia and hepatic disease.
○ Increased band cells and a low total WBC count, known as a *degenerative shift*, indicate bone marrow depression (as in typhoid fever).
○ Increased band cells, metamyelocytes, and myelocytes and a high WBC count, known as a *regenerative shift*, indicate stimulation of the bone marrow (as in pneumonia and appendicitis).

Interfering factors

None known

Nuclear medicine scans

Overview

○ Imaging of specific body organs or systems by a scintillating scanning camera after I.V. injection, inhalation, or oral ingestion of a radioactive tracer compound

Purpose

○ To produce tissue analysis and images not readily seen on standard X-rays
○ To detect or rule out malignant lesions when X-ray findings are normal or questionable

Procedure

Preparation

○ Make sure the patient has signed an appropriate consent form.
○ Note and report all allergies.
○ Note any prior nuclear medicine procedures.
○ Make sure the patient isn't scheduled for more than one radionuclide scan on the same day.
○ Advise the patient that he'll be asked to take various positions on a scanner table.
○ Stress the importance that the patient remain still during the procedure.
○ Explain that the study takes about 1½ hours, but the time varies depending on the specific nuclear medicine scan.

Implementation

○ If the patient will receive an I.V. tracer isotope, an I.V. line is started.
○ The detector of a scintillation camera is directed at the area being scanned and displays the image on a monitor.
○ Scintigraphs are obtained and reviewed for clarity.
○ If necessary, additional views are obtained.

Patient care

○ Tell the patient to resume his normal diet and activities.
○ Monitor vital signs.
○ Observe the injection site.
○ Watch the patient for infection and orthostatic hypotension.

Complications

○ Infection
○ Orthostatic hypotension

Interpretation

Normal results

○ See the specific nuclear medicine scan.

Abnormal results

○ See the specific nuclear medicine scan.

Interfering factors

○ See the specific nuclear medicine scan

5'-nucleotidase

Overview

- More difficult than the alkaline phosphatase (ALP) assay; measures level of serum 5'-nucleotidase (5'NT), a phosphatase formed almost entirely in the hepatobiliary tract.
- Unlike ALP, 5'NT hydrolyzes nucleoside 5'-phosphate groups only.
- Helps to determine whether ALP elevation is caused by skeletal or hepatic disease.
- Because 5'NT remains normal in skeletal disease and pregnancy, it's more specific for assessing hepatic dysfunction than ALP or leucine aminopeptidase.
- Not widely used as a liver function study but may be more sensitive than ALP to diagnose cholangitis, biliary cirrhosis, and malignant infiltrations of the liver.
- Usually used to determine if ALP elevation is caused by skeletal or hepatic disease.

Purpose

- To distinguish between hepatobiliary and skeletal disease when the source of increased ALP levels is uncertain
- To help differentiate biliary obstruction from acute hepatocellular damage
- To detect hepatic metastasis in the absence of jaundice

Procedure

Preparation

- Explain to the patient that this test evaluates liver function.
- Tell the patient that the test requires a blood sample. Explain who will perform the venipuncture and when.
- Explain to the patient that he may experience slight discomfort from the needle puncture and the tourniquet.
- Tell the patient that he need not restrict food and fluids.

Implementation

- Perform a venipuncture and collect the sample in a 4-ml tube without additives.
- Handle the sample gently to prevent hemolysis.

Patient care

- Apply direct pressure to the venipuncture site until bleeding stops.

Complications

- Hematoma at the venipuncture site

Interpretation

Normal results

- Adult serum 5'NT values range from 2 to 17 units/L (SI, 0.03 to 0.29 µkat/L); values for children are lower.

Abnormal results

- Extremely high levels of 5'NT occur in common bile duct obstruction by calculi or tumors in diseases that cause severe intrahepatic cholestasis such as neoplastic infiltrations of the liver.
- Slight to moderate increases may reflect acute hepatocellular damage or active cirrhosis.

Interfering factors

- Hemolysis from rough handling of the sample
- Cholestatic drugs, such as phenothiazines, morphine, meperidine, and codeine as well as aspirin, acetaminophen, and phenytoin (increase)

Ocular ultrasonography

Overview

- Transmits high-frequency sound waves through the eye and measures their reflection from ocular structures.
- A-scan converts echoes into waveforms whose crests represent the positions of different structures, providing a one-dimensional picture.
- B-scan converts echoes into patterns of dots that form a two-dimensional, cross-sectional image of the ocular structure.
- A-scan is more valuable in measuring eye's axial length and characterizing tissue texture of abnormal lesions.
- B-scan is easier to interpret than A-scan, so it's used more often to evaluate structures of the eye and to diagnose abnormalities.
- Combination of A- and B-scans produces most useful test results.
- Especially helpful in evaluating a fundus clouded by an opaque medium such as a cataract.
- May be performed before cataract removal to ensure integrity of the retina or to measure length of eye and curvature of cornea if implanting an intraocular lens.
- Readily available and provides information immediately.
- Identifies intraocular foreign bodies and determines their position in relation to ocular structures as well as assessing severity of resulting ocular damage.

Purpose

- To aid in evaluating the fundus in an eye with opacity such as a cataract
- To aid in the diagnosis of vitreous disorders and retinal detachment
- To diagnose and differentiate between intraocular and orbital lesions and to follow their progression through serial examinations
- To locate intraocular foreign bodies
- To measure the dimensions of other tumors detectable by ophthalmoscopy

Procedure

Preparation

- Describe the procedure to the patient and explain that ocular ultrasonography evaluates the eye's structures.
- Inform the patient that he need not restrict food and fluids.
- Tell the patient that a small transducer will be placed on his closed eyelid and that the transducer transmits high-frequency sound waves that are reflected by the structures in the eye.
- Inform the patient that he may be asked to move his eyes or change his gaze during the procedure and

that his cooperation is required to ensure accurate test results.

Implementation

- The patient is placed in the supine position on an X-ray table.
- For the B-scan, the patient is asked to close his eyes, and a water-soluble gel (such as Goniosol) is applied to his eyelid. The transducer is then placed on the eyelid.
- For the A-scan, anesthetizing drops are instilled in the patient's eye, and a clear plastic eye cup is placed directly on the eyeball.
- A water-soluble gel is then applied to the eye cup, and the transducer is positioned on the medium.
- The transducer then transmits high-frequency sound waves into the patient's eye, and the resulting echoes are transformed into images or waveforms on the oscilloscope screen.

Patient care

- After the test, remove the water-soluble gel from the patient's eyelid.

Complications

None known

Interpretation

Normal results

- The optic nerve and the posterior lens capsule produce echoes that take on characteristic forms on A- and B-scan images.
- The posterior wall of the eye appears as a smooth, concave curve; retrobulbar fat is also visible.
- The lens and vitreous humor are also visible.
- Normal orbital echo patterns depend on the position of the transducer and the position of the patient's gaze during the procedure.

Abnormal results

- Eyes clouded by a vitreous hemorrhage: Organization of the hemorrhage is identifiable by the degree of density that appears on the image. The cause, prognosis, and associated abnormalities can sometimes be determined.
- Massive vitreous organization and vitreous bands.
- Retinal detachment: characteristically produces a dense, sheetlike echo on a B-scan and is commonly found in a patient with an opacity.
- Intraocular tumors: possible to diagnose and differentiate according to size, shape, location, and texture.
- Melanomas, metastatic tumors, hemangiomas, retinoblastomas, and cystic lesions may be present.
- Evidence of meningiomas, neurofibromas, gliomas, neurilemomas, or the inflammatory changes associated with Graves' disease.

Interfering factors

None known

Oculoplethysmography

Overview

○ Noninvasive procedure that indirectly measures blood flow in the ophthalmic artery.
○ Reflects carotid blood flow and cerebral circulation; not a reliable screening or diagnostic test for carotid artery disease.
○ Also called *OPG*.
○ Ocular pneumoplethysmography (OPG-Gee) used to indirectly measure ophthalmic artery pressures.

Purpose

○ To aid in the detection and evaluation of carotid artery disease
○ To evaluate symptoms of transient ischemic attacks
○ To evaluate asymptomatic carotid bruits
○ To evaluate nonhemispheric neurologic symptoms (dizziness, ataxia, or syncope)

Procedure

Preparation

○ Make sure the patient has signed an appropriate consent form.
○ Note and report all allergies.
○ Tell the patient he need not restrict food and fluids.
○ Ask the patient to remove his contact lenses.
○ Advise the patient that he may take the usual glaucoma medications and eyedrops.
○ Advise the patient that his eyes may burn slightly after the anesthetic eye drops are instilled.
○ Warn that if OPG-Gee is scheduled, he may experience transient loss of vision when his eyes receive suction.
○ Instruct the patient to avoid blinking or moving during the procedure.
○ Explain that the test takes only a few minutes.

Implementation

OPG
○ Anesthetic eyedrops are instilled and small photo-electric cells are attached to the patient's earlobes.
○ Tracings for both ears are taken and compared.
○ Eyecups resembling contact lenses are applied to the corneas and held in place with light suction (40 to 50 mm Hg).
○ Tracings of the pulsations within each eye are compared with each other and with right ear tracings.
OPG-Gee
○ Anesthetic eyedrops are instilled.
○ Eyecups are attached to the sclerae.
○ A vacuum of 300 mm Hg is applied to each eye, corresponding to a mean pressure of 100 mm Hg in the ophthalmic artery.
○ When suction is applied, the pulse in both eyes disappears.

○ The pressure is gradually released.
○ The eye pulses should return simultaneously.
○ Pulse arrival times are converted to ophthalmic artery pressures and then compared.
○ Both brachial pressures are taken.
○ The higher systolic pressure is compared with the ophthalmic artery pressures.
○ Pulse arrival times in the eyes and ears are measured and compared.
○ If indicated, cerebral angiography may follow.

Patient care

○ Instruct the patient not to rub his eyes for 2 hours to prevent corneal abrasions.
○ Advise the patient that mild burning is normal as the eyedrops wear off, but to report severe burning.
○ Instruct him not to reinsert contact lenses for about 2 hours after OPG.
○ Observe for and immediately report symptoms of corneal abrasion, such as pain and photophobia.

Complications

○ Corneal abrasion
○ Scleral hematoma

Interpretation

Normal results

○ In OPG, all pulses occur simultaneously.
○ In OPG-Gee, the difference between ophthalmic artery pressures should be less than 5 mm Hg.
○ Ophthalmic artery pressure divided by the higher brachial systolic pressure should exceed 0.67.

Abnormal results

OPG
○ Reduced rate of blood flow during systole and delayed arrival of a pulse in the ipsilateral eye suggest carotid occlusive disease.
○ Reveals only severe narrowing or occlusion and can't be used as a reliable screening or diagnostic test for carotid artery disease.
OPG-Gee
○ A difference between ophthalmic artery pressures of more than 5 mm Hg suggests the presence of carotid occlusive disease on the side with the lower pressure.
○ A ratio between the ophthalmic artery pressure and the higher brachial systolic pressure of less than 0.67 reinforces the diagnosis of carotid occlusive disease.
○ The lower the ratio, the more severe the stenosis.

Interfering factors

○ Hypertension; OPG-Gee test results may be more difficult to interpret because of elevated ophthalmic artery pressures
○ Constant blinking or nystagmus; may cause artifact, making interpretation of tracings difficult
○ Severe cardiac arrhythmias

Ophthalmoscopy, handheld

Overview

- Magnified examination of living vascular and nerve tissue of the fundus, including the optic disk, retinal vessels, macula, and retina
- Used directly or indirectly

Purpose

- To detect and evaluate eye disorders
- To detect and evaluate ocular manifestations of systemic disease
- To identify opacities and lesions

Procedure

Preparation

- Note and report all allergies.
- Advise the patient that eyedrops may be instilled to dilate the pupils.
- Check patient's history for angle-closure glaucoma and previous use of dilating eyedrops.
- Don't give dilating eyedrops to a patient who has angle-closure glaucoma or a history of hypersensitivity reactions to the drops. Don't dilate the patient's pupils if head trauma or acute disease of the central nervous system is suspected.

Implementation

- The patient sits upright in the examination chair.
- Darken the room.
- The right eye is examined with the ophthalmoscope.
- The patient looks straight ahead at a specific object 20′ (6 m) away and is told not to move his eyes.
- The light beam of the ophthalmoscope is directed into the pupil.
- The examiner slowly approaches the patient at an angle of about 15 degrees temporal to the patient's line of vision.
- The red reflex is observed.
- The optic disk is examined.
- The physiologic cup is located.
- The retinal vessels emerging from the optic disk are examined.
- The macula and fovea are examined.
- As the patient looks up, down, and to each side, the extreme periphery is examined.
- The superior, inferior, temporal, and nasal portions of the retina are examined.
- The patient's left eye is examined in the same way.

Patient care

- If the patient's eyes are dilated, protect them from bright lights and explain the need to avoid driving or operating machinery until vision returns to normal.

Complications

- Adverse reaction to mydriatics, if used, including photophobia and increased intraocular pressure

Interpretation

Normal results

- A visible red reflex is found.
- A slightly oval optic disk, measuring 5 mm vertically, lies to the nasal side of the fundus center. It's usually pink with darker edges at its nasal border.
- The physiologic cup varies in size and tends to be larger in myopia and smaller in hyperopia; it appears as a central depression in the surface of the disc.
- A semitransparent retina surrounds the optic disk.
- Retinal vessels branch out from the disk, including venules and the slightly smaller arterioles.
- Vessel diameter progressively decreases with distance from the optic disk.
- Retinal arterioles are medium red; venules appear dark red or blue.
- The macula, a small avascular area, appears darker than the surrounding retina, is located about 2½ disk diameters temporal from the optic disk, and may appear slightly yellow because of the xanthophyll pigment in the retina.
- In the macula's center lies a small, darker spot, the fovea.
- A tiny light reflex is visible at the fovea center.

Abnormal results

- An absent or diminished red reflex suggests possible gross corneal lesions, dense opacities of the aqueous or vitreous humor, cataracts, or a detached retina.
- A cloudy vitreous humor suggests possible inflammatory disease of the optic disk, retina, or uvea.
- An elevated, increased vascular optic disk suggests possible optic neuritis.
- A white disk suggests possible optic nerve atrophy.
- Abnormal elevation of the disk, blurring of disk margins, engorged vessels, and hemorrhages suggest papilledema.
- An enlarged physiologic cup appearing gray with white edges suggests glaucoma.
- A milky-white retina suggests the acute phase of central retinal artery occlusion.
- Widespread retinal hemorrhage, patches of white exudate, and disk elevation suggest central retinal vein occlusion.
- Gray, elevated areas suggest retinal detachment.
- A dark lesion suggests a possible choroidal tumor.
- Vasospasm, sclerosis, and eventual occlusion of retinal arterioles, leading to retinal edema and hemorrhage, and papilledema suggest hypertension.
- Retinal fibroses, patches of white exudate, and microaneurysms suggest complications of diabetes mellitus.

Interfering factors

None known

Oral glucose tolerance

Overview

○ The most sensitive method of evaluating borderline cases of diabetes mellitus
○ Involves monitoring of plasma and urine glucose levels for 3 hours after ingestion of a challenge dose of glucose to assess insulin secretion and the body's ability to metabolize glucose

Purpose

○ To confirm diabetes mellitus in selected patients
○ To aid in the diagnosis of hypoglycemia and malabsorption syndrome

Procedure

Preparation

○ Explain to the patient that the oral glucose tolerance test evaluates glucose metabolism.
○ Notify the laboratory and physician of drugs the patient is taking that may affect test results; it may be necessary to restrict them.
○ Instruct the patient to maintain a high-carbohydrate diet for 3 days and then to fast for 10 to 16 hours before the test.
○ Tell the patient not to smoke, drink coffee or alcohol, or exercise strenuously for 8 hours before or during the test.
○ Tell the patient that this test requires five blood samples and usually five urine samples.
○ The procedure usually takes 3 hours but can last as long as 6 hours.
○ Alert the patient to the symptoms of hypoglycemia (weakness, restlessness, nervousness, hunger, and sweating) and tell him to report such symptoms immediately.

Implementation

○ Between 7 a.m. and 9 a.m., perform a venipuncture to obtain a fasting blood sample in a 7-ml clot-activator tube.
○ A saline lock may be inserted and used to collect the multiple blood samples per facility protocol.
○ Collect a urine sample at the same time if your facility includes this as part of the test.
○ After collecting these samples, give the test load of oral glucose and record the time of ingestion. Encourage the patient to drink the entire glucose solution within 5 minutes.
○ Encourage the patient to drink water throughout the test to promote adequate urine excretion.
○ Draw blood samples 30 minutes, 1 hour, 2 hours, and 3 hours after giving the loading dose, using 7-ml clot-activator tubes.
○ Collect urine samples at the same intervals.

○ Send blood and urine samples to the laboratory immediately or refrigerate them.
○ Specify when the patient last ate and the blood and urine sample collection times.
○ Record the time the patient received his last pretest dose of insulin or oral antidiabetic drug.
○ Tell the patient to lie down if he feels faint.

Patient care

○ Apply direct pressure to the venipuncture site until bleeding stops.

Complications

○ Hematoma at a venipuncture site.

▷ *ALERT For severe hypoglycemia, notify the physician; draw a blood sample, record the time on the laboratory request, and stop the test (have the patient drink a glass of orange juice with sugar added or give I.V. glucose to reverse the reaction).*

Interpretation

Normal results

○ Plasma glucose levels peak at 160 to 180 mg/dl (SI, 8.8 to 9.9 mmol/L) within 30 minutes to 1 hour after the patient receives an oral glucose test dose; they return to fasting levels or lower within 2 to 3 hours.
○ Urine glucose tests negative throughout.

Abnormal results

○ Decreased glucose tolerance, in which levels peak sharply before falling slowly to fasting levels, may confirm diabetes mellitus or may result from Cushing's disease, hemochromatosis, pheochromocytoma, or central nervous system lesions.
○ Increased glucose tolerance, in which levels may peak at less than normal levels, may indicate insulinoma, malabsorption syndrome, adrenocortical insufficiency (Addison's disease), hypothyroidism, or hypopituitarism.

Interfering factors

○ Recent infection, fever, pregnancy, or acute illness such as myocardial infarction (possible increase)
○ Failure to observe pretest restrictions
○ Carbohydrate deprivation before the test (causing a diabetic response [abnormal increase with a delayed decrease] because the pancreas is unaccustomed to responding to a high-carbohydrate load)
○ Chlorthalidone, thiazide diuretics, furosemide, triamterene, hormonal contraceptives, benzodiazepines, phenytoin, phenothiazines, lithium, epinephrine, phenolphthalein, caffeine, arginine, dextrothyroxine, diazoxide, corticosteroids, large doses of nicotinic acid, and recent I.V. glucose infusions (possible increase)
○ Beta blockers, amphetamines, ethanol, clofibrate, insulin, oral antidiabetic drugs, and monoamine oxidase inhibitors (possible decrease)

Oral lactose tolerance

Overview

○ Measures plasma glucose levels after ingestion of a challenge dose of lactose.
○ Screens for lactose intolerance caused by lactase deficiency.
○ Absence or deficiency of lactase causes undigested lactose to remain in the intestinal lumen, producing such symptoms as abdominal cramps and watery diarrhea.
○ True congenital lactase deficiency is rare.
○ Usually, lactose intolerance develops because lactase levels generally decrease with age.

Purpose

○ To detect lactose intolerance

Procedure

Preparation

○ Explain to the patient that this test determines if his symptoms are caused by an inability to digest lactose.
○ Notify the laboratory and physician of drugs the patient is taking that may affect test results; it may be necessary to restrict them.
○ Instruct the patient to fast and to avoid strenuous activity for 8 hours before the test.
○ Inform the patient that this test requires four blood samples. Tell the patient who will be performing the venipunctures and when.
○ Explain to the patient that he may experience slight discomfort from the needle punctures and the tourniquet. Tell the patient that the entire procedure may take up to 2 hours.

Implementation

○ After the patient has fasted for 8 hours, perform a venipuncture and collect a blood sample in a 4-ml tube with sodium fluoride and potassium oxalate added.
○ Give the test load of lactose: for an adult, 50 g of lactose dissolved in 400 ml of water; for a child, 50 g/m² of body surface area. Record the time of ingestion.
○ Draw a blood sample 30, 60, and 120 minutes after giving the loading dose. Use a 4-ml tube with sodium fluoride and potassium oxalate added.
○ If ordered, collect a feces sample 5 hours after giving the loading dose.
○ Send blood and feces samples to the laboratory immediately or refrigerate them if transport is delayed.
○ Specify the collection time on the laboratory requests.
○ Watch for symptoms of lactose intolerance — abdominal cramps, nausea, bloating, flatulence, and watery diarrhea — caused by the loading dose.

Patient care

○ Apply direct pressure to the venipuncture site until bleeding stops.
○ Instruct the patient to resume his usual diet, medications, and activity stopped before the test.

Complications

○ Hematoma at a venipuncture site

Interpretation

Normal results

○ Plasma glucose levels rise over 20 mg/dl (SI, > 1.1 mmol/L) over fasting levels within 15 to 60 minutes after ingestion of the lactose loading dose.

Abnormal results

○ A rise in plasma glucose of less than 20 mg/dl (SI, < 1.1 mmol/L) indicates lactose intolerance, as does feces acidity (pH of 5.5 or less) and high glucose content (> 1+ on the dipstick).
○ Accompanying signs and symptoms provoked by the test also suggest, but don't confirm, the diagnosis because such symptoms may appear in the patient with normal lactase activity after a loading dose of lactose.
○ Small-bowel biopsy with lactase assay may be necessary to confirm the diagnosis.

Interfering factors

○ Failure to observe pretest restrictions
○ Thiazide diuretics, hormonal contraceptives, benzodiazepines, propranolol, and insulin (possible false-low)
○ Delayed emptying of stomach contents (possible decrease)
○ Glycolysis (possible false-negative)

Orbital computed tomography

Overview

○ Orbital computed tomography (CT) test shows abnormalities not readily seen on standard X-rays, delineating their size, position, and relationship to adjoining structures.
○ A series of tomograms reconstructed by a computer and displayed as anatomic slices on a monitor, the orbital CT scan identifies space-occupying lesions earlier and more accurately than other radiographic techniques and provides three-dimensional images of orbital structures, especially the ocular muscles and the optic nerve.

Purpose

○ To evaluate pathologies of the orbit and eye — especially expanding lesions and bone destruction
○ To evaluate fractures of the orbit and adjoining structures, showing a complete three-dimensional view
○ To determine the cause of unilateral exophthalmos

Procedure

Preparation

○ Describe the procedure to the patient and explain that the orbital CT scan shows the anatomy of the eye and its surrounding structures.
○ Make sure the patient or a responsible family member has signed an appropriate consent form, if required.
○ Check the patient's history for hypersensitivity reactions to iodine, shellfish, or contrast media, and notify the physician of the sensitivities.
○ Instruct the patient to remove jewelry, hairpins, or other metal objects in the X-ray field to allow for precise imaging of the orbital structures.
○ If the patient won't be receiving contrast enhancement, tell him he need not restrict food and fluids. If he'll be receiving contrast enhancement, withhold food and fluids from him for 4 hours before the test.
○ Tell the patient that a series of X-rays will be taken.
○ Tell the patient that he'll lie on an X-ray table and that the head of the table will be moved into the scanner, which will rotate around his head and make loud clacking sounds.
○ If the patient will receive a contrast medium, tell him that he may feel flushed and warm and may experience a transient headache, a salty or metallic taste, and nausea or vomiting after the injection.

Implementation

○ Assist the patient into a supine position on the X-ray table with his head immobilized by straps, if required. Ask him to lie still.
○ The head of the table is moved into the scanner, which rotates around the patient's head, taking X-rays.
○ Information from the scan is stored on magnetic tapes, and the images are displayed on a monitor. It's possible to make photographs if a permanent record is needed.
○ When this series of X-rays is complete, contrast enhancement is performed.
○ The contrast medium is injected intravenously, and a second series of scans is recorded.

Patient care

○ If the patient received a contrast medium, watch for its residual adverse effects, including headache, nausea, or vomiting.
○ Tell the patient that he may resume his usual diet.

Complications

○ Adverse reaction to the contrast medium

Interpretation

Normal results

○ Dense orbital bone provides a marked contrast to less dense periocular fat.
○ The optic nerve and the medial and lateral rectus muscles are clearly defined.
○ The rectus muscles appear as thin dense bands on each side, behind the eye.
○ The optic canals appear equal in size.

Abnormal results

○ Intraorbital and extraorbital space-occupying lesions that obscure the normal structures or cause orbital enlargement, indentation of the orbital walls, or bone destruction.
○ Infiltrative lesions, such as lymphomas and metastatic carcinomas, appear as irregular areas of density.
○ Encapsulated tumors, such as benign hemangiomas and meningiomas, appear as clearly defined masses of consistent density.
○ Intracranial tumors may invade the orbit; thickening of the optic nerve may occur with gliomas, meningiomas, and secondary tumors that may cause enlargement of the optic canal.
○ Early erosion or expansion of the medial orbital wall may arise from lesions in the ethmoidal cells (determines the cause of unilateral exophthalmos).
○ Space-occupying lesions appear in the orbit or paranasal sinuses (causes exophthalmos).
○ Thickening of the medial and lateral rectus muscles in proptosis (resulting from Graves' disease).
○ Contrast medium may provide information about the circulation through abnormal ocular tissues.

Interfering factors

○ Head movement
○ Failure to remove metallic objects from the examination field

Orbital radiography

Overview

○ Involves X-rays of the orbital structures, eyebrow, bridge of the nose, and cheekbone.
○ Tomograms may be taken with standard X-rays.

Purpose

○ To identify orbital fractures and pathology
○ To locate intraorbital or intraocular foreign bodies and changes to the structure of the eye, which may indicate various diseases
○ To detect problems resulting from injury and trauma to the eye

Procedure

Preparation

○ Make sure the patient has signed an appropriate consent form.
○ Note and report all allergies.
○ Screen women for pregnancy.
○ Have the patient remove any jewelry or metal objects that may interfere with a clear image.
○ Advise the patient that positioning may cause some discomfort.
○ Explain that the test takes about 15 minutes.

Implementation

○ Assist the patient into a supine position on the radiographic table, or seat him in a chair.
○ If the patient is in severe pain from injury or trauma, give him an analgesic.
○ A series of orbital X-rays is taken, including projections of the optical canal.
○ Images of the unaffected eye may also be taken to compare its shapes and structures to those of the affected eye.
○ Films are developed and checked for quality.

Patient care

○ Monitor the patient's response to the test.

Complications

None known

Interpretation

Normal results

○ Each orbit is composed of a roof, floor, and medial and lateral walls.
○ The medial walls of both orbits are parallel to each other.
○ The lateral walls of both orbits project toward each other.

○ The superior orbital fissure lies in the back of the orbit, between the lateral wall and the roof.

Abnormal results

○ Enlargement of an orbit suggests the presence of a lesion.
○ Superior orbital fissure enlargement suggests possible orbital meningioma, intracranial conditions (such as pituitary tumors), or vascular anomalies.
○ Optic canal enlargement suggests possible extraocular extension of a retinoblastoma, or indicates irritation from an injury or foreign body.
○ Destruction of the orbital walls suggests possible malignant neoplasm or infection.

✷ *AGE AWARE A child's orbit is more likely to be enlarged by a fast-growing lesion because the orbital bones aren't fully developed.*

○ Clear-cut local indentations of the orbital wall suggest a benign tumor or cyst.
○ Increased bone density suggests possible conditions, such as osteoblastic metastasis, sphenoid ridge meningioma, or Paget's disease.

Interfering factors

None known

Osmotic fragility

Overview

- Measures red blood cell (RBC) resistance to hemolysis when exposed to a series of increasingly dilute saline solutions.
- The sooner hemolysis occurs, the greater the osmotic fragility of the cells.
- Osmotic fragility is based on *osmosis* — movement of water across a membrane from a less-concentrated liquid, in a natural tendency to correct the imbalance.
- RBCs suspended in an isotonic saline solution — one with the same salt concentration (osmotic pressure) as normal plasma (0.85 g/dl) — keep their shape.
- If RBCs are added to a less-concentrated (hypotonic) solution, they take up water until they burst; if placed in a hypertonic solution, they shrink.
- Degree of hypotonicity needed to produce hemolysis varies inversely with the RBC's osmotic fragility; the closer the saline tonicity is to normal physiologic values when hemolysis occurs, the more fragile the cells.
- In some cases, RBCs don't hemolyze immediately, and their incubation in solution for 24 hours improves test sensitivity.
- Osmotic fragility offers quantitative confirmation of RBC morphology and should supplement the stained cell examination.

Purpose

- To aid in the diagnosis of hereditary spherocytosis
- To confirm morphologic RBC abnormalities

Procedure

Preparation

- Explain to the patient that the osmotic fragility test identifies the cause of anemia.
- Inform the patient that he need not restrict food and fluids.
- Tell the patient that the test requires a blood sample. Explain who will perform the venipuncture and when.
- Explain to the patient that he may feel slight discomfort from the needle puncture and the tourniquet.

Implementation

- Perform a venipuncture, collecting the sample in a 4.5-ml heparinized tube.
- Completely fill the collection tube and invert it gently several times to mix the sample and the anticoagulant thoroughly.
- Handle the sample gently to prevent accidental hemolysis.

Patient care

- Apply direct pressure to the venipuncture site until bleeding stops.

Complications

- Hematoma at the venipuncture site

Interpretation

Normal results

- Osmotic fragility values (percentage of RBCs hemolyzed) that have been obtained photometrically are plotted against decreasing saline tonicity to produce an S-shaped curve with a slope characteristic of the disorder. Reference values differ with tonicities.

Abnormal results

- Low osmotic fragility (increased resistance to hemolysis) is characteristic of thalassemia, iron deficiency anemia, sickle cell anemia, and other RBC disorders in which target cells are found.
- Low osmotic fragility also occurs after splenectomy.
- High osmotic fragility (increased tendency to hemolyze) occurs in hereditary spherocytosis; and in spherocytosis associated with autoimmune hemolytic anemia, severe burns, or chemical poisoning.
- High osmatic fragility may also be found in hemolytic disease of the neonate (erythroblastosis fetalis).

Interfering factors

- Failure to use the proper anticoagulant in the collection tube, to fill the tube completely, or to adequately mix the sample and the anticoagulant
- Hemolysis from rough handling of the sample
- Presence of hemolytic organisms in the sample
- Conditions, such as severe anemia, that provide fewer RBCs for testing
- Recent blood transfusion

Otoacoustic emissions

Overview

○ Rapid screening method to assess the function of outer hair cells of the cochlea; shows abnormalities that may precede hearing loss
○ Screens for cochlear hearing loss because outer hair cells are usually lost before inner cells are damaged
○ Shows absent emissions when hearing loss is more than slight to mild
○ Shows subtle changes in otoacoustic emissions in those with normal hearing who are carriers of recessive hearing loss genes
○ Provides a cost-effective method of neonatal screening because patient need not participate
○ Measures outer hair cell function, assists in patient triage during diagnostic testing, and provides a rapid indication of whether the outer hair cells are intact
○ Helps detect nonorganic hearing loss (hearing loss that develops after birth, such as from maternal cytomegalovirus infection, and some genetic hearing losses may not be identified)
○ May not detect slight (minimal) hearing loss

Purpose

○ To screen and assess the health of the outer hair cells of the cochlea
○ To screen the hearing of neonates

Procedure

Preparation

○ Remove significant cerumen accumulation from the patient's ear canals.
○ Inform the patient that the test requires about 1 minute per ear, or slightly longer if findings aren't immediately found to be normal.

Implementation

○ In screening, the technician places the probe in the patient's ear after having cleared it of debris, such as vernix, which is present in the neonate's ear.
○ The audiologist adjusts signal levels and, in the case of distortion-product otoacoustic emissions, the frequency characteristics.
○ The emission level is monitored and compared with the background noise level.

Patient care

○ Answer the patient's questions about the test.

Complications

None known

Interpretation

Normal results

○ 500 to 6,000 Hz, with signal-to-noise ratios of at least 5 dB.
○ Emissions sufficiently higher than the background physiologic and ambient noise levels.
○ Results are frequency specific.

Abnormal results

○ An absence of otoacoustic emissions at any test frequency suggests outer hair cell dysfunction and hearing loss of at least 25 dB hearing loss.
○ The presence of otoacoustic emissions at traditional screening levels indicates no more than a slight cochlear hearing disorder.
○ A reduction in size or elimination of the otoacoustic emission can occur because of significant conductive hearing loss.

Interfering factors

○ Screening by inexperienced technicians in the technique, possibly leading to high false-positive rates. Retesting is usually routinely done in screening programs.
○ Significant conductive hearing loss, which can cause a patient to fail the screening test or receive a referral. Although this means that some children with transient conductive loss won't pass the screening otoacoustic emissions test, it reveals most congenital conductive losses.
○ Presence of cerumen obstruction.
○ Auditory dyssynchrony, sometimes called *auditory neuropathy*, such as from hyperbilirubinemia or kernicterus, undetected with this procedure: If outer hair cells function, but the disorder is such that a neural signal isn't transmitted to the brain, otoacoustic emissions will be normal and the hearing deficit won't be discovered.

Otoscopy

Overview

- Shows the external auditory canal and tympanic membrane by use of an otoscope
- Indirectly provides information about the eustachian tube and middle ear cavity

Purpose

- To detect foreign bodies, cerumen, or stenosis in the external canal
- To detect external or middle ear pathology (infection or perforation)
- To evaluate integrity and appearance of the tympanic membrane

Procedure

Preparation

- Make sure the patient has signed a consent form.
- Warn the patient that with pneumatic otoscopy, he may experience dizziness with nystagmus.
- Explain that the test lasts less than 5 minutes.

Implementation

- The patient's head is tilted slightly away from the examiner with the ear to be examined pointed up.
- The auricle is pulled up, back, and away from the head to straighten an adult's ear canal; to straighten a child's canal, the auricle is pulled down.
- The largest speculum that will comfortably fit is selected.
- If the patient has ear pain, the unaffected ear is assessed first; then the affected ear is assessed.
- The otoscope is gently inserted into the ear canal with a downward and forward motion.
- The tympanic membrane is located and examined.
- The malleus is located; it should be partially visible through the translucent tympanic membrane.
- The tympanic membrane and surrounding fibrous rim (annulus) are examined.

Patient care

- Answer the patient's questions about the test.

Complications

- Perforation of the tympanic membrane

Interpretation

Normal results

- The tympanic membrane is thin, translucent, shiny, and slightly concave. It appears pearl gray or pale pink, and reflects light in its inferior portion (cone of light) with clearly defined landmarks.
- The short process of the malleus, manubrium, and umbo are visible but not prominent.
- Blood vessels should be visible only in the periphery.

Abnormal results

- Scarring, discoloration, retraction, or bulging of the tympanic membrane as well as the presence of drainage and scaly surface areas suggests pathology.
- Movement of the tympanic membrane in tandem with respiration suggests abnormal patency of the eustachian tube.
- A dry, flaky auditory canal lining may suggest eczema.
- An inflamed, swollen, and narrowed auditory canal, possibly with discharge, suggests otitis externa. (See *Common abnormalities of the tympanic membrane.*)

Interfering factors

- Obstruction of the ear canal by cerumen or foreign matter obscures the tympanic membrane.

Common abnormalities of the tympanic membrane

Visual examination of the tympanic membrane may reveal abnormal findings. This table lists some of the more common findings and their typical causes.

Abnormal findings	Usual cause
Bright red color	Inflammation (otitis media)
Yellowish color	Pus or serum behind the tympanic membrane (acute or chronic otitis media)
Bubble behind the tympanic membrane	Serous fluid in the middle ear (serous otitis media)
Absent light reflection	Bulging tympanic membrane (acute otitis media)
Absent or diminishing landmarks	Thickened tympanic membrane (chronic otitis media, otitis externa, or tympanosclerosis)
Oval-dark areas	Perforated or scarred tympanic membrane (otitis media or trauma)
Prominent malleus	Retracted tympanic membrane (nonfunctional eustachian tube)
Reduced mobility	Stiffened middle ear system (serous otitis media or, less commonly, middle ear adhesions)

Papanicolaou test

Overview

○ Widely used for early detection of cervical cancer
○ Permits cytologic evaluation of the vaginal pool, prostatic secretions, urine, gastric secretions, cavity fluids, bronchial aspirates, sputum, and solid tumor cells obtained by fine-needle aspiration
○ Also known as a *Pap test* or *ThinPrep Pap test* (new variation)

Purpose

○ To detect malignant cells
○ To detect inflammatory changes in tissue
○ To assess response to chemotherapy and radiation therapy
○ To detect viral, fungal, and, occasionally, parasitic invasion

Procedure

Preparation

○ Make sure the patient has signed an appropriate consent form.
○ Note and report all allergies.
○ Schedule the study for the middle of the menstrual cycle.
○ Advise the patient that she may experience slight discomfort from the speculum.
○ Explain the need to avoid activities that can wash away cellular deposits and change vaginal pH, including sexual intercourse for 24 hours, douching for 48 hours, and using vaginal creams or medications for 1 week.
○ Explain that the test takes 5 to 10 minutes.

Implementation

○ The patient is assisted into the lithotomy position with her feet in stirrups.
○ An unlubricated speculum is inserted into the vagina.
○ The cervix is located.
○ Secretions from the cervix and material from the endocervical canal are collected with an endocervical brush and a wooden spatula.
○ Specimens are spread on slides and immediately immersed in a fixative or sprayed with a fixative.
○ Specimens are appropriately labeled with date of last menses, collection site, and method.
○ If vaginal or vulval lesions are present, scrapings taken directly from the lesion are preferred.
○ The slides are preserved immediately.

Patient care

○ If patient bleeds, give her a sanitary napkin.
○ Schedule a return appointment for the patient's next Pap test.

Complications

○ Bleeding

Interpretation

Normal results

○ No malignant cells or abnormalities are present.

Abnormal results

○ Cells with relatively large nuclei, only small amounts of cytoplasm, abnormal nuclear chromatin patterns, and marked variation in size, shape, and staining properties, with prominent nucleoli, suggest malignancy.
○ Atypical but nonmalignant cells suggest a benign abnormality.
○ Atypical cells may suggest dysplasia.

Interfering factors

○ Douching within 24 hours of testing
○ Excessive use of lubricating jelly on the slide
○ Collection of specimen during menstruation
○ Delay in fixing the specimen
○ Consistency of specimen too thin or too thick

Paracentesis

Overview

- Obtains samples of ascitic fluid for diagnostic and therapeutic purposes by insertion of a trocar and cannula through the abdominal wall
- May be performed using image-guidance
- In four-quadrant tap, aspirates fluid from each quadrant of the abdomen to verify abdominal trauma and the need for surgery
- In peritoneal fluid analysis, assesses gross appearance, red blood cell (RBC) and white blood cell (WBC) counts, cytologic studies, microbiological studies for bacteria and fungi, and determinations of protein, glucose, amylase, ammonia, and alkaline phosphatase levels

Purpose

- To determine the cause of ascites
- To detect abdominal trauma
- To remove accumulated ascitic fluid

Procedure

Preparation

- Make sure the patient has signed an appropriate consent form.
- Note and report all allergies.
- Tell the patient that he need not restrict food or fluids before the test.
- Inform the patient that he'll receive a local anesthetic.
- If the patient has severe ascites, inform him that the procedure will relieve his discomfort and allow him to breathe easier.
- Explain that a blood sample may be taken for analysis.
- Explain that the test takes 45 to 60 minutes.

Implementation

- Obtain baseline vital signs, weight, and abdominal girth measurement.
- Assist the patient onto a bed or chair.
- If the patient can't tolerate being out of bed, assist him into high Fowler's position.
- Prepare and drape the puncture site.
- Local anesthetic is injected.
- The needle or trocar and cannula are inserted, usually 1″ to 2″ (2.5 to 5 cm) below the umbilicus, or in each quadrant of the abdomen.
- Fluid samples are aspirated.
- Specimens are placed in appropriately labeled containers.
- The trocar or needle is removed and a dressing applied.

Patient care

- Instruct the patient to resume his previous activity.
- Give I.V. infusions and albumin.
- Monitor vital signs and intake and output.
- Observe the puncture site and drainage for bleeding and infection.
- Obtain the patient's daily weight and daily abdominal girth measurement.
- Observe the patient for hematuria, which may indicate bladder trauma.
- Monitor serum electrolyte (especially sodium) and protein levels.
- If a large amount of fluid was removed, watch for signs of vascular collapse (tachycardia, tachypnea, hypotension, dizziness, and mental status changes).
- Watch for signs and symptoms of hemorrhage and shock and for increasing pain and abdominal tenderness. These may indicate a perforated intestine or, depending on the site of the tap, puncture of the inferior epigastric artery, hematoma of the anterior cecal wall, or rupture of the iliac vein or bladder.
- Observe the patient with severe hepatic disease for signs of hepatic coma, which may result from loss of sodium and potassium accompanying hypovolemia. Watch for mental status changes, drowsiness, and stupor. Such a patient is also prone to uremia, infection, hemorrhage, and protein depletion.

Complications

- Bleeding, hemorrhage
- Infection
- Bladder trauma
- Shock
- Perforated intestine
- Inferior epigastric artery puncture
- Anterior cecal wall hematoma
- Iliac vein rupture

Interpretation

Normal results

- Fluid is odorless, clear to pale yellow.

Abnormal results

- Milk-colored fluid may indicate chylous ascites.
- Bloody fluid may indicate benign or malignant tumor, hemorrhagic pancreatitis, or perforated intestine or duodenal ulcer.
- Cloudy or turbid fluid may indicate peritonitis or an infectious process.
- RBC count greater than 100/µl suggests possible neoplasm or tuberculosis.
- RBC count greater than 100,000/µl suggests intra-abdominal trauma.
- WBC count greater than 300/µl, with more than 25% neutrophils, suggests spontaneous bacterial peritonitis or cirrhosis.

- A high percentage of lymphocytes suggests tuberculous peritonitis or chylous ascites.
- A protein ascitic fluid–serum ratio of 0.5 or greater, a lactate dehydrogenase (LD) ascitic fluid–serum ratio greater than 0.6, and an LD ascitic fluid level greater than 400 µ/ml suggest malignant, tuberculous, or pancreatic ascites.
- Albumin gradient between ascitic fluid and serum greater than 1 g/dl indicates chronic hepatic disease.
- Gram-positive cocci commonly indicate primary peritonitis; gram-negative organisms indicate secondary peritonitis.
- Fungi may indicate histoplasmosis, candidiasis, or coccidioidomycosis.

Interfering factors
- Contamination of the specimen or improper collection technique

Paranasal sinus radiography

Overview

○ Film image differentiates sinus structures.
○ Formed by X-rays or electromagnetic waves that penetrate the paranasal sinuses.
○ Air normally fills the paranasal sinuses and appears black on film.
○ Fluid appears as a cloudy or opaque density.

Purpose

○ To detect and monitor unilateral or bilateral abnormalities
○ To confirm diagnosis of neoplastic or inflammatory paranasal sinus disease
○ To determine the location and size of an abnormality such as a tumor

Procedure

Preparation

○ Make sure the patient has signed an appropriate consent form.
○ Note and report all allergies.
○ Explain the need to remove dentures, jewelry, and any metal objects in the X-ray field.
○ Explain to the patient the need for possible immobilization of his head in a foam vise to help maintain correct position. Provide reassurance that this won't hurt.
○ Explain that the test usually takes 10 to 15 minutes.

Implementation

○ The patient sits upright between the X-ray tube and a film cassette.
○ A lead-lined apron should be placed to protect the gonads.
○ To avoid radiation exposure, leave the immediate area during the test or wear a lead-lined apron.
○ The X-ray tube is positioned at specific angles, and the patient's head is placed in various standard positions.
○ The paranasal sinuses are filmed from different angles.

Patient care

○ Answer the patient's questions about the test.

Complications

○ None known

Interpretation

Normal results

○ The radiolucent paranasal sinuses are filled with air.

Abnormal results

○ Linear, radiolucent defects may suggest bone fractures.
○ Soft-tissue masses projecting into the sinus may suggest cysts, polyps, and tumors.

Interfering factors

○ If surrounding facial structures interfere with visualization of relevant areas, computed tomography scans may be indicated for further evaluation and diagnosis.

Parathyroid hormone

Overview

- Evaluates parathyroid function
- Parathyroid hormone (PTH), also known as *parathormone,* regulates calcium and phosphorus levels
- Measures serum calcium, phosphorus, and creatinine levels with serum PTH to understand the causes and effects of pathologic parathyroid function
- PTH release is regulated by a negative feedback mechanism involving calcium level
- Normal or elevated circulating calcium (especially ionized) level inhibits PTH release; decreased level stimulates PTH release
- Circulating PTH exists in three molecular forms: the intact PTH molecule, which originates in the parathyroid glands, and two smaller circulating forms, N-terminal fragments and C-terminal fragments

Purpose

- To aid in the differential diagnosis of hyperparathyroidism and hypoparathyroidism
- C-terminal PTH assay: to diagnose chronic disturbances in PTH metabolism, such as secondary and tertiary hyperparathyroidism; to differentiate ectopic from primary hyperparathyroidism
- Intact PTH and the N-terminal fragment assays: to reflect acute changes in PTH metabolism and monitor a patient's response to PTH therapy

Procedure

Preparation

- Explain to the patient that this test helps evaluate parathyroid function.
- Instruct the patient to observe an overnight fast because food may affect PTH levels and interfere with results.
- Tell the patient that the test requires a blood sample. Explain who will perform the venipuncture and when.
- Explain to the patient that he may experience slight discomfort from the tourniquet and the needle puncture.

Implementation

- Perform a venipuncture and collect 3 ml of blood into two separate 7-ml clot-activator tubes.
- Handle the sample gently to prevent hemolysis.
- Send the sample to the laboratory immediately so the serum can be separated and frozen for assay.

Patient care

- Apply direct pressure to the venipuncture site until bleeding stops.
- Instruct the patient that he may resume his usual diet.

Complications

- Hematoma at the venipuncture site

Interpretation

Normal results

- Levels vary, depending on the laboratory; they must be interpreted depending on calcium levels.
- Intact PTH levels are 10 to 50 pg/ml (SI, 1.1 to 5.3 pmol/L).
- N-terminal fraction is 8 to 24 pg/ml (SI, 0.8 to 2.5 pmol/L).
- C-terminal fraction is 0 to 340 pg/ml (SI, 0 to 35.8 pmol/L).

Abnormal results

- Measured along with serum calcium levels, abnormally elevated PTH values may indicate primary, secondary, or tertiary hyperparathyroidism.
- Abnormally low PTH levels may result from hypoparathyroidism and from certain malignant diseases.

Interfering factors

- Failure to fast overnight before the test
- Hemolysis from rough handling of the sample

Partial thromboplastin time

Overview

○ Used to evaluate all the clotting factors of the intrinsic pathway — except platelets — by measuring the time required for formation of a fibrin clot after the addition of calcium and phospholipid emulsion to a plasma sample
○ Used with an activator, such as kaolin, to shorten clotting time

Purpose

○ To screen for deficiencies of the clotting factors in the intrinsic pathways
○ To monitor response to heparin therapy

Procedure

Preparation

○ Explain to the patient that the partial thromboplastin time (PTT) test determines whether blood clots normally.
○ Inform the patient that he need not restrict food and fluids.
○ Tell the patient that the test requires a blood sample. Explain who will perform the venipuncture and when.
○ Explain to the patient that he may feel slight discomfort from the tourniquet and the needle puncture.
○ When appropriate, tell the patient receiving heparin therapy that this test may be repeated at regular intervals to assess his response to treatment.

Implementation

○ Perform a venipuncture and collect the sample in a 7-ml tube with sodium citrate added.
○ Completely fill the collection tube, invert it gently several times, and send it to the laboratory on ice.
○ To prevent hemolysis, avoid excessive probing at the venipuncture site and handle the sample gently.

Patient care

○ Apply direct pressure to the venipuncture site until bleeding stops.
○ Make sure that subdermal bleeding has stopped before removing pressure.
○ For a patient on anticoagulant therapy, it may be necessary to use additional pressure at the venipuncture site to control bleeding.
○ If a large hematoma develops at the venipuncture site, monitor pulses distal to the site.

Complications

○ Hematoma at the venipuncture site

Interpretation

Normal results

○ A fibrin clot forms 21 to 35 seconds (SI, 21 to 35 s) after adding reagents.
○ For a patient receiving an anticoagulant, ask the physician to specify the reference values for the therapy being delivered.

Abnormal results

○ A prolonged PTT may indicate a deficiency of certain plasma clotting factors, the presence of heparin, or the presence of fibrin split products, fibrinolysins, or circulating anticoagulants that are antibodies to specific clotting factors.

Interfering factors

○ Failure to fill the collection tube completely, to use the proper anticoagulant, or to adequately mix the sample and the anticoagulant
○ Hemolysis from rough handling of the sample or from excessive probing at the venipuncture site
○ Failure to send the sample to the laboratory immediately or to place it on ice

Parvovirus B-19 antibodies

Overview

○ Parvovirus B-19, a small, single-stranded deoxyribonucleic acid virus belonging to the family *Parvoviridae,* destroys red blood cell (RBC) precursors and interferes with normal RBC production.
○ Linked to erythema infectiosum (a self-limiting, low-grade fever and rash in young children) and aplastic crisis (in patients with chronic hemolytic anemia and immunodeficient patients with bone marrow failure).
○ Immunoglobulin (Ig) G and IgM antibodies are detectable with enzyme-linked immunosorbent assay and immunofluorescence.

Purpose

○ To detect parvovirus B-19 antibody, especially in prospective organ donors
○ To diagnose erythema infectiosum, parvovirus B-19, aplastic crisis, and related parvovirus B-19 diseases

Procedure

Preparation

○ Explain the test purpose and procedure to the patient.
○ To a potential organ donor, explain that the test is part of a panel of tests that occur before organ donation to protect the organ recipient from potential infection.
○ Tell the patient that the test requires a blood sample.
○ Explain to the patient that he may experience slight discomfort from the tourniquet and the needle puncture.

Implementation

○ Perform a venipuncture, collect the blood sample in a 5-ml clot-activator tube, and store it on ice.
○ Handle the sample gently to prevent hemolysis.

Patient care

○ Apply direct pressure to the venipuncture site until bleeding stops.

Complications

○ Hematoma at the venipuncture site

Interpretation

Normal results

○ Test is negative for IgG- and IgM-specific antibodies to parvovirus B-19.

Abnormal results

○ About 50% of all adults lack immunity to parvovirus B-19; up to 20% of susceptible adults become infected after exposure.
○ Positive results for IgG and IgM-specific antibodies to parvovirus B-19 are linked to joint arthralgia, hydrops fetalis, fetal loss, transient aplastic anemia, chronic anemia in immunocompromised patients, and bone marrow failure.
○ A positive result for parvovirus B-19 should be confirmed using the Western blot test.

Interfering factors

○ Failure to put the sample on ice
○ Hemolysis from rough handling of the sample

Percutaneous renal biopsy

Overview

○ Needle excision of a core of kidney tissue for histologic examination
○ May help assess histologic changes caused by acute or chronic glomerulonephritis, pyelonephritis, renal vein thrombosis, amyloid infiltration, and systemic lupus erythematosus
○ Can differentiate a primary renal cancer from a metastatic lesion in patients with a mass

Purpose

○ To aid in the diagnosis of renal parenchymal disease
○ To monitor the progression of renal disease and assess the effectiveness of therapy

Procedure

Preparation

○ Explain that this test diagnoses kidney disorders.
○ Instruct the patient to restrict food and fluids for 8 hours before the test.
○ Make sure that blood samples and urine specimens are collected and tested before the biopsy and that results of other tests are available.
○ Check the patient's history for hemorrhagic tendencies and hypersensitivity to the local anesthetic.
○ Give a mild sedative 30 minutes to 1 hour before the biopsy to help the patient relax.
○ Inform the patient that he may experience a pinching sensation when the needle is inserted through his back into the kidney.
○ Check the patient's vital signs, and tell him to void just before the test.

Implementation

○ Assist the patient into a prone position on a firm surface with a sandbag beneath his abdomen.
○ Tell him to take a deep breath while his kidney is being palpated.
○ A 7″, 20G needle is used to inject the local anesthetic into the skin at the biopsy site.
○ Instruct the patient to hold his breath and remain still as the needle is inserted.
○ After the needle is inserted, tell the patient to take several deep breaths. If the needle swings smoothly during deep breathing, it has penetrated the kidney capsule.
○ After the penetration depth is marked on the needle shaft, instruct the patient to hold his breath and remain as still as possible while the needle is withdrawn.
○ After a small incision is made in the anesthetized skin, instruct the patient to hold his breath and re-

main still while the Vim-Silverman needle with stylet is inserted to the measured depth.
○ Tell the patient to breathe deeply. Then tell him to remain still while the tissue specimen is obtained.
○ The tissue is examined immediately under a hand lens to ensure that the specimen contains tissue from the cortex and medulla.
○ Next it's placed on a saline-soaked gauze pad and placed in a properly labeled container.
○ If an adequate tissue specimen hasn't been obtained, the procedure is repeated immediately.

Patient care

○ After an adequate specimen is secured, apply pressure to the biopsy site for 3 to 5 minutes to stop superficial bleeding, then apply a pressure dressing.
○ Instruct the patient to lie flat on his back without moving for at least 12 hours to prevent bleeding. Check his vital signs every 15 minutes for 4 hours, every 30 minutes for the next 4 hours, every hour for the next 4 hours, and finally, every 4 hours. Report any changes.
○ Examine the patient's urine for blood; small amounts may be present after the biopsy but should disappear within 8 hours.
○ Hematocrit may be monitored after the procedure.
○ Encourage the patient to drink fluids.
○ Discourage the patient from engaging in strenuous activities for several days after the procedure.

Complications

○ Bleeding or infection

Interpretation

Normal results

○ Bowman's capsule in a section of kidney (the area between two layers of flat epithelial cells) the glomerular tuft, and the capillary lumen.
○ One layer of epithelial cells with microvilli (the proximal tubule) that form a brush border.
○ Flat, squamous epithelial cells in the descending loop of Henle.
○ The ascending loop is distally convoluted, with collecting tubules lined with squamous epithelial cells.

Abnormal results

○ Cancer or renal disease
○ Malignant tumors (including Wilms' tumor and renal cell carcinoma)
○ Disseminated lupus erythematosus, amyloid infiltration, acute or chronic glomerulonephritis, renal vein thrombosis, and pyelonephritis

Interfering factors

○ Failure to obtain an adequate tissue specimen
○ Failure to store the specimen properly
○ Failure to send the specimen to the laboratory immediately

Percutaneous transhepatic cholangiography

Overview

- Fluoroscopic examination of the biliary ducts after injection of an iodinated contrast medium directly into a biliary radicle
- Used in patients with previous GI surgery and endoscopically inaccessible bilioenteric anastomosis to perform a contrast study of the biliary ducts
- May be performed for unsuccessful endoscopic cholangiopancreatography
- Also called *PTHC*

Purpose

- To evaluate upper abdominal pain after cholecystectomy
- To evaluate patients with severe jaundice
- To distinguish between obstructive and nonobstructive jaundice
- To determine location, extent, and, in many cases, cause of mechanical obstruction

Procedure

Preparation

- Make sure the patient has signed a consent form.
- Note and report all allergies.
- Check the patient's history for abnormal coagulation study results.
- Check the patient's history for hypersensitivity to iodine, seafood, the local anesthetic, and iodinated contrast media.
- Instruct the patient to fast for 8 hours before the test.
- Explain the possible need for a laxative the night before and a cleansing enema the morning of the test.
- Tell the patient that he'll receive a local anesthetic and I.V. sedation.
- Inform the patient that he may feel transient pain as the liver capsule is entered.
- Warn the patient that injection of the contrast medium may cause a sensation of pressure and epigastric fullness.
- Explain that the test takes about 1 to 2 hours.

Implementation

- The patient is given preprocedure antibiotics.
- The patient is given a sedative and analgesic.
- The patient is placed in the supine position on the table.
- The right upper quadrant of the abdomen is draped.
- The skin, subcutaneous tissue, and liver capsule are infiltrated with local anesthetic.

- A flexible needle is inserted under fluoroscopic guidance through the 10th or 11th intercostal space at the right midclavicular line.
- A contrast medium is injected.
- Spot films of significant findings are taken in various views.
- A drainage tube may be inserted to allow percutaneous drainage of bile, if dilated ducts are caused by obstruction.
- An internal stent may be inserted to allow bile drainage into the bowel, when the dilation and inflammation have diminished.

Patient care

- Enforce bed rest.
- Instruct the patient to resume his usual diet.
- Monitor vital signs and intake and output.
- Check the access site for bleeding, swelling, and tenderness.
- Watch for signs and symptoms of peritonitis: chills, temperature between 102° and 103° F (38.9° to 39.4° C), and abdominal pain, tenderness, and distention.

Complications

- Adverse effects of iodinated contrast media
- Adverse effects of sedation
- Pneumothorax
- Vasovagal reactions
- Peritonitis
- Bleeding
- Infection or sepsis
- Bile leakage

Interpretation

Normal results

- Biliary ducts are of normal diameter and appear as regular channels homogeneously filled with the contrast medium.

Abnormal results

- Dilated biliary ducts may suggest cholelithiasis, biliary tract cancer, cancer of the pancreas, or cancer of the ampulla of Vater.
- Persistent filling defects may suggest calculi.
- A short and irregular stricture with a rat-tail appearance and gross dilation of the proximal ducts may suggest pancreatic or biliary carcinoma.
- Diffuse intrahepatic and extrahepatic stricture may suggest advanced sclerosing cholangitis or infiltrating cholangiocarcinoma.
- Ducts filled with debris, with possible abscesses of various sizes in communication with the ducts, may suggest acute supportive cholangitis.

Interfering factors

None known

Pericardial fluid analysis

Overview

○ Analyzes pericardial fluid for the patient with pericardial effusion (an accumulation of excess pericardial fluid), which may result from inflammation (as in pericarditis), rupture, or penetrating trauma.
○ If possible, echocardiography should determine the effusion site before pericardiocentesis to minimize the risk of complications.

Purpose

○ To help identify the cause of pericardial effusion and to help determine appropriate therapy

Procedure

Preparation

○ Check the patient's history for current antimicrobial usage and record such usage on the test request form.
○ Tell the patient he need not restrict food and fluids.
○ Tell the patient that an I.V. line will be started at a slow rate in case he needs to receive medications.

○ Inform the patient that he'll receive a local anesthetic before the aspiration needle is inserted.
○ Warn him that although fluid aspiration isn't painful, he may experience pressure upon needle insertion into the pericardial sac.
○ Advise him that he may be asked to hold his breath briefly to aid needle insertion and placement.
○ Explain the test to the family if pericardiocentesis is performed to relieve cardiac tamponade and the patient is in shock.

Implementation

○ Assist the patient into a supine position with the thorax elevated 60 degrees.
○ When the patient is comfortable and well supported, instruct him to remain still during the procedure.
○ A local anesthetic is given at the insertion site after the skin is prepared with alcohol or povidone-iodine solution from the left costal margin to the xiphoid process.
○ With the three-way stopcock open, a 50-ml syringe is aseptically attached to one end and the cardiac needle to the other end.
○ The electrocardiogram (ECG) lead wire is attached to the needle hub with an alligator clip. The ECG is set to lead V and turned on (or the patient is connected to a bedside monitor). (See *Aspirating pericardial fluid.*)

Aspirating pericardial fluid

In pericardiocentesis, a needle and syringe assembly is inserted through the chest wall into the pericardial sac, as illustrated here. Electrocardiographic (ECG) monitoring with a leadwire attached to the needle and electrodes placed on the limbs (right arm [RA], right leg [RL], left arm [LA], and left leg [LL]) helps to ensure proper needle placement and to avoid damage to the heart

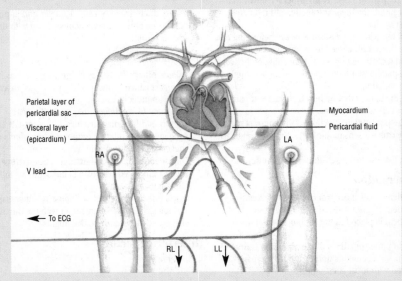

- The needle is inserted through the chest wall into the pericardial sac, maintaining gentle aspiration until fluid appears in the syringe.
- The needle is angled 35 to 45 degrees toward the tip of the right scapula between the left costal margin and the xiphoid process. A Kelly clamp is attached at the skin surface after the needle is properly positioned so it won't advance further.
- While the fluid is being aspirated, label and number the specimen tubes.
- Watch for grossly bloody aspirate — a sign of inadvertent puncture of a cardiac chamber.
- Be sure to use specimen tubes with the proper additives.
- If the patient will receive bacterial culture and sensitivity tests, record antimicrobial therapy the patient is receiving on the laboratory request.
- If anaerobic organisms are suspected, consult the laboratory concerning the proper collection technique to avoid exposing the aspirate to air.

Patient care

- When the needle is withdrawn, apply pressure *immediately* with sterile gauze pads for 3 to 5 minutes. Then apply a bandage.
- Check blood pressure readings, pulse, respiration, and heart sounds every 15 minutes until stable, every 1½ hours for 2 hours, every hour for 4 hours, and then every 4 hours thereafter.

▽ *ALERT Watch for signs of cardiac tamponade: muffled and distant heart sounds, distended neck veins, paradoxical pulse, and shock.*

Complications

- Inadvertent puncture of a cardiac chamber

Interpretation

Normal results

- 10 to 50 ml of sterile fluid in the pericardium.
- Pericardial fluid is clear or straw-colored, without evidence of pathogens, blood, or malignant cells.
- Fewer than 1,000/µl (SI, $< 1.0 \times 10^9$/L) white blood cells (WBCs).
- Level in glucose equals level in whole blood.

Abnormal results

- Transudates are protein-poor effusions that arise from mechanical factors altering fluid formation or resorption, such as increased hydrostatic pressure, decreased plasma oncotic pressure, or obstruction of the pericardial lymphatic drainage system by a tumor.
- Exudate effusions may occur in pericarditis, neoplasms, acute myocardial infarction, tuberculosis (TB), rheumatoid disease, and systemic lupus erythematosus.
- An elevated WBC count or neutrophil fraction may also accompany inflammatory conditions; a high lymphocyte fraction may indicate fungal or tuberculous pericarditis.
- Turbid or milky effusions may result from lymph or pus accumulation in the pericardial sac or TB or rheumatoid disease.
- Bloody pericardial fluid may indicate hemopericardium, hemorrhagic pericarditis, or a traumatic tap.
- Hemorrhagic effusions may indicate a malignant tumor, closed chest trauma, Dressler's syndrome, or postcardiotomy syndrome.
- Glucose level below whole blood levels may reflect increased local metabolism because of malignancy, inflammation, or infection.

Interfering factors

- Failure to use aseptic collection technique
- Failure to use proper additives in test tubes
- Antimicrobial therapy

Peritoneal fluid analysis

Overview

- Assesses a specimen of peritoneal fluid obtained by paracentesis.
- Requires inserting a trocar and cannula through the abdominal wall while patient receives a local anesthetic.
- In the four-quadrant tap, fluid is aspirated from each quadrant of the abdomen to verify abdominal trauma and confirm the need for surgery.

Purpose

- To determine the cause of ascites
- To detect abdominal trauma

Procedure

Preparation

- Explain to the patient that peritoneal fluid analysis helps determine the cause of ascites or detects abdominal trauma.
- Make sure that the patient or a responsible family member has signed an informed consent form.
- Record baseline vital signs, weight, and abdominal girth.
- Tell the patient to void just before the test.
- X-rays may be performed before peritoneal analysis.
- Tell the patient that the test requires a peritoneal fluid specimen, that he'll receive a local anesthetic to minimize discomfort, and that the procedure takes about 45 minutes to perform.

Implementation

- Have the patient sit on a bed or in a chair with his feet flat on the floor and his back well-supported. If he can't tolerate being out of bed, place him in high Fowler's position and make him as comfortable as possible.
- Shave the puncture site, prepare the skin, and drape the area.
- A local anesthetic is injected.
- The examiner inserts the needle or trocar and cannula 1″ to 2″ (2.5 to 5 cm) below the umbilicus (or through the flank, iliac fossa, or border of the rectus, or at each quadrant of the abdomen).
- If a trocar and cannula are used, a small incision is made to facilitate insertion. When the needle pierces the peritoneum, a sound can be heard when it "gives." The trocar is removed and a sample of fluid is aspirated with a 50-ml Luer-Lok syringe.
- Check the patient's vital signs every 15 minutes during the procedure. Watch for deviations from baseline findings. Observe for dizziness, pallor, perspiration, and increased anxiety.

- If additional fluid is to be drained, assist in attaching one end of an I.V. tube to the cannula and the other end to a collection bag.
- The fluid is then aspirated (no more than 1,500 ml). If aspirating is difficult, reposition the patient.
- After aspiration, the trocar needle is removed and a pressure dressing is applied. Occasionally, the wound may be sutured first.
- Label the specimens in the order they were drawn. If the patient has received antibiotic therapy, note this on the laboratory request.

Patient care

- Apply gauze dressing to the puncture site. Check the dressing frequently and reinforce or apply a pressure dressing, if needed.
- Monitor the patient's vital signs until they're stable.
- Weigh him and measure his abdominal girth; compare these with his baseline values.
- Monitor the patient's urine output for at least 24 hours, and watch for hematuria, which may indicate bladder trauma.
- Watch the patient for signs of hemorrhage or shock and for increasing pain or abdominal tenderness.
- If a large amount of fluid was aspirated, watch the patient for signs of vascular collapse. Give fluids orally if the patient is alert and can accept them.
- If rapid fluid aspiration induces hypovolemia and shock, reduce the vertical distance between the trocar and the collection bag to slow the drainage rate.
- Observe the patient with severe hepatic disease for signs of hepatic coma, which may result from sodium and potassium loss accompanying hypovolemia. Watch him for mental changes, drowsiness, and stupor.
- Give I.V. infusions and albumin. Check the laboratory report for electrolyte and serum protein levels.

Complications

- Hypovolemia and shock caused by rapid fluid aspiration

Interpretation

Normal results

See *Normal findings in peritoneal fluid analysis.*

Abnormal results

- Milk-colored peritoneal fluid may result from chyle or lymph fluid escaping from a thoracic duct that's damaged or blocked by a malignant tumor, lymphoma, tuberculosis, parasitic infestation, adhesion, or hepatic cirrhosis; a pseudochylous condition may result from the presence of leukocytes or tumor cells.
- Differential diagnosis of true chylous ascites depends on the presence of elevated triglyceride levels ($\geq$ 400 mg/dl [SI, $\geq$ 4.36 mmol/L]) and microscopic fat globules.

Normal findings in peritoneal fluid analysis

Use this table to determine normal findings in peritoneal fluid.

Element	Normal value or finding
Gross appearance	Sterile, odorless, clear to pale yellow color; scant amount (< 50 ml)
Red blood cells	None
White blood cells	$< 300/\mu l$ (SI, $< 300 \times 10^9$/L)
Protein	0.3 to 4.1 g/dl (SI, 3 to 41 g/L)
Glucose	70 to 100 mg/dl (SI, 3.5 to 5 mmol/L)
Amylase	138 to 404 units/L (SI, 138 to 404 U/L)
Ammonia	< 50 µg/dl (SI, < 29 µmol/L)
Alkaline phosphatase	Males over age 18: 90 to 239 units/L (SI, 90 to 239 U/L) Females under age 45: 76 to 196 units/L (SI, 76 to 196 U/L) Females over age 45: 87 to 250 units/L (SI, 87 to 250 U/L)
Cytology	No malignant cells present
Bacteria	None
Fungi	None

○ Cloudy or turbid fluid may indicate peritonitis from primary bacterial infection, a ruptured bowel (after trauma), pancreatitis, a strangulated or an infarcted intestine, or an appendicitis.

○ Bloody fluid may result from a benign or malignant tumor, hemorrhagic pancreatitis, or a traumatic tap; if the fluid fails to clear on continued aspiration, a traumatic tap isn't the cause.

○ Bile-stained green fluid may indicate a ruptured gallbladder, acute pancreatitis, or a perforated intestine or duodenal ulcer.

○ A red blood cell count over $100/\mu l$ (SI, >100/L) indicates neoplasm or tuberculosis; a count over $100,000/\mu l$ (SI, $>100,000$/L) indicates intra-abdominal trauma.

○ An elevated white blood cell count with more than 25% neutrophils occurs in 90% of patients with spontaneous bacterial peritonitis and in 50% of those with cirrhosis.

○ A high percentage of lymphocytes suggests tuberculous peritonitis or chylous ascites. Numerous mesothelial cells indicate tuberculous peritonitis.

○ Protein levels rise above 3 g/dl in malignancy (SI, > 3 g/L) and above 4 g/dl (SI, > 4 g/L) in tuberculosis.

○ Peritoneal fluid glucose levels fall in the patient with tuberculous peritonitis or peritoneal carcinomatosis.

○ Amylase levels rise with pancreatic trauma, pancreatic pseudocyst, or acute pancreatitis and may also rise in intestinal necrosis or strangulation.

○ Peritoneal alkaline phosphatase levels rise to more than twice the normal serum levels in the patient with ruptured or strangulated small intestines.

○ Peritoneal ammonia levels also exceed twice the normal serum levels in ruptured or strangulated large and small intestines and in a ruptured ulcer or an appendix.

○ A protein ascitic fluid to serum ratio of 0.5 or greater may suggest a malignancy or tuberculous or pancreatic ascites. The presence of this finding indicates a nonhepatic cause; its absence suggests uncomplicated hepatic disease.

○ An albumin gradient between ascitic fluid and serum greater than 1 g/dl (SI, > 1 g/L) indicates chronic hepatic disease; a lesser value suggests malignancy.

○ Cytologic examination of peritoneal fluid accurately detects malignant cells.

○ Microbiological examination can reveal coliforms, anaerobes, and enterococci, which can enter the peritoneum from a ruptured organ or from infections accompanying appendicitis, pancreatitis, tuberculosis, or ovarian disease.

○ Gram-positive cocci commonly indicate primary peritonitis; gram-negative organisms, secondary peritonitis.

○ The presence of fungi may indicate histoplasmosis, candidiasis, or coccidioidomycosis.

Interfering factors

○ Unsterile collection technique or failure to send the specimen to the laboratory immediately after collection

○ Contamination of the specimen with blood, bile, urine, or feces because of injury to underlying structures during paracentesis

Persantine thallium imaging

Overview

○ An alternative method of assessing coronary vessel function for the patient who can't tolerate exercise or stress electrocardiography (ECG).
○ Dipyridamole (Persantine) infusion simulates the effects of exercise by increasing blood flow to the collateral circulation and away from the coronary arteries, inducing ischemia.
○ Thallium infusion allows the examiner to evaluate the cardiac vessel response.
○ The heart is scanned immediately after the thallium infusion and again 2 to 4 hours later (diseased vessels can't deliver thallium to the heart, and thallium lingers in diseased areas of the myocardium).

Purpose

○ To identify exercise- or stress-induced arrhythmias
○ To assess the presence and degree of cardiac ischemia

Procedure

Preparation

○ Tell the patient that a painless, 5- to 10-minute baseline ECG will precede Persantine thallium imaging.
○ Explain to the patient that he'll need to restrict food and fluids before the test. Tell him to avoid caffeine and other stimulants (which may cause arrhythmias).
○ Instruct the patient to continue taking all his regular medications, with the possible exception of beta blockers.
○ Make sure that the patient or a responsible family member has signed an informed consent form.
○ Explain to the patient that an I.V. line infuses the medications for the study. Tell him who will start the I.V. and when. Explain that he may experience slight discomfort from the needle insertion and the tourniquet.
○ Inform the patient that he may experience mild nausea, headache, dizziness, or flushing after Persantine administration.
○ Reassure him that these adverse reactions are usually temporary and rarely need treatment.

Implementation

○ The patient reclines or sits while a resting ECG is performed. Persantine is either given orally or infused I.V. over 4 minutes. Monitor blood pressure, pulse rate, and cardiac rhythm continuously.
○ After Persantine administration, the patient is asked to get up and walk. After it takes effect, thallium is injected.

○ The patient is placed in the supine position for about 40 minutes while the scan is performed. The scan is then reviewed. If necessary, a second scan is performed.

Patient care

○ If the patient must return for further scanning, tell him to rest and to restrict food and fluids in the interim.

▽ *ALERT The patient may experience arrhythmias, angina, ST-segment depression, or bronchospasm. Make sure resuscitation equipment is readily available.*

Complications

○ Adverse reactions including nausea, headache, flushing, dizziness, and epigastric pain

Interpretation

Normal results

○ Distribution of the isotope throughout the left ventricle is characteristic and with no visible defects.

Abnormal results

○ The presence of ST-segment depression, angina, and arrhythmias strongly suggests coronary artery disease (CAD).
○ Persistent ST-segment depression usually indicates a myocardial infarction. In contrast, transient ST-segment depression indicates ischemia from CAD.
○ Cold spots usually indicate CAD but may result from sarcoidosis, myocardial fibrosis, cardiac contusion, attenuation because of soft tissue (for example, breast and diaphragm), apical cleft, and coronary spasm.
○ The absence of cold spots in the presence of CAD may result from insignificant obstruction, single-vessel disease, or collateral circulation.

Interfering factors

○ Failure to observe pretest restrictions
○ Artifacts, such as implants and electrodes (possible false-positive)
○ Absence of cold spots with CAD (possible delay in imaging)

pH test, 24-hour

Overview

○ Most sensitive indicator of gastric reflux
○ Considered the "gold standard" to diagnose gastro-esophageal reflux disease
○ Also known as a *24-hour ambulatory pH monitoring study*

Purpose

○ To measure esophageal pH for a total of 24 hours, while a probe is in place
○ To determine the presence of gastroesophageal reflux
○ To evaluate control of gastroesophageal reflux while on proton pump inhibition
○ To determine if reflux episodes correlate with symptoms such as chest pain

Procedure

Preparation

○ Make sure the patient has signed an appropriate consent form.
○ Note and report all allergies.
○ Explain the need for fasting and the avoidance of cigarette smoking after midnight the night before testing.
○ Explain the need for possible withholding of certain GI medications.
○ For documenting reflux, Explain the need for withholding certain medications including all proton pump inhibitors (generally for 7 days before the procedure). It may also be necessary to withhold histamine-2 receptor antagonists, calcium channel blockers, beta blockers, metoclopramide, erythromycin, nitroglycerin, belladonna/phenobarbital (Donnatal), chlordiazepoxide/clidinium (Librax), hyoscyamine sulfate (Levsin), and bethanechol. These medications are generally stopped for at least 48 hours before the procedure.
○ For documenting adequacy of control with proton pump inhibition (PPI): Explain the need for fasting after midnight and resumption of routine medications including PPI after probe placement.
○ Advise the patient that he may experience slight discomfort and possible gagging or coughing during probe insertion.
○ Explain that the test takes up to 15 minutes.
○ Explain to the patient the need for his keeping a diary while the probe is in place.

Implementation

○ The patient is placed in high Fowler's position.
○ A probe, with a pH electrode, is inserted gently into one of the patient's nostrils.
○ The probe is advanced to the lower esophageal sphincter.
○ After it's appropriately placed, the probe is taped to the patient's cheek and placed behind his ear with the unit attached to the recorder.
○ Probe may inadvertently enter the trachea; if respiratory distress or paroxysmal coughing occurs, the catheter is removed immediately.

Patient care

○ Have the patient resume his usual diet and medications.
○ Schedule a return visit in 24 hours to remove the probe.

Complications

○ Catheter inadvertently entering the trachea
○ Epistaxis (rare)

Interpretation

Normal results

○ pH < 4.0 before 4% of the 24 hours

Abnormal results

○ pH < 4.0 occurs during more than 4% of the 24 hours, suggesting gastroesophageal reflux disease.

Interfering factors

○ Failure to withhold certain drugs

pH, urine

Overview

- Measures how acidic or alkaline (basic) the urine is; may range from 0 (most acidic) to 14 (most basic).
- Certain types of treatment may adjust the pH of urine.
- Urine that is either acidic or alkaline can help to prevent the formation of certain types of kidney calculi.

Purpose

- To measure the acidic or alkaline value of urine

Procedure

Preparation

- Tell the patient to avoid foods that will alter pH, such as dairy products and citrus foods.
- Tell the patient to avoid medications such as antacids that will alter pH.

Implementation

- Collect a urine sample.
- Test the sample with litmus paper test strips or reagent test strips.

Patient care

- Answer the patient's questions about the test.

Complications

None known

Interpretation

Normal results

- 4.5 to 8.0

Abnormal results

- 4.0 (strongly acidic)
- 9.0 (strongly alkaline)
- Alkaline pH can be caused by Fanconi's syndrome, metabolic or respiratory alkalosis, prolonged vomiting, kidney disease, urinary tract infection caused by urea-splitting bacteria (*Proteus* and *Pseudomonas*), and asthma.
- Acidic pH may be a sign of severe lung disease (emphysema), uncontrolled diabetes, aspirin overdose, prolonged diarrhea, dehydration, starvation, drinking an excessive amount of alcohol or antifreeze (ethylene glycol), renal tuberculosis, pyrexia, phenylketonuria, alkaptonuria, and acidosis.

Interfering factors

- Citrus fruit and dairy products
- Antacids

Phenolsulfonphthalein excretion

Overview

- Evaluates kidney function
- Should be performed in the patient with abnormal results in the urine concentration test, an early sign of renal dysfunction
- Also called *PSP*

Purpose

- To determine renal plasma flow
- To evaluate tubular function

Procedure

Preparation

- Explain to the patient that this test evaluates kidney function.
- Inform the patient that he need not restrict food before the test.
- Encourage him to drink fluids before and during the test to maintain adequate urine flow.
- Tell the patient the test requires an I.V. injection and collection of urine specimens 15 minutes, 30 minutes, 1 hour, and possibly 2 hours after the I.V. injection.
- Tell the patient who will give the I.V. injection and when.
- Explain to the patient that he may experience slight discomfort from the tourniquet and the needle puncture and that the dye temporarily turns the urine red.
- If the patient can't void and requires catheterization, tell him that he may have the urge to void when the catheter is in place.
- Notify the laboratory and physician of drugs the patient is taking that may affect test results; it may be necessary to restrict them. If the patient must continue them, note this on the laboratory request.

Implementation

- Instruct the patient to empty his bladder and discard the urine.
- The physician will give 1 ml of PSP, which equals 6 mg of dye, I.V.
- Collect a urine specimen at 15 minutes, 30 minutes, 1 hour, and, possibly, 2 hours after the injection.
- Encourage the patient to drink fluids because 40 ml of urine is necessary for each specimen.
- Don't use the urine in the drainage bag if the patient already has a catheter in place.
- Empty the bag and clamp the catheter for 1 hour before the test.
- Record the PSP dosage on the laboratory request.
- Properly label each specimen and include the collection time.

- Send the specimen to the laboratory immediately after collection.
- Refrigerate the specimen if more than 10 minutes will elapse before transport.

Patient care

- Monitor the I.V. site for signs of infiltration.
- If the patient is catheterized, make sure he voids within 8 hours after the catheter is removed.
- Inform the patient that he may resume his usual medications.
- Keep epinephrine, histamine-1 receptor antagonists (diphenhydramine), and a glucocorticoid (methylprednisolone) available due to the possibility of allergic reactions to PSP.
- Elevate the arm and apply warm soaks if phlebitis develops at the I.V. site.

Complications

- Phlebitis at the I.V. site
- Allergic reaction to PSP

Interpretation

Normal results

- In adults, 25% of the PSP dose is excreted in 15 minutes, 50% to 60% in 30 minutes, 60% to 70% in 1 hour, and 70% to 80% in 2 hours.
- In children (excluding infants), results should be 5% to 10% higher than those in adults.

Abnormal results

- The 15-minute value is the most sensitive indicator of tubular function and renal plasma flow because depressed excretion at this interval, with normal excretion later, suggests relatively mild or early-stage bilateral renal disease.
- A depressed 2-hour value may reveal moderate to severe renal impairment.
- Depressed PSP excretion is also characteristic in renal vascular disease, urinary tract obstruction, heart failure, and gout.
- Elevated PSP excretion is characteristic in hypoalbuminemia, hepatic disease, and multiple myeloma.

Interfering factors

- Failure to collect an adequate specimen at required times
- Radiographic contrast media, aspirin, chlorothiazide, salicylates, sulfonamides, penicillin, cascara sagrada, ethanol, indomethacin, nitrofurantoin, phenylbutazone, probenecid, and vitamins (possible increase or decrease)
- Beets, carrots, and rhubarb (possible increase or decrease)
- Incorrect PSP dosage (possible increase or decrease)
- High serum protein levels (decrease)
- Severe hypoalbuminemia, excessive albuminuria, or severe liver disease (possible effect on excretion)

Phenylalanine

Overview

○ Screens infants for elevated serum phenylalanine levels, an indication of phenylketonuria (PKU).
○ Also called the *Guthrie screening test*.
○ A naturally occurring amino acid essential to growth and nitrogen balance; an accumulation of this amino acid may indicate a serious enzyme deficiency.
○ Detects abnormal phenylalanine levels through the growth rate of *Bacillus subtilis,* an organism that needs phenylalanine to thrive.
○ To ensure accurate results, performed after 3 full days (preferably 4 days) of milk or formula feeding.

Purpose

○ To screen the infant for PKU

Procedure

Preparation

○ Explain to the parents that this test is a routine screening measure for possible PKU and is required in many states.
○ Tell the parents that a small amount of blood will be drawn from the infant's heel, and that collecting the sample only takes a few minutes.

Implementation

○ Perform a heelstick and collect three drops of blood—one in each circle—on the filter paper.
○ Note the infant's name and birth date and the date of the first milk or formula feeding on the laboratory request.
○ Send the sample to the laboratory immediately.

Patient care

○ Reassure the parents of a child who may have PKU that although this disease is a common cause of congenital mental deficiency, early detection and continuous treatment with a low-phenylalanine diet can prevent permanent mental retardation.
○ Apply direct pressure to the heelstick site until bleeding stops.

Complications

None known

Interpretation

Normal results

○ A negative test result, indicating normal phenylalanine levels (< 2 mg/dl [SI, < 121 μmol/L]) and no appreciable danger of PKU

Abnormal results

○ At birth, a neonate with PKU usually has normal phenylalanine levels, but after milk or formula feeding begins, levels gradually increase because of a deficiency of the liver enzyme that converts phenylalanine to tyrosine.
○ A positive test result suggests the *possibility* of PKU.
○ A definitive diagnosis requires exact serum phenylalanine measurement and urine testing.
○ A positive test result may also indicate hepatic disease, galactosemia, or delayed development of certain enzyme systems.

Interfering factors

○ Performing the test before the infant has received at least 3 full days of milk or formula feeding (false-negative)

Phosphate, serum

Overview

○ Measures levels of phosphate, the primary anion in intracellular fluid.
○ Phosphates are needed for storing and using energy, regulating calcium levels, and for red blood cell function, acid-base balance, bone formation, and the metabolism of carbohydrates, protein, and fat.
○ The intestines absorb most phosphates from dietary sources; the kidneys excrete phosphates and serve as a regulatory mechanism.
○ Abnormal phosphate levels usually result from improper excretion rather than faulty ingestion or absorption from dietary sources.
○ Normally, calcium and phosphate levels have an inverse relationship; if one is increased, the other is decreased.

Purpose

○ To aid in the diagnosis of renal disorders and acid-base imbalance
○ To detect endocrine, skeletal, and calcium disorders

Procedure

Preparation

○ Explain to the patient that the serum phosphate test measures phosphate levels in the blood.
○ Tell the patient that the test requires a blood sample. Explain who will perform the venipuncture and when.
○ Explain to the patient that he may experience slight discomfort from the tourniquet and the needle puncture.
○ Inform the patient that he need not restrict food and fluids.
○ Notify the laboratory and physician of drugs the patient is taking that may affect test results; it may be necessary to restrict them.

Implementation

○ Perform a venipuncture without using a tourniquet, if possible, and collect the sample in 3- or 4-ml clot-activator tube.
○ Handle the sample gently to prevent hemolysis.

Patient care

○ Apply pressure to the venipuncture site until bleeding stops.
○ Instruct the patient that he may resume any medications stopped before the test.

Complications

○ Hematoma at the venipuncture site

Interpretation

Normal results

○ In adults, 2.7 to 4.5 mg/dl (SI, 0.87 to 1.45 mmol/L)
○ In children, 4.5 to 6.7 mg/dl (SI, 1.45 to 1.78 mmol/L)

Abnormal results

○ Decreased phosphate levels (hypophosphatemia) may result from malnutrition, malabsorption syndromes, hyperparathyroidism, renal tubular acidosis, and treatment of diabetic ketoacidosis (DKA).
○ In children, hypophosphatemia can suppress normal growth.
○ Symptoms of hypophosphatemia include anemia, prolonged bleeding, bone demineralization, decreased white blood cell count, and anorexia.
○ Increased levels (hyperphosphatemia) may result from skeletal disease, healing fractures, hypoparathyroidism, acromegaly, DKA, high intestinal obstruction, lactic acidosis (because of hepatic impairment), and renal failure.
○ Hyperphosphatemia is seldom clinically significant, but it can alter bone metabolism in prolonged cases.
○ Symptoms of hyperphosphatemia include tachycardia, muscular weakness, diarrhea, cramping, and hyperreflexia.

Interfering factors

○ Venous stasis from tourniquet use
○ Sample obtained above an I.V. site that's receiving a solution containing phosphate
○ Excessive vitamin D intake or therapy with anabolic steroids or androgens (possible increase)
○ Use of acetazolamide, insulin, epinephrine, or phosphate-binding antacids; excessive excretion from prolonged vomiting or diarrhea; vitamin D deficiency; and extended I.V. infusion of dextrose 5% in water (possible decrease)
○ Hemolysis of the sample (false-high)

Phosphate, urine

Overview

- Determines whether urine calcium and phosphate levels parallel serum levels.
- Calcium and phosphates, absorbed in the upper intestine and excreted in feces and urine, aid carbohydrate metabolism and help maintain tissue and fluid pH, electrolyte balance in cells and extracellular fluids, and permeability of cell membranes.

Purpose

- To evaluate calcium and phosphate metabolism and excretion
- To monitor the treatment of calcium or phosphate deficiency

Procedure

Preparation

- Explain to the patient that the urine calcium and phosphates test measures the amount of calcium and phosphates in the urine.
- Provide a diet that contains about 130 mg of calcium/24 hours for 3 days before the test or provide a copy of the diet for the patient to follow at home.
- Notify the laboratory and physician of drugs the patient is taking that may affect test results; it may be necessary to restrict them.
- Encourage the patient to be as active as possible before the test.
- Tell the patient that the test requires urine collection over a 24-hour period. If the patient is to collect the specimen, teach him the proper technique.

Implementation

- Collect the patient's urine over a 24-hour period, discarding the first specimen and retaining the last.
- Tell the patient not to contaminate the specimen with toilet tissue or feces.

Patient care

- Inform the patient that he may resume his usual diet, activities, and medications.

Complications

None known

Interpretation

Normal results

- Results depend on dietary intake.
- Excretion of phosphate is < 1,000 mg/24 hours.

Abnormal results

- Many disorders may affect calcium and phosphate levels.
- Excretion of phosphate is ≥ 1,000 mg/24 hours.

Interfering factors

- Failure to collect all urine during the test period
- Parathyroid hormones (increase phosphates excretion)
- Vitamin D (increases phosphate absorption and excretion)

Phospholipids

Overview

○ Quantitative analysis of phospholipids, the major form of lipids in cell membranes, which aid in cellular membrane composition and permeability and help control enzyme activity within the membrane, help transport fatty acids and lipids across the intestinal barrier and from the liver and other fat stores to other body tissues, and are essential for pulmonary gas exchange

Purpose

○ To aid in the evaluation of fat metabolism
○ To aid in the diagnosis of hypothyroidism, diabetes mellitus, nephrotic syndrome, chronic pancreatitis, obstructive jaundice, and hypolipoproteinemia

Procedure

Preparation

○ Explain to the patient that the phospholipid test is used to determine how the body metabolizes fats.
○ Tell the patient that the test requires a blood sample. Explain who will perform the venipuncture and when.
○ Explain to the patient that he may experience slight discomfort from the tourniquet and the needle puncture.
○ Instruct the patient to abstain from drinking alcohol for 24 hours before the test and not to eat or drink anything after midnight before the test.
○ Notify the laboratory and physician of drugs the patient is taking that may affect test results; they may need to be restricted.

Implementation

○ Perform a venipuncture and collect the sample in a 10- to 15-ml tube without additives.
○ Send the sample to the laboratory immediately because spontaneous redistribution may occur among plasma lipids.

Patient care

○ Apply direct pressure to the venipuncture site until bleeding stops.
○ Instruct the patient that he may resume his usual diet and medications stopped before the test, as ordered.

Complications

○ Hematoma at the venipuncture site

Interpretation

Normal results

○ 180 to 320 mg/dl (SI, 1.8 to 3.2 g/L)

○ Men usually have higher levels than women, unless the woman is pregnant; values in pregnant women exceed those of men.

Abnormal results

○ Elevated phospholipid levels may indicate hypothyroidism, diabetes mellitus, nephrotic syndrome, chronic pancreatitis, or obstructive jaundice.
○ Decreased levels may indicate primary hypolipoproteinemia.

Interfering factors

○ Failure to observe pretest restrictions
○ Antilipemics (possible decrease)
○ Estrogens, epinephrine, and some phenothiazines (increase)

Plasma amino acid screening

Overview

○ Qualitative screen for inborn errors of metabolism of amino acids, the chief component of all proteins and polypeptides.
○ The body contains at least 20 amino acids; 10 of these aren't formed in the body and must be acquired by diet.
○ Certain congenital enzyme deficiencies interfere with normal metabolism of these amino acids, resulting in amino acid accumulation or deficiency.

Purpose

○ To screen for inborn errors of amino acid metabolism

Procedure

Preparation

○ Explain to the parents that plasma and amino acid screening determines how well their infant metabolizes amino acids.
○ Instruct the parents that the infant must fast for 4 hours before the test.
○ Tell the parents that a small amount of blood will be drawn from the infant's heel, but that collecting the sample takes only a few minutes.

Implementation

○ Perform a heelstick and collect 0.1 ml of blood in a heparinized capillary tube.
○ Handle the sample gently to prevent hemolysis.

Patient care

○ Apply direct pressure to the venipuncture site until bleeding stops.
○ Tell the parents to resume the feeding of their infant's usual diet.

Complications

○ Hematoma at the heelstick site

Interpretation

Normal results

○ Chromatography shows a normal plasma amino acid pattern.

Abnormal results

○ Excessive accumulation of amino acids typically produces overflow aminoaciduria.

○ Congenital abnormalities of the amino acid transport system in the kidneys produce a second group of disorders called *renal aminoaciduria*.
○ Comparisons of blood and urine chromatography can help distinguish between the two types of aminoaciduria.
○ The plasma amino acid pattern is normal in renal aminoaciduria and abnormal in overflow aminoaciduria.

Interfering factors

○ Failure to observe pretest restrictions
○ Hemolysis from rough handling of the sample

Plasma calcitonin

Overview

○ A radioimmunoassay that measures calcitonin levels (*thyrocalcitonin*).
○ The role of calcitonin in normal human physiology is not fully defined, but calcitonin can act as an antagonist to parathyroid hormone and may lower calcium levels.
○ Usual clinical indication for this test is suspected medullary carcinoma of the thyroid, which causes hypersecretion of calcitonin (without associated hypocalcemia).
○ Equivocal results require provocative testing with I.V. pentagastrin or calcium to rule out disease

Purpose

○ To aid in the diagnosis of thyroid medullary carcinoma and ectopic calcitonin-producing tumors (rare)

Procedure

Preparation

○ Explain to the patient that this test helps evaluate thyroid function.
○ Instruct the patient to fast overnight because food may interfere with calcium homeostasis and, subsequently, calcitonin levels.
○ Tell the patient that the test requires a blood sample. Explain who will perform the venipuncture and when.
○ Explain to the patient that he may experience slight discomfort from the tourniquet and the needle puncture.
○ Tell him that the laboratory requires several days to complete the analysis.

Implementation

○ Perform a venipuncture and collect the sample in a 7-ml heparinized tube.
○ Handle the sample gently to prevent hemolysis.
○ Send the sample to the laboratory immediately.

Patient care

○ Apply direct pressure to the venipuncture site until bleeding stops.
○ Instruct the patient that he may resume his usual diet.

Complications

○ Hematoma at the venipuncture

Interpretation

Normal results

○ Serum basal calcitonin levels in men are 40 pg/ml (SI, 40 ng/L); in women, 20 pg/ml (SI, 20 ng/L).
○ After 4-hour calcium infusion, in men they rise to 190 pg/ml (SI, 190 ng/L); in women, 130 pg/ml (SI, 130 ng/L).
○ After testing with pentagastrin infusion, in men they should be 110 pg/ml (SI, 110 ng/L); in women, 30 pg/ml (SI, 30 ng/L).

Abnormal results

○ Elevated serum calcitonin levels in the absence of hypocalcemia usually indicate medullary carcinoma of the thyroid.
○ Transmitted as an autosomal dominant trait, thyroid medullary carcinoma may occur as part of multiple endocrine neoplasia.
○ Increased calcitonin levels may be caused by ectopic calcitonin production by oat cell carcinoma of the lung or by breast carcinoma.

Interfering factors

○ Failure of patient to fast overnight before the test
○ Hemolysis from rough handling of the sample

Plasma catecholamines

Overview

○ A total or fractionated analysis of plasma catechol-amine (including hormones epinephrine, norepi-nephrine, and dopamine) levels for the hypertensive patient with signs of adrenal medullary tumor or the patient with a neural tumor that affects endocrine function.
○ Elevated plasma catecholamine levels necessitate supportive confirmation by urinalysis.
○ Catecholamines prepare the body for the fight-or-flight response, increasing heart rate and contractili-ty, constricting blood vessels, redistributing blood to-ward the skeletal and coronary muscles, mobilizing carbohydrate and lipid reserves, and sharpening alertness.
○ Plasma levels commonly fluctuate in response to temperature, stress, postural change, diet, smoking, anoxia, volume depletion, renal failure, obesity, and many drugs.

Purpose

○ To rule out pheochromocytoma (adrenal medullary or extra-adrenal) in the patient with hypertension
○ To help identify neuroblastoma, ganglioneuroblas-toma, and ganglioneuroma
○ To distinguish between adrenal medullary tumors through fractional analysis
○ To aid in the diagnosis of autonomic nervous system dysfunction such as idiopathic orthostatic hypoten-sion

Procedure

Preparation

○ Explain to the patient that this test helps determine if hypertension or other symptoms are related to im-proper hormonal secretion.
○ Instruct the patient to refrain from using self-prescribed medications, especially cold and allergy remedies that may contain sympathomimetics, for 2 weeks before the test.
○ If the patient is in your facility, withhold drugs that affect catecholamine levels, such as amphetamines, phenothiazines (chlorpromazine), sympathomimet-ics, and tricyclic antidepressants.
○ Tell the patient to exclude amine-rich foods and bev-erages, such as bananas, avocados, cheese, coffee, tea, cocoa, beer, and Chianti, from his diet for 48 hours; to maintain vitamin C intake, which is nec-essary for formation of catecholamines; to abstain from smoking for 24 hours; and to fast for 10 to 12 hours before the test.
○ Tell the patient that the test requires one or two blood samples.

○ Explain who will perform the venipuncture and when.
○ Explain to the patient that he may experience slight discomfort from the tourniquet and the needle punc-ture.
○ Insert an indwelling venous catheter (heparin lock) 24 hours before the test because the stress of the venipuncture itself may significantly raise cate-cholamine levels.
○ Make sure the patient is relaxed and recumbent for 45 to 60 minutes before the test.
○ If necessary, provide blankets to keep the patient warm; low temperatures stimulate catecholamine se-cretion.

Implementation

○ Perform a venipuncture between 6 a.m. and 8 a.m.
○ Collect the sample in a 10-ml chilled ethylenedia-minetetraacetic acid tube (EDTA) (sodium metabi-sulfite solution), which can be obtained from the lab-oratory on request.
○ If a second sample is requested, have the patient stand for 10 minutes and draw the sample into an-other tube exactly like the first.
○ If a heparin lock is used, it may be necessary to dis-card the first 1 or 2 ml of blood. Check with the lab-oratory for the preferred procedure.
○ After collecting each sample, roll the tube slowly be-tween your palms to distribute the EDTA without agi-tating the blood.
○ Pack the tube in crushed ice to minimize deactivation of catecholamines and send it to the laboratory im-mediately.
○ Indicate on the laboratory request whether the pa-tient was supine or standing during the venipuncture and the time the sample was drawn.

Patient care

○ Apply direct pressure to the venipuncture site until bleeding stops.
○ Instruct the patient that he may resume his usual diet and medications stopped before the test.

Complications

○ Hematoma at the venipuncture site

Interpretation

Normal results

○ In fractional analysis, catecholamine supine levels are: epinephrine, undetectable to 110 pg/ml (SI, un-detectable to 600 pmol/L); norepinephrine, 70 to 750 pg/ml (SI, 413 to 4,432 pmol/L).
○ In fractional analysis, standing catecholamine levels are: epinephrine, undetectable to 140 pg/ml (SI, un-detectable to 764 pmol/L); norepinephrine, 200 to 1,700 pg/ml (SI, 1,182 to 10,047 pmol/L).

Abnormal results

○ High catecholamine levels may indicate pheochromocytoma, neuroblastoma, ganglioneuroblastoma, ganglioneuroma, thyroid disorders, hypoglycemia, and cardiac disease; may also result from electroconvulsive therapy, shock resulting from hemorrhage, endotoxins, and anaphylaxis.

○ Excessive catecholamine secretion by tumors causes hypertension, weight loss, episodic sweating, headache, palpitations, and anxiety.

○ Fractional analysis helps identify the cause of elevated catecholamine levels. For example, adrenal medullary tumors secrete epinephrine, whereas ganglioneuromas, ganglioblastomas, and neuroblastomas secrete norepinephrine.

○ In the patient with normal or low baseline catecholamine levels, failure to show an increase in the sample taken after standing suggests autonomic nervous system dysfunction.

Interfering factors

○ Failure to observe pretest restrictions
○ Epinephrine, levodopa, amphetamines, phenothiazines, sympathomimetics, decongestants, and tricyclic antidepressants (increase)
○ Reserpine (decrease)
○ Radioactive scan performed within 1 week before the test

Plasma cortisol

Overview

- Quantitative analysis of plasma cortisol levels for patients with signs of adrenal dysfunction.
- Dynamic tests, suppression tests for hyperfunction, and stimulation tests for hypofunction confirm the diagnosis.
- Cortisol helps metabolize nutrients, mediate physiologic stress, and regulate the immune system, with levels rising in the morning, peaking around 8 a.m., and declining in the evening and during sleep.
- Intense heat or cold, infection, trauma, exercise, obesity, and debilitating disease influence cortisol secretion.

Purpose

- To aid in the diagnosis of Cushing's disease, Cushing's syndrome, Addison's disease, and secondary adrenal insufficiency

Procedure

Preparation

- Explain to the patient that this test helps determine if his symptoms are caused by improper hormonal secretion.
- Instruct the patient to maintain a normal salt diet (2 to 3 g/day) for 3 days before the test and to fast and limit physical activity for 10 to 12 hours before the test.
- Withhold all drugs that may interfere with plasma cortisol levels, such as estrogens, androgens, and phenytoin, for 48 hours before the test.
- Tell the patient that the test requires a blood sample. Explain who will perform the venipuncture and when.
- Explain to the patient that he may experience slight discomfort from the tourniquet and the needle puncture.
- If the patient is receiving replacement therapy and is dependent on exogenous steroids for survival, note this on the laboratory request along with other drugs that he must continue.
- Make sure the patient is relaxed and recumbent for at least 30 minutes before the test.

Implementation

- Perform a venipuncture between 6 a.m. and 8 a.m.
- Collect the sample in a 7-ml heparinized tube, label it appropriately, and send it to the laboratory immediately.
- For diurnal variation testing, draw another sample between 4 p.m. and 6 p.m.
- Collect the second sample in a 7-ml heparinized tube, label it appropriately, and send it to the laboratory immediately.
- Handle the sample gently to prevent hemolysis.
- Record the collection time on the laboratory request.

Patient care

- Apply direct pressure to the venipuncture site until bleeding stops.
- Instruct the patient that he may resume his usual diet, activities, and medications stopped before the test.

Complications

- Hematoma at the venipuncture site

Interpretation

Normal results

- 9 to 35 µg/dl (SI, 250 to 690 nmol/L) in the morning; 3 to 12 µg/dl (SI, 80 to 330 nmol/L) in the afternoon.

Abnormal results

- Increased plasma cortisol levels may indicate adrenocortical hyperfunction in Cushing's disease (a rare disease caused by basophilic adenoma of the pituitary gland) or Cushing's syndrome (glucocorticoid excess from any cause).
- In most patients with Cushing's syndrome, the adrenal cortex secretes independently of a natural rhythm; absence of diurnal variation in cortisol secretion is a significant finding in almost all patients with Cushing's syndrome; in these patients, little difference in values is found between morning and afternoon samples.
- Diurnal variations may also be absent in otherwise healthy people who are under considerable emotional or physical stress.
- Decreased cortisol levels may indicate primary adrenal hypofunction (Addison's disease), usually caused by idiopathic glandular atrophy (a presumed autoimmune process).
- Adrenocortical destruction can result from tuberculosis, fungal invasion, and hemorrhage.
- Low cortisol levels resulting from secondary adrenal insufficiency may occur in conditions of impaired corticotropin secretion, such as hypophysectomy, postpartum pituitary necrosis, craniopharyngioma, and chromophobe adenoma.

Interfering factors

- Failure to observe pretest restrictions
- Hemolysis from rough handling of the sample
- Pregnancy or use of hormonal contraceptives because of increase in cortisol-binding plasma proteins (false-high)
- Obesity, stress, and severe hepatic or renal disease (possible increase)
- Androgens and phenytoin caused by decrease in cortisol-binding plasma proteins (possible decrease)
- Radioactive scan performed within 1 week before the test

Plasma fibrinogen

Overview

○ Fibrinogen (factor I) originates in the liver and is converted to fibrin by thrombin during clotting.
○ Because fibrin is necessary for clot formation, fibrinogen deficiency can produce mild to severe bleeding disorders.

Purpose

○ To aid in the diagnosis of suspected clotting or bleeding disorders caused by fibrinogen abnormalities

Procedure

Preparation

○ Explain to the patient that the plasma fibrinogen test determines if blood clots normally.
○ Tell the patient that a blood sample will be taken. Explain who will perform the venipuncture and when.
○ Explain to the patient that he may feel slight discomfort from the tourniquet and the needle puncture.
○ Notify the laboratory and physician of drugs the patient is taking that may affect test results; it may be necessary to restrict them.
○ Inform the patient that he need not restrict food and fluids.

Implementation

○ Perform a venipuncture and collect the sample in a 3- or 4.5-ml tube with sodium citrate added.
○ Completely fill the collection tube, invert it gently several times, and send it to the laboratory immediately or place it on ice.

Patient care

○ Apply direct pressure to venipuncture site until bleeding stops.
○ Make sure that subdermal bleeding has stopped before removing pressure.
○ Instruct the patient that he may resume any medications stopped before the test.
○ If a large hematoma develops at the venipuncture site, monitor pulses distal to the site.

Complications

○ Hematoma at the venipuncture site

Interpretation

Normal results

○ 200 to 400 mg/dl (SI, 2 to 4 g/L)

Abnormal results

○ Depressed fibrinogen levels may indicate congenital afibrinogenemia; hypofibrinogenemia or dysfibrino-genemia; disseminated intravascular coagulation; fibrinolysis; severe hepatic disease; cancer of the prostate, pancreas, or lung; or bone marrow lesions.
○ Obstetric complications or trauma may cause low levels.
○ Markedly decreased fibrinogen levels impede the accurate interpretation of coagulation tests that have a fibrin clot as an end point.
○ Elevated levels may indicate cancer of the stomach, breast, or kidney or inflammatory disorders, such as pneumonia or membranoproliferative glomerulonephritis.
○ Prolonged partial thromboplastin time, prothrombin time, and thrombin time may also indicate a fibrinogen deficiency.

Interfering factors

○ Failure to fill the collection tube completely, to adequately mix the sample and anticoagulant, or to send the sample to the laboratory promptly
○ Hemolysis from excessive probing at the venipuncture site or from rough handling of the sample
○ Heparin or hormonal contraceptives
○ Third trimester of pregnancy and postoperative status (possible increase)

Plasma glucagons

Overview

- Quantitative analysis of plasma glucagon by radio-immunoassay that evaluates patients suspected of having glucagonoma (alpha cell tumor) or hypoglycemia caused by idiopathic glucagon deficiency or pancreatic dysfunction.
- Glucagon, which promotes glucose production and controls its storage, is secreted during hypoglycemia; the other pancreatic hormones, insulin and somatostatin, inhibit its secretion (these hormone levels are normally balanced, to ensure an adequate and constant fuel supply while keeping glucose levels relatively stable).
- Glucagon level is usually measured along with glucose and insulin levels because these influence glucagon secretion.

Purpose

- To aid in the diagnosis of glucagonoma and hypoglycemia caused by chronic pancreatitis or idiopathic glucagon deficiency

Procedure

Preparation

- Explain to the patient that this test helps to evaluate pancreatic function.
- Instruct the patient to fast for 10 to 12 hours before the test.
- Withhold insulin, catecholamines, and other drugs that could influence the test results. If the patient must continue them, note this on the laboratory request.
- Tell the patient that the test requires a blood sample. Explain who will perform the venipuncture and when.
- Have the patient lie down and relax for 30 minutes before the test.
- Explain to the patient that he may experience slight discomfort from the tourniquet and the needle puncture.

Implementation

- Perform a venipuncture and collect the sample in a chilled 10-ml ethylenediaminetetraacetic acid tube.
- Place the sample on ice and send it to the laboratory immediately.
- Handle the sample gently to prevent hemolysis.

Patient care

- Apply direct pressure to the venipuncture site until bleeding stops.
- Instruct the patient that he may resume his usual diet and medications stopped before the test.

Complications

- Hematoma at the venipuncture site

Interpretation

Normal results

- Less than 60 pg/ml (SI, < 60 ng/L)

Abnormal results

- Elevated fasting levels (900 to 7,800 pg/ml [SI, 900 to 7,800 ng/L]) can occur in glucagonoma, diabetes mellitus, acute pancreatitis, and pheochromocytoma.
- Abnormally low glucagon levels are linked to idiopathic glucagon deficiency and hypoglycemia caused by chronic pancreatitis.

Interfering factors

- Failure to observe pretest restrictions
- Hemolysis from rough handling of the sample
- Failure to pack the sample in ice and send it to the laboratory immediately
- Exercise, stress, prolonged fasting, insulin, or catecholamines (increase)
- Radioactive scans and tests performed within 48 hours of the test

Plasma luteinizing hormone

Overview

- Quantitative analysis of plasma luteinizing hormone (LH) or interstitial cell-stimulating hormone levels to test for anovulation and infertility in women.
- For accurate diagnosis, results are evaluated in light of findings obtained from related hormone tests (follicle-stimulating hormone [FSH], estrogen, and testosterone, for example).
- LH is a glycoprotein secreted by basophilic cells of the anterior pituitary gland.
- In women, cyclic LH secretion (with FSH) causes ovulation and transforms the ovarian follicle into the corpus luteum, which in turn secretes progesterone.
- In men, continuous LH secretion stimulates the interstitial (*Leydig*) cells of the testes to release testosterone, which stimulates and maintains spermatogenesis (with FSH).

Purpose

- To detect ovulation
- To assess male or female infertility
- To evaluate amenorrhea
- To monitor therapy designed to induce ovulation

Procedure

Preparation

- Explain to the female patient that this test helps determine if her secretion of female hormones is normal.
- Tell the patient that this test requires a blood sample. Explain who will perform the venipuncture and when.
- Because there's no evidence that plasma LH levels are affected by fasting, eating, or exercise, such pretest restrictions may be unnecessary.
- Withhold drugs that may interfere with plasma LH levels, such as steroids (including estrogens and progesterone), for 48 hours before the test, as ordered. If the patient must continue them, note this on the laboratory request.
- Inform the patient that she may experience slight discomfort from the tourniquet and the needle puncture.

Implementation

- Perform a venipuncture, and collect the sample in a 7-ml clot-activator tube.
- Handle the sample gently to prevent hemolysis.
- If the patient is a woman, indicate the phase of her menstrual cycle on the laboratory request. Make a note if the patient is menopausal.

Patient care

- Apply direct pressure to the venipuncture site until bleeding stops.
- Instruct the patient that she may resume medications stopped before the test.

Complications

- Hematoma at the venipuncture site

Interpretation

Normal results

- In women in the follicular phase, 5 to 15 mIU/ml (SI, 5 to 15 IU/L); ovulatory phase, 30 to 60 mIU/ml (SI, 30 to 60 IU/L); luteal phase, 5 to 15 mIU/ml (SI, 5 to 15 IU/L)
- In postmenopausal women, 50 to 100 mIU/ml (SI, 50 to 100 IU/L)
- In men, 5 to 20 mIU/ml (SI, 5 to 20 IU/L)
- In children, 4 to 20 mIU/ml (SI, 4 to 20 IU/L)

Abnormal results

- In women, absence of a midcycle peak in plasma LH levels may indicate anovulation.
- Decreased or low-normal plasma LH levels may indicate hypogonadism; these findings are often linked to amenorrhea.
- High plasma LH levels may indicate congenital absence of ovaries or ovarian failure from Stein-Leventhal syndrome (polycystic ovary syndrome), Turner's syndrome (ovarian dysgenesis), menopause, or early-stage acromegaly.
- Infertility can result from primary or secondary gonadal dysfunction.
- In men, low plasma LH values may indicate secondary gonadal dysfunction (of hypothalamic or pituitary origin); high values may indicate testicular failure (primary hypogonadism) or destruction, or congenital absence of testes.

Interfering factors

- Failure to observe pretest restrictions
- Hemolysis from rough handling of the sample
- Steroids, including estrogens, progesterone, and testosterone (possible decrease)
- Radioactive scan performed within 1 week before the test

Plasma renin activity

Overview

- Screening procedure for renovascular hypertension; doesn't unequivocally confirm diagnosis.
- Supplemented with other tests, it helps establish the cause of hypertension.
- Can categorize essential hypertension according to renin levels (low, normal, or high) to allow for appropriate therapy.
- Indexing renin levels against urinary sodium excretion can help identify primary aldosteronism (sodium-depleted result can confirm this).
- Renin secretion from the kidneys is the first stage of the renin-angiotensin-aldosterone cycle, which controls the body's sodium-potassium balance, fluid volume, and blood pressure.
- Renin is released into renal veins in response to sodium depletion and blood loss.
- Renin catalyzes the conversion of angiotensinogen to angiotensin I, which in turn is converted to angiotensin II, a vasoconstrictor that stimulates aldosterone production in the adrenal cortex.
- When present in excessive amounts, angiotensin II causes renal hypertension.
- Plasma renin activity (PRA) is measured by radio-immunoassay of a peripheral or renal blood sample; results are expressed as the rate of angiotensin I formation per unit of time.
- Patient preparation is crucial; may take up to 1 month.

Purpose

- To screen for renal origin of hypertension
- To help plan treatment of essential hypertension, a genetic disease commonly aggravated by excess sodium intake
- To help identify hypertension linked to unilateral (sometimes bilateral) renovascular disease by renal vein catheterization
- To help identify primary aldosteronism (Conn's syndrome) resulting from an aldosterone-secreting adrenal adenoma
- To confirm primary aldosteronism (sodium-depleted plasma renin test)

Procedure

Preparation

- Explain to the patient that this test helps determine the cause of hypertension.
- Tell the patient that the test requires a blood sample. Explain who will perform the venipuncture and when.
- Tell the patient that the procedure will occur in the X-ray department and that he'll receive a local anesthetic.

- Notify the laboratory and physician of drugs the patient is taking that may affect test results; it may be necessary to restrict them.
- The patient shouldn't receive radioactive treatments for several days before the test.
- Tell the patient to maintain a normal sodium diet (3 g/day) during this period.
- For the sodium-depleted plasma renin test, tell the patient that he'll receive furosemide (or, if he has angina or cerebrovascular insufficiency, chlorothiazide) and will follow a specific low-sodium diet for 3 days.
- If the patient is to receive a recumbent sample, instruct him to remain in bed at least 2 hours before the test. (Posture influences renin secretion.)
- If the patient is to receive an upright sample, instruct him to stand or sit upright for 2 hours before the test.
- If the patient is to receive renal vein catheterization, make sure he has signed an informed consent form.
- Explain to the patient that he may experience slight discomfort from the tourniquet and the needle puncture. Collect a morning sample, if possible.

Implementation

- For a peripheral vein sample, perform a venipuncture and collect the sample in a 4-ml ethylenediaminetetraacetic acid tube.
- Note on the laboratory request whether the patient was fasting and whether he was upright or supine during peripheral vein sample collection.
- Because renin is unstable, the sample must be drawn into a chilled syringe and collection tube, placed on ice, and sent to the laboratory immediately.
- Completely fill the collection tube and invert it gently several times to mix the sample and the anticoagulant.
- In renal vein catheterization, a catheter is advanced to the kidneys through the femoral vein under fluoroscopic control, and samples are obtained from the renal veins and vena cava.

Patient care

- Apply direct pressure to the peripheral venipuncture site until bleeding stops.
- After renal vein catheterization, apply pressure to the catheterization site for 10 to 20 minutes to prevent extravasation.

> ◢ *ALERT Monitor vital signs and check the catheterization site every 30 minutes for 2 hours and then every hour for 4 hours to ensure that the bleeding has stopped. Check the patient's distal pulse for signs of thrombus formation and arterial occlusion (cyanosis, loss of pulse, cool skin).*

- Both methods: Instruct the patient that he may resume his usual diet and medications stopped before the test.

Complications

- Hematoma at the venipuncture site

Interpretation

Normal results

○ PRA and aldosterone levels decrease with age.

Sodium-depleted, upright, peripheral vein

○ For ages 18 to 39, 2.9 to 24 nanograms/ml/hour; mean, 10.8 nanograms/ml/hour

○ For age 40 and over, 2.9 to 10.8 nanograms/ml/hour; mean, 5.9 nanograms/ml/hour

Sodium-replete, upright, peripheral vein

○ For ages 18 to 39, less than or equal to 0.6 to 4.3 nanograms/ml/hour; mean, 1.9 nanograms/ml/hour

○ For age 40 and over, less than or equal to 0.6 to 3.0 nanograms/ml/hour; mean, 1 nanogram/ml/hour

Renal vein catheterization

○ The renal venous–renin ratio (the renin level in the renal vein compared with the level in the inferior vena cava) is less than 1.5 to 1.

Abnormal results

○ Elevated renin levels may occur in essential hypertension (uncommon), malignant and renovascular hypertension, cirrhosis, hypokalemia, hypovolemia caused by hemorrhage, renin-producing renal tumors (Bartter syndrome), and adrenal hypofunction (Addison's disease).

○ High renin levels may also be found in chronic renal failure with parenchymal disease, end-stage renal disease, and transplant rejection.

○ Decreased renin levels may indicate hypervolemia caused by a high-sodium diet, salt-retaining steroids, primary aldosteronism, Cushing's syndrome, licorice ingestion syndrome, or essential hypertension with low renin levels.

○ High serum and urine aldosterone levels with low plasma renin activity help identify primary aldosteronism.

○ In the sodium-depleted renin test, low plasma renin confirms this and differentiates it from secondary aldosteronism (characterized by increased renin).

Interfering factors

○ Failure to observe pretest restrictions

○ Improper patient position

○ Failure to use the proper anticoagulant in the collection tube, to completely fill it, or to adequately mix the sample and the anticoagulant (ethylenediaminetetraacetic acid helps preserve angiotensin I, but heparin doesn't)

○ Failure to chill the collection tube, syringe, and sample or to send the sample to the laboratory immediately

○ Salt intake, severe blood loss, licorice ingestion, hormonal contraceptives, pregnancy, and therapy with diuretics, antihypertensives, or vasodilators (increase)

○ Salt-retaining corticosteroid therapy and antidiuretic therapy (decrease)

○ Radioisotope use within several days before the test

Plasma thrombin time

Overview

○ Measures how quickly a clot forms when a standard amount of bovine thrombin is added to a platelet-poor plasma sample from the patient and to a normal plasma control sample
○ Allows a quick but imprecise estimation of plasma fibrinogen levels, which are a function of clotting time
○ Also called *thrombin clotting time*

Purpose

○ To detect a fibrinogen deficiency or defect
○ To aid in the diagnosis of disseminated intravascular coagulation (DIC) and hepatic disease
○ To monitor the effectiveness of treatment with heparin or thrombolytic agents

Procedure

Preparation

○ Explain to the patient that the plasma thrombin time test determines whether blood clots normally.
○ Notify the laboratory and physician of drugs the patient is taking that may affect test results; it may be necessary to restrict them.
○ Tell the patient that the test requires a blood sample. Explain who will perform the venipuncture and when.
○ Explain to the patient that he may feel slight discomfort from the tourniquet and the needle puncture.
○ Inform the patient that he need not restrict food and fluids.

Implementation

○ Perform a venipuncture and collect the sample in a 3- to 4.5-ml siliconized tube.
○ Completely fill the collection tube and invert it gently several times to mix the sample and the anticoagulant thoroughly. If the tube isn't filled to the correct volume, an excess of citrate appears in the sample.
○ To prevent hemolysis, avoid excessive probing during venipuncture and rough handling of the sample.
○ Immediately put the sample on ice and send it to the laboratory.

Patient care

○ Make sure that bleeding has stopped before removing pressure.
○ Tell the patient that he may resume medications stopped before the test.
○ If a large hematoma develops at the venipuncture site, monitor pulses distal to the site.

Complications

○ Hematoma at the venipuncture site

Interpretation

Normal results

○ 10 to 15 seconds (SI, 10 to 15 s)

Abnormal results

○ A prolonged thrombin time may indicate heparin therapy, hepatic disease, DIC, hypofibrinogenemia, or dysfibrinogenemia.
○ The patient with a prolonged thrombin time may require measurement of fibrinogen levels; in suspected DIC, the test for fibrin split products is also necessary.

Interfering factors

○ Failure to use the proper anticoagulant, to mix the sample and the anticoagulant adequately, or to send the sample to the laboratory properly
○ Hemolysis from rough handling of the sample or from excessive probing at the venipuncture site
○ Heparin, fibrinogen, or fibrin degradation products (possible increase)

Platelet count

Overview

- Tests function of platelets, or *thrombocytes,* which promote coagulation and formation of a hemostatic plug in vascular injury
- Determines ability of patient's blood to clot normally

Purpose

- To evaluate platelet production
- To assess the effects of chemotherapy or radiation therapy on platelet production
- To diagnose and monitor severe thrombocytosis or thrombocytopenia
- To confirm a visual estimate of platelet number and morphology from a stained blood film

Procedure

Preparation

- Explain to the patient that the platelet count test determines whether the patient's blood clots normally.
- Tell the patient that the test requires a blood sample. Explain who will perform the venipuncture and when.
- Notify the laboratory and physician of drugs the patient is taking that may affect test results; it may be necessary to restrict them.
- Inform the patient that he need not restrict food and fluids.
- Explain to the patient that he may feel slight discomfort from the tourniquet and the needle puncture.

Implementation

- Perform a venipuncture and collect the sample in a 3- or 4.5-ml ethylenediaminetetraacetic acid tube.
- To prevent hemolysis, avoid excessive probing at the venipuncture site and handle the sample gently.
- Completely fill the collection tube and invert it gently several times to mix the sample and the anticoagulant thoroughly.

Patient care

- Make sure that subdermal bleeding has stopped before removing pressure.
- Tell the patient that he may resume any medications stopped before the test.
- If a large hematoma develops, monitor pulses distal to the venipuncture site.

Complications

- Hematoma at the venipuncture site

Interpretation

Normal results

- Adults, 140,000 to 400,000/µl (SI, 140 to 400 $\times$ 10^9/L)
- Children, 150,000 to 450,000/µl (SI, 150 to 450 $\times$ 10^9/L)

Abnormal results

- A count below 50,000/µl can cause spontaneous bleeding; when the count is below 5,000/µl, fatal central nervous system bleeding or massive GI hemorrhage is possible.
- A decreased count (thrombocytopenia, 80 to 100 million platelets per ml) can result from aplastic or hypoplastic bone marrow; infiltrative bone marrow disease, such as leukemia, or disseminated infection; megakaryocytic hypoplasia; ineffective thrombopoiesis caused by folic acid or vitamin B$_{12}$ deficiency; pooling of platelets in an enlarged spleen; increased platelet destruction caused by drugs or immune disorders; disseminated intravascular coagulation; Bernard-Soulier syndrome; or mechanical injury to platelets.
- An increased count (thrombocytosis) can result from hemorrhage, infectious disorders, iron deficiency anemia, recent surgery, pregnancy, splenectomy, or inflammatory disorders. In such cases, the platelet count returns to normal after the patient recovers from the primary disorder.
- An increased count remains elevated in primary thrombocythemia, myelofibrosis with myeloid metaplasia, polycythemia vera, and chronic myelogenous leukemia.
- Whenever the platelet count is abnormal, diagnosis usually requires complete blood count, bone marrow biopsy, direct antiglobulin test (direct Coombs' test), and serum protein electrophoresis for confirmation.

Interfering factors

- Failure to use the proper anticoagulant or to mix the sample and anticoagulant promptly and adequately
- Hemolysis from rough handling of the sample or excessive probing at the venipuncture site
- Heparin (decrease)
- Acetazolamide, acetohexamide, antineoplastics, brompheniramine maleate, carbamazepine, chloramphenicol, ethacrynic acid, furosemide, gold salts, hydroxychloroquine, indomethacin, isoniazid, mephenytoin, mefenamic acid, methazolamide, methimazole, methyldopa, oral diazoxide, penicillamine, penicillin, phenylbutazone, phenytoin, pyrimethamine, quinidine sulfate, quinine, salicylates, streptomycin, sulfonamides, thiazide and thiazide-like diuretics, and tricyclic antidepressants (possible decrease)
- High altitudes, persistent cold temperatures, strenuous exercise, or excitement (increase)

Pleural fluid analysis

Overview

○ Analyzes a specimen of pleural fluid collected during pleural fluid aspiration (*thoracentesis*)

Purpose

○ To determine the cause and nature of pleural effusion
○ To permit better radiographic visualization of a lung with large effusions

Procedure

Preparation

○ Explain to the patient that this test assesses the space around the lungs for fluid.
○ Inform the patient that he need not restrict food and fluids.
○ Check the patient's history for hypersensitivity to local anesthetics.
○ Warn the patient that he may feel a stinging sensation on injection of the anesthetic and some pressure during withdrawal of the fluid.

Implementation

○ Shave the area around the needle insertion site.
○ Position the patient to widen the intercostal spaces and to allow easier access to the pleural cavity.
○ Make sure that the patient is well-supported and comfortable, preferably seated at the edge of the bed with a chair or stool supporting his feet, and his head and arms resting on a padded overbed table.
○ If the patient can't sit up, position him on his unaffected side, with the arm on the affected side elevated above his head.
○ Remind the patient not to cough, breathe deeply, or move suddenly during the procedure.
○ After positioning, the physician disinfects the skin, drapes the area, injects a local anesthetic into the subcutaneous tissue, and inserts the thoracentesis needle above the rib to avoid lacerating intercostal vessels.
○ When the needle reaches the pocket of fluid, the 50-ml syringe is attached and the stopcock and clamps are opened on the tubing to aspirate the fluid into the container.
○ During aspiration, observe for signs of respiratory distress.
○ After the needle is withdrawn, apply slight pressure and a small adhesive bandage to the puncture site.
○ Label the specimen container and record the date and time of the test; the amount, color, and character of the fluid; and the exact location from which fluid was removed.

○ Note the patient's temperature and whether he's receiving antimicrobial therapy on the laboratory request.

Patient care

○ Reposition the patient comfortably on the affected side. Tell him to remain on this side for at least 1 hour to seal the puncture site.
○ Elevate the head of the bed to facilitate breathing.
○ Monitor vital signs every 30 minutes for 2 hours and then every 4 hours until stable.
○ Tell the patient to call a nurse immediately if he experiences difficulty breathing.
○ Watch for signs of pneumothorax, tension pneumothorax, fluid reaccumulation, and — if a large amount of fluid was withdrawn — pulmonary edema or cardiac distress caused by mediastinal shift.
○ The patient receives a posttest X-ray to detect these complications before clinical symptoms appear.
○ Check the puncture site for fluid leakage.

Complications

○ Pneumothorax; tension pneumothorax

Interpretation

Normal results

○ Pressure is negative and less than 20 ml of serous fluid.

Abnormal results

○ Exudate is a protein-rich fluid leaked from blood vessels with increased permeability.
○ Pleural fluid may contain blood (hemothorax), chyle (chylothorax), or pus (empyema) and necrotic tissue.
○ Blood-tinged fluid may indicate a traumatic tap; the fluid should clear as aspiration progresses.
○ Transudative effusion usually results from diminished colloidal pressure, increased negative pressure within the pleural cavity, ascites, systemic and pulmonary venous hypertension, heart failure, hepatic cirrhosis, and nephritis.
○ Exudative effusion results from disorders that increase pleural capillary permeability, lymphatic drainage interference, infections, pulmonary infarctions, and neoplasms.
○ Exudative effusion with depressed glucose levels, elevated lactate dehydrogenase (LD) isoenzymes, rheumatoid arthritis cells, and negative smears, cultures, and cytologic examination may indicate pleurisy linked to rheumatoid arthritis.
○ Cultures are usually positive during the early stages of infection.
○ Empyema may result from complications of pneumonia, pulmonary abscess, perforation of the esophagus, or penetration from mediastinitis.
○ High percentage of neutrophils suggests septic inflammation.

- Lymphocytes suggest tuberculosis or fungal or viral effusions.
- Serosanguineous fluid suggests pleural extension of a malignant tumor.
- Elevated LD in a nonpurulent, nonhemolyzed, non-bloody effusion may also suggest malignancy.
- Pleural fluid glucose levels 30 to 40 mg/dl lower than blood glucose levels may indicate a malignant tumor, a bacterial infection, nonseptic inflammation, or metastasis.
- Increased amylase levels occur in pleural effusions associated with pancreatitis.

Interfering factors

- Antimicrobial therapy before fluid aspiration for culture

Potassium, serum

Overview

- Measures serum levels of potassium, a major intracellular cation that helps maintain cellular osmotic equilibrium; regulates muscle activity, enzyme activity, and acid-base balance; and influences renal function.
- Kidneys excrete nearly all ingested potassium, even when the body's supply is depleted; potassium deficiency can develop rapidly and is quite common.
- Potassium levels are affected by variations in secretions of adrenal steroid hormones and by fluctuations in pH, serum glucose levels, and serum sodium levels.
- Reciprocal relationship exists between potassium and sodium; a substantial intake of one element causes a corresponding decrease in the other.
- Dietary potassium intake of at least 40 mEq/day is essential; average diet usually includes 60 to 100 mEq of potassium.

Purpose

- To evaluate clinical signs of potassium excess (*hyperkalemia*) or potassium depletion (*hypokalemia*)
- To monitor renal function, acid-base balance, and glucose metabolism
- To evaluate neuromuscular and endocrine disorders
- To detect the origin of arrhythmias

Procedure

Preparation

- Explain to the patient that the serum potassium test determines the potassium content of blood.
- Tell the patient that the test requires a blood sample. Explain who will perform the venipuncture and when.
- Explain to the patient that he may experience slight discomfort from the tourniquet and the needle puncture.
- Inform the patient that he need not restrict food and fluids.
- Notify the laboratory and physician of drugs the patient is taking that may affect test results; it may be necessary to restrict them.

Implementation

- Perform a venipuncture and collect the sample in a 3- or 4-ml clot-activator tube.
- Draw the sample immediately after applying the tourniquet because a delay may increase the potassium level by allowing intracellular potassium to leak into the serum.
- Handle the sample gently to prevent hemolysis.

Patient care

- Apply direct pressure to the venipuncture site until bleeding stops.
- Instruct the patient to resume any medications stopped before the test.
- Observe the patient with hyperkalemia for weakness, malaise, nausea, diarrhea, colicky pain, muscle irritability progressing to flaccid paralysis, oliguria, and bradycardia. The electrocardiogram (ECG) reveals flattened P waves; a prolonged PR interval; a wide QRS complex; tall, tented T waves; and ST-segment depression. Cardiac arrest may occur without warning.

> *ALERT Observe the patient with hypokalemia for decreased reflexes; a rapid, weak, irregular pulse; mental confusion; hypotension; anorexia; muscle weakness; and paresthesia. The ECG shows a flattened T wave, ST-segment depression, and U-wave elevation. In severe cases, ventricular fibrillation, respiratory paralysis, and cardiac arrest can develop.*

Complications

- Hematoma at the venipuncture site

Interpretation

Normal results

- 3.5 to 5 mEq/L (SI, 3.5 to 5 mmol/L)

Abnormal results

- Hyperkalemia develops when excess cellular potassium enters the blood, such as in burn injuries, crush injuries, diabetic ketoacidosis, transfusions of large amounts of blood, and myocardial infarction; or when sodium excretion is reduced, possibly because of renal failure (preventing normal exchange of sodium and potassium) or Addison's disease (because of potassium buildup and sodium depletion).
- Hypokalemia may occur in aldosteronism or Cushing's syndrome, loss of body fluids (such as long-term diuretic therapy, vomiting, or diarrhea), and excessive licorice ingestion.
- Although serum values and clinical symptoms can indicate a potassium imbalance, an ECG allows a definitive diagnosis.

Interfering factors

- Repeated clenching of the fist before venipuncture (possible increase)
- Delay in drawing blood after applying a tourniquet or excessive hemolysis of the sample (increase)
- Excessive or rapid potassium infusion, spironolactone or penicillin G potassium therapy, and renal toxicity from administration of amphotericin B, methicillin, or tetracycline (increase)
- Insulin and glucose administration; diuretic therapy (especially with thiazides but not with triamterene, amiloride, or spironolactone); and I.V. infusions without potassium (decrease)

Potassium, urine

Overview

○ Quantitative measurement of urine levels of potassium, a major intracellular cation that helps regulate acid-base balance and neuromuscular function.
○ Potassium imbalance may cause muscle weakness, nausea, diarrhea, confusion, hypotension, and electrocardiogram changes; severe imbalance may lead to cardiac arrest.
○ May be performed to evaluate abnormally low potassium levels (*hypokalemia*) discovered by serum potassium test results, if cause of imbalance is still unknown.
○ If results suggest a renal disorder, additional renal function tests may be necessary.

Purpose

○ To determine whether hypokalemia is caused by renal or extrarenal disorders

Procedure

Preparation

○ Explain to the patient that the urine potassium test evaluates kidney function.
○ Advise the patient that no special dietary restrictions are necessary.
○ Tell the patient that the test requires urine collection over a 24-hour period.
○ If the patient is to collect the specimen at home, teach him the correct collection technique.
○ Notify the laboratory and physician of drugs the patient is taking that may affect test results; it may be necessary to restrict them.

Implementation

○ Collect the patient's urine over a 24-hour period, discarding the first specimen and retaining the last.
○ Give the patient potassium supplements and monitor serum levels as appropriate.
○ Instruct the patient not to use a metallic bedpan for collection.
○ Tell the patient not to contaminate the specimen with toilet tissue or feces.
○ Refrigerate the specimen or place it on ice during the collection period.
○ Send the specimen to the laboratory immediately after the collection is complete, or refrigerate it.

Patient care

○ Provide dietary supplements and nutritional counseling as necessary.
○ Replace fluid volume loss with I.V. or oral fluids as necessary.
○ Instruct the patient that he may resume his usual medications.

Complications

None known

Interpretation

Normal results

○ In adults, 25 to 125 mmol/24 hours (SI, 25 to 125 mmol/d), varying with diet
○ In children, 22 to 57 mmol/24 hours (SI, 22 to 57 mmol/d)

Abnormal results

○ In a patient with hypokalemia, a potassium level less than 10 mmol/24 hours (SI, < 10 mmol/d) suggests normal renal function, indicating that potassium loss is most likely the result of a GI disorder such as malabsorption syndrome.
○ In a patient with hypokalemia lasting more than 3 days, urine potassium level above 10 mmol/24 hours (SI, >10 mmol/d) indicates renal loss of potassium.
○ Renal potassium losses may result from such disorders as aldosteronism, renal tubular acidosis, or chronic renal failure.
○ Extrarenal disorders, such as dehydration, starvation, Cushing's disease, or salicylate intoxication, may elevate urine potassium levels.

Interfering factors

○ Excess dietary potassium (increase)
○ Contamination of the specimen with toilet tissue or feces
○ Failure to collect all urine and send the specimen to the laboratory immediately after collection or to refrigerate it
○ Potassium-wasting drugs, such as ammonium chloride, thiazide diuretics, and acetazolamide (increase)
○ Excess vomiting or stomach suctioning

Proctosigmoidoscopy

Overview

○ Endoscopic examination of the lining of the distal sigmoid colon, the rectum, and the anal canal.
○ Three separate steps: digital examination, sigmoidoscopy, and proctoscopy.
○ Specimens obtained from suspicious areas of the mucosa by biopsy, lavage or cytology brush, or culture swab.

Purpose

○ To aid in the diagnosis of inflammatory, infectious, and ulcerative bowel disease
○ To diagnose hemorrhoids, hypertrophic anal papilla, polyps, fissures, fistulas, and abscesses within the rectum and anal canal
○ To evaluate recent changes in bowel habits, lower abdominal and perineal pain, prolapse on defecation, pruritus ani, or passage of mucus, blood, or pus in feces

Procedure

Preparation

○ Make sure the patient has signed an appropriate consent form.
○ Note and report all allergies.
○ Check the patient's history for barium tests within the past week.
○ Instruct the patient to maintain a clear liquid diet for 24 to 48 hours before the test as ordered.
○ Explain the need for fasting the morning of the procedure.
○ Explain the need for administration of an enema 3 to 4 hours before the procedure.
○ Explain the need for sedation to help the patient relax.
○ Warn about a possible urge to defecate during insertion of the scope.
○ Advise the patient that air may be introduced through the endoscope to distend the walls of the intestine. Flatus may escape around the endoscope, and he shouldn't attempt to control it.
○ Warn about possible blood in the feces if a biopsy or polypectomy is performed.

Implementation

○ The patient is placed in a knee-to-chest or left lateral position with his knees flexed.
○ The patient is asked to breathe deeply and slowly through his mouth.
○ A well-lubricated, gloved index finger is inserted into the anus.
○ Anal canal is palpated for induration and tenderness.
○ The rectal mucosa is palpated.

○ The sigmoidoscope is inserted into the anus and passed through the anal sphincters, anal canal, and into the rectum.
○ At the rectosigmoid junction, a small amount of air may be insufflated to open the bowel lumen.
○ The scope is advanced to its full length into the distal sigmoid colon.
○ As the sigmoidoscope is slowly withdrawn, air is carefully insufflated and the intestinal mucosa is thoroughly examined.
○ Specimens may be obtained from a suspicious area of the intestinal mucosa.
○ Polyps may be removed for histologic examination by insertion of an electrocautery snare through the sigmoidoscope.
○ After the sigmoidoscope is withdrawn, the proctoscope is inserted through the anus and gently advanced to its full length.
○ After examination, the proctoscope is withdrawn.

Patient care

○ Instruct the patient to resume his previous diet and activities when fully awake.
○ Monitor vital signs and intake and output.
○ Observe the patient closely for signs of bowel perforation (abdominal distention and pain, nausea, vomiting, and fever) and for vasovagal reaction (hypotension, pallor, diaphoresis, and bradycardia).

Complications

○ Rectal bleeding
○ Bowel perforation

Interpretation

Normal results

○ Mucosa of the sigmoid colon is light pink-orange and marked by semilunar folds and deep tubular pits.
○ The rectal mucosa appears redder because of its rich vascular network, deepens to purple at the pectinate line (the anatomic division between the rectum and anus), and has three distinct valves.
○ The lower two-thirds of the anus (anoderm) is lined with smooth gray-tan skin and joins with the hair-fringed perianal skin.

Abnormal results

○ Biopsy results may suggest the presence of malignant tumors.
○ Inflammatory changes suggest possible ulcerative and ischemic colitis.
○ Visual examination and palpation may disclose possible abnormalities of the anal canal and rectum, including internal and external hemorrhoids, hypertrophic anal papillae, anal fissures and fistulas, or anorectal abscesses.

Interfering factors

○ Barium in the colon from previous barium studies

Progesterone, plasma

Overview

- This radioimmunoassay is a quantitative analysis of plasma progesterone levels and provides reliable information about corpus luteum function in fertility studies and placental function in pregnancy.
- Serial determinations are recommended.
- Although plasma levels provide accurate information, progesterone can also be monitored by measuring urine pregnanediol, a catabolite of progesterone.
- Progesterone, an ovarian steroid hormone secreted by the corpus luteum, causes thickening and secretory development of the endometrium in preparation for implantation of the fertilized ovum.
- Progesterone levels, therefore, peak during the mid-luteal phase of the menstrual cycle; if implantation doesn't occur, progesterone (and estrogen) levels drop sharply and menstruation begins about 2 days later.
- During pregnancy, the placenta releases about 10 times the normal monthly amount of progesterone to maintain the pregnancy; increased secretion begins toward the end of the first trimester and continues until delivery.
- Progesterone prevents abortion by decreasing uterine contractions.
- Along with estrogen, progesterone helps prepare the breasts for lactation.

Purpose

- To assess corpus luteum function as part of infertility studies
- To evaluate placental function during pregnancy
- To aid in confirming ovulation; test results support basal body temperature readings

Procedure

Preparation

- Explain to the patient that this test helps determine if her female sex hormone secretion is normal.
- Inform the patient that she need not restrict food and fluids.
- Tell the patient that the test requires a blood sample. Explain who will perform the venipuncture and when.
- Explain to the patient that she may experience slight discomfort from the tourniquet and the needle puncture.
- Inform the patient that the test may be repeated at specific times coinciding with phases of her menstrual cycle or with each prenatal visit.
- Check the patient's history to determine if she's taking drugs that may interfere with test results, including progesterone and estrogen. Note your findings on the laboratory request.

Implementation

- Perform a venipuncture and collect the sample in a 7-ml heparinized tube.
- Handle the sample gently to prevent hemolysis.
- Completely fill the collection tube; then invert it gently at least 10 times to mix the sample and the anticoagulant adequately.
- Indicate the date of the patient's last menses and the phase of her cycle on the laboratory request. If the patient is pregnant, also indicate the month of gestation.
- Send the sample to the laboratory immediately.

Patient care

- Apply direct pressure to the venipuncture site until bleeding stops.

Complications

- Hematoma at the venipuncture site

Interpretation

Normal results

- During menstruation, follicular phase, < 150 nanograms/dl (SI, < 5nmol/L); luteal phase, 300 to 1,200 nanograms/dl (SI, 10 to 40 nmol/L)
- During pregnancy, first trimester, 1,500 to 5,000 nanograms/dl (SI, 50 to 160 nmol/L); second and third trimesters, 8,000 to 20,000 nanograms/dl (SI, 250 to 650 nmol/L)
- In menopausal women, 10 to 22 nanograms/dl (SI, 0 to 2 nmol/L)

Abnormal results

- Elevated progesterone levels may indicate ovulation, luteinizing tumors, ovarian cysts that produce progesterone, or adrenocortical hyperplasia and tumors that produce progesterone along with other steroidal hormones.
- Low progesterone levels are associated with amenorrhea because of several causes (such as panhypopituitarism and gonadal dysfunction), eclampsia, threatened abortion, and fetal death.

Interfering factors

- Hemolysis from rough handling of the sample
- Progesterone or estrogen therapy
- Radioactive scans performed within 1 week of the test

Prolactin, serum

Overview

○ Quantitative radioimmunoassay to analyze serum levels of prolactin, a polypeptide hormone secreted by the anterior pituitary gland, which normally rise 10- to 20-fold during pregnancy, corresponding to accompanying elevations in human placental lactogen levels.
○ Used in patients who may have pituitary tumors, which secrete excessive amounts of prolactin.
○ Evaluates hypothalamic dysfunction, like the thyrotropin-releasing hormone (TRH) stimulation test.
○ Prolactin acts directly on tissues, its levels rising in response to sleep and physical or emotional stress.
○ Prolactin is essential for develop the mammary glands to develop during pregnancy for breast-feeding and for stimulating and maintaining lactation postpartum.
○ After delivery, prolactin secretion falls to basal levels in mothers who don't breast-feed; however, prolactin secretion increases during breast-feeding, apparently as a result of a stimulus triggered by suckling that curtails the release of prolactin-inhibiting factor by the hypothalamus.
○ This, in turn, allows transient elevations of prolactin secretion by the pituitary gland.

Purpose

○ To facilitate diagnosis of pituitary dysfunction, possibly caused by pituitary adenoma
○ To aid in the diagnosis of hypothalamic dysfunction regardless of cause
○ To evaluate secondary amenorrhea and galactorrhea

Procedure

Preparation

○ Tell the patient that this test helps evaluate hormonal secretion.
○ Advise the patient to restrict food and fluids and limit physical activity for 12 hours before the test. Encourage her to relax for about 30 minutes before the test.
○ Tell the patient the test requires a blood sample. Explain who will perform the venipuncture and when.
○ Explain to the patient that she may experience slight discomfort from the tourniquet and the needle puncture.
○ Withhold drugs that may interfere with test results. If the patient must continue them, note this on the laboratory request.

Implementation

○ Perform a venipuncture at least 3 hours after the patient wakes; samples collected earlier are likely to show sleep-induced peak levels.
○ Collect the sample in a 7-ml clot-activator tube.
○ Handle the sample gently to prevent hemolysis.
○ Confirm slight elevations with repeat measurements on two other occasions.

Patient care

○ Apply direct pressure to the venipuncture site until bleeding stops.
○ Instruct the patient that she may resume her usual diet, activities, and medications stopped before the test.

Complications

○ Hematoma at the venipuncture site

Interpretation

Normal results

○ Levels are undetectable to 23 nanograms/ml (SI, 23 µg/L) in nonlactating women.
○ Levels normally rise 10- to 20-fold during pregnancy and, after delivery, fall to basal levels in mothers who don't breast-feed.
○ Prolactin secretion increases during breast-feeding.

Abnormal results

○ Abnormally high levels (100 to 300 nanograms/ml [SI, 100 to 300 µg/L]) suggest autonomous prolactin production by a pituitary adenoma, especially when amenorrhea or galactorrhea is present (Forbes-Albright syndrome).
○ Rarely, hyperprolactinemia may also result from severe endocrine disorders such as hypothyroidism.
○ Idiopathic hyperprolactinemia may be linked to anovulatory infertility.
○ Slight elevations require repeat measurements on two other occasions.
○ Decreased prolactin levels in a lactating mother cause failure of lactation and may be associated with postpartum pituitary infarction (Sheehan's syndrome).
○ Abnormally low prolactin levels have also occurred in the patient with empty sella syndrome. In these cases, a flattened pituitary gland makes the pituitary fossa look empty.

Interfering factors

○ Failure to take into account physiologic variations related to sleep or stress
○ Ethanol, morphine, methyldopa, and estrogens (increase)
○ Apomorphine, ergot alkaloids, and levodopa (decrease)
○ Radioactive scan performed within 1 week before the test or recent surgery
○ Breast stimulation
○ Hemolysis from rough handling of the sample

Prostate gland biopsy

Overview

○ Needle excision of a prostate tissue specimen for histologic examination
○ Three possible approaches: perineal, transrectal, or transurethral
○ Transrectal approach usually for high prostatic lesions

Purpose

○ To confirm prostate cancer
○ To determine cause of prostatic hypertrophy

Procedure

Preparation

○ Depending on the approach used, the patient may need to fast for 6 to 8 hours before the test.
○ Make sure the patient has signed an appropriate consent form.
○ Note and report all allergies.
○ For a transrectal approach, give enemas until the return is clear.
○ Give the patient antibiotics.
○ Give the patient a sedative before the study.
○ Explain the need to use a local anesthetic.
○ Explain that the test takes less than 30 minutes.

Implementation

Perineal approach
○ The patient is placed in the left lateral, knee-chest, or lithotomy position.
○ The perineal skin is cleaned and prepared; a 2-mm incision is made into the perineum.
○ The biopsy needle is introduced into a prostate lobe.
○ Specimens are obtained from several different areas of the prostate.
○ Specimens are placed immediately in a labeled specimen bottle containing 10% formalin solution.
○ Hemostasis is obtained, and a dressing applied.
Transrectal approach
○ The patient is placed in the left lateral position.
○ A curved needle guide (or a spring-powered device for cone biopsy) is attached to the finger palpating the rectum.
○ The biopsy needle is pushed along the guide, into the prostate.
○ The needle is rotated to cut the tissue and is then withdrawn.
Transurethral approach
○ An endoscopic instrument with a cutting loop is passed through the urethra.
○ The endoscope permits direct viewing of the prostate and passage of a cutting loop.

○ Specimens are obtained and placed immediately in a labeled specimen bottle containing 10% formalin solution.

Patient care

○ Give the patient an analgesic.
○ Instruct the patient to gradually resume his normal diet and activity, as tolerated.
○ Monitor vital signs and intake and output.
○ Watch for urinary retention and hematuria.
○ Observe the biopsy site for and immediately report hematoma and signs of infection, such as redness, swelling, and pain.

Complications

○ Bleeding into the prostatic urethra and bladder
○ Infection
○ Urinary retention

Interpretation

Normal results

○ A thin, fibrous capsule surrounds the stroma, which is made up of elastic and connective tissues and smooth-muscle fibers.
○ Epithelial glands that drain into the chief excreting ducts are evident.
○ No cancer cells are found.

Abnormal results

○ Increased acid phosphatase levels suggest possible metastatic prostate cancer.
○ Low acid phosphatase levels suggest possible cancer that is confined to the prostatic capsule.
○ Histologic examination of the tissue reveals various possible disorders, including prostate, rectal, and bladder cancer, benign prostatic hyperplasia, prostatitis, tuberculosis, or lymphomas.

Interfering factors

○ Failure to obtain an adequate tissue specimen may affect accuracy of results

Prostate-specific antigen

Overview

○ Measures level of prostate-specific antigen (PSA), which appears in normal, benign hyperplastic and malignant prostatic tissue, as well as in metastatic prostate cancer.
○ Measures PSA levels to monitor the spread or recurrence of stage B3 to D1 prostate cancer and evaluate the patient's response to treatment.
○ PSA level measurement and a digital rectal examination are recommended to screen men over age 50 for prostate cancer.

Purpose

○ To screen for prostate cancer in men over age 50
○ To monitor the course of prostate cancer and evaluate treatment

Procedure

Preparation

○ Explain to the patient that this test screens for prostate cancer or, if appropriate, monitors the course of treatment.
○ Tell the patient that this test requires a blood sample.
○ Explain to the patient that he may experience slight discomfort from the tourniquet and the needle puncture.
○ Inform the patient that he need not restrict food and fluids.

Implementation

○ Perform a venipuncture and collect the sample in a 7-ml clot-activator tube.
○ Collect the sample either before digital prostate examination or at least 48 hours after examination to avoid falsely elevated PSA levels.
○ Handle the sample gently to prevent hemolysis.
○ Immediately put the sample on ice and send it to the laboratory.

Patient care

○ Apply direct pressure to the venipuncture site until bleeding stops.

Complications

○ Hematoma at the venipuncture site

Interpretation

Normal results

○ Ages 40 to 50: 2 to 2.8 nanograms/ml (SI, 2 to 2.8 µg/L)
○ Ages 51 to 60: 2.9 to 3.8 nanograms/ml (SI, 2.9 to 3.8 µg/L)
○ Ages 61 to 70: 4 to 5.3 nanograms/ml (SI, 4 to 5.3 µg/L)
○ Ages 71 and older: 5.6 to 7.2 nanograms/ml (SI, 5.6 to 7.2 µg/L)

Abnormal results

○ About 80% of patients with prostate cancer have pretreatment PSA values greater than 4 nanograms/ml.
○ About 20% of patients with benign prostatic hyperplasia also have levels greater than 4 nanograms/ml.
○ PSA results alone don't confirm a diagnosis of prostate cancer. Further assessment and testing, including tissue biopsy, are necessary to confirm cancer.

Interfering factors

○ Hemolysis from rough handling of the sample
○ Excessive doses of chemotherapeutic drugs, such as cyclophosphamide, diethylstilbestrol, and methotrexate (possible increase or decrease)

Protein C

Overview

○ Measures the level of vitamin K–dependent protein C, which is produced in the liver and circulates in the plasma.
○ Deficiencies may be acquired or congenital; as a potent anticoagulant, protein C suppresses activated factors V and VIII. Once identified, a deficiency is further investigated to determine its type.
○ Identifying the role of protein C deficiency in idiopathic venous thrombosis may help prevent thromboembolism.

Purpose

○ To investigate the mechanism of idiopathic venous thrombosis
○ To prevent thromboembolism

Procedure

Preparation

○ Explain to the patient that the protein C test evaluates blood clotting.
○ Tell the patient that the test requires a blood sample. Explain who will perform the venipuncture and when.
○ Explain to the patient that he may feel slight discomfort from the tourniquet and the needle puncture.
○ Inform the patient that he need not restrict food and fluids.
○ Notify the laboratory and physician of drugs the patient is taking that may affect test results; it may be necessary to restrict them.

Implementation

○ Perform a venipuncture. Collect a 3-ml sample in a siliconized vacuum specimen tube or in a special syringe with anticoagulant provided by the laboratory.
○ Completely fill the collection tube and invert it several times to mix the sample and anticoagulant thoroughly; handle the sample gently.
○ Send the sample to the laboratory immediately.

Patient care

○ Tell the patient that he may resume any medications stopped before the test.
○ Apply direct pressure to the venipuncture site until bleeding stops.

Complications

○ Hematoma at the venipuncture site

Interpretation

Normal results

○ 70% to 140% (SI, 0.7 to 1.4)

Abnormal results

○ Rare, homozygous protein C deficiency is characterized by rapidly fatal thrombosis in the perinatal period, a condition known as *purpura fulminans*.
○ The more common heterozygous deficiency causes genetic susceptibility to venous thromboembolism before age 30 and throughout life. The patient may require long-term treatment with warfarin therapy or protein C supplements from plasma fractions.
○ Protein C deficiency is also seen in those with liver cirrhosis and vitamin K deficiency or taking warfarin.

Interfering factors

○ Hemolysis from excessive probing at the venipuncture site or from rough handling of the sample
○ Anticoagulant therapy

Prothrombin time

Overview

○ Measures the time required for a fibrin clot to form in a citrated plasma sample after addition of calcium ions and tissue thromboplastin (factor III)

Purpose

○ To evaluate the extrinsic coagulation system (factors V, VII, and X and prothrombin and fibrinogen)
○ To monitor response to oral anticoagulant therapy

Procedure

Preparation

○ Explain to the patient that the prothrombin time (PT) test determines whether the blood clots normally.
○ Notify the laboratory and physician of drugs the patient is taking that may affect test results; it may be necessary to restrict them.
○ Inform the patient that he need not restrict food and fluids.
○ Tell the patient that the test requires a blood sample. Explain who will perform the venipuncture and when.
○ Explain to the patient that he may feel slight discomfort from the tourniquet and the needle puncture.
○ When appropriate, explain that this test monitors the effects of oral anticoagulants; the test will occur daily when therapy begins and will be repeated at longer intervals when medication levels stabilize.

Implementation

○ Perform a venipuncture and collect the sample in a 3- or 4.5-ml siliconized tube.
○ Completely fill the collection tube and invert it gently several times to mix the sample and the anticoagulant thoroughly. If the tube isn't filled to the correct volume, an excess of citrate will appear in the sample.
○ To prevent hemolysis, avoid excessive probing during venipuncture and handle the sample gently.

Patient care

○ Make sure subdermal bleeding has stopped before removing pressure.
○ Instruct the patient that he may resume his usual diet and medications discontinued before the test.
○ If a large hematoma develops at the venipuncture site, monitor pulses distal to the site.

Complications

○ Hematoma at the venipuncture site

Interpretation

Normal results

○ PT should be 10 to 14 seconds (SI, 10 to 14 s), depending on the source of tissue thromboplastin and the type of sensing devices used to measure clot formation.
○ In a patient receiving oral anticoagulants, PT should be from 1 to 2½ times the normal control value.

Abnormal results

○ Prolonged PT may indicate deficiencies in fibrinogen, prothrombin, factors V, VII, or X (specific assays can pinpoint such deficiencies), or vitamin K. It may also result from ongoing oral anticoagulant therapy.
○ A prolonged PT that exceeds 2½ times the control value usually indicates abnormal bleeding.

Interfering factors

○ Failure to fill the collection tube completely (possible false-high)
○ Failure to adequately mix the sample and the anticoagulant or to send the sample to the laboratory promptly
○ Hemolysis from rough handling of the sample
○ Salicylates, more than 1 g/day (increase)
○ Fibrin or fibrin split products in the sample or plasma fibrinogen levels >100 mg/dl (possible prolonged PT)
○ Antihistamines, chloral hydrate, corticosteroids, digoxin, diuretics, glutethimide, griseofulvin, progestin-estrogen combinations, pyrazinamide, vitamin K, and xanthines, such as caffeine and theophylline (possible decrease)
○ Corticotropin, anabolic steroids, cholestyramine resin, heparin I.V. (within 5 hours of sample collection), indomethacin, mefenamic acid, para-aminosalicylic acid, methimazole, oxyphenbutazone, phenylbutazone, phenytoin, propylthiouracil, quinidine, quinine, thyroid hormones, vitamin A, or alcohol in excess (prolonged PT)
○ Antibiotics, barbiturates, hydroxyzine, sulfonamides, mineral oil, or clofibrate (possible increase or decrease)

Pulmonary angiography

Overview

○ Radiographically examines the pulmonary circulation after injection of a radiopaque contrast medium into the pulmonary artery or one of its branches
○ May diagnose pulmonary embolism (PE) when lung ventilation perfusion scans are indeterminate
○ May give local thrombolytic therapy in patients with PE
○ Also known as *pulmonary arteriography*

Purpose

○ To detect pulmonary embolism in a symptomatic patient with an equivocal lung scan
○ To evaluate pulmonary circulation abnormalities
○ To provide accurate preoperative evaluation of patients with shunt physiology caused by congenital heart disease
○ To treat identified PE with thrombolysis

Procedure

Preparation

○ Make sure the patient has signed an appropriate consent form.
○ Note and report all allergies.
○ Check the patient's history for hypersensitivity to iodine, seafood, or iodinated contrast media.
○ Check for and report history of anticoagulation.
○ Check for and report history of renal insufficiency.
○ Note and inform the physician of any abnormal laboratory results.
○ Instruct the patient to fast for 8 hours before the test.
○ Stop heparin infusion 3 to 4 hours before the test.
○ Explain the need to use a local anesthetic.
○ Warn the patient that he may have a possible urge to cough, a flushed feeling, or a salty taste for 3 to 5 minutes after the injection.
○ Explain that the test takes about 1½ to 2 hours
○ Explain that the patient will be monitored during the study.

Implementation

○ The patient is placed in the supine position.
○ The access site is cleaned and prepared, usually the right groin.
○ A local anesthetic is injected.
○ The vein is accessed and a catheter is introduced under image-guidance.
○ The catheter is advanced through the right atrium, the right ventricle, and into the pulmonary artery.
○ Pulmonary artery pressures are measured and blood samples may be drawn from various regions of the pulmonary circulation.
○ The contrast medium is injected and images are obtained.

○ Thrombolysis is initiated, if indicated.
○ After the catheter is removed, hemostasis is obtained.
○ The access site is cleaned and dressed.

Patient care

○ Maintain bed rest.
○ Have the patient resume his usual diet.
○ Restart anticoagulation.
○ Encourage the patient to drink fluids, or give I.V. fluids to help eliminate the contrast medium.
○ Monitor vital signs and intake and output.
○ Monitor renal function studies.
○ Monitor the patient for adverse reaction to the contrast medium.

▼ *ALERT Observe the site for bleeding and swelling. If these occur, maintain pressure at the insertion site for at least 10 minutes and notify the radiologist.*

Complications

○ Myocardial perforation or rupture
○ Ventricular arrhythmias and conduction defects
○ Acute renal failure
○ Bleeding and hematoma formation
○ Infection
○ Adverse reaction to the contrast medium
○ Cardiac valve damage
○ Right-sided heart failure

Interpretation

Normal results

○ The contrast medium flows symmetrically and without interruption through the pulmonary circulation.

Abnormal results

○ Interruption of blood flow and filling defects suggest possible acute pulmonary embolism.
○ Arterial webs, stenoses, irregular occlusions, wall-scalloping, and "pouching" defects (a concave edge of thrombus facing the opacified lumen) suggest chronic pulmonary embolism.

Interfering factors

None known

Pulmonary artery catheterization

Overview

○ Using a balloon-tipped, flow-directed catheter to provide intermittent occlusion of the pulmonary artery, permitting measurement of pulmonary artery pressure (PAP) and pulmonary artery wedge pressure (PAWP), which accurately reflects left atrial pressure and left ventricular end-diastolic pressure
○ Also known as *Swan-Ganz catheterization*

Purpose

○ To assess right- and left-sided heart failure
○ To monitor therapy for complications of acute myocardial infarction
○ To monitor fluid status in patients with serious burns, renal disease, noncardiogenic pulmonary edema, or adult respiratory distress syndrome
○ To establish baseline pressures preoperatively in patients with existing cardiac disease
○ To differentiate between noncardiac and cardiac pulmonary edema

Procedure

Preparation

○ Make sure the patient has signed an appropriate consent form.
○ Note and report all allergies.
○ Instruct the patient to restrict food and fluids before the test.
○ Explain the use of a local anesthetic.
○ Explain that the catheter will remain in place, causing little or no discomfort, for 48 to 72 hours.
○ Explain that the test takes about 30 minutes.

Implementation

○ The patient is placed in the supine position with his head and shoulders slightly lower than his trunk.
○ The catheter is introduced into the vein percutaneously.
○ The catheter is directed into the right atrium.
○ The catheter balloon is partially inflated.
○ Venous flow carries the catheter tip through the right atrium and tricuspid valve into the right ventricle and into the pulmonary artery.
○ The monitor is observed for characteristic pressure waveform changes as the catheter enters each heart chamber.
○ As the catheter is passed into the chambers on the right side of the heart, the monitor screen is observed for frequent premature ventricular contractions, ventricular tachycardia, and other arrhythmias. If arrhythmias occur, the catheter may be partially

withdrawn or medication given to suppress the arrhythmias.
○ For recording PAWP, the catheter balloon is carefully inflated with the specified amount of air (no more than 1.5 cc), until a PAWP waveform is obtained.
○ After PAWP is recorded, the air from the balloon is allowed to return to the syringe.
○ The monitor screen is observed for a pulmonary artery waveform.
○ The catheter may be sutured to the skin and a dressing applied.

⚠ *ALERT The balloon catheter shouldn't be overinflated, which could distend the pulmonary artery, causing vessel rupture. If the balloon can't be fully deflated after recording the PAWP, it shouldn't be reinflated unless the physician is present; balloon rupture can cause a life-threatening air embolism.*

Patient care

○ Obtain a chest X-ray to verify proper catheter placement and to assess for complications such as pneumothorax.
○ Monitor the patient's vital signs.
○ Watch for cardiac arrhythmias.
○ Monitor PAP and PAWP pressures and waveforms.
○ Monitor right atrial and right ventricular pressures and waveforms.
○ Monitor cardiac output.
○ Watch for infection of the insertion site and bleeding.
○ Watch for signs and symptoms of pulmonary emboli, pulmonary artery perforation, and arrhythmias.
○ Maintain 300 mm Hg pressure in the pressure bag to permit 3 to 6 ml/hour fluid flow to flush the system continuously.
○ Notify the physician if there is difficulty in flushing the system.
○ If a damped waveform occurs, it may be necessary to slightly withdraw the catheter; pulmonary infarct can occur if the catheter remains in a wedged position.

Complications

○ Pulmonary infarction
○ Ventricular arrhythmias
○ Air emboli
○ Infection and sepsis

Interpretation

Normal results

○ Right atrial (RA) pressure is 1 to 6 mm Hg.
○ Right ventricular (RV) systolic pressure is 20 to 30 mm Hg.
○ RV diastolic pressure is less than 5 mm Hg.
○ Systolic PAP is 20 to 30 mm Hg.
○ Diastolic PAP is 10 to 15 mm Hg.
○ Mean PAP is less than 20 mm Hg.
○ PAWP is 6 to 12 mm Hg.

Abnormal results

○ Elevated RA pressures may suggest pulmonary disease, right-sided heart failure, fluid overload, or cardiac tamponade.
○ Elevated RV pressures may suggest pulmonary hypertension, pulmonary valvular stenosis, right-sided heart failure, pericardial effusion, or ventricular septal defects.
○ Elevated PAP may suggest atrial or ventricular septal defects, pulmonary hypertension, mitral stenosis, chronic obstructive pulmonary disease, pulmonary edema or embolus, or left-sided heart failure.
○ Elevated PAWP may suggest left-sided heart failure or cardiac tamponade.
○ Decreased PAWP may suggest hypovolemia.

Interfering factors

○ Improper insertion

Pulmonary function tests

Overview

○ Evaluates pulmonary function through a series of spirometric measurements
○ Also known as *PFTs*

Purpose

○ To assess effectiveness of a specific therapeutic regimen
○ To evaluate pulmonary status

Procedure

Preparation

○ Make sure the patient has signed an appropriate consent form.
○ Note and report all allergies.
○ Stress the need for the patient to avoid smoking for 12 hours before the tests.
○ Withhold bronchodilators for 8 hours.
○ Stress the need to avoid a heavy meal before the tests.

Implementation

○ For tidal volume (V_T), the patient breathes normally into the mouthpiece 10 times.
○ For expiratory reserve volume (ERV), the patient breathes normally for several breaths and then exhales as completely as possible.
○ For vital capacity (VC), the patient inhales as deeply as possible and exhales into the mouthpiece as completely as possible. This is repeated three times, and the largest volume is recorded.
○ For inspiratory capacity (IC), the patient breathes normally for several breaths and inhales as deeply as possible.
○ For functional residual capacity (FRC), the patient breathes normally into a spirometer. After a few breaths, the levels of gas in the spirometer and in the lungs reach equilibrium. FRC is calculated by subtracting the spirometer volume from the original volume.
○ For forced vital capacity (FVC) and forced expiratory volume (FEV), the patient inhales as slowly and deeply as possible and then exhales into the mouthpiece as quickly and completely as possible. This is repeated three times, and the largest volume is recorded. The volume of air expired at 1 second (FEV_1), at 2 seconds (FEV_2), and at 3 seconds (FEV_3) during all three repetitions is recorded.
○ For maximal voluntary ventilation, the patient breathes into the mouthpiece as quickly and deeply as possible for 15 seconds.
○ For diffusing capacity for carbon monoxide, the patient inhales a gas mixture with a low level of carbon monoxide and holds his breath for 10 to 15 seconds before exhaling.

Patient care

○ Pulmonary function tests may be contraindicated in patients with acute coronary insufficiency, angina, or recent myocardial infarction. Watch for respiratory distress, changes in pulse rate and blood pressure, coughing, and bronchospasm in these patients.

Complications

○ Respiratory distress
○ Bronchospasm
○ Physical exhaustion

Interpretation

Normal results

○ Results are based on age, height, weight, and sex; values expressed as a percentage.
○ V_T is 5 to 7 mg/kg of body weight.
○ ERV is 25% of VC.
○ IC is 75% of VC.
○ FEV_1 is 83% of VC after 1 second.
○ FEV_2 is 94% of VC after 2 seconds.
○ FEV_3 is 97% of VC after 3 seconds.

Abnormal results

○ FEV_1 less than 80% suggests obstructed pulmonary disease.
○ FEV_1-to-FVC ratio greater than 80% suggests restrictive pulmonary disease.
○ Decreased V_T suggests possible restrictive disease.
○ Decreased minute volume (MV) suggests possible disorders such as pulmonary edema.
○ Increased MV suggests possible acidosis, exercise, or low compliance states.
○ Reduced CO_2 response suggests possible emphysema, myxedema, obesity, hypoventilation syndrome, or sleep apnea.
○ Residual volume greater than 35% of total lung capacity after maximal expiratory effort suggests obstructive disease.
○ Decreased IC suggests restrictive disease.
○ Increased FRC suggests possible obstructive pulmonary disease.
○ Low total lung capacity (TLC) suggests restrictive disease.
○ High TLC suggests obstructive disease.
○ Decreased FVC suggests flow resistance from obstructive disease or from restrictive disease.
○ Low forced expiratory flow suggests obstructive disease of the small and medium-sized airways.
○ Decreased peak expiratory flow rate suggests upper airway obstruction.
○ Decreased diffusing capacity for carbon monoxide suggests possible interstitial pulmonary disease.

Interfering factors

○ Chest pain, abdominal pain, or cough

Pure tone audiometry

Overview

○ Records lowest intensity levels at which a patient can hear a set of test tones about 50% of the time.
○ Test tones are introduced through earphones or a bone conduction vibrator.
○ Pure tones have energy concentrated at discrete frequencies and are compared with established norms of various frequencies.
○ Octave frequencies obtain air conduction thresholds.
○ Comparison of air and bone conduction thresholds suggests possible conductive, sensorineural, or mixed hearing loss but not its cause.
○ Pure tone average suggests need for referral to evaluate communication difficulties.

Purpose

○ To document a patient's auditory acuity
○ To determine the presence, type, and degree of hearing loss
○ To assess communication abilities and rehabilitation needs
○ To accurately determine pure tone and speech reception threshold

Procedure

Preparation

○ Make sure the patient has signed an appropriate consent form.
○ Note and report all allergies.
○ Obtain and document a complete aural history, including possible hearing loss, noise exposure, and use of hearing protection.
○ Instruct the patient to remove all potential obstructions (such as earrings) to permit proper earphone placement.
○ Explain the importance of responding to even faint tones.
○ Explain that the test takes about 20 minutes.

Implementation

○ The ear canal is checked for impacted cerumen.
○ The earphones are positioned and the headband tightened.
○ The examiner familiarizes the patient with the test tone by presenting it to his better ear at a level 15 to 25 dB above the expected threshold to avoid cross-hearing.
○ If the patient responds to the tone, air conduction testing begins.
○ After testing the better ear, the poorer ear is tested.
○ In each ear, test or retest differences may be ± 5 dB.
○ For bone conduction testing, the earphones are removed and a small plastic vibrator is placed on the mastoid process.

○ Ascending and descending tones are used as in air conduction testing, using 250 Hz, 500 Hz, 1,000 Hz, 2,000 Hz, and 4,000 Hz and 8,000 Hz.
○ An audiogram displays frequency on the x-axis (horizontal) and dB of hearing loss on the y-axis (vertical).

Patient care

○ Answer the patient's questions about the test.

Complications

None known

Interpretation

Normal results

○ Adults, -10 to $+15$ dB
○ Children, 0 to $+15$ dB

Abnormal results

○ Depressed threshold responses for air and bone conduction tones suggest sensorineural loss.
○ Depressed threshold responses for air and unchanged bone thresholds suggest conductive loss.
○ Abnormal threshold responses for air and bone conduction tones, with air conduction more depressed than bone conduction, suggest mixed hearing loss.

Interfering factors

○ False responses (including failure to indicate when a tone has been heard or responding when no tone has been heard)
○ A patient exposed to noises within the past 16 hours loud enough to cause tinnitus or make face-to-face communication difficult
○ Alcohol and other drugs
○ Faking results to get compensation

Pyruvate kinase

Overview

- Assay to confirm pyruvate kinase (PK) deficiency when red blood cell (RBC) enzyme deficiency may be causing a patient's anemia.
- Abnormally low PK level is an inherited autosomal recessive trait that may cause an RBC membrane defect resulting in congenital hemolytic anemia.
- PK helps in the anaerobic metabolism of glucose.

Purpose

- To differentiate PK-deficient hemolytic anemia from other congenital hemolytic anemias or from acquired hemolytic anemia
- To detect PK deficiency in asymptomatic, heterozygous inheritance

Procedure

Preparation

- Explain to the patient that this test detects inherited enzyme deficiencies.
- Inform the patient that he need not restrict food and fluids.
- Check the patient's history for recent blood transfusion and note it on the laboratory request.
- Tell the patient that the test requires a blood sample. Explain who will perform the venipuncture and when.
- Explain to the patient that he may experience slight discomfort from the tourniquet and the needle puncture.

Implementation

- Perform a venipuncture and collect the sample in a 4-ml ethylenediaminetetraacetic acid tube.
- Completely fill the collection tube and invert it gently several times to mix the sample and the anticoagulant.
- Handle the sample gently to prevent hemolysis.
- Send the sample to the laboratory immediately; otherwise, refrigerate it.

Patient care

- Apply direct pressure to the venipuncture site until bleeding stops.

Complications

- Hematoma at the venipuncture site

Interpretation

Normal results

- 9 to 22 units/g of hemoglobin (Hb); in the low substrate assay, 1.7 to 6.8 units/g of Hb

Abnormal results

- Low serum PK levels confirm a diagnosis of PK deficiency and allow differentiation between PK-deficient hemolytic anemia and other inherited disorders.

Interfering factors

- Hemolysis from rough handling of the sample

Quantitative immunoglobulins G, A, and M

Overview

- Measures levels of immunoglobulins (Igs) G, A, and M, proteins that function as specific antibodies in response to antigen stimulation, are responsible for the humoral aspects of immunity, and are normally present in serum in predictable percentages
- Detects deviations from normal immunoglobulin percentages, which may occur in many immune disorders, including cancer, hepatic disorders, rheumatoid arthritis, and systemic lupus erythematosus
- Using immunoelectrophoresis, identifies IgG, IgA, and IgM in a serum sample; measures the level of each by radial immunodiffusion or nephelometry (or by indirect immunofluorescence and radioimmunoassay)

Purpose

- To diagnose paraproteinemias, such as multiple myeloma and Waldenström's macroglobulinemia
- To detect hypogammaglobulinemia and hypergammaglobulinemia as well as nonimmunologic diseases, such as cirrhosis and hepatitis, that are linked to abnormally high immunoglobulin levels
- To assess the effectiveness of chemotherapy and radiation therapy

Procedure

Preparation

- Explain to the patient that this test measures antibody levels.
- If appropriate, tell the patient that the test evaluates the effectiveness of treatment.
- Check the patient's history for drugs that may affect test results.
- Be aware that alcohol or narcotic abuse may affect results.
- Instruct the patient to restrict food and fluids, except for water, for 12 to 14 hours before the test.
- Tell the patient that the test requires a blood sample.
- Explain to the patient that he may experience slight discomfort from the needle puncture and the tourniquet.

Implementation

- Perform a venipuncture and collect the sample in a 7-ml clot-activator tube.
- Send the sample to the laboratory immediately to prevent immunoglobulin deterioration.

Patient care

- Apply direct pressure to the venipuncture site until bleeding stops.
- Instruct the patient that he may resume his usual diet and medications stopped before the test.
- Advise the patient with abnormally low immunoglobulin levels (especially IgG or IgM) to protect himself against bacterial infection. When caring for such a patient, watch for signs of infection, such as fever, chills, rash, and skin ulcers.
- Instruct the patient with abnormally high immunoglobulin levels and symptoms of monoclonal gammopathies to report bone pain and tenderness. Such a patient has numerous antibody-producing malignant plasma cells in bone marrow, which hamper production of other blood components. Watch for signs of hypercalcemia, renal failure, and spontaneous pathologic fractures.

Complications

- Hematoma at the venipuncture site

Interpretation

Normal results

- With nephelometry, in adults, IgG: 800 to 1,800 mg/dl (SI, 8 to 18 g/L); IgA, 100 to 400 mg/dl (SI, 1 to 4 g/L); IgM, 55 to 150 mg/dl (SI, 0.55 to 1.5 g/L)
- IgG is 75% of serum immunoglobulins, including the warm-temperature type; IgA, about 15% of the total; IgM, 5% to 7%, including cold agglutinins, rheumatoid factor, and ABO blood group isoagglutinins.

Abnormal results

- In congenital and acquired hypogammaglobulinemias, myelomas, and macroglobulinemia, the findings confirm the diagnosis.
- In hepatic and autoimmune diseases, leukemias, and lymphomas, such findings are less important, but they can support the diagnosis based on other tests, such as biopsies and white blood cell differential, and on the physical examination.

Interfering factors

- Radiation therapy or chemotherapy (possible decrease caused by suppressive effects on bone marrow)
- Aminophenazone, anticonvulsants, asparaginase, hydralazine, hydantoin derivatives, hormonal contraceptives, and phenylbutazone (possible increase)
- Methotrexate and severe hypersensitivity to bacille Calmette-Guérin vaccine (possible decrease)
- Dextrans and methylprednisolone (decrease in IgM levels)
- Dextrans and high doses of methylprednisolone and phenytoin (decrease in IgG and IgA levels)
- Methadone (increase in IgA levels)

Radioactive iodine uptake test

Overview

○ Evaluates thyroid function by measuring the amount of orally ingested iodine-123 (^{123}I) or iodine-131 (^{131}I) that accumulates in the thyroid gland after 2, 6, and 24 hours
○ Measures (using an external single counting probe) the radioactivity in the thyroid as a percentage of the original dose, thus indicating its ability to trap and retain iodine
○ Accurately diagnoses hyperthyroidism, but is less accurate for hypothyroidism
○ Performed with radionuclide thyroid imaging and the T_3 resin uptake test; helps differentiate Grave's disease from hyperfunctioning toxic adenoma
○ Indicated by abnormal results of chemical tests used to evaluate thyroid function
○ If Hashimoto's disease suspected, may add the perchlorate suppression test for verification of diagnosis

Purpose

○ To evaluate thyroid function
○ To help diagnose hyperthyroidism or hypothyroidism
○ To help distinguish between primary and secondary thyroid disorders (in combination with other tests)

Procedure

Preparation

○ Tell the patient that the radioactive iodine uptake test assesses thyroid function.
○ Instruct the patient to begin fasting at midnight the night before the test.
○ Explain to the patient that he'll receive radioactive iodine (capsule or liquid) and that he'll then be scanned after 2 hours, 6 hours, and 24 hours.
○ Assure the patient that the test is painless and that the small amount of radioactivity is harmless.
○ Check the patient's history for iodine exposure, which may interfere with test results.
○ Note previous radiologic tests using contrast media, nuclear medicine procedures, or current use of iodine preparations or thyroid drugs on the film request slip.
○ Iodine hypersensitivity isn't considered a contraindication because the amount of iodine used is similar to the amount consumed in a normal diet.
○ Make sure the patient or a responsible family member has signed an informed consent form, if required.

Implementation

○ After ingesting an oral dose of radioactive iodine, the patient has his thyroid scanned at 2 hours, 6 hours,

and 24 hours by placing the anterior portion of his neck in front of an external single counting probe.
○ The amount of radioactivity detected by the probe is compared with the amount of radioactivity contained in the original dose to determine the percentage of radioactive iodine retained by the thyroid.

Patient care

○ Instruct the patient to resume a light diet 2 hours after taking the oral dose of radioactive iodine. When the study is complete, the patient may resume his usual diet.

Complications

None known

Interpretation

Normal results

○ At 2 hours, 4% to 12% of the radioactive iodine accumulates in the thyroid; after 6 hours, 5% to 20%; at 24 hours, 8% to 29%.
○ The remaining radioactive iodine is excreted in the urine. Local variations in the normal range of iodine uptake may occur because of regional differences in dietary iodine intake and procedural differences among laboratories.

Abnormal results

○ Below-normal iodine uptake may indicate hypothyroidism, subacute thyroiditis, or iodine overload.
○ Above-normal uptake may indicate hyperthyroidism, early Hashimoto's thyroiditis, hypoalbuminemia, lithium ingestion, or iodine-deficient goiter.
○ In hyperthyroidism, the rate of turnover may be so rapid that a falsely normal measurement occurs at 24 hours.

Interfering factors

○ Renal failure; diuresis; severe diarrhea; X-ray contrast media studies; ingestion of iodine preparations, including iodized salt, cough syrups, and some multivitamins (decrease)
○ Thyroid hormones, thyroid hormone antagonists, salicylates, penicillins, antihistamines, anticoagulants, corticosteroids, and phenylbutazone (decrease)
○ Phenothiazines or an iodine-deficient diet (increase)

Radioallergosorbent test

Overview

○ Measures immunoglobulin (Ig) E antibodies in serum by radioimmunoassay and identifies specific allergens that cause rash, asthma, hay fever, drug reactions, and other atopic complaints.
○ Compares test results with control values to represent the patient's reactivity to a specific allergen.
○ Easier to perform, more specific, less painful, and less dangerous than skin testing.
○ Careful selection of specific allergens, based on the patient's history, crucial for result effectiveness.
○ May be more useful than skin testing when a skin disorder makes accurate reading of skin tests difficult, when a patient requires continual antihistamine therapy, or when skin test results are negative but the patient's history supports IgE-mediated hypersensitivity.
○ Exposes a sample of the patient's serum to a panel of allergen particle complexes (APCs) on cellulose disks.
○ After the patient's IgE reacts with APCs to which it's sensitive, radiolabeled anti-IgE antibody is added, which binds to the IgE-APC complexes; after centrifugation, the amount of radioactivity in the particulate material is directly proportional to the amount of IgE antibodies present.

Purpose

○ To identify allergens to which the patient has an immediate (IgE-mediated) hypersensitivity
○ To monitor the patient's response to therapy

Procedure

Preparation

○ Explain to the patient that this test may detect the cause of allergy or monitor the effectiveness of allergy treatment.
○ Inform the patient that he need not restrict food and fluids.
○ Tell the patient that the test requires a blood sample.
○ Explain to the patient that he may experience slight discomfort from the needle puncture and the tourniquet.
○ If the patient is to receive a radioactive scan, make sure the blood sample is collected before the scan.

Implementation

○ Perform a venipuncture and collect the sample in a 7-ml clot-activator tube.
○ Usually, 1 ml of serum is sufficient for five allergen assays.

○ Note on the laboratory request the specific allergens to be tested.

Patient care

○ Apply direct pressure to the venipuncture site until bleeding stops.

Complications

○ Hematoma at the venipuncture site

Interpretation

Normal results

○ Results depend on the relation to a control serum value that differs among laboratories.

Abnormal results

○ Elevated serum IgE levels suggest hypersensitivity to the specific allergen or allergens used.

Interfering factors

○ Radioactive scan within 1 week before sample collection

Radionuclide renal imaging

Overview

- Assesses renal blood flow, renal structure, and nephron and collecting system function.
- Injected radioisotope depends on specific information required and examiner's preference.

Purpose

- To detect and assess functional and structural renal abnormalities and acute or chronic disease
- To assess renal transplantation or renal injury caused by trauma to the urinary tract or obstruction.

Procedure

Preparation

- Make sure the patient has signed an appropriate consent form.
- Inform the patient that he'll receive an injection of a radionuclide; tell him he may experience transient flushing and nausea.
- Emphasize that only a small amount of radionuclide is given and that it's usually excreted within 24 hours.
- If the patient receives antihypertensive medication, ask the physician if it should be withheld before the test.
- A pregnant patient or a young child may receive a supersaturated solution of potassium iodide 1 to 3 hours before the test to block thyroid uptake of iodine.

Implementation

- The patient is placed prone for posterior views. If the test is to evaluate transplantation, the patient is placed supine for anterior views.
- Instruct the patient not to change position.
- A perfusion study (radionuclide angiography) is performed first to evaluate renal blood flow. The I.V. ^{99m}Tc is given, and rapid-sequence (one per second) photographs are taken for 1 minute.
- Next, a function study is performed to measure the transit time of the radionuclide through the kidneys' functional units.
- After I.V. iodine-131 (Hippuran) is given, images are obtained at a rate of one per minute for 20 minutes. Or, this entire procedure can be recorded on computer-compatible magnetic tape, and concurrent renogram curves plotted.
- Static images are obtained 4 or more hours later, after the radionuclide has drained through the pelvi-caliceal system.

Patient care

- Instruct the patient to flush the toilet immediately after each voiding for 24 hours as a radiation precaution.
- Monitor the infection site for signs of hematoma, infection, and discomfort. Apply warm compresses for comfort.
- Monitor the patient's intake and output; monitor electrolyte, acid-base, blood urea nitrogen, and creatinine levels, as indicated.

Complications

- Hematoma at the venipuncture site

Interpretation

Normal results

- Renal perfusion is seen immediately after uptake of the ^{99m}Tc in the abdominal aorta.
- Within 1 to 2 minutes, a normal renal circulation appears.
- Kidneys are delineated simultaneously, symmetrically, and with equal intensity.
- Kidneys are normal in size, shape, and position.
- Maximum counts of the radionuclide in the kidneys occur within 5 minutes after injection (and within 1 minute of each other) and fall to one-third or less of the maximum counts in the same kidney within 25 minutes.
- Within this time, kidney function can be evaluated as the level of radionuclide shifts from the cortex to the pelvis and, finally, to the bladder.
- In normal total function, the effective renal plasma flow is 420 ml/minute or greater, and more than 66% of the dose is excreted in the urine at 30 to 35 minutes.

Abnormal results

- Renal circulation is impeded, such as that caused by trauma and renal artery stenosis or renal infarction.
- Perfusion is abnormal (possible obstruction of the vascular grafts in patients with a kidney transplant).
- Abnormalities of the collecting system and urine extravasation.
- Reduced radionuclide activity in the collecting system (caused by markedly decreased tubular function); decreased radionuclide activity in the tubules, with increased activity in the collecting system (caused by outflow obstruction).
- Defined level of ureteral obstruction.
- Lesions, congenital abnormalities, and traumatic injury.
- Space-occupying lesions within or surrounding the kidney, such as tumors, infarcts, and inflammatory masses; congenital disorders.
- Infarction, rupture, or hemorrhage after trauma.
- Lower-than-normal total concentration of the radionuclide (possible diffuse renal disorder, such as

acute tubular necrosis, severe infection, or ischemia).
○ Radionuclide uptake is decreased (general indication of organ rejection in a patient with a kidney
transplant).
○ Failure of visualization (possible congenital ectopia
or aplasia).

Interfering factors

○ Antihypertensives (possible masking of abnormalities)
○ Scans of different organs performed on the same day
(possible poor imaging)

Radionuclide thyroid imaging

Overview

○ Studies the thyroid by gamma camera after the patient receives iodine-123 (^{123}I), technetium-99m (^{99m}Tc) pertechnetate, or iodine-131 (^{131}I)
○ Usually follows discovery of a palpable mass, an enlarged gland, or an asymmetrical goiter and is performed along with thyroid uptake tests and measurements of serum triiodothyronine (T_3) and serum thyroxine (T_4) levels

Purpose

○ To assess the size, structure, position, and function of the thyroid gland

Procedure

Preparation

○ Tell the patient that radionuclide thyroid imaging helps determine the cause of thyroid dysfunction.
○ Explain to the patient that after he receives the radiopharmaceutical, a gamma camera will produce an image of his thyroid.
○ Check the patient's diet and drug history. Instruct him to stop taking drugs, such as thyroid hormones, thyroid hormone antagonists, and iodine preparations (Lugol's solution, some multivitamins, and cough syrups), 2 to 3 weeks before the test. Instruct him to stop taking phenothiazines, corticosteroids, salicylates, anticoagulants, and antihistamines 1 week before the test.
○ Instruct the patient to stop consuming iodized salt, iodinated salt substitutes, and seafood for 14 to 21 days before the test.
○ Tell him to stop T_4 10 days before the test, and to stop liothyronine, propylthiouracil, and methimazole 3 days before the test.
○ If the patient is to receive ^{123}I or ^{131}I, tell him to fast after midnight the night before the test. Fasting isn't required if he is to receive an I.V. injection of ^{99m}Tc pertechnetate.
○ Ask the patient if he has undergone tests that used radiographic contrast media within the past 60 days. Note previous radiographic contrast media exposure on the X-ray request.
○ Make sure the patient or a responsible family member has signed a consent form, if required.
○ Just before the test, tell the patient to remove dentures, jewelry, and other materials that may interfere with the imaging process.
○ The patient receives ^{123}I or ^{131}I (oral) or ^{99m}Tc pertechnetate (I.V.). Record the date and the time of administration.

○ The patient receiving an oral radioisotope should fast for another 2 hours after administration.

Implementation

○ The test is performed 24 hours after oral administration of ^{123}I or ^{131}I or 20 to 30 minutes after I.V. injection of ^{99m}Tc pertechnetate.
○ The patient is placed in the supine position with his neck extended; the thyroid gland is palpated.
○ The gamma camera is positioned above the anterior portion of his neck.
○ Images of the patient's thyroid gland are projected on a monitor and are recorded on X-ray film.
○ Three views of the thyroid are obtained: a straight-on anterior view and two bilateral oblique views.

Patient care

○ Tell the patient that he may resume his usual diet and medications.

Complications

○ Adverse reaction to the radioisotope

Interpretation

Normal results

○ The thyroid gland is about 2″ (5 cm) long and 1″ (2.5 cm) wide, with a uniform uptake of the radioisotope and without tumors.
○ The gland is butterfly-shaped, with the isthmus located at the midline. Occasionally, a third lobe called the *pyramidal lobe* may be present.

Abnormal results

○ Hyperfunctioning nodules (areas of excessive iodine uptake) appear as black regions called *hot spots.*
○ The presence of hot spots requires a follow-up T_3 thyroid suppression test to determine if the hyperfunctioning areas are autonomous.
○ Hypofunctioning nodules (areas of little or no iodine uptake) appear as white or light gray regions called *cold spots.* If a cold spot appears, subsequent thyroid ultrasonography may be performed to rule out cysts; in addition, fine-needle aspiration and biopsy of such nodules may be performed to rule out malignancy.

Interfering factors

○ An iodine-deficient diet and phenothiazines (increase)
○ Decreased uptake of radioactive iodine caused by renal disease; ingestion of iodized salt, iodine preparations, iodinated salt substitutes, or seafood; and use of thyroid hormones, thyroid hormone antagonists, aminosalicylic acid, corticosteroids, multivitamins, or cough syrups containing inorganic iodine (decrease)
○ Severe diarrhea and vomiting, impairing GI absorption of radioiodine (decrease)

Raji cell assay

Overview

- Detects the presence of circulating immune complexes; studies the Raji lymphoblastoid cell line.
- Identifying these cells, which have receptors for immunoglobulin G complement, helps to evaluate autoimmune disease.

Purpose

- To detect circulating immune complexes
- To aid in the study of autoimmune disease

Procedure

Preparation

- Explain to the patient the purpose of the test, as appropriate.
- Tell the patient that the test requires a blood sample.
- Explain to the patient that he may experience slight discomfort from the needle puncture and the tourniquet.

Implementation

- Perform a venipuncture, collect a sample in a clot-activator tube, and promptly send it to the laboratory.
- Handle the sample gently to prevent hemolysis.

Patient care

- Apply direct pressure to the venipuncture site until bleeding stops.

Complications

- Hematoma at the venipuncture site

Interpretation

Normal results

- Raji cells aren't present.

Abnormal results

- A positive Raji cell assay can detect immune complexes, including those found in viral, microbial, and parasitic infections; metastasis; autoimmune disorders; and drug reactions.
- The test may also detect immune complexes associated with celiac disease, cirrhosis of the liver, Crohn's disease, cryoglobulinemia, dermatitis herpetiformis, sickle cell anemia, and ulcerative colitis.

Interfering factors

- Hemolysis from rough handling of the sample

Rapid corticotropin

Overview

○ Also known as the *cosyntropin test*; gradually replacing the 8-hour corticotropin stimulation test as the most effective diagnostic tool for evaluating adrenal hypofunction.
○ Using cosyntropin, the rapid corticotropin test provides faster results and causes fewer allergic reactions than the 8-hour test, which uses natural corticotropin from animal sources.
○ Requires prior determination of baseline cortisol levels to evaluate the effect of cosyntropin administration on cortisol secretion.
○ An unequivocally high morning cortisol level rules out adrenal hypofunction and makes further testing unnecessary.

Purpose

○ To aid in the identification of primary and secondary adrenal hypofunction

Procedure

Preparation

○ Explain to the patient that this test helps determine if his condition is caused by a hormonal deficiency.
○ Inform him that he may need to fast for 10 to 12 hours before the test and must be relaxed and resting quietly for 30 minutes before the test.
○ Tell him that the test takes at least 1 hour to perform.
○ If the patient is an inpatient, withhold corticotropin and all steroid drugs, as ordered.
○ If he's an outpatient, tell him to refrain from taking these drugs, if instructed by his physician. If he must continue taking them, note this on the laboratory request.
○ Explain to the patient that he may experience slight discomfort from the needle puncture and the tourniquet.

Implementation

○ Draw 5 ml of blood for a baseline value. Collect the sample in a 5-ml heparinized tube. Label this sample "preinjection" and send it to the laboratory.
○ Inject 250 µg (0.25 mg) of cosyntropin I.V. or I.M. (I.V. administration provides more accurate results because ineffective absorption after I.M. administration may cause wide variations in response.)
○ Direct I.V. injection should take about 2 minutes.
○ Draw another 5 ml of blood at 30 and 60 minutes after the cosyntropin injection.
○ Collect the samples in 5 ml heparinized tubes. Label the samples "30 minutes postinjection" and "60 minutes postinjection" and send them to the laboratory. Include the collection times on the laboratory request.

○ Handle the samples gently to prevent hemolysis. They require no special precautions other than avoiding stasis.

Patient care

○ Apply direct pressure to the venipuncture site until bleeding stops.
○ Observe the patient for signs of a rare allergic reaction to cosyntropin, such as hives, itching, and tachycardia.
○ Instruct the patient that he may resume his usual diet, activities, and medications stopped before the test.

Complications

Hematoma at the venipuncture site

Interpretation

Normal results

○ Cortisol levels rise after 30 to 60 minutes to a peak of 18 mg/dl (SI, 500 mmol/L) or more 60 minutes after the cosyntropin injection.
○ Generally, doubling the baseline value indicates a normal response.

Abnormal results

○ A normal result excludes adrenal hypofunction (insufficiency).
○ In the patient with primary adrenal hypofunction (Addison's disease), cortisol levels remain low.
○ If test results show subnormal increases in cortisol levels, prolonged stimulation of the adrenal cortex may be necessary to differentiate between primary and secondary adrenal hypofunction.

Interfering factors

○ Failure to observe pretest restrictions
○ Hemolysis from rough handling of the sample
○ Estrogens and amphetamines (increase in plasma cortisol)
○ Smoking and obesity (possible increase in plasma cortisol)
○ Lithium carbonate (decrease in plasma cortisol)
○ Radioactive scan performed within 1 week before the test

Rapid monoclonal test for cytomegalovirus

Overview

○ Cytomegalovirus (CMV), a member of the herpes virus group, can cause systemic infection in congenitally infected infants and in immunocompromised patients, such as transplant recipients, patients receiving chemotherapy for neoplastic disease, and those with acquired immunodeficiency syndrome (AIDS).
○ In the past, CMV infections were detected in the laboratory by recognizing the distinctive cytopathic effects (CPE) that the virus produced in conventional tube cell cultures.
○ In this slow method of detecting CMV, CPE cultures grow in about 9 days.
○ The faster shell vial assay (rapid monoclonal test) is based on the availability of a monoclonal antibody specific for the 72 kD protein of CMV synthesized during the immediate early stage of viral replication.
○ Through indirect immunofluorescence, CMV-infected fibroblasts are recognized by their dense, homogeneous staining confined to the nucleus.
○ Because of the smooth, regular shape of the nucleus and the surrounding nuclear membrane, infected cells are readily differentiated from nonspecific background fluorescence that may be present in some specimens.

Purpose

○ To obtain rapid laboratory diagnosis of CMV infection, especially in the immunocompromised patient who currently has, or is at risk for developing, systemic infections caused by this virus

Procedure

Preparation

○ Explain the purpose of the test and describe the procedure for collecting the specimen, which will depend on the laboratory used.

Implementation

○ Specimens should be collected during the prodromal and acute stages of clinical infection to maximize the chances of detecting CMV.
○ Each type of specimen requires a specific collection device.
○ For throat, use a microbiologic transport swab.
○ For urine or cerebrospinal fluid, use a sterile screw-capped tube or vial.
○ For bronchoalveolar lavage tissue, use a sterile screw-capped jar.
○ For blood, use a sterile tube with anticoagulant (heparin).

○ Transport the specimen to the laboratory as soon as possible after the collection. If the anticipated time between collection and inoculation into shell vial cell cultures is longer than 3 hours, store the specimen at 39.2° F (4° C). Don't freeze the specimen or allow it to become dry.
○ Use gloves when obtaining and handling all specimens.

Patient care

○ Answer the patient's questions about the test.

Complications

None known

Interpretation

Normal results

○ CMV shouldn't appear in a culture specimen.

Abnormal results

○ CMV is detectable in urine and throat specimens from an asymptomatic patient. Detection from these sites indicates active, asymptomatic infection, which may herald symptomatic involvement, especially in the immunocompromised patient.
○ Detection of CMV in specimens of blood, tissue, and bronchoalveolar lavage generally indicates systemic infection and disease.

Interfering factors

○ Administration of antiviral drugs before collecting the specimen

Red blood cell count

Overview

- Also called an *erythrocyte count,* part of a complete blood count
- Detects the number of red blood cells (RBCs) in a microliter (μl), or cubic millimeter (mm^3), of whole blood
- Can't give information about the size, shape, or concentration of hemoglobin (Hb) in the corpuscles but may calculate mean corpuscular volume (MCV) and mean corpuscular hemoglobin (MCH)

Purpose

- To provide data for calculating MCV and MCH, which reveal RBC size and Hb content
- To support other hematologic tests for diagnosing anemia or polycythemia

Procedure

Preparation

- Explain to the patient that the RBC count evaluates the number of blood cells and detects possible blood disorders.
- Inform the patient that he need not restrict food and fluids.
- Tell the patient that the test requires a blood sample. Explain who will perform the venipuncture and when.
- Explain to the patient that he may feel slight discomfort from the needle puncture and the tourniquet.
- If the patient is a child who's old enough to understand, explain to him and his parents that a small amount of blood will be taken from his finger or earlobe.

Implementation

- For adults and older children, draw venous blood into a 3- or 4.5-ml ethylenediaminetetraacetic acid sodium metabisulfite solution tube.
- For younger children, collect capillary blood in a microcollection device.
- Fill the collection tube completely.
- Invert the tube gently several times to mix the sample and the anticoagulant.
- Handle the sample gently to prevent hemolysis.

Patient care

- Ensure that subdermal bleeding has stopped before removing pressure.

Complications

- Hematoma at the venipuncture site

Interpretation

Normal results

- In men, 4.5 to 5.5 million RBCs/μl (SI, 4.5 to 5.5 × 10^{12}/L) of venous blood.
- In women, 4 to 5 million RBCs/μl (SI, 4 to 5 × 10^{12}/L) of venous blood.
- In full-term neonates, 4.4 to 5.8 million/μl (SI, 4.4 to 5.8 × 10^{12}/L) of capillary blood at birth, decreasing to 3 to 3.8 million/μl (SI, 3 to 3.8 × 10^{12}/L) at age 2 months, and increasing slowly thereafter.
- In children, 4.6 to 4.8 million/μl (SI, 4.6 to 4.8 × 10^{12}/L) of venous blood.
- RBCs may exceed these levels in patients who live at high altitudes or are very active.

Abnormal results

- A high RBC count may indicate absolute or relative polycythemia.
- A low RBC count may indicate anemia, fluid overload, or hemorrhage beyond 24 hours.
- Further tests, such as stained cell examination, hematocrit, Hb, RBC indices, and white blood cell (WBC) studies, are needed to confirm a diagnosis.

Interfering factors

- Failure to use the proper anticoagulant or to adequately mix the sample and the anticoagulant
- Hemoconcentration from prolonged tourniquet constriction
- Hemodilution from drawing the sample from the same arm used for I.V. infusion of fluids
- High WBC count (false-high test results in semiautomated and automated counters)
- Diseases that cause RBCs to agglutinate or form rouleaux (false decrease)
- Hemolysis from rough handling of the sample or drawing the blood through a small-gauge needle for venipuncture

Red blood cell indices

Overview

○ Evaluates mean corpuscular volume (MCV), mean corpuscular hemoglobin (MCH), and mean corpuscular hemoglobin concentration (MCHC)
○ Often follows the red blood cell (RBC) count and hematocrit (HCT) and total hemoglobin (Hb) tests and provides important information about the size, Hb concentration, and Hb weight of an average RBC

Purpose

○ To aid in the diagnosis and classification of anemias

Procedure

Preparation

○ Explain to the patient that RBC indices help determine if he has anemia.
○ Tell the patient that the test requires a blood sample. Explain who will perform the venipuncture and when.
○ Explain to the patient that he may feel slight discomfort from the needle puncture and the tourniquet.

Implementation

○ Perform a venipuncture and collect the sample in a 3- or 4.5-ml ethylenediaminetetraacetic acid tube.
○ Completely fill the collection tube and invert it gently several times to adequately mix the sample and the anticoagulant.
○ Handle the sample gently to prevent hemolysis.

Patient care

○ Ensure subdermal bleeding has stopped before removing pressure.
○ If a large hematoma develops, monitor pulses distal to the site.

Complications

○ Hematoma at the venipuncture site

Interpretation

Normal results

○ MCV, the HCT (packed cell volume)-to-RBC count ratio, expresses the average size of the erythrocytes and indicates whether they're undersized (microcytic), oversized (macrocytic), or normal (normocytic).
○ MCH (the Hb-to-RBC count ratio) gives the weight of Hb in an average RBC.
○ MCHC (the Hb weight-to-HCT ratio) defines the concentration of Hb in 100 ml of packed RBCs. It helps to distinguish normally colored (normochromic) RBCs from paler (hypochromic) RBCs.
○ MCV, 84 to 99 μm^3.

○ MCH, 26 to 32 pg/cell.
○ MCHC, 30 to 36 g/dl.

Abnormal results

○ Low MCV and MCHC indicate microcytic, hypochromic anemias caused by iron-deficiency anemia, pyridoxine-responsive anemia, or thalassemia.
○ A high MCV suggests macrocytic anemias caused by megaloblastic anemias, folic acid or vitamin B_{12} deficiency, inherited disorders of deoxyribonucleic acid synthesis, or reticulocytosis.
○ Because the MCV reflects the average volume of many cells, a value within the normal range can encompass RBCs of varying size, from microcytic to macrocytic.

Interfering factors

○ Failure to use the proper anticoagulant or to adequately mix the sample and the anticoagulant
○ Hemolysis from rough handling of the sample or use of a small-gauge needle for blood aspiration
○ Hemoconcentration from prolonged tourniquet constriction
○ High white blood cell count (false-high RBC count in semiautomated and automated counters, invalidating MCV and MCHC results)
○ Falsely elevated Hb values, invalidating MCH and MCHC results
○ Diseases that cause RBCs to agglutinate or form *rouleaux* (false-low RBC count)

Red blood cell survival time

Overview

○ Measures the survival time of red blood cells (RBCs) circulating in the bloodstream and identifies sites where they are being destroyed, if RBC survival time is decreased.
○ RBCs are normally destroyed as they age, but in hemolytic anemia, they're destroyed randomly, regardless of age.

Purpose

○ To evaluate unexplained anemias, especially those caused by excessive destruction of RBCs
○ To identify the site of abnormal RBC creation and destruction

Procedure

Preparation

○ Explain to the patient that this test requires a blood sample.
○ Tell the patient that he may feel discomfort from the needle puncture and the tourniquet.
○ Inform the patient that he need not fast before testing.

Implementation

○ Perform a venipuncture and collect a 30 ml blood sample.
○ Blood in the sample is mixed with radioactive chromium (^{51}Cr).
○ The mixture is then injected into the patient.
○ A blood sample is drawn again in 30 minutes.
○ Radioactivity per milliliter of the sample is calculated.
○ Gamma camera scans of the patient's chest, back, liver, and spleen detect radioactivity at sites that show an abnormal increase in volume of RBCs in a limited area.

Patient care

○ Apply direct pressure to the venipuncture site until bleeding stops.
○ Inform the patient that follow-up blood samples are collected every 3 days for 3 to 4 weeks.

Complications

○ Hematoma at the venipuncture site

Interpretation

Normal results

○ Results are determined by measuring radioactive chromium that has been mixed with a measured blood sample and reinjected into the patient.

Abnormal results

○ Decreased RBC survival time indicates a hemolytic disease, such as chronic lymphocytic leukemia, congenital non-spherocytic hemolytic anemia, hemoglobin C disease, hereditary spherocytosis, paroxysmal nocturnal hemoglobinuria, pernicious anemia, sickle-cell anemia, elliptocytosis, idiopathic-acquired hemolytic anemia.

Interfering factors

○ Dehydration
○ Overhydration
○ Blood loss (from severe bleeding or blood samples drawn for other tests)
○ Blood transfusions during the test period

Refraction

Overview

○ Enables images to focus on the retina and directly affects visual acuity
○ Done routinely during an eye examination or whenever a patient complains of a change in vision; defines refractive error and determines the degree of correction required to improve visual acuity with corrective lenses
○ Performed objectively, by using a retinoscope, and subjectively, by asking the patient about his visual acuity while placing trial lenses before his eyes

Purpose

○ To diagnose refractive error and prescribe corrective lenses, if necessary

Procedure

Preparation

○ Explain to the patient that the refraction test helps determine whether he needs corrective lenses.
○ Tell the patient that eyedrops may be instilled to dilate his pupils and that the test takes 10 to 20 minutes.
○ Check the patient's history for angle-closure glaucoma and for previous use of and hypersensitivity to dilating eyedrops. Don't give dilating eyedrops to a patient with either.

Implementation

○ After short-acting mydriatic eyedrops are given, the examiner directs the light of the retinoscope at the pupillary opening.
○ Through the aperture at the top of the instrument, the examiner looks for an orange glow — the retinoscopic, or red, reflex, which represents the reflection of light from the retinoscope — and notes its brightness, clarity, and uniformity.
○ Moving the retinoscope light across the pupil, the examiner observes the reflex for any movement.
○ The examiner then places trial lenses before the patient's eyes and adjusts the lens power to make the reflex clear, bright, and uniform and to neutralize its motion. The lens power necessary to make this adjustment is recorded.
○ Objective findings can be refined by altering the trial lenses and having the patient read lines on a standardized visual chart. This helps determine which lens or combination of lenses provides the best correction of his visual acuity.

Patient care

○ If corrective lenses are prescribed, advise the patient that images may appear blurred the first time he wears the lenses.

○ If the patient has worn glasses or contact lenses previously, he should wear only his new prescription lenses because changing back and forth from the old prescription to the new one will prevent his eyes from making the required adjustment to the new lenses.
○ Instruct the patient to report ocular discomfort or redness immediately.

Complications

○ Hypersensitivity reactions
○ Ocular discomfort

Interpretation

Normal results

○ Refractive power, measured in diopters, is greatest at the cornea (about 44 diopters) because of its curvature.
○ The aqueous humor has the same refractive power as the cornea and is considered to be the same medium.
○ The lens, normally a convex structure, has a refractive power of about 10 to 14 diopters but can alter this power by changing its shape. This phenomenon is known as *accommodation* and occurs when the eye views objects closer than 20′ (6 m).
○ The vitreous humor, a gelatinous medium, has little refractive power and mainly transmits light.
○ In the absence of accommodation, the average refractive power of the human eye is 58 diopters.
○ Ideally, the eyes have no refractive error (*emmetropia*). Parallel light rays emanating from a point source can be focused directly on the retina to produce a clear image.

Abnormal results

○ Most patients show some degree of refractive error (*ametropia*). *Hyperopia*, or farsightedness, occurs when the eyeball is too short and parallel light rays focus behind the retina.
○ Retinoscopic examination shows a red reflex moving in the same direction as the retinoscope's light. A patient with hyperopia sees distant objects clearly but experiences blurring of near objects.
○ *Myopia*, or nearsightedness, occurs when the eyeball is too long and parallel light rays focus in front of the retina.
○ Retinoscopic examination shows reflex motion opposite to movement of the retinoscope's light. A patient with myopia sees near objects clearly but experiences blurring of distant objects.
○ When light rays entering the eye aren't refracted uniformly and a clear focal point on the retina isn't attained, the patient has *astigmatism*.

Interfering factors

○ Inadequate paralysis of accommodation or pupil dilation or the patient's failure to cooperate

Renal angiography

Overview

- Permits radiographic examination of the renal vasculature and parenchyma
- Requires arterial injection of a contrast medium

Purpose

- To demonstrate the configuration of total renal vasculature before surgical procedures
- To determine the cause of renovascular hypertension
- To evaluate chronic renal disease or renal failure
- To investigate renal masses and renal trauma
- To detect complications following kidney transplantation
- To differentiate highly vascular tumors from avascular cysts

Procedure

Preparation

- Instruct the patient to fast for 8 hours before the test and to drink extra fluids the day before the test. Or, start an I.V. line, if needed.
- Tell the patient he may continue oral drugs; a patient with diabetes requires a special order.
- Check the patient's history for hypersensitivity to iodine-based contrast media or iodine-containing foods such as shellfish.
- Instruct the patient to remove all metallic objects that may interfere with test results.
- Ask the patient to void before leaving the unit.
- Verify adequate renal function and adequate clotting ability.
- Evaluate peripheral pulse sites and mark them for easy access.

Implementation

- The patient is placed in the supine position and a peripheral I.V. infusion is started. The skin over the arterial puncture site is cleaned with antiseptic solution and a local anesthetic is injected.
- The femoral artery is punctured and cannulated under fluoroscopic visualization.
- After the flexible guide wire is passed through the artery, the cannula is withdrawn, leaving several inches of wire in the lumen.
- A polyethylene catheter is passed over the wire and advanced, under fluoroscopic guidance, up the femoroiliac vessels to the aorta.
- The guide wire is removed, and the catheter is flushed with heparin flush solution. The contrast medium is injected, and screening aortograms are taken before proceeding.
- On completion of the aortographic study, a renal catheter is exchanged for the vascular catheter.
- To determine the position of the renal arteries and ensure that the tip of the catheter is in the lumen, a test bolus (3 to 5 ml) of contrast medium is injected immediately.
- If the patient has no adverse reaction to the contrast medium, 20 to 25 ml of the substance is injected just below the origin of the renal arteries.
- A series of rapid-sequence X-ray films of the filling of the renal vascular tree is exposed.
- If additional selective studies are required, the catheter remains in place. If the films are satisfactory, the catheter is removed.

Patient care

- Apply a sterile pad firmly to the puncture site for 15 minutes.
- Observe the puncture site for a hematoma.
- Keep the patient flat in bed and instruct him to keep the punctured leg straight for at least 6 hours or as otherwise needed.
- Check vital signs every 15 minutes for 1 hour, every 30 minutes for 2 hours, and then every hour until they stabilize.
- Monitor popliteal and dorsalis pedis pulses for adequate perfusion at least every hour for 4 hours.
- Note the color and temperature of the involved extremity and compare it with the uninvolved extremity.
- Watch for signs of pain or paresthesia in the involved limb.
- Watch for bleeding or hematomas at the injection site. Keep the pressure dressing in place and check for bleeding.
- Apply cold compresses to the puncture site.
- Provide extra fluids (2,000 to 3,000 ml) in the 24-hour period after the test to prevent nephrotoxicity from the contrast medium.

▼ ALERT *Monitor the patient for anaphylaxis from the contrast medium. Signs include cardiorespiratory distress, renal failure, and shock.*

- Monitor for atrial arrhythmias and evaluate aspartate aminotransferase and lactate dehydrogenase activity.

Complications

- Adverse reaction to the contrast medium
- Hematoma at the venipuncture site

Interpretation

Normal results

- Normal arborization of the vascular tree and architecture of the renal parenchyma.

Abnormal results

- Renal tumors usually show hypervascularity; renal cysts typically appear as clearly delineated, radiolucent masses.
- Renal artery stenosis caused by arteriosclerosis produces a noticeable constriction in the blood vessels, usually within the proximal portion of its length.

- In renal infarction, blood vessels may appear to be absent or cut off, with the normal tissue replaced by scar tissue.
- Appearance of triangular areas of infarcted tissue near the periphery of the affected kidney. The kidney may appear shrunken.
- Detect renal artery aneurysms (saccular or fusiform) and renal arteriovenous fistula with abnormal widening of and direct passage between the renal artery and renal vein.
- Destruction, distortion, and fibrosis of renal tissue with areas of reduced and tortuous vascularity in severe or chronic pyelonephritis may be visible; an increase in capsular vessels with abnormal intrarenal circulation indicates renal abscesses or inflammation.
- In renal trauma, intrarenal hematoma, a parenchymal laceration, shattered kidneys, and areas of infarction may be visible.

Interfering factors

- Recent contrast studies such as barium enema or an upper GI series
- Presence of feces or gas in the GI tract (possible poor imaging)

Renal venography

Overview

- Allows radiographic examination of the main renal veins and their tributaries
- Requires injection of contrast medium by percutaneous catheter passed through the femoral vein and inferior vena cava into the renal vein

Purpose

- To detect renal vein thrombosis
- To evaluate renal vein compression caused by extrinsic tumors or retroperitoneal fibrosis
- To assess renal tumors and detect invasion of the renal vein or inferior vena cava
- To detect venous anomalies and defects
- To differentiate renal agenesis from a small kidney
- To collect renal venous blood samples for evaluation of renovascular hypertension

Procedure

Preparation

- Make sure the patient has signed an appropriate consent form.
- Notify the physician of drugs the patient is taking that may affect test results; it may be necessary to restrict them.
- If prescribed, instruct the patient to fast for 4 hours before the test.
- Check the patient's history for hypersensitivity to contrast media, iodine, or iodine-containing foods such as shellfish.
- Check the patient's history and any coagulation studies for indications of bleeding disorders.
- If the patient will receive renin assays, check his diet and drugs and consult with the health care team.
- Make sure pretest blood urea nitrogen and urine creatinine levels are adequate.

Implementation

- The patient is placed in the supine position on the X-ray table, with his abdomen centered over the film.
- The skin over the right femoral vein near the groin is cleaned with antiseptic solution and draped. (The left femoral vein or jugular veins may be used.)
- A local anesthetic is injected; the femoral vein is then cannulated.
- Under fluoroscopic guidance, a guide wire is threaded a short distance through the cannula, which is then removed. A catheter is passed over the wire into the inferior vena cava.
- When catheterization of the femoral vein is contraindicated, the right antecubital vein is punctured, and the catheter is inserted and advanced through the right atrium of the heart into the inferior vena cava.

- A test bolus of contrast medium is injected to determine whether the vena cava is patent. If so, the catheter is advanced into the right renal vein, and contrast medium (usually 20 to 40 ml) is injected.
- When studies of the right renal vasculature are complete, the catheter is withdrawn into the vena cava, rotated, and guided into the left renal vein.
- If visualization of the renal venous tributaries is indicated, epinephrine can be injected into the ipsilateral renal artery by catheter before contrast medium is injected into the renal vein.
- Epinephrine temporarily blocks arterial flow and allows filling of distal intrarenal veins. Obstructing the artery briefly with a balloon catheter produces the same effect.
- After anteroposterior films are made, the patient lies prone for posteroanterior films.
- For renin assays, blood samples are withdrawn under fluoroscopy within 15 minutes after venography.

Patient care

- After catheter removal, apply pressure for 15 minutes and apply a dressing.
- Check vital signs and distal pulses every 15 minutes for the first hour, every 30 minutes for the second hour, and then every 2 hours for 24 hours. Keep the patient on bed rest for 2 hours.
- Observe the puncture site for bleeding or a hematoma.
- Report signs of vein perforation, embolism, and extravasation.
- Report complaints of paresthesia or pain in the catheterized limb — symptoms of nerve irritation or vascular compromise.
- Instruct the patient to increase fluid intake to clear the contrast medium.

Complications

- Hypersensitivity to the contrast medium
- Paresthesia, vein perforation, embolism

Interpretation

Normal results

- After injection of the contrast medium, immediate opacification of the renal vein and tributaries
- Normal renin content of venous blood in a supine adult, 1.5 to 1.6 nanograms/ml/hour

Abnormal results

- Renal vein occlusion near the inferior vena cava or the kidney indicates renal vein thrombosis.
- A clot is usually identifiable because it's within the lumen and less sharply outlined than a filling defect.
- A filling defect of the renal vein may indicate obstruction or compression by an extrinsic tumor or retroperitoneal fibrosis. A renal tumor that invades the renal vein or inferior vena cava usually produces a filling defect with a sharply defined border.

- Absence of a renal vein differentiates renal agenesis from a small kidney.
- Elevated renin content in renal venous blood usually indicates essential renovascular hypertension when assay results correspond for both kidneys.
- Elevated renin levels in one kidney indicate a unilateral lesion and usually require further evaluation by arteriography.

Interfering factors

- Recent contrast studies or feces or gas in the bowel
- Failure to restrict salt, antihypertensive drugs, diuretics, estrogen, and hormonal contraceptives

Reticulocyte count

Overview

○ Counts reticulocytes in a whole blood sample and expresses the value as a percentage of the total red blood cell (RBC) count.
○ Usually larger than mature RBCs, reticulocytes are nonnucleated, immature RBCs that remain in the peripheral blood for 24 to 48 hours while maturing.
○ Because the manual method of reticulocyte counting uses only a small sample, values may be imprecise and should be compared with the RBC count or hematocrit.
○ The reticulocyte count is useful for evaluating anemia and is an index of effective erythropoiesis and bone marrow response to anemia.

Purpose

○ To aid in distinguishing between hypoproliferative and hyperproliferative anemias
○ To help assess blood loss, bone marrow response to anemia, and therapy for anemia

Procedure

Preparation

○ Explain to the patient that the reticulocyte count is used to detect anemia or to monitor its treatment.
○ Tell the patient that the test requires a blood sample.
○ Notify the laboratory and physician of drugs the patient is taking that may affect test results; it may be necessary to restrict them.
○ Inform the patient that he need not restrict food and fluids.
○ Explain to the patient that he may feel slight discomfort from the needle puncture and the tourniquet.
○ If the patient is an infant or child, explain to the parents that a small amount of blood will be taken from his finger or earlobe.

Implementation

○ Perform a venipuncture and collect the sample in a 3- or 4.5-ml ethylenediaminetetraacetic acid tube.
○ Completely fill the collection tube and invert it gently several times to mix the sample and the anticoagulant.
○ Handle the sample gently.

Patient care

○ Ensure that subdermal bleeding has stopped before removing pressure.
○ If a hematoma develops at the venipuncture site, apply warm soaks.
○ If the hematoma is large, monitor pulses distal to the phlebotomy site.
○ Instruct the patient that he may resume medications stopped before the test.

○ Monitor the patient with an abnormal reticulocyte count for trends or significant changes in repeated tests.

Complications

○ Hematoma at the venipuncture site

Interpretation

Normal results

○ 0.5% to 2.5% (SI, 0.005 to 0.025) of the total RBC count
○ In neonates, 2% to 6% (SI, 0.002 to 0.006) at birth, decreasing to adult levels in 1 to 2 weeks

Abnormal results

○ A low reticulocyte count indicates hypoproliferative bone marrow (*hypoplastic anemia*) or ineffective erythropoiesis (*pernicious anemia*).
○ A high reticulocyte count indicates a bone marrow response to anemia caused by hemolysis or blood loss.
○ The reticulocyte count may also increase after therapy for iron deficiency anemia or pernicious anemia.

Interfering factors

○ Failure to use the proper anticoagulant or to adequately mix the sample and the anticoagulant
○ Prolonged tourniquet constriction
○ Azathioprine, chloramphenicol, dactinomycin, and methotrexate (possible false-low)
○ Corticotropin, antimalarials, antipyretics, furazolidone (in infants), levodopa (possible false-high)
○ Sulfonamides (possible false-low or false-high)
○ Recent blood transfusion
○ Hemolysis from rough handling of the sample or use of a small-gauge needle for blood aspiration

Retrograde cystography

Overview

○ Involves the instillation of a contrast medium into the bladder, followed by radiographic examination
○ Diagnoses bladder rupture without urethral involvement because it can determine the location and extent of the rupture
○ Indicated in patients with neurogenic bladder; recurrent urinary tract infections (UTIs), especially in children; suspected vesicoureteral reflux; and vesical fistulas, diverticula, and tumors
○ Performed when cystoscopic examination is impractical, as in male infants, or when excretory urography hasn't adequately shown the bladder

Purpose

○ To evaluate the structure and integrity of the bladder

Procedure

Preparation

○ Explain to the patient that retrograde cystography permits radiographic examination of the bladder.
○ Inform the patient that he need not restrict food and fluids.
○ Check the patient's history for hypersensitivity to contrast media, iodine, or shellfish; mark it on the chart and inform the physician.
○ Inform the patient that he may experience some discomfort when the catheter is inserted and when the contrast medium is instilled through the catheter.
○ Tell the patient that he may hear loud, clacking sounds as the X-ray films are made.

Implementation

○ The patient is placed in the supine position on the X-ray table; a preliminary kidney-ureter-bladder X-ray is taken.
○ The X-ray is developed immediately and scrutinized for renal shadows, calcifications, contours of the bone and psoas muscles, and gas patterns in the lumen of the GI tract.
○ The bladder is catheterized and 200 to 300 ml of sterile contrast medium (50 to 100 ml for an infant) is instilled by gravity or gentle syringe injection. The catheter is then clamped.
○ With the patient in a supine position, an anteroposterior film is taken. The patient is then tilted to one side, then the other, and two posterior oblique (and sometimes lateral) views are taken.
○ If the patient's condition permits, he's assisted into the jackknife position. A posteroanterior film is taken. A space-occupying vesical lesion may require additional exposures. Rarely, to enhance visualization, 100 to 300 ml of air may be insufflated into the blad-der by syringe after removal of the contrast medium (double-contrast technique).
○ The catheter is then unclamped, the bladder fluid is allowed to drain, and an X-ray is obtained to detect urethral diverticula, reflux into the ureters, fistulous tracts into the vagina, or intraperitoneal or extraperitoneal extravasation of the contrast medium.

Patient care

○ Monitor the patient's vital signs every 15 minutes for the first hour, every 30 minutes during the second hour, and then every 2 hours for up to 24 hours.
○ Record the time of the patient's voidings and the color and volume of the urine. Observe for hematuria that persists after the third voiding and notify the physician.
○ Watch for signs of urinary sepsis from UTIs or similar signs related to extravasation of contrast medium into the general circulation.
○ Prepare the patient for surgery and urinary diversion, if indicated. Strain urine if calculi are detected.
○ Monitor for retention or distention if neurogenic bladder is diagnosed and give drugs (baclofen for spasms; bethanechol chloride for hypotonic bladder).
○ Discuss the use of a percutaneous stimulator if one is being contemplated. Teach self-catheterization, if indicated for neurogenic bladder.

Complications

○ Hematuria
○ Urinary sepsis

Interpretation

Normal results

○ The bladder appears with normal contours, capacity, integrity, and urethrovesical angle, and no evidence of a tumor, diverticula, or a rupture.
○ No vesicoureteral reflux is apparent.
○ The bladder appears without displacement or external compression with a bladder wall that is smooth and not thick.

Abnormal results

○ Vesical trabeculae or diverticula, space-occupying lesions (tumors), calculi or gravel, blood clots, high- or low-pressure vesicoureteral reflux, and a hypotonic or hypertonic bladder

Interfering factors

○ Gas, feces, or residual barium from recent diagnostic tests in the bowel (possible poor imaging)

Retrograde ureteropyelography

Overview

○ Allows radiographic examination of the renal collecting system after injection of a contrast medium through a ureteral catheter during cystoscopy.
○ Contrast medium is usually iodine-based, and although some of it may be absorbed through the mucous membranes, this test is preferred for the patient with hypersensitivity to iodine.
○ Isn't influenced by impaired renal function and is therefore indicated when visualization of the renal collecting system by excretory urography is inadequate because of inferior films or marked renal insufficiency.

Purpose

○ To assess the structure and integrity of the renal collecting system

Procedure

Preparation

○ Explain to the patient that retrograde ureteropyelography shows the urinary collecting system.
○ If the patient is to receive a general anesthetic, instruct him to fast for 8 hours before the test. Usually, he should be well hydrated to ensure adequate urine flow.
○ If the patient will be awake throughout the procedure, tell him that he may feel pressure as the catheter is inserted and a pressure sensation in the kidney area when the contrast medium is introduced. Also, he may feel an urgency to void.
○ Give the patient prescribed premedication just before the procedure.

Implementation

○ Assist the patient into the lithotomy position.
○ After the patient is anesthetized, the urologist first performs a cystoscopic examination.
○ After visual inspection of the bladder, one or both ureters are catheterized with opaque catheters, depending on the condition or abnormality suspected. Radiographic monitoring allows correct positioning of the catheter tip in the renal pelvis.
○ The renal pelvis is emptied by gravity drainage or aspiration.
○ About 5 ml of contrast medium is then slowly injected through the catheter, using the syringe with the special adapter.
○ When adequate filling and opacification have occurred, anteroposterior radiographic films are taken and immediately developed. Lateral and oblique films can be taken, as needed, after the injection of more contrast medium.
○ After the X-rays of the renal pelvis are examined, a few more milliliters of contrast medium are injected to outline the ureters as the catheter is slowly withdrawn.
○ Delayed films are then taken to check for contrast medium retention, indicating urinary stasis.
○ If ureteral obstruction is present, the ureteral catheter may be kept in place and, together with an indwelling urinary catheter, connected to a gravity drainage system until posttest urinary flow is corrected or returns to normal.

Patient care

○ Check the patient's vital signs every 15 minutes for the first hour, every 30 minutes for 1 hour, every hour for the next 2 hours, and then every 4 hours for 24 hours.
○ Monitor the patient's fluid intake and urine output for 24 hours.
○ Observe each specimen for hematuria. Gross hematuria or hematuria after the third voiding is abnormal and should be reported. If the patient doesn't void for 8 hours after the procedure or if the patient immediately feels distress and his bladder is distended, urethral catheterization may be necessary.
○ Be especially attentive to catheter output if ureteral catheters have been left in place because inadequate output may reflect catheter obstruction, requiring irrigation. Protect ureteral catheters from dislodgment. Note output amounts for each catheter (indwelling, urinary, urethral) separately; this helps determine the location of an obstruction that's causing reduced output.
○ Give prescribed analgesics and tub baths, and increase fluid intake for dysuria.
○ Watch for and report severe pain in the area of the kidneys as well as any signs of sepsis (such as chills, fever, and hypotension).
○ If irrigation is necessary, never use more than 10 ml of sterile saline solution.

Complications

○ Hematuria

Interpretation

Normal results

○ Opacification of the pelvis and calyces should occur immediately.
○ Normal structures should be outlined clearly and should appear symmetrical in bilateral testing.
○ Ureters should fill uniformly and appear normal in size and course.
○ Inspiratory and expiratory exposures, when superimposed, normally create two outlines of the renal pelvis ¾″ (2 cm) apart.

Abnormal results

○ Incomplete or delayed drainage reflects an obstruction, most commonly at the ureteropelvic junction.
○ Enlargement of the components of the collecting system or delayed emptying of contrast medium may indicate obstruction caused by a tumor, a blood clot, a stricture, or calculi.
○ Perinephric inflammation or suppuration commonly causes fixation of the kidney on the same side, resulting in a single sharp radiographic outline of the collecting system when inspiratory and expiratory exposures are superimposed.
○ Upward, downward, or lateral renal displacement can result from a renal abscess or tumor or from a perinephric abscess.
○ Neoplasms can cause displacement of either pole or the entire kidney.

Interfering factors

○ Previous contrast studies or presence of feces or gas in the bowel

Retrograde urethrography

Overview

○ Used almost exclusively in men, requires instillation or injection of a contrast medium into the urethra and shows its membranous, bulbar, and penile portions
○ May be used together with voiding cystourethrography if the posterior portion must be viewed more clearly

Purpose

○ To diagnose urethral strictures, diverticula, and congenital anomalies
○ To assess urethral lacerations or other trauma
○ To assist with follow-up examination after surgical repair of the urethra

Procedure

Preparation

○ Explain to the patient that retrograde urethrography diagnoses urethral structural problems. Inform him that he need not restrict food and fluids.
○ Check the patient's history for hypersensitivity to iodine-containing foods, such as shellfish, or contrast media.
○ Give any prescribed sedatives just before the procedure and instruct the patient to void before leaving the unit.
○ Inform the patient that he may experience some discomfort when the catheter is inserted and when the contrast medium is instilled through the catheter.
○ Tell the patient that he may hear loud, clacking sounds as the X-ray films are made.

Implementation

For men
○ The patient is placed into a recumbent position on the examining table. Anteroposterior exposures of the bladder and urethra are made, and the resulting films are studied for radiopaque densities, foreign bodies, or calculi.
○ The glans and meatus are cleaned with an antiseptic solution.
○ The catheter is filled with the contrast medium before insertion to eliminate air bubbles.
○ Although no lubricant should be used, the tip of the catheter may be dipped in sterile water to facilitate insertion.
○ The catheter is inserted until the balloon portion is inside the meatus; the balloon is then inflated with 1 to 2 ml of water, which prevents the catheter from slipping during the procedure.

○ The patient then assumes the right posterior oblique position, with his right thigh drawn up to a 90-degree angle and the penis placed along its axis. The left thigh is extended.
○ The contrast medium is injected through the catheter. After three-fourths of the contrast medium has been injected, the first X-ray film is exposed while the remainder of the contrast medium is being injected. Left lateral oblique views may also be taken.
○ Fluoroscopic control may be helpful, especially for evaluating urethral injury.

For women
○ Used when urethral diverticula are suspected, a double-balloon catheter is inserted, which occludes the bladder neck from above and the external meatus from below.

For children
○ The same procedure is used as for adults except with a smaller catheter.

Patient care

○ Watch for chills and fever related to extravasation of the contrast medium into the general circulation for 12 to 24 hours after retrograde urethrography.
○ Observe for signs of sepsis and allergic manifestations.
○ Monitor the patient for a urinary tract infection.
○ If urethral trauma is present, monitor for stricture, infection, and urinary extravasation.

Complications

○ Infection
○ Extravasation of contrast medium

Interpretation

Normal results

○ The membranous, bulbar, and penile portions of the urethra — and occasionally the prostatic portion — are normal in size, shape, and course.

Abnormal results

○ X-rays obtained during retrograde urethrography may show the following abnormalities: urethral diverticula, fistulas, strictures, false passages, calculi, and lacerations; congenital anomalies, such as urethral valves and perineal hypospadias; and, rarely, tumors (in less than 1% of cases).

Interfering factors

None known

Rhesus blood group system

Overview

○ Classifies blood according to the presence or absence of rhesus (Rh) antigen, screens all prospective donors for the weak D antigen, and rarely tests for other antigens to establish paternity, determine family studies, or distinguish between heterozygous and homozygous Rh-positive factors.

○ In 15% or less of the population, people lack the Rh antigen — known as $Rh_o(D)$ factor — in their red blood cells, and their blood is typed *Rh-negative*.

○ An Rh-negative mother and an Rh-positive father may have a baby at risk for developing hemolytic disease of the neonate (HDN).

○ The Rh-negative mother is given an injection of Rh immunoglobulin (RhIg) at 28 weeks' gestation and again after delivery if the baby is Rh positive.

○ The Rh antigen is highly immunogenic — that is, it's more likely to stimulate antigen formation than other known antigen.

○ The Rh-positive weak D antigen is less immunogenic than $Rh_o(D)$ and may not provoke antibody production in persons who lack it.

Purpose

○ To classify blood according to the presence or absence of Rh antigen

○ To screen all prospective donors for the weak D antigen, which is more common in blacks than in whites

○ To test for other antigens, such as rh8 (C), rh9 (F), hr8 (c), and hr9 (e) — done only in special cases, to establish paternity, determine family studies, or distinguish between heterozygous and homozygous Rh-positive factors

○ To prevent HDN in pregnancy or a reaction after a transfusion

Procedure

Preparation

○ Explain to the patient that this test classifies blood according to the Rh antigen that is found.

○ Tell the patient that this test requires a blood sample.

○ Inform the patient that she may feel slight discomfort from the needle puncture and the tourniquet.

Implementation

○ A venipuncture is performed and a blood sample collected.

○ For the pregnant patient, at the first prenatal visit, her blood is tested to determine whether she has been previously sensitized to Rh-positive blood. If test results show that the patient wasn't sensitized, a repeat test is scheduled at 28 weeks.

Patient care

○ Apply direct pressure to the venipuncture site until bleeding stops.

○ Answer the patient's questions about the test and the results.

Complications

○ Hematoma at the venipuncture site

Interpretation

Normal results

○ If the D antigen is present, that person is Rh-positive.

○ If the D antigen is absent, that person is Rh-negative.

○ Antibodies to Rh antigens develop only as an immune response after a transfusion or during pregnancy.

Abnormal results

○ Rh incompatibility is the most common and severe cause of HDN, possible when an Rh-negative woman and an Rh-positive man produce an Rh-positive baby.

Interfering factors

None known

Rheumatoid factor

Overview

○ Rheumatoid factor (RF) is an antibody that is measurable in the blood.
○ The RF test is the most useful immunologic test for confirming rheumatoid arthritis (RA).
○ Sheep cell agglutination and latex fixation techniques uncover the RF, even though this autoantibody may not be the cause of RA.
○ In RA, "renegade" immunoglobulin (Ig) G antibodies, produced by lymphocytes in the synovial joints, react with IgM antibody to produce immune complexes, complement activation, and tissue destruction.
○ Unknown how IgG molecules become antigenic, but they may be altered by aggregating with viruses or other antigens.

Purpose

○ To confirm RA when diagnosis is uncertain

Procedure

Preparation

○ Explain to the patient that this test helps confirm RA.
○ Inform the patient that he need not restrict food and fluids.
○ Tell the patient that the test requires a blood sample. Explain who will perform the venipuncture and when.
○ Explain to the patient that he may experience slight discomfort from the needle puncture and the tourniquet.

Implementation

○ Perform a venipuncture and collect the sample in a 7-ml clot-activator tube.

Patient care

○ Apply direct pressure to the venipuncture site until bleeding stops.
○ Check regularly for signs of infection.
○ Because a patient with RA may be immunologically compromised, keep the venipuncture site clean and dry for 24 hours.

Complications

○ Hematoma at the venipuncture site

Interpretation

Normal results

○ RF titer is less than 1:20; rheumatoid screening test is nonreactive.

Abnormal results

○ Non-RA and RA populations aren't clearly separated with regard to the presence of RF: 25% of patients with RA have a nonreactive titer; 8% of non-RA patients are reactive at greater than 39 IU/ml, and only 3% of non-RA patients are reactive at greater than 80 IU/ml.
○ Patients with various non-RA diseases characterized by chronic inflammation may test positive for RF. These diseases include systemic lupus erythematosus, polymyositis, tuberculosis, infectious mononucleosis, syphilis, viral hepatic disease, and influenza.

Interfering factors

○ Inadequately activated complement (possible false-positive)
○ Serum with high lipid or cryoglobulin levels (possible false-positive, requiring a repeat test after restricting fat intake)
○ Serum with high IgG levels (possible false-negative because of competition with IgG on the surface of latex particles or sheep RBCs used as substrate)

Rubella antibodies

Overview

- Because rubella infection normally induces immunoglobulin (Ig) G and IgM antibody production, measuring rubella antibodies can determine present infection as well as immunity resulting from past infection.
- Hemagglutination inhibition test is the most commonly used serologic test for rubella antibodies.
- Suspected cases of congenital rubella may be confirmed if rubella-specific IgM antibodies are present in the infant's serum.
- Immune status in adults can be confirmed by an existing IgG-specific titer.
- Exposure risk (when the immunity status is unknown) may be evaluated using two serum samples.
- First sample should be drawn in the acute phase of clinical symptoms; if clinical symptoms aren't apparent, the sample should be drawn as soon as possible after the suspected exposure.
- Second sample should be drawn 3 to 4 weeks later during the convalescent phase.
- Although rubella (German measles) is generally a mild viral infection in children and young adults, it can produce severe infection in the fetus, resulting in spontaneous abortion, stillbirth, or congenital rubella syndrome.

Purpose

- To diagnose rubella infection, especially congenital infection
- To determine susceptibility to rubella in children and in women of childbearing age

Procedure

Preparation

- Explain to the patient that this test diagnoses or evaluates susceptibility to rubella.
- Inform the patient that she need not restrict food and fluids.
- Tell the patient that this test requires a blood sample and that if a current infection is suspected, a second blood sample will be necessary in 2 to 3 weeks to identify a rise in the titer.
- Explain to the patient that she may experience slight discomfort from the needle puncture and the tourniquet.

Implementation

- Perform a venipuncture and collect the sample in a 7-ml clot-activator tube.
- Handle the specimen gently to prevent hemolysis.

Patient care

- Apply direct pressure to the venipuncture site until bleeding stops.
- Instruct the patient to return for an additional blood test, when appropriate.
- If a woman of childbearing age is found to be susceptible to rubella, explain that vaccination can prevent rubella and that she must wait at least 3 months after the vaccination to become pregnant or risk permanent damage or death to the fetus.
- If the pregnant patient is found to be susceptible to rubella, instruct her to return for follow-up rubella antibody tests to detect possible subsequent infection.
- If the test confirms rubella in a pregnant patient, provide emotional support. Refer her for appropriate counseling, as needed.

Complications

- Hematoma at the venipuncture site

Interpretation

Normal results

- A titer of 1:8 or less indicates little or no immunity against rubella; titer more than 1:10 indicates adequate protection against rubella.
- IgM results are reported as positive or negative.

Abnormal results

- Hemagglutination inhibition antibodies normally appear 2 to 4 days after the onset of the rash, peak in 3 to 4 weeks, and then slowly decline but remain detectable for life.
- A fourfold or greater rise from the acute to the convalescent titer indicates a recent rubella infection.
- The presence of rubella-specific IgM antibodies indicates recent infection in an adult and congenital rubella in an infant.

Interfering factors

- Hemolysis from rough handling of the sample

Schirmer's tearing

Overview

○ Assesses the function of the major lacrimal glands, which are responsible for reflex tearing in response to stressful situations such as the presence of a foreign body; both eyes tested at once.
○ Involves stimulating tearing by inserting a strip of filter paper into the lower conjunctival sac; then measuring the amount of moisture absorbed by the paper.
○ A variation of this test evaluates the function of the accessory lacrimal glands of Krause and Wolfring by instilling a topical anesthetic before inserting the filter papers.
○ The anesthetic inhibits reflex tearing by the major lacrimal glands, ensuring measurement of only the basic tear film normally produced by the accessory glands.
○ This tear film usually maintains adequate corneal moisture under normal circumstances.

Purpose

○ To measure tear secretion in a patient with suspected tearing deficiency

Procedure

Preparation

○ Tell the patient that this test requires that a strip of filter paper be placed in the lower part of each eye for 5 minutes.
○ Reassure the patient that the procedure is painless.
○ If the patient wears contact lenses, ask him to remove them before the test. If an anesthetic is instilled, tell him he won't be able to reinsert the lenses for 2 hours after the test.

Implementation

○ Assist the patient into the examining chair with his head against the headrest.
○ To remove the test strip from the wrapper, bend the rounded wick end at the indentation and cut open the envelope at the other end.
○ Tell the patient to look up, and then gently lower the inferior eyelid.
○ Hook the bent end of the strip over the inferior eyelid at the junction of the medial and nasal segments.
○ Insert one strip in each eye and note the time of insertion. Tell the patient not to squeeze or rub his eyes, but to blink normally or to keep his eyes closed lightly.
○ After 5 minutes, remove the strips from the patient's eyes and measure the length of the moistened area from the indentation, using the millimeter scale on the envelope.

○ Report the results as a fraction: the numerator is the length of the moistened area, and the denominator is the time the strips were left in place. Note which eye was tested — if a strip inserted in the right conjunctival sac for 5 minutes shows 8 mm of moisture, the correct notation is OD (*oculus dexter,* or right eye), 8 mm/5 minutes.
○ To measure the function of the accessory lacrimal glands of Krause and Wolfring, instill one drop of topical anesthetic into each conjunctival sac before inserting the test strips.
○ To prevent patient discomfort, be careful not to touch the cornea while inserting the test strip.

Patient care

○ If a topical anesthetic was instilled, advise the patient not to rub his eyes for at least 30 minutes after instillation because this can cause a corneal abrasion.
○ The patient who wears contact lenses shouldn't reinsert them for at least 2 hours.

Complications

None known

Interpretation

Normal results

○ The test strip shows at least 15 mm of moisture after 5 minutes. Both eyes usually secrete the same amount of tears.
○ Because tear production decreases with age, normal test results in a patient over age 40 range from 10 to 15 mm.

Abnormal results

○ Up to 15% of the patients tested have false-positive or false-negative results.
○ Because the test is rapid and simple, it may be repeated and findings compared.
○ Additional testing, such as a slit-lamp examination with fluorescein or rose Bengal stain, is necessary to corroborate results.
○ A positive result confirmed by additional testing indicates a definite tearing deficiency, which may result from aging or, more seriously, from Sjögren's syndrome, a systemic disease of unknown origin most common among postmenopausal women.
○ A tearing deficiency may also arise secondarily to systemic diseases, such as lymphoma, leukemia, and rheumatoid arthritis.
○ Regardless of the cause, a tearing deficiency is a matter of clinical concern because it can lead to corneal erosions, scarring, and secondary infection.

Interfering factors

○ The patient closing his eyes too tightly during the test
○ Reflex tearing caused by contact of the test strip with the cornea

Screening test for congenital hypothyroidism

Overview

- Measures serum thyroxine (T_4) levels in the neonate to detect congenital hypothyroidism; mandatory in some states.
- Characterized by low or absent levels of T_4, congenital hypothyroidism affects roughly 1 in 5,000 neonates, occurring in females three times more often than in males.
- Congenital hypothyroidism can result from thyroid dysgenesis or hypoplasia, congenital goiter, or maternal use of thyroid inhibitors during pregnancy.
- If untreated, can lead to irreversible brain damage by age 3 months.
- Radioimmunoassays for T_4 and thyroid-stimulating hormone (TSH) are effective in screening neonates for congenital hypothyroidism.

Purpose

- To screen neonates for congenital hypothyroidism

Procedure

Preparation

- Explain to the parents that although hypothyroidism is uncommon in infants, this screening test detects the disorder early enough to begin therapy before irreversible brain damage occurs.
- Tell the parents that the test will occur before the infant is discharged from the facility and again 4 to 6 weeks later.
- Emphasize the importance of the screening and the need for following the test protocol.
- Because false-positive findings can result from variations in the test procedure or from a congenital thyroxine-binding globulin (TBG) defect, inform the parents that a second test may be necessary before the infant is discharged.

Implementation

- Wipe the infant's heel with an alcohol or a povidone-iodine swab, and then dry it thoroughly with a gauze pad.
- Perform a heelstick.
- Squeeze the heel gently and fill the circles on the filter paper with blood. Make sure the blood saturates the paper.
- When the filter paper is dry, label it appropriately and send it to the laboratory.

Patient care

- Apply gentle pressure with a gauze pad until bleeding stops at the puncture site.
- If results of the screening test indicate congenital hypothyroidism, tell the parents that additional testing is necessary to determine the cause of the disorder.
- If the sample isn't processed in the facility's laboratory, make sure to notify the parents when test results are available.

Complications

None known

Interpretation

Normal results

- Immediately after birth, T_4 levels are higher than adult levels.
- By the end of the first week, T_4 values decrease markedly.
- 1 to 5 days, 4.9 µg/dl (SI, 58.8 nmol/L).
- 6 to 8 days, 4 µg/dl (SI, 48 nmol/L).
- 9 to 11 days, 3.5 µg/dl (SI, 42 nmol/L).
- 12 to 120 days, 3 µg/dl (SI, 36 nmol/L).

Abnormal results

- Low serum T_4 levels in the neonate require TSH testing for clarification of the diagnosis.
- Decreased T_4 levels accompanied by elevated TSH readings (> 25 µU/ml [SI, 300 nmol/L]) indicate primary congenital hypothyroidism (thyroid gland dysfunction).
- If T_4 and TSH levels are depressed, secondary congenital hypothyroidism (resulting from pituitary or hypothalamic dysfunction) should be suspected.
- If T_4 levels are subnormal in the presence of normal TSH readings, further testing is required.
- Serum TBG levels must be analyzed to identify infants with hypothyroidism resulting from congenital defects in TBG.
- This low T_4–normal TSH pattern also occurs in a transient form of congenital hypothyroidism, which may accompany prematurity, or prenatal hypoxia.
- A complete thyroid workup, including serum T_3, TBG, and free T_4 levels, is necessary for unequivocal diagnosis of congenital hypothyroidism before treatment begins.

Interfering factors

- Failure to allow the filter paper to dry completely
- Failure to follow special directions for obtaining the sample

Semen analysis

Overview

○ A simple, inexpensive, and reasonably definitive test that's used in many applications, including evaluating a man's fertility.
○ Usually includes measuring seminal fluid volume, performing sperm counts, and microscopically examining spermatozoa.
○ Sperm are counted in semen in much the same way that white blood cells, red blood cells, and platelets are counted in a blood sample.
○ Motility and morphology are studied microscopically after staining a drop of semen.
○ This test can also detect semen on a rape victim, identify the blood group of an alleged rapist, or prove sterility in a paternity suit. (See *Identifying semen for medicolegal purposes.*)

Purpose

○ To evaluate male fertility in an infertile couple
○ To substantiate the effectiveness of a vasectomy
○ To detect semen on the body or clothing of a suspected rape victim or elsewhere at a crime scene
○ To identify blood group substances to exonerate or incriminate a criminal suspect
○ To rule out paternity on grounds of complete sterility

Procedure

Preparation

○ For fertility evaluation, provide the patient with written instructions, and inform him that the most desirable specimen requires masturbation, ideally in a physician's office or laboratory.
○ Tell the patient to follow the written instructions regarding the period of sexual continence before the test because this may increase his sperm count.
○ If the patient prefers to collect the specimen at home, emphasize the importance of delivering the specimen to the laboratory within 1 hour after collection. Warn him not to expose the specimen to extreme temperatures or to direct sunlight.
○ Ideally, the specimen should remain at body temperature until liquefaction is complete (about 20 minutes). To deliver a semen specimen during cold weather, suggest that the patient keep the specimen container in a coat pocket on the way to the laboratory to protect the specimen from exposure to cold.
○ Alternatives to collection by masturbation include coitus interruptus or the use of a condom.
○ For collection by coitus interruptus, instruct the patient to withdraw immediately before ejaculation and to deposit the ejaculate in a suitable specimen container.
○ For collection by condom, tell the patient to first wash the condom with soap and water, rinse it thor-

oughly, and allow it to dry completely. (Powders or lubricants applied to the condom may be spermicidal.)
○ Special sheaths that don't contain spermicide are also available for semen collection. Instruct the patient to tie the condom after collection, place it in a glass jar, and promptly deliver it to the laboratory.
○ It's also possible to determine fertility by collecting semen from the woman after coitus to assess the ability of the spermatozoa to penetrate the cervical mucus and remain active.
○ For the postcoital cervical mucus test, instruct the patient to report for examination 1 to 2 days before ovulation as determined by basal temperature records.
○ Instruct the couple to abstain from intercourse for 2 days and then to have sexual intercourse 2 to 8 hours before the examination. Remind them to avoid using lubricants.
○ Explain to the patient that she'll be placed in the lithotomy position and that a speculum will be inserted into the vagina to collect the specimen. Tell her that she may feel some pressure but no pain.
○ For semen collection from a rape victim, explain to the patient that the examiner will try to obtain a semen specimen from her vagina.
○ Prepare the victim for insertion of the speculum as you would the patient scheduled for postcoital examination.
○ Handle the victim's clothes as little as possible. If her clothes are moist, put them in a paper bag — not a plastic bag (which causes seminal stains and secretions to mold). Label the bag properly, and send it to the laboratory immediately.
○ Provide emotional support by speaking to the patient calmly and reassuringly. Encourage her to express her fears and anxieties. Listen sympathetically.
○ If the patient is scheduled for vaginal lavage, tell the rape victim to expect a cold sensation when saline solution is instilled to wash out the specimen.
○ Help the patient relax by instructing her to breathe deeply and slowly through her mouth.
○ Instruct the victim to urinate just before the test, but warn her not to wipe the vulva afterward because this may remove semen.

Implementation

○ Obtain a semen specimen for a fertility study by asking the patient to collect semen in a clean plastic specimen container.
○ Before postcoital examination, the examiner wipes excess mucus from the external cervix and collects the specimen by direct aspiration of the cervical canal using a 1-ml tuberculin syringe without a cannula or needle.
○ A specimen is obtained from the vagina of a rape victim by direct aspiration, saline lavage, or a direct smear of vaginal contents using a Pap stick or, less desirably, a cotton applicator stick.
○ Never lubricate the vaginal speculum. Oil or grease hinders examination of spermatozoa by interfering

with smear preparation and staining and by inhibiting sperm motility through toxic ingredients. Instead, moisten the speculum with water or physiologic saline solution.
- Dried smears are usually collected from the suspected rape victim's skin by gently washing the skin with a small piece of gauze moistened with physiologic saline solution.
- Prepare direct smears on glass microscopic slides after labeling the frosted end. Immediately place smeared slides in Coplin jars containing 95% ethanol.

Patient care

- Inform a patient who's undergoing infertility studies that test results should be available in 24 hours.
- Refer the patient to an appropriate specialist for counseling.

Complications

None known

Interpretation

Normal results

- 0.7 to 6.5 ml
- The semen volume of many men in infertile couples is increased, compared to the normal range.
- Abstinence for 1 week or more increases semen volume. (With abstinence of up to 10 days, sperm counts increase, sperm motility progressively decreases, and sperm morphology stays the same.)
- Liquefied semen is generally highly viscid, translucent, and gray-white, with a musty or acrid odor. After liquefaction, specimens of normal viscosity can be poured in drops.
- Normally, semen is slightly alkaline with a pH of 7.3 to 7.9.
- Semen coagulates immediately and liquefies within 20 minutes; the normal sperm count is 20 to 150 million/ml and can be greater; 40% of spermatozoa have normal morphology; and 20% or more of spermatozoa show progressive motility within 4 hours of collection.
- The normal postcoital cervical mucus test shows 10 to 20 motile spermatozoa per microscopic high-power field and spinnbarkeit (a measurement of the tenacity of the mucus) of at least 4″ (10 cm). These findings indicate adequate spermatozoa and receptivity of the cervical mucus. Shaking or dead sperm may indicate antisperm antibodies.

Abnormal results

- Abnormal semen is *not* synonymous with infertility.
- Only one viable spermatozoon is needed to fertilize an ovum.
- Only men who can't deliver *any* viable spermatozoa in their ejaculate during sexual intercourse are absolutely sterile.

Identifying semen for medicolegal purposes

Spermatozoa (or their fragments) persist in the vagina for more than 72 hours after sexual intercourse. This allows detection and positive identification of semen from vaginal aspirates or smears or from stains on clothing, other fabrics, skin, or hair, which is usually necessary for medicolegal purposes, most often in connection with rape or homicide investigations. Identification of spermatozoa taken from the vagina of an exhumed body is also possible if the body has been properly embalmed and remains reasonably intact.

To determine which stains or fluids require further investigation, clothing or other fabrics can be scanned with ultraviolet light to detect the typical green-white fluorescence of semen. Soaking appropriate samples of clothing, fabric, or hair in physiologic saline solution extracts the semen and spermatozoa. Deposits of dried semen can be gently sponged from the victim's skin.

The two most common ways to identify semen are testing for *acid phosphatase concentration* (the more sensitive test) and a *microscopic examination* for the presence of spermatozoa. Acid phosphatase appears in semen in significantly greater levels than in other body fluids. In microscopic examination, spermatozoa or head fragments can be identified on stained smears prepared directly from vaginal scrapings or aspirates or from the concentrated sediment of eluates or lavages.

Like other body fluids, semen contains the soluble A, B, and H blood group substances in about 80% of men who are genetically determined secretors (men who have the dominant secretor gene in a homozygous or heterozygous state). Thus, the man who has group A blood and is a secretor has soluble blood group A substance in his seminal fluid and group A substance on the surface of his red blood cells. This fact can be of considerable medicolegal importance. Semen analysis can demonstrate that the semen of a rape or homicide investigation suspect is different from or consistent with semen found in or on the victim's body.

- Subnormal sperm counts, decreased sperm motility, and abnormal morphology usually indicate decreased fertility.

Interfering factors

- Poor timing of test within the menstrual cycle
- Previous cervical conization or cryotherapy and some drugs such as clomiphene citrate
- Delayed transport of the specimen, exposure to extreme temperatures or direct sunlight, or the presence of toxic chemicals in the container or the condom
- An incomplete specimen (decrease in specimen volume)

Sentinel lymph node biopsy

Overview

- Identifies sentinel lymph node, the first node in the lymphatic basin into which a primary tumor site drains.
- Uses lymphoscintigraphy and blue dye injection to increase chances of locating node.
- The histology of the sentinel node reflects the histology of the other nodes in that basin.

Purpose

- To identify the sentinel lymph node and evaluate it for the presence or absence of tumor cells indicating nodal metastasis

Procedure

Preparation

- Make sure the patient has signed an appropriate consent form.
- Note and report all allergies.
- Tell the patient that he will receive a radioactive substance injected under the skin.
- Explain that the test usually accompanies lumpectomy or mastectomy.

Implementation

- The patient is placed onto the table in the nuclear medicine suite.
- A standard dose of technetium-99m (^{99m}Tc) pyro phosphate is injected circumferentially around the margins of a palpable mass, using a 25G needle.
- For a nonpalpable mass, injections are guided with ultrasound or mammographic techniques.
- Images of the axilla are taken with a gamma camera. The location of the sentinel node is marked on the skin in indelible ink and noted on a data sheet.
- The patient is transported to the operating room and placed under appropriate anesthesia.
- Blue dye is injected circumferentially in the tissue immediately surrounding the biopsy site using a 25G needle.
- A small incision is made in the axilla over the suspected location of the sentinel lymph node.
- The node having the highest radioactivity is deemed the sentinel node and is removed.
- The axilla is then checked for remaining radioactivity; if none is noted, the surgical procedure concludes.
- Because of the radioactivity, the sentinel lymph node is maintained in formalin for 24 to 48 hours before it's processed.

Patient care

- Provide the patient with routine postoperative care.
- Observe for allergic reaction to ^{99m}Tc or blue dye, such as skin changes and respiratory difficulties.

Complications

- Adverse reaction to ^{99m}Tc or blue dye (rare)

Interpretation

Normal results

- Normal findings are the same as for a normal lymph node biopsy.

Abnormal results

- Abnormal pathology indicates the presence of melanoma or breast cancer cells.
- Presence of cancer cells suggests lymph node metastasis.

Interfering factors

- Inability of the patient to raise his arm, allowing access to the axilla
- Inability to obtain an adequate specimen
- Improper specimen storage

Sex chromosome tests

Overview

○ Indicated for abnormal sexual development, ambiguous genitalia, amenorrhea, and suspected chromosomal abnormalities
○ Screens for abnormalities in the number of sex chromosomes; the faster, simpler, more accurate full karyotype (chromosome analysis) has nearly replaced these tests

Purpose

○ To quickly screen for abnormal sexual development (X and Y chromatin tests)
○ To aid in the assessment of an infant with ambiguous genitalia (X chromatin test)
○ To determine the number of Y chromosomes in an individual (Y chromatin test)

Procedure

Preparation

○ Explain to the patient or his parents, if appropriate, why the sex chromosome test is necessary.
○ Tell the patient that this test requires that the inside of his cheek be scraped to obtain a specimen. Tell him who will perform the test.
○ Assure the patient that the test takes only a few minutes but may require a follow-up chromosome analysis.
○ Inform the patient that the laboratory generally requires as long as 4 weeks to complete the analysis.

Implementation

○ Scrape the buccal mucosa firmly with a wooden or metal spatula at least twice to obtain a specimen of healthy cells (vaginal mucosa is occasionally used in young women).
○ Rub the spatula over the glass slide, making sure the cells are evenly distributed.
○ Spray the slide with a cell fixative and send it to the laboratory with a brief patient history and indications for the test.
○ Make sure the buccal mucosa is scraped firmly to ensure a sufficient number of cells.
○ Check that the specimen isn't saliva, which contains no cells.

Patient care

○ Answer the patient's questions about the test.
○ The patient or his parents will require genetic counseling after identification of the cause of chromosomal abnormal sexual development.

Complications

None known

Interpretation

Normal results

○ A normal female (XX) has only one X chromatin mass (the number of X chromatin masses discernible is one less than the number of X chromosomes in the cells examined).
○ An X chromatin mass is ordinarily discernible in only 20% to 50% of the buccal mucosal cells of a normal woman.
○ A normal male (XY) has only one Y chromatin mass (the number of Y chromatin masses equals the number of Y chromosomes in the cells examined).

Abnormal results

○ If less than 20% of the cells in a buccal smear contain an X chromatin mass, some cells are presumed to contain only one X chromosome, necessitating full karyotyping.
○ A person with a female phenotype and a positive Y chromatin mass runs a high risk of developing a malignancy in the intra-abdominal gonads. In such cases, removal of these gonads is indicated and should generally be performed before age 5.
○ A medical team composed of physicians, psychologists, psychiatrists, and educators must decide the child's sex if a child is phenotypically of one sex and genotypically of the other. This careful evaluation should be made early to prevent developmental problems related to incorrect gender identification.

Interfering factors

○ Obtaining saliva instead of buccal cells (false specimen)
○ Cell deterioration caused by failure to apply cell fixative to the slide
○ Presence of bacteria or wrinkles in the cell membrane, analysis of degenerative cells, or use of an outdated stain

Sickle cell

Overview

- The sickle cell test, also known as the *hemoglobin (Hb) S test*, detects sickle cells (severely deformed, rigid erythrocytes that may slow blood flow).
- The sickle cell trait (characterized by heterozygous Hb S) exists almost exclusively in blacks — 0.2% of blacks born in the United States have sickle cell disease. (See *Inheritance patterns in sickle cell anemia.*)
- Although the sickle cell test is useful as a rapid screening procedure, it may produce erroneous results.
- Hb electrophoresis can confirm the diagnosis if sickle cell disease is strongly suspected.

Purpose

- To identify sickle cell disease and sickle cell trait

Procedure

Preparation

- Explain to the patient that the sickle cell test detects sickle cell disease.
- Tell the patient that the test requires a blood sample.
- Explain to the patient that he may feel slight discomfort from the tourniquet and the needle puncture.
- If the patient is an infant or child, explain to his parents that a small amount of blood will be taken from his finger or earlobe.
- Check the patient's history for a blood transfusion within the past 3 months.
- Inform the patient that he need not restrict food and fluids.

Inheritance patterns in sickle cell anemia

When both parents have sickle cell anemia (left), child-bearing — if possible at all — is dangerous for the mother, and all offspring will have sickle cell anemia. When one parent has sickle cell anemia and one does not (right), all offspring will be carriers of sickle cell anemia.

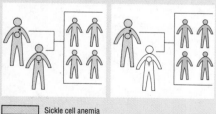

- Sickle cell anemia
- Sickle cell trait
- Normal

Implementation

- Perform a venipuncture and collect the sample in a 3- or 4.5-ml ethylenediaminetetraacetic acid tube.
- For young children, collect capillary blood in a microcollection device.
- Completely fill the collection tube and invert it gently several times to thoroughly mix the sample and the anticoagulant.

Patient care

- Apply direct pressure to the venipuncture site until bleeding stops.
- Provide genetic counseling referral to the parents if needed.

Complications

- Hematoma at the venipuncture site; if large, monitor pulses distal to the phlebotomy site.

Interpretation

Normal results

- A negative result suggests the absence of Hb S.

Abnormal results

- A positive result may indicate the presence of sickle cells, but Hb electrophoresis is necessary to further diagnose the sickling tendency of cells.
- Rarely, in the absence of Hb S, other abnormal Hb may cause sickling.

Interfering factors

- Failure to fill the tube completely, to use the proper anticoagulant in the collection tube, or to adequately mix the sample and the anticoagulant
- Hemolysis from rough handling of the sample or use of a small-gauge needle for blood aspiration
- Hb level < 10%, elevated Hb S levels in infants under age 6 months, or transfusion within 3 months of the test (possible false-negative)

Sigmoidoscopy, flexible

Overview

- An endoscopic examination of the lining of the descending colon, sigmoid colon, rectum, and anal canal, using a flexible sigmoidoscope
- Allows several methods for obtaining specimens from suspicious areas of the mucosa: biopsy, cytology brush, or aspirate
- Used in colorectal screening (starting at age 50 for normal risk individuals without family history of colorectal cancer or adenomatous colon polyps)

Purpose

- To aid in the diagnosis of acute or chronic diarrhea and rectal bleeding
- To evaluate changes in bowel habits or feces characteristics
- To aid in the assessment of known ulcerative colitis

Procedure

Preparation

- Note and report all allergies.
- Check the patient's history for barium tests within the last week because barium in the colon makes accurate examination impossible.
- Advise the patient about whether or not he must fast before the procedure.
- Tell the patient that he may receive a laxative or enema before the examination.
- Discuss the possible use of sedation to help the patient relax.
- Warn the patient about a possible urge to defecate during the procedure.
- Advise the patient that air may be introduced through the endoscope to distend the walls of the colon, which causes flatus.
- Explain that the test takes 10 to 30 minutes.

Implementation

- The patient is placed in the Sims' position on the examination table.
- Before the procedure, the endoscopist visually inspects the anus and perineum.
- Digital rectal examination is performed.
- The flexible sigmoidoscope is slowly advanced to the splenic flexure, if possible, or as far as the patient can tolerate with only mild discomfort.
- Specimens may be obtained from any suspicious area of the intestinal mucosa.
- Polyps may be biopsied for histologic diagnosis or removed by the insertion of an electrocautery snare through the endoscope and submitted for histological examination.
- Feces aspirate may be obtained when indicated for laboratory analysis.

- Before withdrawal of the scope, retroflexion is performed, allowing examination of the internal anal verge and the adjacent rectal mucosa.
- The scope is withdrawn, the lining of the colon is thoroughly examined, and air is removed.

Patient care

- Have the patient resume his previous diet.
- If the patient has received sedation, don't resume diet and activity until the patient is fully awake.
- Encourage the patient to expel flatus.
- If the patient received a biopsy or polypectomy, tell him that he may notice a minute amount of blood in his feces.
- Monitor the patient's vital signs.
- Monitor feces and bowel sounds.
- Observe the patient for bleeding.
- Observe closely for any signs of bowel perforation (abdominal distention and pain, nausea, vomiting, and fever).
- Observe for vasovagal reaction (hypotension, pallor, diaphoresis, and bradycardia).

Complications

- Rectal bleeding
- Bowel perforation
- Vasovagal reaction
- Adverse reaction to sedation

Interpretation

Normal results

- Mucosa of the anal canal is pearly white or pigmented, depending on the patient's race.
- Mucosa of the rectum is pink and may appear velvety because of the prevalence of lymphoid tissue.
- The rich vascular network becomes less prominent at the rectosigmoid junction.
- Three semilunar valves (Houston's valves) are present in the proximal half of the rectum.
- Mucosa of the sigmoid and descending colon is light pink-orange.

Abnormal results

- Biopsy results suggest possible benign, precancerous, or malignant polyps or tumors and various forms of colitis.
- Visual inspection of the anus and perineum may disclose abnormalities, such as external hemorrhoids, anal fissure, anorectal cellulitis or abscess, and perirectal skin tag.
- Digital rectal examination may disclose rectal mass, internal hemorrhoids, or anorectal abscess.
- Inflammatory change suggests possible diverticulitis.
- *Melanosis coli* (a brownish discoloration of the colon) suggests possible chronic laxative use.

Interfering factors

- Barium in the colon makes accurate examination impossible

Site-of-lesion tests

Overview

○ Identify the location of a lesion suggested by patient history or pure tone audiometry
○ Indicated for those having difficulty understanding speech, disproportionate to the degree of pure tone loss; dizziness, tinnitus, or sudden or fluctuating hearing loss; or other neural symptoms; or a difference between sensorineural components in each ear
○ Distinguish cochlear from retrocochlear lesions and localize lesions in the retrocochlear system at the eighth nerve, in the extra-axial (peripheral) or intra-axial brain stem, and in the cortex

Purpose

○ To distinguish cochlear from retrocochlear hearing loss
○ To localize lesions in the retrocochlear component of the auditory system

Procedure

Preparation

○ Note and report all allergies.
○ Tell the patient that the tests take about 90 minutes.

Implementation

○ Earphones are applied to the patient.

Alternate binaural loudness

○ A tone is presented alternately to one ear and then the other. The tone in one ear is held at a constant intensity of 90 dB hearing level (HL); the other tone is varied.
○ The patient indicates when the tones sound equally loud to both ears.

Simultaneous binaural midplane localization

○ A 90-dB HL tone is presented to one ear, and tones of varying intensity are presented simultaneously to the other ear.
○ The patient indicates when he perceives a single tone in the center of his head.

Rosenburg tone decay

○ A tone is presented at or near threshold; the patient indicates how long he can hear it.
○ If the tone becomes inaudible or changes to a buzzing or hissing sound, the tone is raised 5 dB, to produce a tone that the patient should again be able to hear.
○ The process is repeated until the patient hears the tone continuously for 60 seconds.

Suprathreshold Adaptation Test

○ A tone is presented at 110 dB sensation level, rounded to 100 dB HL at 500 and 2,000 Hz and to 105 dB HL at 1,000 Hz.

Békésy audiometry

○ The patient controls the tone intensity by depressing a response button whenever he hears a tone. When the tone softens and disappears, he releases the button; the tone then becomes louder.
○ The patient repeats this procedure for several minutes, and the resulting audiometric tracing shows excursions above and below the actual threshold.
○ Tracings are obtained for pulsed and continuous tones. The relationship between these two categories can be grouped into diagnostic patterns.

Masking level differences

○ A 500-Hz tone and a narrow-band masking noise are presented to both ears at the same time. The noise is held at a constant intensity, and the patient's threshold for the tonal stimulus in that noise is determined. Then the phase of the tone is changed to one ear by 180 degrees, and the difference is tested.

Difficult speech discrimination tasks

○ To gauge the patient's ability to discriminate speech in white noise, a speech stimulus is presented to one ear; the result is scored.
○ White noise and a speech stimulus are presented simultaneously to the same ear, and the result is scored. The two scores are then compared.
○ The task is repeated for the other ear and the scored are compared. Finally, each ear's score is compared with the other and with normal range.

Auditory brain stem electrical response measures

○ Electrodes are placed at the vertex of the patient's scalp (active), the mastoid process or earlobe of the stimulated ear (reference), and the mastoid process or earlobe of the opposite ear (ground).
○ Stimuli are presented in the form of clicks or rapid rise time (1 millisecond) tone pips at 10 per second until 2,000 time-locked responses are collected and averaged. This tests mainly the 1,000- to 4,000-Hz frequency.

Competing message tasks

○ A different message is presented to each ear, and the patient is asked to discriminate between the messages.
○ In a gross measure test, such as the Northwestern University Test #20, speech discrimination words are presented to one ear, and the patient is asked to repeat them. Then speech discrimination words are presented to the same ear, and short sentences are simultaneously presented to the other ear; the patient is asked to repeat the words and ignore the sentences. The patient's scores on each task are then compared.

Precise message test

○ An example of this type of test is the dichotic nonsense syllables test.
○ Carefully aligned nonsense syllables are presented to both ears at once, and the patient is asked to repeat or write both syllables. The number of syllables correctly identified in one ear is compared with the number of syllables correctly identified in the other ear, as well as with a normal range.

Patient care

○ Answer the patient's questions about the tests.

Complications

None known

Interpretation

Normal results

○ Sensory and neural deficits are absent.

Abnormal results

○ Sensory deficits suggest lesions of the auditory portions of the inner ear (*cochlea*).
○ Neural deficits suggest lesions beyond the inner ear (*retrocochlear*).
○ Abnormal adaptation to a continuous tone in tone decay tests suggests the presence of retrocochlear lesions.

Interfering factors

None known

Skin biopsy

Overview

○ Removal of a small piece of tissue, under local anesthesia, from lesion suspected of being malignant.
○ Specimen for histologic examination may be obtained by shave, punch, or excision biopsy.
○ Fully developed lesions are selected for biopsy whenever possible because they provide more diagnostic information than resolving lesions or those in early developing stages.

Purpose

○ To allow differential diagnosis of basal cell carcinoma, squamous cell carcinoma, malignant melanoma, and benign growths
○ To diagnose chronic bacterial or fungal skin infections

Procedure

Preparation

○ Make sure the patient has signed an appropriate consent form.
○ Note and report all allergies.
○ Tell the patient that he need not restrict food and fluids.
○ Inform the patient that he will receive a local anesthetic to minimize pain during the procedure.
○ Explain that the biopsy takes about 15 minutes.

Implementation

○ Position the patient comfortably and clean the biopsy site.
○ The patient is given a local anesthetic.
Shave biopsy
○ The protruding growth is cut off at the skin line with a #15 scalpel, and the tissue placed immediately in a properly labeled specimen bottle containing 10% formalin solution.
○ Pressure is applied to the area to stop the bleeding.
Punch biopsy
○ The skin surrounding the lesion is pulled taut, and the punch is firmly introduced into the lesion and rotated to obtain a tissue specimen.
○ The plug is lifted with forceps or a needle and is severed as deeply into the fat layer as possible.
○ The specimen is placed in a properly labeled specimen bottle containing 10% formalin solution or, if indicated, in a sterile container.
○ The method used to close the wound depends on the size of the punch.
Excision biopsy
○ A #15 scalpel is used to excise the lesion completely; the incision is made as wide and as deep as necessary.

○ The examiner removes the tissue specimen and places it immediately in a properly labeled specimen bottle containing 10% formalin solution.
○ Pressure is applied to the site to stop the bleeding. The wound is closed, and if the incision is large, a skin graft may be required.

Patient care

○ If the patient experiences pain at the biopsy site, give an analgesic.
○ Advise the patient with sutures to keep the area clean and as dry as possible. Facial sutures are removed in 3 to 5 days; trunk sutures, in 7 to 14 days.
○ Instruct the patient with adhesive strips to leave them in place for 14 to 21 days or until they fall off.
○ Monitor the patient for bleeding and infection.

Complications

○ Bleeding
○ Infection

Interpretation

Normal results

○ Normal skin consists of squamous epithelium (*epidermis*) and fibrous connective tissue (*dermis*).

Abnormal results

○ Histologic examination of the tissue specimen suggests possible benign lesions such as dermatofibromas, or malignant lesions such as malignant melanoma.

Interfering factors

○ Improper selection of a biopsy site
○ Failure to use appropriate fixative or sterile container

Skull radiography

Overview

- Noninvasive neurologic test (use has declined with increased use of other diagnostic studies, such as computed tomography and magnetic resonance imaging)
- Complete skull examination (because bones of the skull form a complex anatomic structure, requires several radiologic views of each area)
- For head injuries, offers limited information about skull fractures
- Extremely valuable for studying abnormalities of the base of the skull and the cranial vault, neoplasms, congenital and perinatal anomalies, and many metabolic and endocrinologic diseases that produce bone defects of the skull

Purpose

- To detect fractures in patients with head trauma
- To aid in the diagnosis of pituitary tumors
- To detect congenital anomalies
- To detect metabolic and endocrinologic disorders

Procedure

Preparation

- Make sure the patient has signed an appropriate consent form.
- Note and report all allergies.
- Tell the patient that he need not restrict food and fluids.
- Advise the patient to remove glasses, dentures, jewelry, and metal objects in the radiographic field.
- Explain that the procedure causes no discomfort and takes about 15 minutes.

Implementation

- The patient is placed in the supine position on an X-ray table or seated in a chair. Instruct him to keep still while the X-rays are taken.
- A headband, foam pads, or sandbags are used to immobilize the patient's head and increase his comfort.
- Routinely, five views of the skull are taken: left and right lateral, anteroposterior Towne's, postero-anterior Caldwell's, and axial (or base).

Patient care

- Answer the patient's questions about the test.

Complications

None known

Interpretation

Normal results

- Size, shape, thickness, and position of cranial bones and vascular markings, sinuses, and sutures are normal.

Abnormal results

- Structural abnormalities suggest possible fractures of the vault or base of the skull or congenital anomalies.
- Erosion, enlargement, or decalcification of the sella turcica suggests possible increased intracranial pressure.
- Areas of calcification suggest possible conditions, such as osteomyelitis, or the presence of neoplasms within the brain substance that contain calcium, such as oligodendrogliomas or meningiomas.
- Midline shifting of a calcified pineal gland suggests a possible space-occupying lesion.
- Changes in bone structure suggest possible metabolic disorders, such as acromegaly or Paget's disease.

Interfering factors

- Improper positioning of the patient
- Failure to remove radiopaque objects from the X-ray field

Sleep studies

Overview

- Also known as *polysomnography*
- Helps in the differential diagnosis of sleep-disordered breathing
- Parameters evaluated for sleep disorder: cardiac rate and rhythm, chest and abdominal wall movement, nasal and oral airflow, oxygen saturation, muscle activity, retinal function, and brain activity during the sleep phase

Purpose

- To diagnose a breathing disorder in a person with a history of excessive snoring, narcolepsy, excessive daytime sleepiness, insomnia, cardiac rhythm disorders, or restless leg spasms

Procedure

Preparation

- Make sure the patient has signed an appropriate consent form.
- Note and report all allergies.
- Schedule the tests for the evening and night hours, usually from 10 p.m. to 6 a.m.
- Instruct the patient to abstain from using products that contain caffeine and from taking naps for 2 to 3 days before the test.
- Advise the patient to maintain a normal sleep schedule so that he's neither deprived of sleep nor over-rested.
- Tell the patient that he may bathe or shower before the test.

Implementation

- Electrodes are secured to the patient's skin, depending on the type of monitoring being used.
- The patient is made comfortable and told that normal body movements won't interfere with the electrodes.
- The lights are turned off and the EEG monitored for a baseline reading before the patient falls asleep.
- The recording and video equipment record the sleep events as they occur.
- Monitoring of the patient during sleep continues until the test is complete.
- For the patient with known sleep apnea, split-night studies may be necessary, such as monitoring the patient for the first half of the night, then using continuous positive airway pressure or nasal ventilation to open the obstructed airway during the second half of the night.

Patient care

- Monitor the patient for respiratory distress during the study.

Complications

- Respiratory distress

Interpretation

Normal results

- A respiratory disturbance index (or apnea-hypopnea index) of fewer than 5 to 10 episodes per study period
- No ischemic change or arrhythmia (electrocardiogram)
- Normal impedance (chest and abdominal wall motion)
- Normal airway (nasal and oral airflow)
- Normal arterial oxygen saturation (oximetry)
- Normal leg electromyogram (for muscle activity)
- Normal electro-oculogram (for retinal function)
- Normal EEG (for brain activity)

Abnormal results

- Abnormal recordings suggest possible obstructive sleep apnea syndrome.
- Abnormal movement during sleep suggests a possible seizure or movement disorder.

Interfering factors

- Improper electrode placement

Slit-lamp examination

Overview

○ Examines the eye using an instrument comprising a special lighting system and a binocular microscope
○ Allows ophthalmologist to view the anterior segment of the eye, including eyelids, eyelashes, conjunctiva, sclera, cornea, tear film, anterior chamber, iris, crystalline lens, and vitreous face
○ Evaluates transparent ocular fluids and tissues

Purpose

○ To detect and evaluate abnormalities of the anterior segment tissues and structures

Procedure

Preparation

○ Make sure the patient has signed an appropriate consent form.
○ Note and report all allergies.
○ Instruct the patient to remove his contact lenses before the test, unless the test is to evaluate the fit of the contact lenses.
○ Explain to the patient the need to remain still during the test.
○ Mydriatics aren't used for a routine eye examination because the slit lamp's bright light would hurt the dilated eyes.
○ Some diseases, such as iritis, require pupillary dilation to alleviate pain and allow the ophthalmologist to examine the eyes with adequate illumination.
○ Explain that the test takes 5 to 10 minutes
○ Explain that the examination is painless.
○ Don't instill mydriatic drops into the eyes of a patient with angle-closure glaucoma or the eyes of a patient who has had a hypersensitivity reaction to the drops.

Implementation

○ The patient is placed into the examining chair with both feet on the floor.
○ The patient is assessed before the examination for the presence of obvious signs, such as different corneal diameters or heterochromia.
○ The patient is asked to place his chin on the rest and his forehead against the bar.
○ The room lights are dimmed.
○ The ophthalmologist examines the patient's eyes — starting with the lids and lashes and progressing to the vitreous face — altering light and magnification as necessary.
○ A special camera may be attached to the slit lamp to photograph portions of the eye.
○ If a corneal abrasion or ulcer is detected, a fluorescein stain allows better viewing of the area.
○ If a tearing deficiency is suspected, the ophthalmologist may examine the eye after applying a fluorescein

or rose Bengal stain; he may also perform the Schirmer tearing test.

Patient care

○ If dilating drops were instilled, tell the patient that his near vision will be blurred for 40 minutes to 2 hours.

Complications

○ Increased intraocular pressure when mydriatic drops are used in patients with angle-closure glaucoma
○ Hypersensitivity reaction to eyedrops

Interpretation

Normal results

○ Normal anterior segment tissues and structures

Abnormal results

○ Irregular corneal shape suggests possible keratoconus.
○ A parchmentlike consistency of the lid skin, with redness, minor swelling, and moderate itching, suggests a possible hypersensitivity reaction.
○ Early-stage lens opacities suggest the possible development of cataracts.
○ Fluorescein stain suggests possible corneal abrasion or ulcer.
○ A Schirmer's tearing test suggests a possible tearing deficiency.

Interfering factors

○ Patient's inability to cooperate

Small-bowel biopsy

Overview

- Uses a capsule to obtain larger tissue samples for histologic analysis than in endoscopic biopsy
- Allows removal of tissue from areas beyond the reach of an endoscope
- Causes little pain and few complications

Purpose

- To evaluate diseases of the intestinal mucosa, which may cause malabsorption or diarrhea
- To confirm the diagnosis of some diseases, such as Whipple's disease and tropical sprue

Procedure

Preparation

- Make sure the patient has signed an appropriate consent form.
- Note and report all allergies.
- Ensure that the patient received coagulation tests and abnormal results were reported to the physician.
- Withhold aspirin and anticoagulants.
- Tell the patient to restrict food and fluids for at least 8 hours before the test.
- Explain that the biopsy takes 45 to 60 minutes but causes little discomfort.

Implementation

- The tubing and capsule are lightly lubricated with a water-soluble lubricant and the mercury bag moistened with water.
- The back of the patient's throat is sprayed with a local anesthetic to decrease gagging during passage of the tube.
- With the patient seated upright, the capsule is placed in his pharynx, and he is asked to flex his neck and swallow as the physician advances the tube about 20″ (50 cm). (If a local anesthetic is used to control the gag reflex, the patient must not receive any fluids to help him swallow the capsule.)
- The patient is positioned on his right side; the tube is advanced another 20″.
- The tube position is checked by fluoroscopy or by instilling air through the tube and listening with a stethoscope for air to enter the stomach.
- Next, the tube is advanced 2″ to 4″ (5 to 10 cm) at a time to pass the capsule through the pylorus.
- Food is discussed with the patient to stimulate the pylorus and help the capsule pass.
- When fluoroscopy confirms that the capsule has passed the pylorus, the patient is kept on his right side to allow the capsule to move into the second and third portions of the small bowel.

- The patient is instructed that he may hold the tube loosely to one side of his mouth if it makes him more comfortable.
- Capsule position is rechecked by fluoroscopy, and the biopsy site determined.
- The patient is placed in the supine position so the capsule position can be verified fluoroscopically.
- A glass syringe is placed on the end of the tube, and steady suction is applied to close the capsule and cut off a tissue specimen.
- Suction is maintained on the syringe as the tube and capsule are removed; then the suction is released.
- The specimen is gently removed with forceps, placed mucosal side up on a piece of mesh, and placed in a biopsy bottle with the required fixative.
- The specimen is sent to the laboratory immediately.

Patient care

- Tell the patient to resume his diet after his gag reflex returns.
- Instruct the patient to report abdominal pain or bleeding.
- Monitor vital signs.
- Observe the patient for infection, aspiration, and abdominal distention.
- Monitor bowel sounds.
- Watch for and immediately report signs and symptoms of hemorrhage, bacteremia, and bowel perforation.
- Keep suction equipment nearby in case aspiration occurs.

Complications

- Hemorrhage
- Bacteremia
- Bowel perforation

Interpretation

Normal results

- Normal small-bowel biopsy specimen consisting of fingerlike villi, crypts, columnar epithelial cells, and round cells

Abnormal results

- Histologic changes in cell structure suggest Whipple's disease; abetalipoproteinemia; lymphoma; lymphangiectasia; eosinophilic enteritis; parasitic infections, such as giardiasis and coccidiosis; celiac disease; tropical sprue; infectious gastroenteritis; intraluminal bacterial overgrowth; folate and vitamin B_{12} deficiency; radiation enteritis; and malnutrition, requiring further investigation.

Interfering factors

- Failure to fast before the biopsy
- Mechanical failure of the biopsy capsule or hole in the tubing

Small-bowel enema

Overview

- Also called *enteroclysis*, a fluoroscopic examination of the small bowel using a contrast medium
- Uses a small-lumen catheter inserted through the nose or mouth and passed through the stomach into the distal duodenum or jejunum
- May involve inflating a small balloon at the tip of the catheter to prevent reflux of the contrast medium into the stomach
- Allows evaluation and diagnosis when the contrast medium distends and opacifies the bowel loops

Purpose

- To diagnose and evaluate Crohn's disease
- To diagnose Meckel's diverticulum
- To aid in the diagnosis of small-bowel obstruction
- To detect tumors

Procedure

Preparation

- Tell the patient that a contrast medium will be instilled into his bowel and that X-ray films will be taken to track the flow of the medium and allow the evaluation of small-bowel function.
- Inform the patient that he'll receive a laxative (such as bisacodyl) the afternoon before the examination, and then he'll receive nothing by mouth until the test. (If the test is being done on an emergency basis, no preparation is required.)
- Inform the patient that he shouldn't take peristalsis-inhibiting drugs (such as meperidine or oxycodone and aspirin) on the day of the test.
- Tell the patient that the examination will take about 45 minutes and that just before the test, he'll be asked to change into a gown, remove his undergarments and jewelry, and empty his bladder.
- Inform the patient that he'll receive an I.V. line for medication.
- Explain to the patient that he may receive an I.V. sedative, if needed, and that a local anesthetic will be injected inside his nose to make the catheter insertion more comfortable. A GI stimulant (such as metoclopramide) will be given to aid passage of the tube and to speed the flow of barium by increasing peristalsis.
- Tell the patient that he'll be asked to turn from side to side and sometimes onto his abdomen during the procedure. Inform the patient that his cooperation will help the test proceed smoothly.
- After the test is completed, tell the patient that he'll go to a recovery area until he's ready for discharge.
- If the patient is having the procedure as an outpatient, make sure that he has someone to drive him home if he receives I.V. sedation.
- Make sure that the patient or a responsible family member has signed an informed consent form.

Implementation

- Assist the patient into a supine position on the X-ray table with his neck slightly extended.
- Give the patient I.V. medication to help him relax and to aid in the tube passage.
- The local anesthetic is given nasally; the patient is instructed to swallow if he feels it at the back of his throat.
- The tube is passed through the nose into the nasopharynx, and the patient's chin is brought down to the chest; the tube is advanced into the stomach and duodenum and, if possible, into the jejunum.
- A small balloon is inflated at the catheter tip to prevent reflux of the contrast medium into the patient's stomach.
- The barium contrast is given by infusion pump.
- Methylcellulose is then given to help propel the barium into the distal bowel. This double-contrast administration distends the bowel walls and opacifies the bowel loops, allowing clearer evaluation.
- Spot films and overhead films are then taken. Barium flow is followed on fluoroscopy.
- The physician examines individual bowel loops, as they are opacified, and compresses the abdomen to better evaluate the loops.
- The patient is asked to turn from side to side during the examination.
- After the examination, the balloon is deflated and the catheter is removed.

Patient care

- Observe the patient in the recovery area until he's ready for discharge.
- Monitor the patient's vital signs until he's alert.
- The patient may experience discomfort with the passage of the catheter. Provide reassurance as well as the prescribed anesthetic and sedative when needed.

Complications

- Adverse reaction to barium

Interpretation

Normal results

- Visible bowel loops and walls with no tumors, ulcers, or constrictions

Abnormal results

- By observing Kerckring's folds, lumen diameters, and wall thickness, Crohn's disease, tumors, partial or complete bowel obstruction, Meckel's diverticula, or congenital disorders may be indicated.

Interfering factors

- Complete gastric or duodenal obstruction

Sodium, serum

Overview

○ Measures serum levels of sodium in relation to amount of water in the body.
○ Sodium, the major extracellular cation, affects body water distribution, maintains osmotic pressure of extracellular fluid, helps promote neuromuscular function, helps maintain acid-base balance, and influences chloride and potassium levels.
○ Because extracellular sodium level helps the kidneys to regulate body water (decreased sodium levels promote water excretion and increased levels promote retention), serum sodium levels are evaluated in relation to the amount of water in the body.
○ Body normally regulates this sodium-water balance through aldosterone, which inhibits sodium excretion and promotes its resorption (with water) by the renal tubules to maintain balance.
○ Low sodium levels stimulate aldosterone secretion; elevated sodium levels depress it.

Purpose

○ To evaluate fluid-electrolyte and acid-base balance and related neuromuscular, renal, and adrenal functions

Procedure

Preparation

○ Explain to the patient that the serum sodium test determines the sodium content of the blood.
○ Tell the patient that this test requires a blood sample. Explain who will perform the venipuncture and when.
○ Explain to the patient that he may experience slight discomfort from the needle puncture and the tourniquet.
○ Inform the patient that he need not restrict food and fluids.
○ Notify the laboratory and physician of drugs the patient is taking that may affect test results; it may be necessary to restrict them.

Implementation

○ Perform a venipuncture and collect the sample in a 3- or 4-ml clot-activator tube.
○ Handle the sample gently to prevent hemolysis

Patient care

○ Apply direct pressure to the venipuncture site until bleeding stops.
○ Instruct the patient to resume any medications stopped before the test.
○ In the patient with increased sodium levels (*hypernatremia*) and loss of water, observe for signs of thirst, restlessness, dry and sticky mucous membranes, flushed skin, oliguria, and diminished reflexes.
○ If increased total body sodium causes water retention, observe for hypertension, dyspnea, edema, and heart failure.
○ In the patient with decreased sodium levels (*hyponatremia*), watch for apprehension, lassitude, headache, decreased skin turgor, abdominal cramps, and tremors that may progress to seizures.

Complications

○ Hematoma at the venipuncture site

Interpretation

Normal results

○ 135 to 145 mEq/L (SI, 135 to 145 mmol/L)

Abnormal results

○ Increased or decreased sodium level or altered state of hydration may be found.
○ Hypernatremia may be caused by excessive sodium intake, inadequate water intake, water loss in excess of sodium (such as diabetes insipidus, impaired renal function, prolonged hyperventilation and, occasionally, severe vomiting or diarrhea), and sodium retention (such as aldosteronism).
○ Hyponatremia may be caused by inadequate sodium intake or excessive sodium loss because of profuse sweating, GI suctioning, diuretic therapy, diarrhea, vomiting, adrenal insufficiency, burns, and chronic renal insufficiency with acidosis.

Interfering factors

○ Hemolysis from rough handling of the sample
○ Most diuretics (decrease by promoting sodium excretion)
○ Lithium, chlorpropamide, and vasopressin (decrease by inhibiting water excretion)
○ Corticosteroids (increase by promoting sodium retention)
○ Antihypertensives, such as methyldopa, hydralazine, and reserpine (possible increase caused by sodium and water retention)

Sodium, urine

Overview

- Determines urine levels of sodium, the major extracellular cation
- Less significant than serum sodium levels, so performed less frequently
- Evaluates renal conservation of sodium and chloride and confirms their levels in the serum

Purpose

- To help evaluate fluid and electrolyte imbalance
- To monitor the effects of a low-salt diet
- To help evaluate renal and adrenal disorders

Procedure

Preparation

- Explain to the patient that the urine sodium and chloride test helps determine the balance of salt and water in the body.
- Advise the patient that he need not restrict food or fluids.
- Tell the patient that the test requires urine collection over a 24-hour period.
- If the specimen is to be collected at home, instruct the patient on the proper collection technique.
- Notify the laboratory and physician of drugs the patient is taking that may affect test results; it may be necessary to restrict them.

Implementation

- Collect the patient's urine over a 24-hour period, discarding the first specimen and retaining the last.
- Tell the patient not to contaminate the specimen with toilet tissue or feces.
- Tell the patient not to use a metallic bedpan for specimen collection.

Patient care

- Instruct the patient that he may resume his usual medications.

Complications

None known

Interpretation

Normal results

- Results depend on dietary salt intake and perspiration.
- In adults, 40 to 220 mEq/L/24 hours (SI, 40 to 220 mmol/d)
- In children, 41 to 115 mEq/L/24 hours (SI, 41 to 115 mmol/d)

Abnormal results

- Most commonly, urine sodium and urine chloride levels are parallel, rising and falling in tandem.
- Abnormal levels of both minerals may indicate the need for more specific testing.
- Elevated urine sodium levels may reflect increased salt intake, adrenal failure, salicylate toxicity, diabetic acidosis, salt-losing nephritis, and water-deficient dehydration.
- Decreased urine sodium levels suggest decreased salt intake, primary aldosteronism, acute renal failure, and heart failure.
- To evaluate fluid-electrolyte imbalance, results must be correlated with findings of serum electrolyte studies.

Interfering factors

- Failure to collect all urine during the test period
- Sodium bicarbonate and thiazide diuretics (increase in sodium)
- Steroids (decrease in sodium)

Soluble amyloid beta protein precursor

Overview

○ Assesses the extracellular deposition of amyloid beta-peptide (in the form of cerebrovascular amyloid and extracellular plaques), a major neuropathologic sign of Alzheimer's disease (AD)
○ Amyloid beta-peptide is generated proteolytically from the large beta-amyloid precursor protein (APP).
○ APP is the major protein subunit of the vascular and plaque amyloid filaments in individuals with Alzheimer's disease and in elderly patients with trisomy 21 (Down syndrome).

Purpose

○ To diagnose AD
○ To monitor the progression of AD and the effectiveness of its treatment

Procedure

Preparation

○ Explain the purpose of this test to the patient and his family.

Implementation

○ Testing can be performed with plasma and cerebrospinal fluid.

Patient care

○ Answer the patient's questions about the test.
○ Provide referral for counseling and support groups.

Complications

None known

Interpretation

Normal results

○ Establish the patient's baseline level; then track his levels over time to help determine if he will develop AD.

Abnormal results

○ Mutations in the beta-amyloid precursor protein gene on chromosome 21 cause a small proportion of Alzheimer's disease cases.
○ Abnormal cerebrovascular levels of beta-amyloid protein (low level for the patient's age) and tau protein (high level for the patient's age) confirm the diagnosis of Alzheimer's disease; this measurement isn't reliable for asymptomatic patients.

Interfering factors

None known

Speech

Overview

○ Uses speech signals to determine the lowest level at which a patient can hear words and his ability to correctly recognize words presented above the threshold level
○ Degrades speech signal by using interfering speech, filtered speech that removes frequencies, and speech that's delivered at a faster rate
○ Stresses the auditory processing system to determine the patient's function in challenging conditions

Purpose

○ To determine the degree of hearing loss for speech recognition

Procedure

Preparation

○ Review any educational materials given to the patient by the audiologist.
○ Remove significant cerumen accumulation from the patient's ear canals.

Implementation

○ To obtain the threshold of speech reception, the audiologist presents two-syllable words (*spondee* words) to the patient, decreasing the intensity until the threshold is obtained.
○ Threshold testing results are reported as spondee thresholds, or *speech reception thresholds (SRTs)*.
○ Children may be asked to point to pictures representing the words. Very young children who lack the vocabulary to identify pictures are asked to point to body parts, such as eyes, nose, and mouth.
○ *Speech awareness thresholds* are used in lieu of SRTs to assess the lowest level at which a patient can detect speech (usually 10 dB below the SRT).
○ Speech awareness threshold testing may substitute for the SRT test in a young child and for someone who speaks a foreign language.
○ To estimate the patient's ability to understand speech, lists of one-syllable words are presented, typically in quiet and at an intensity that's comfortable for the patient.
○ The *speech discrimination test* or *word recognition test* assesses word understanding. Given at the level of typical conversational speech (40 to 50 dB hearing level [HL]), this test estimates the impact of hearing loss on communication in ideal environments. Given at an intensity level that's comfortable for the patient, it provides limited prognostic information about probable benefit from amplification. A percentage correct score is obtained.
○ When there's a suspicion of cranial nerve VIII or other retrocochlear involvement, the speech under-

standing testing may be repeated at a very high intensity. This form of testing is referred to as *rollover testing*.

Patient care

○ Answer questions about the tests for the patient or his parents.

Complications

None known

Interpretation

Normal results

○ A normal speech threshold (spondee threshold, SRT) is −10 to 15 dB HL for children ages 2 and older and −10 to 25 dB HL for adults.
○ Word recognition scores are 100%. Speech tests for auditory processing are interpreted by comparing the patient's score to age-appropriate norms.

Abnormal results

○ Abnormal auditory processing test results are those significantly below the expected level when compared to age-appropriate norms.
○ SRTs higher than 25 dB HL indicate that the patient can't hear a whispered sound.
○ Thresholds that range up to 40 dB HL suggest that the patient has difficulty hearing faint or distant speech.
○ If the person doesn't wear a hearing aid and has an SRT of 30 to 40 dB HL, make sure that you speak to the patient in a quiet environment from a distance of no more than 6′ (1.8 m).
○ Speech reception thresholds above 40 dB HL indicate increasing difficulty understanding speech.
○ When thresholds exceed 50 dB HL, the patient can't be expected to understand you without amplification.
○ The audiologist will compare the SRT with the pure tone average to cross-check test reliability.
○ The patient whose SRT and pure tone average differ by 10 dB may have misunderstood test instructions.
○ The patient with nonorganic loss (exaggeration of hearing thresholds) commonly has a better SRT than pure tone testing would predict.
○ Word understanding scores below 90% indicate that the patient has some degree of communication difficulty.
○ The audiologist uses the score, interpreted in conjunction with the presentation level and the audiometric configuration, as a prognostic indicator of potential for success with amplification.
○ The audiologist's finding of decreased word understanding at a high intensity level indicates rollover, which, if significant, is an indicator of possible retrocochlear involvement.

Interfering factors

○ Failure to consider receptive vocabulary when interpreting test results

Sputum culture

Overview

○ Bacteriologic examination of sputum, collected by expectoration or tracheal suctioning
○ Acid-fast sputum smear: may disclose evidence of mycobacterial infection such as tuberculosis (TB)

Purpose

○ To isolate and identify causes of pulmonary infections
○ To aid diagnosis of respiratory diseases, such as bronchitis, TB, lung abscess, and pneumonia

Procedure

Preparation

○ Inform the patient that this test requires a sputum specimen.
○ Explain that specimens may be collected on at least three consecutive mornings if the suspected organism is *Mycobacterium tuberculosis.*
○ Inform the patient that results for TB cultures take up to 2 months.

Implementation

○ Maintain asepsis; wear personal protective equipment.

Expectoration

○ Instruct the patient to cough deeply and expectorate into the container.
○ A Gram's stain of expectorated sputum must be examined to ensure that it's a representative specimen of secretions from the lower respiratory tract (many white blood cells [WBCs], few epithelial cells) rather than one contaminated by oral flora (few WBCs, many epithelial cells).
○ If the cough is nonproductive, use chest physiotherapy or nebulization to induce sputum.
○ Don't use more than 20% propylene glycol with water as an inducer for a specimen scheduled for TB culturing, since higher concentrations inhibit the growth of *M. tuberculosis.* (If propylene glycol isn't available, use 10% to 20% acetylcysteine with water or sodium chloride.)
○ Close the container securely.
○ Dispose of equipment properly; seal the container in a leak-proof bag before sending it to the laboratory.

Tracheal suctioning

○ Give oxygen to the patient before and after the procedure as necessary.
○ Attach the sputum trap to the suction catheter.
○ Lubricate the catheter with normal saline solution and pass the catheter through the patient's nostril without suction.
○ Advance the catheter into the trachea; apply suction while withdrawing the catheter, not during catheter insertion.

○ Suction for only 5 to 10 seconds at a time.
○ Stop suction and remove the catheter.
○ Discard the catheter in the proper receptacle.
○ Detach the in-line sputum trap from the suction apparatus and cap the opening.
○ During passage through the throat and oropharynx, sputum specimens are commonly contaminated with indigenous bacterial flora.
○ Label the container with the patient's name, the nature and origin of the specimen, the date and time of collection, the initial diagnosis, and any current antimicrobial therapy.
○ Send the specimen to the laboratory immediately after collection.

Patient care

○ Provide mouth care for the patient.
○ Monitor his vital signs and respiratory status.
○ Monitor oxygen saturations with a pulse oximeter.
○ If the patient becomes hypoxic or cyanotic during suctioning, remove the catheter immediately and give oxygen while monitoring pulse oximetry.

Complications

○ Hypoxemia
○ Cardiac arrhythmias
○ Laryngospasm
○ Bronchospasm
○ Pneumothorax
○ Perforation of the trachea or bronchus
○ Trauma to respiratory structures
○ Bleeding

Interpretation

Normal results

○ Common flora includes alpha-hemolytic streptococci, *Neisseria* species, and diphtheroid.
○ Presence of common flora doesn't rule out infection.

Abnormal results

○ Because sputum is invariably contaminated with normal oropharyngeal flora, a culture isolate must be interpreted in light of the patient's overall clinical condition.
○ Isolation of *M. tuberculosis* suggests TB.
○ Isolation of pathogenic organisms most often includes *Streptococcus pneumoniae, M. tuberculosis, Klebsiella pneumoniae* (and other Enterobacteriaceae), *Haemophilus influenzae, Staphylococcus aureus,* and *Pseudomonas aeruginosa.*

Interfering factors

○ Contaminated or inadequate sample

Sputum examination

Overview

- Evaluates sputum for presence of parasitic infestation, which may rarely result from exposure to *Entamoeba histolytica, Ascaris lumbricoides, Echinococcus granulosus, Strongyloides stercoralis, Paragonimus westermani*, or *Necator americanus*
- Involves obtaining a sputum specimen by expectoration or tracheal suctioning to evaluate for parasites

Purpose

- To identify pulmonary parasites

Procedure

Preparation

- Explain to the patient that this test helps identify parasitic pulmonary infection.
- Tell the patient that the test requires a sputum specimen or, if necessary, tracheal suctioning.
- Inform the patient that early morning collection is preferred because secretions accumulate overnight.
- Encourage the patient to help sputum production by drinking fluids the night before collection.
- Teach the patient how to expectorate by taking three deep breaths and forcing a deep cough.
- Tell the patient that he'll experience some discomfort from the catheter during tracheal suctioning.
- Notify the laboratory and physician of drugs the patient is taking that may affect test results; it may be necessary to restrict them.

Implementation

Expectoration
- Instruct the patient to breathe deeply a few times and then to cough deeply and expectorate into the container.
- Use chest physiotherapy, or heated aerosol spray (nebulization), if the patient's cough is unproductive.
- Use proper precautions in sending the specimen to the laboratory.

Tracheal suctioning
- Don't perform tracheal suctioning on the patient with esophageal varices.
- Give oxygen before and after the procedure, if necessary.
- Attach a sputum trap to the suction catheter.
- Wearing a sterile glove, lubricate the tip of the catheter and then pass the catheter through the patient's nostril without suction. (He'll cough when the catheter passes into the larynx.)
- Advance the catheter into the trachea.
- Apply suction for no longer than 15 seconds to obtain the specimen.
- Stop suctioning and gently remove the catheter.
- Discard the catheter and glove in a proper receptacle.
- Detach the sputum trap from the suction apparatus and cap the opening.
- Label all specimens carefully.

Patient care

- Provide proper mouth care. After suctioning, offer the patient water.
- Monitor the patient's vital signs every hour until he's stable.

Complications

- If the patient has asthma or chronic bronchitis, watch for aggravated bronchospasms with use of more than 10% concentration of sodium chloride or acetylcysteine in an aerosol.
- If the patient shows signs of hypoxia or cyanosis during suctioning, remove the suctioning catheter immediately and give oxygen.

Interpretation

Normal results

- No parasites or ova are present in sputum.

Abnormal results

- *E. histolytica* trophozoites indicates pulmonary amebiasis.
- *A. lumbricoides* larvae and adults indicate pneumonitis.
- *E. granulosus* cysts of larvae indicate hydatid disease.
- *S. stercoralis* larvae indicate strongyloidiasis.
- *P. westermani* ova indicate paragonimiasis.
- *N. americanus* larvae indicate hookworm disease.

Interfering factors

- Improper collection technique or failure to send the specimen to the laboratory immediately after collection
- Recent therapy with anthelmintics or amebicides

Stool examination for ova and parasites

Overview

○ Examines a stool specimen to assess for intestinal parasites, both nonpathogenic and disease-causing
○ May reveal roundworms *Ascaris lumbricoides* and *Necator americanus* (commonly called *hookworm*); tapeworms *Diphyllobothrium latum, Taenia saginata,* and, rarely, *T. solium;* amoeba *Entamoeba histolytica;* flagellate *Giardia lamblia,* or *Cyclospora*

Purpose

○ To confirm or rule out intestinal parasitic infection and disease

Procedure

Preparation

○ Explain to the patient that this test detects intestinal parasitic infection.
○ Instruct the patient to avoid treatments with castor or mineral oil, bismuth, magnesium or antidiarrheal compounds, barium enemas, and antibiotics for 7 to 10 days before the test.
○ Tell the patient that the test requires three stool specimens — one every other day or every third day. Up to six specimens may be necessary to confirm the presence of *E. histolytica.*
○ If the patient has diarrhea, record recent dietary and travel history.
○ Check the patient's history for use of antiparasitic drugs, such as tetracycline, paromomycin, metronidazole, and iodoquinol, within 2 weeks of the test.

Implementation

○ Put on gloves and collect a stool specimen directly in the container.
○ If the patient is bedridden, collect the specimen in a clean, dry bedpan; then, using a tongue blade, transfer it into a properly labeled container.
○ Send the specimen to the laboratory immediately. If a liquid or soft stool specimen can't be examined within 30 minutes of passage, place some of it in a preservative; if a formed stool specimen can't be examined immediately, refrigerate it or place it in preservative.
○ If the entire stool can't be sent to the laboratory, include macroscopic worms or worm segments as well as bloody and mucoid portions of the specimen.
○ Note on the laboratory request the date and time of collection and the specimen consistency. Also record recent or current antimicrobial therapy and any pertinent travel or dietary history.

Patient care

○ Tell the patient that he may resume his usual medications.

Interpretation

Normal results

○ No parasites or ova are present in stool.

Abnormal results

○ *E. histolytica* confirms amebiasis; *G. lamblia,* giardiasis (extent of infection depends on degree of tissue invasion).
○ If amebiasis is suspected but stool examination result is negative, specimen collection after saline catharsis using buffered sodium biphosphate or during sigmoidoscopy may be necessary.
○ If giardiasis is suspected but stool examination result is negative, examination of duodenal contents may be necessary.
○ Because injury to the host is difficult to detect — even when helminth ova or larvae appear — the number of worms is usually correlated with the patient's clinical symptoms to distinguish between helminth infestation and helminth diseases.
○ Eosinophilia may also indicate parasitic infection.
○ Helminths may migrate from the intestinal tract, producing pathologic changes in other parts of the body. For example, the roundworm *Ascaris* may perforate the bowel wall, causing peritonitis, or may migrate to the lungs, causing pneumonitis.
○ Hookworms can cause hypochromic microcytic anemia secondary to bloodsucking and hemorrhage, especially in the patient with an iron-deficient diet.
○ The tapeworm *D. latum* may cause megaloblastic anemia by removing vitamin B_{12}.

Interfering factors

○ Improper collection technique, not enough specimens, or the presence of urine (false-negative results)
○ Failure to transport the specimen promptly or to refrigerate or preserve it if transport is delayed
○ Excessive heat or cold
○ Failure to observe pretest drug restrictions
○ Stool collected from a toilet bowl; water is toxic to trophozoites and may contain organisms that interfere with test results

Stool examination for rotavirus antigen

Overview

○ Detects human rotaviruses using sensitive, specific enzyme immunoassays that provide results within minutes or hours (depending on the assay) because human rotaviruses don't replicate efficiently in laboratory cell cultures.
○ Rotavirus infection is most common cause of infectious diarrhea (with vomiting, fever, and abdominal pain) in infants (especially those in group settings like hospitals, preschools, and day-care centers) and young children ages 3 months to 2 years, usually in winter; it can infect all age-groups but is usually more severe in young children.
○ Transmission is probably by the fecal-oral route, from person to person. In a facility setting, nosocomial spread of this viral infection can cause significant harm.

Purpose

○ To obtain a laboratory diagnosis of rotavirus gastroenteritis

Procedure

Preparation

○ Explain the purpose of the test to the patient or his parents if the patient is a child.
○ Inform the patient that the test requires a stool specimen.

Implementation

○ Collect the specimens during the prodromal and acute stages of clinical infection to ensure detection of the viral antigens by enzyme immunoassay.
○ Usually, a stool specimen (1 g in a screw-capped tube or vial) is used to detect rotaviruses. If a microbiological transport swab is used, it must be heavily stained with stool to be diagnostically productive for rotavirus.
○ Avoid using collection containers with preservatives, metal ions, detergents, and serum, which may interfere with the assay.
○ Store feces specimens for up to 24 hours at 35.6° to 46.4° F (2° to 8° C). If a longer period of storage or shipment is necessary, freeze specimens at –4° F (–20° C) or colder. Repeated freezing and thawing will cause the specimen to deteriorate and yield misleading results.
○ Don't store the specimen in a self-defrosting freezer.

Patient care

○ Monitor the patient's intake and output and provide him with fluids to avoid dehydration caused by vomiting and diarrhea.

Complications

None known

Interpretation

Normal results

○ No rotavirus appears in the specimen.

Abnormal results

○ Rotavirus detected by enzyme immunoassay confirms current infection with the organism.

Interfering factors

○ Collection of a specimen in containers with preservatives, such as metal ions, detergents, or serum (decreased number of pathogens)

Sweat test

Overview

○ Quantitative measurement of electrolyte concentrations (primarily sodium and chloride) in sweat, usually through pilocarpine iontophoresis (pilocarpine is a sweat inducer)
○ Used almost exclusively in children to confirm cystic fibrosis, a congenital condition that increases sodium and chloride electrolyte levels in sweat

Purpose

○ To confirm cystic fibrosis
○ To exclude the diagnosis in siblings of those with cystic fibrosis

Procedure

Preparation

○ Make sure the patient, or parent if the patient is a minor, has signed an appropriate consent form.
○ Note and report all allergies.
○ No restrictions of diet, medications, or activity are necessary before the test.
○ Warn the patient that he may experience a slight tickling sensation during the procedure.

Implementation

○ The area to be tested (flexor surface of the right forearm or, if the arm is too small to secure electrodes, as with an infant, the right thigh) is cleaned using distilled water and dried thoroughly.

▼ *ALERT Never perform iontophoresis on the chest, especially in a child, because the current can induce cardiac arrest.*

○ A gauze pad saturated with premeasured pilocarpine solution is placed on the positive electrode; another pad saturated with normal saline solution is placed on the negative electrode.
○ Both electrodes are applied to the area to be tested and secured with straps.
○ Lead wires to the analyzer are given a current of 4 mA in 15 to 20 seconds. This process (iontophoresis) is continued at 15- to 20-second intervals for 5 minutes.
○ Stop the test immediately if the patient complains of a burning sensation, which usually indicates that the positive electrode is exposed or positioned improperly. Adjust the electrode and continue the test.
○ After iontophoresis, both electrodes are removed.
○ The pads are discarded, and the patient's skin is cleaned with distilled water and dried.
○ Using forceps, a dry gauze pad or filter paper (previously weighed on a gram scale) is placed on the area where the pilocarpine was used.

○ Cover the pad or filter paper with a slightly larger piece of plastic and seal the edges of the plastic with waterproof adhesive tape.
○ The gauze pad or filter paper is left in place for about 45 minutes. (The appearance of droplets on the plastic usually indicates induction of an adequate amount of sweat.)
○ The pad or filter paper is removed with the forceps and place it immediately in the weighing bottle.
○ Carefully seal the gauze pad or filter paper in the weighing bottle and send the bottle to the laboratory at once.
○ The difference between the first and second weights indicates the weight of the sweat specimen collected.
○ Make sure at least 100 mg of sweat is collected in 45 minutes.

Patient care

○ Wash the tested area with soap and water, and dry it thoroughly.
○ If the area looks red, reassure the patient that this is normal and that the redness will disappear within a few hours.
○ Tell the patient that he may resume his usual activities.

Complications

○ Electric shock if improperly performed

Interpretation

Normal results

○ Sodium, 10 to 30 mEq/L
○ Chloride, 10 to 35 mEq/L
○ In women, sweat electrolyte levels fluctuate cyclically. Chloride levels usually peak 5 to 10 days before onset of menses, and most women retain fluid before menses.

Abnormal results

○ Sodium and chloride levels of 50 to 60 mEq/L strongly suggest cystic fibrosis.
○ Elevated sweat electrolyte levels may also suggest untreated adrenal insufficiency, type I glycogen storage disease, vasopressin-resistant diabetes insipidus, meconium ileus, and renal failure.

Interfering factors

○ Dehydration or edema, especially in the collection area
○ Failure to obtain an adequate amount of sweat
○ Presence of pure salt depletion
○ Failure to clean the skin thoroughly or to use sterile gauze pads
○ Failure to seal gauze pad or filter paper carefully

Synovial membrane biopsy

Overview

○ Needle excision of a tissue specimen of the thin epithelial layer lining the diarthrodial joint capsules for histologic examination.
○ Performed when analysis of synovial fluid (a viscous, lubricating fluid contained within the synovial membrane) is nondiagnostic or fluid is absent.
○ Preliminary arthroscopy performed, to aid selection of biopsy site in a large joint such as the knee.

Purpose

○ To diagnose gout, pseudogout, bacterial infections and lesions, and granulomatous infections
○ To aid in the diagnosis of rheumatoid arthritis, systemic lupus erythematosus, or Reiter syndrome
○ To monitor joint pathology

Procedure

Preparation

○ Make sure the patient has signed an appropriate consent form.
○ Note and report all allergies.
○ Give the patient a sedative if needed.
○ Tell the patient that he need not restrict food or fluids.
○ Provide reassurance that he'll receive a local anesthetic to minimize discomfort.
○ Warn the patient about transient pain when the needle enters the joint.
○ Tell him that the test takes about 30 minutes
○ Explain which site was selected for biopsy (usually, the most symptomatic joint): knee (most common), elbow, wrist, ankle, or shoulder.
○ Explain that test results are usually available in 1 or 2 days.
○ Explain that complications are rare but may include infection and bleeding into the joint.

Implementation

○ The patient is positioned properly.
○ The biopsy site is prepared and draped.
○ Local anesthetic is injected into the joint space.
○ The trocar is forcefully thrust into the joint space, away from the site of anesthetic infiltration.
○ The biopsy needle is inserted through the trocar.
○ While the trocar is held stationary, the biopsy needle is twisted to cut off a tissue segment.
○ The needle is then withdrawn, and the specimen is placed in a properly labeled sterile container or a specimen bottle containing heparin or absolute ethyl alcohol.

○ It's possible to obtain several specimens without reinserting the trocar.
○ After the trocar is removed, the biopsy site is cleaned and a dressing applied.

Patient care

○ Give the patient analgesics.
○ Instruct the patient to rest the joint from which the tissue specimen was removed for 1 day before resuming normal activities.
○ Monitor vital signs.
○ Watch the patient for bleeding into the joint.
○ Observe the biopsy site for infection.

Complications

○ Bleeding into the joint
○ Infection

Interpretation

Normal results

○ Synovial membrane contains cells identical to those found in other connective tissue and is relatively smooth, except for villi, folds, and fat pads that project into the joint cavity.
○ Synovial membrane tissue produces synovial fluid and contains a capillary network, lymphatic vessels, and a few nerve fibers.

Abnormal results

○ Histologic examination of synovial tissue can diagnose coccidioidomycosis, gout, pseudogout, hemochromatosis, tuberculosis, sarcoidosis, amyloidosis, pigmented villonodular synovitis, or synovial tumors.

Interfering factors

○ Failure to obtain several biopsy specimens
○ Failure to obtain the specimens away from the anesthetic's infiltration site
○ Failure to store the specimens in the appropriate solution or to send them to the laboratory immediately

T- and B-lymphocyte assays

Overview

○ Lymphocytes, key cells in the immune system, recognize antigens through special receptors on their surfaces.
○ T and B cells, the two primary kinds of lymphocytes, originate in the bone marrow. T cells mature under the influence of the thymus gland; B cells evolve without thymic influence.
○ Cell separation isolates lymphocytes from other cellular blood elements — a whole blood sample is layered on Ficoll-Hypaque in a narrow tube, which is then centrifuged. Granulocytes and erythrocytes form sediment at the bottom of the tube, and lymphocytes, monocytes, and platelets form a distinct band at the Ficoll-Hypaque plasma interface.
○ This procedure recovers about 80% of the lymphocytes but doesn't differentiate between T and B cells. The percentage of T and B cells is determined by attaching a label or marker and by using different identification techniques.
  – The E rosette test identifies T cells, which tend to form unstable clusterlike shapes (or rosettes) after exposure to sheep red blood cells at 39.2° F (4° C).
  – Direct immunofluorescence detects B cells, which have monoclonal immunoglobulin on their surfaces; unlike T cells, B cells present receptors for complement as well as for Fc portions of immunoglobulin.

Purpose

○ To aid in the diagnosis of primary and secondary immunodeficiency diseases
○ To distinguish between benign and malignant lymphocytic proliferative diseases
○ To monitor the patient's response to therapy

Procedure

Preparation

○ Tell the patient that this test requires a blood sample. Explain who will perform the venipuncture and when.
○ Explain to the patient that he may experience slight discomfort from the tourniquet and the needle puncture.

Implementation

○ Perform a venipuncture and collect the sample in a 7-ml green-top tube.
○ Fill the collection tube completely and invert it gently several times to mix the sample and the anticoagulant adequately.

○ Send the sample to the laboratory immediately to make sure you have viable lymphocytes.
○ If antilymphocyte antibodies are suspected, as in autoimmune disease, notify the laboratory.

Patient care

○ Apply direct pressure to the venipuncture site until bleeding stops.
○ Because the patient may have a compromised immune system, keep the venipuncture site clean and dry.

Complications

○ Hematoma at the venipuncture site

Interpretation

Normal results

○ T-cell and B-cell values may differ from one laboratory to another, depending on test technique.
○ T cells usually constitute 68% to 75% of total lymphocytes; B cells, 10% to 20%; and null cells, 5% to 20%.
○ In adults, the total lymphocyte count is 1,500 to 3,000/µl, the T-cell count is 1,400 to 2,700/µl, and the B-cell count is 270 to 640/µl; these counts are higher in children.
○ Normal T-cell and B-cell counts don't necessarily ensure a competent immune system. In autoimmune diseases, such as systemic lupus erythematosus and rheumatoid arthritis, T and B cells may be present in normal numbers but may not be functionally competent.

Abnormal results

○ An abnormal T-cell or B-cell count suggests, but doesn't confirm, specific diseases.
○ The B-cell count remains normal in many immunoglobulin deficiency diseases, especially if only one immunoglobulin class is deficient.
○ The B-cell count decreases in acute lymphocytic leukemia and in certain congenital or acquired immunoglobulin deficiency diseases.
○ The B-cell count increases in chronic lymphocytic leukemia (thought to be a B-cell malignancy), multiple myeloma, Waldenström's macroglobulinemia, and DiGeorge syndrome (a congenital T-cell deficiency).
○ The T-cell count may increase in infectious mononucleosis, multiple myeloma, and acute lymphocytic leukemia.
○ The T-cell count decreases in congenital T-cell deficiency diseases, such as DiGeorge, Nezelof, and Wiskott-Aldrich syndromes, and in some B-cell proliferative disorders, such as chronic lymphocytic leukemia, Waldenström's macroglobulinemia, and acquired immunodeficiency syndrome.

Interfering factors

○ Exposing the sample to temperature extremes or failure to use the proper collection tube, to mix the sample adequately, or to send the sample to the laboratory

○ Changes in health status from the effects of stress, surgery, chemotherapy, steroid or immunosuppressive therapy, or radiography (possible rapid change in T- and B-cell counts)

○ Immunoglobulins such as autologous antilymphocyte antibodies that sometimes occur in autoimmune disease (possible change in results)

Tangent screen examination

Overview

- Evaluates central visual field in each eye by moving an object across a tangent screen, usually a piece of black felt with concentric circles and lines radiating from a central fixation point, like a spider web
- Detects and follows the progression of ocular diseases, such as glaucoma and optic neuritis, and detects and evaluates neurologic disorders, such as brain tumors and strokes
- Localizes a specific visual field defect, usually pointing to the underlying pathology

Purpose

- To detect central visual field loss and evaluate its progression or regression

Procedure

Preparation

- Explain to the patient that the tangent screen examination takes about 30 minutes to perform.
- Reassure him that it causes no pain but requires his full cooperation.
- If he normally wears corrective lenses, tell him to wear them during the test.

Implementation

- Have the patient sit comfortably about 3′ (1 m) from the tangent screen so that the eye being tested is directly in line with the central fixation target on the screen.
- Occlude the patient's left eye, and tell him that while he fixates on the central target, you'll move a test object into his visual field.
- The test object is white on one side and black on the other; its diameter varies in size from 1 to 10 mm, depending on the patient's visual acuity (for example, if he has 20/20 vision, the test object should have a diameter of 1 mm).
- Tell the patient not to look for the test object but to wait for it to appear and then to signal when he sees it. Stand to the side of the eye being tested.
- Move the test object inward from the periphery of the screen at 30-degree intervals, as represented by the radiating lines on the screen.
- Using black-tipped straight pins, plot the points on the screen at which the patient can see the object. When connected, this becomes the boundary of the areas of equal visual acuity (called an *isopter*).
- To guarantee the adequacy of fixation, the physiologic blind spot should be clearly identified.
- After plotting the boundaries of the patient's central visual field, test how well he can see within his visual field by turning the test object to the black side. Then turn it over within each 30-degree interval, and ask the patient to signal when he sees the test object.
- Plot suspicious areas — those in which the patient has failed to identify the test object — for size, shape, and density.
- Record the patient's visual field on the recording chart, marked in degrees, and note any abnormal areas within the field.
- Because isopters vary with the patient's age, visual acuity, and pupil size; the size and color of the test object; and the distance between the patient and the screen, carefully record all measurements.
- Occlude the patient's right eye and repeat the test.

Patient care

- Explain that repeat tangent screen examinations can help evaluate progression or regression of a diagnosed disorder.

Complications

None known

Interpretation

Normal results

- The central visual field normally forms a circle, extending 25 degrees superiorly, nasally, inferiorly, and temporally.
- The physiologic blind spot lies 12 to 15 degrees temporal to the central fixation point, about 1.5 degrees below the horizontal meridian. It extends about 7.5 degrees in height and 5.5 degrees in width.
- The test object should be visible throughout the patient's entire central visual field, except within the physiologic blind spot.

Abnormal results

- The inability to see the test object within the temporal half of the central visual field may indicate bitemporal hemianopsia, resulting from lesions of the optic chiasm, stroke, craniopharyngiomas in young patients, and meningiomas or an aneurysm of the circle of Willis in adults.
- Bilateral homonymous hemianopsia is uncommon but may follow multiple thrombi in the posterior cerebral circulation. Plotting visual fields after a stroke helps to locate cerebrovascular lesions.
- An enlarged blind spot, a central scotoma, or a centrocecal scotoma may be caused by diseases that involve the optic nerve such as glaucoma.
- Retinitis pigmentosa, a slowly progressive disease that leads to night blindness, causes a ring 10 or more degrees away from the fixation point. The peripheral area beyond this ring is usually spared. Retinal detachment can be outlined as well.

Interfering factors

- An uncooperative patient
- Patient's inability to see even the largest test object

Technetium-99m pyrophosphate scanning

Overview

○ Detects and determines the extent of recent myocardial infarction (MI)
○ I.V. tracer isotope (technetium-99m pyrophosphate) accumulates in damaged myocardial tissue (possibly by combining with calcium in the damaged myocardial cells), where it forms a hot spot on a scan made with a scintillation camera
○ Useful when serum cardiac enzyme tests are unreliable or when patients have equivocal electrocardiograms (ECGs) such as in left bundle-branch block
○ Also known as *hot spot myocardial imaging* and *infarct avid imaging*

Purpose

○ To confirm a recent MI
○ To define the size and location of a recent MI
○ To assess prognosis after an acute MI

Procedure

Preparation

○ Make sure the patient has signed an appropriate consent form.
○ Note and report all allergies.
○ Tell the patient that he need not restrict food and fluids.
○ Reassure the patient that he will feel only transient discomfort during isotope injection and that the scan itself is painless.
○ Stress the need to remain quiet and motionless during scanning.

Implementation

○ Inject technetium-99m pyrophosphate into the antecubital vein.
○ After 2 to 3 hours, assist the patient into a supine position.
○ Attach ECG electrodes for continuous monitoring during the test.
○ Scans are usually taken with the patient in several positions, including anterior, left anterior oblique, right anterior oblique, and left lateral.
○ Each scan takes about 10 minutes.

Patient care

○ Answer the patient's questions about the test.

Complications

None known

Interpretation

Normal results

○ No isotope found in the myocardium

Abnormal results

○ Isotope is taken up by the sternum and ribs, and their activity is compared with that of the heart; 2+, 3+, and 4+ activity (equal to or greater than bone) suggest a positive myocardial scan.
○ Areas of isotope accumulation, or hot spots, suggest damaged myocardium.

Interfering factors

None known

Tensilon test

Overview

○ Involves I.V. administration of edrophonium chloride (Tensilon), a rapid, short-acting anticholinesterase that improves strength of muscles by increasing their response to nerve impulses

Purpose

○ To aid in the diagnosis of myasthenia gravis
○ To differentiate myasthenic from cholinergic crises
○ To monitor oral anticholinesterase therapy

Procedure

Preparation

○ Make sure the patient has signed a consent form.
○ Note and report all allergies.
○ Check the patient's history for use of drugs that affect muscle function.
○ If the patient is receiving anticholinesterase therapy, note this on the requisition form along with the last dose he received and the time it was given.
○ Withhold drugs.
○ Start an I.V. infusion of dextrose 5% in water or normal saline solution.
○ Tell the patient that he need not restrict food and fluids.
○ Warn about possible transient unpleasant effects from the Tensilon, including nausea, dizziness, and blurred vision.
○ Reassure the patient that someone will stay with him at all times.
○ Inform the patient that it may be necessary to repeat the test several times.
○ Explain that the study takes 15 to 30 minutes.

Implementation

○ Give atropine during the test to patients with respiratory disorders such as asthma to minimize Tensilon's adverse effects.

To diagnose myasthenia gravis

○ Give the patient 2 mg of Tensilon initially. Adjust dosage for infants and children.
○ Before giving the rest of the dose, the physician may want to tire the muscles by asking the patient to perform various exercises, such as looking up until ptosis develops or holding his arms above his shoulders until they drop.
○ When the muscles are fatigued, give the remaining 8 mg of Tensilon over 30 seconds.
○ If a placebo is used (to evaluate the patient's muscle response more accurately), observe the patient after its administration.
○ After giving the Tensilon, ask the patient to perform repetitive muscular movements, such as crossing and uncrossing his legs.

○ Observe the patient closely for improved muscle strength.
○ If muscle strength doesn't improve within 3 to 5 minutes, repeat the test.

To differentiate between myasthenic crisis and cholinergic crisis

○ Infuse 1 to 2 mg of Tensilon.
○ After infusion, monitor vital signs continuously.
○ Watch the patient closely for respiratory distress.
○ If muscle strength doesn't improve, infuse more Tensilon cautiously — 1 mg at a time, up to 5 mg — and watch the patient for signs of distress.
○ Give the patient neostigmine immediately if the test demonstrates myasthenic crisis; give atropine for cholinergic crisis.

To evaluate oral anticholinesterase therapy

○ Infuse 2 mg of Tensilon 1 hour after the patient's last dose of the anticholinesterase.
○ Observe the patient carefully for adverse reactions and muscle response.
○ After giving the patient Tensilon, keep the I.V. line open at a rate of 20 ml/hour until all the patient's responses have been evaluated.

Patient care

○ When the test is complete, stop the I.V. infusion.
○ Tell the patient that he may resume medications stopped before the test.
○ Monitor vital signs and respiratory status.
○ Keep resuscitation equipment immediately available in case of respiratory failure.
○ Monitor the patient's muscle strength.
○ Watch for adverse effects of Tensilon.

Complications

○ Seizures
○ Bradycardia, heart block, cardiac arrest
○ Paralysis of respiratory muscles
○ Bronchospasm, laryngospasm
○ Respiratory depression
○ Respiratory arrest

Interpretation

Normal results

○ Development of fasciculations

Abnormal results

○ Improvement in muscle strength (a positive response) suggests myasthenia gravis.
○ A positive response may also suggest motor neuron disease, some neuropathies, and myopathies.
○ Patients in myasthenic crisis show a brief improvement in muscle strength after receiving Tensilon.
○ Patients in cholinergic crisis experience exaggerated muscle weakness after receiving Tensilon.

Interfering factors

○ Myasthenia gravis that affects only ocular muscles

Terminal deoxynucleotidyl transferase

Overview

○ Measures levels of terminal deoxynucleotidyl transferase (TdT), using indirect immunofluorescence

Purpose

○ To help differentiate acute lymphocytic leukemia (ALL) from acute nonlymphocytic leukemia
○ To help differentiate lymphoblastic lymphomas from malignant lymphomas
○ To monitor the patient's response to therapy, help determine his prognosis, or obtain early diagnosis of a relapse

Procedure

Preparation

○ Explain to the patient that this test detects an enzyme that can help classify tissue origin.
For blood test
○ Tell the patient to fast for 12 to 14 hours before the test.
○ Tell the patient who will perform the venipuncture and when.
○ Explain to the patient that he may experience slight discomfort from the tourniquet and the needle puncture.
For bone marrow aspiration
○ Inform the patient that he need not restrict food and fluids.
○ Tell the patient that the biopsy usually takes 5 to 10 minutes.
○ Make sure the patient or a responsible family member has signed an informed consent form.
○ Give a mild sedative 1 hour before the aspiration.
○ Tell the patient which bone will be the biopsy site.
○ Check the patient's history for hypersensitivity to the local anesthetic.
○ Inform the patient that he'll receive a local anesthetic but will feel pressure on insertion of the biopsy needle and a brief, pulling pain when the marrow is withdrawn.

Implementation

○ If the patient is to receive a blood test, perform a venipuncture and collect the sample in one 10-ml heparinized blood tube and one ethylenediaminetetraacetic acid tube.
○ If assisting with bone marrow aspiration, inject 1 ml of bone marrow into a 7-ml heparinized tube and di-

lute it with 5 ml of normal saline solution, or submit four air-dried marrow smears.
○ Send the sample to the laboratory immediately.

Patient care

○ Because the patient may have a compromised immune system, take special care to keep the venipuncture site clean and dry.
○ Because a patient with leukemia may bleed excessively, apply pressure to the venipuncture site until bleeding stops.
○ Check the bone marrow aspiration site for bleeding and inflammation, and observe the patient for signs of hemorrhage and infection.

Complications

○ Hematoma at the venipuncture site

Interpretation

Normal results

○ TdT is present in less than 2% of marrow cells and undetectable in normal peripheral blood.

Abnormal results

○ Positive cells are present in more than 90% of patients with ALL, in 33% of patients with chronic myelogenous leukemia in blast crisis, and in 5% of patients with nonlymphocytic leukemias.
○ TdT-positive cells are absent in patients with ALL who are in remission.

Interfering factors

○ Failure to obtain a representative sample during bone marrow aspiration
○ Performing bone marrow aspiration on a child because of presence of TdT-positive bone marrow during proliferation of prelymphocytes (possible false-positive)
○ Bone marrow regeneration, idiopathic thrombocytopenic purpura, and neuroblastoma, causing TdT-positive bone marrow (possible false-positive)
○ Failure to send the sample to the laboratory immediately

Testosterone

Overview

- Competitive protein-binding test that measures level of testosterone, the main androgen secreted by the interstitial cells of the testes (Leydig cells), which induces puberty in the male and maintains male secondary sex characteristics.
- Evaluates gonadal dysfunction in men and women, when combined with plasma gonadotropin level measurement (follicle-stimulating hormone and luteinizing hormone).
- Prepubertal levels of testosterone are low. Increased testosterone secretion during puberty stimulates growth of the seminiferous tubules and sperm production; it also contributes to the enlargement of external genitalia, accessory sex organs (such as prostate glands), and voluntary muscles and to the growth of facial, pubic, and axillary hair.
- Testosterone production begins to rise at the onset of puberty and continues to rise during adulthood. Production begins to taper at about age 40 and eventually drops to about one-fifth the peak level by age 80. In women, the adrenal glands and ovaries secrete small amounts of testosterone.

Purpose

- To facilitate in the differential diagnosis of male sexual precocity in boys under age 10 (distinguishing true precocious puberty from pseudoprecocious puberty)
- To aid in the differential diagnosis of hypogonadism (distinguishing primary from secondary hypogonadism)
- To evaluate male infertility or other sexual dysfunction
- To evaluate hirsutism and virilization in women

Procedure

Preparation

- Explain to the patient that this test helps determine if male sex hormone secretion is adequate.
- Inform the patient that he need not restrict food and fluids.
- Tell the patient that the test requires a blood sample. Explain who will perform the venipuncture and when.
- Explain to the patient that he may experience slight discomfort from the tourniquet and the needle puncture.

Implementation

- Perform a venipuncture and collect a serum sample in a 7-ml clot-activator tube.
- If plasma is to be collected, use a heparinized tube.

- Indicate the patient's age, sex, and history of hormone therapy on the laboratory request.
- Handle the sample gently to prevent hemolysis, and send it to the laboratory promptly.

Patient care

- Apply direct pressure to the venipuncture site until bleeding stops.

Complications

- Hematoma at the venipuncture site

Interpretation

Normal results

- In men, 300 to 1,200 nanograms/dl (SI, 10.4 to 41.6 nmol/L)
- In women, 20 to 80 nanograms/dl (SI, 0.7 to 2.8 nmol/L)
- In prepubertal children, lower values than adults

Abnormal results

- Increased testosterone levels may occur with a benign adrenal tumor or cancer, hyperthyroidism, and incipient puberty.
- Increased testosterone levels in women with ovarian tumors or polycystic ovary syndrome may rise, leading to hirsutism.
- Increased testosterone levels in prepubertal boys may indicate true sexual precocity caused by excessive gonadotropin secretion or pseudoprecocious puberty caused by male hormone production by a testicular tumor.
- Decreased testosterone levels can indicate primary hypogonadism (as in Klinefelter's syndrome), secondary hypogonadism (hypogonadotropic eunuchoidism) from hypothalamic-pituitary dysfunction.
- Decreased testosterone levels may also follow orchiectomy, testicular or prostate cancer, delayed male puberty, estrogen therapy, and cirrhosis of the liver.
- Decreased testosterone levels may also indicate congenital adrenal hyperplasia, which results in precocious puberty in boys (from ages 2 to 3) and pseudohermaphroditism and milder virilization in girls.

Interfering factors

- Hemolysis from rough handling of the sample
- Exogenous sources of estrogens and androgens, thyroid and growth hormones, and other pituitary-based hormones
- Estrogens (decrease in free testosterone levels, increasing sex hormone-binding globulin, which binds testosterone)
- Androgens (possible increase)

Thallium imaging

Overview

- Evaluates blood flow after I.V. injection of the radio-isotope thallium-201 or Cardiolyte

Cardiolyte
- Has a better energy spectrum for imaging
- Requires living myocardial cells for uptake and allows for imaging the myocardial blood flow both before and after reperfusion

Thallium
- Concentrates in healthy myocardial tissue but not in necrotic or ischemic tissue: taken up rapidly in areas of the heart with normal blood supply and intact cells; fails to be taken up by areas with poor blood flow and ischemic cells, which appear as cold spots on a scan

Rest imaging
- Can disclose acute myocardial infarction (MI) within the first few hours of symptoms but doesn't distinguish an old from a new infarct

Stress imaging
- Performed after exercise stress testing or after pharmacologic stress testing; used to assess known or suspected coronary artery disease (CAD)
- Also known as *cardiac nuclear imaging, cold spot myocardial imaging,* or *myocardial perfusion scan*

Purpose

- To assess myocardial perfusion
- To demonstrate the location and extent of an MI
- To diagnose CAD (stress imaging)
- To evaluate coronary artery patency following surgical revascularization
- To evaluate effectiveness of antianginal therapy or percutaneous revascularization interventions (stress imaging)

Procedure

Preparation

- Make sure the patient has signed a consent form.
- Note and report all allergies.
- For stress imaging: Instruct the patient to wear comfortable walking shoes during the treadmill exercise.
- Inform the patient that he must restrict his use of alcohol, tobacco, and nonprescription medications for 24 hours before the test.
- Tell him to fast after midnight the night before the test.
- Tell the patient to report fatigue, pain, shortness of breath, or other anginal symptoms immediately.

Implementation

- Stress imaging: the patient walks on a treadmill at a regulated pace that's gradually increased while his electrocardiogram (ECG), blood pressure, and heart rate are monitored.
- When the patient reaches peak stress, give him 1.5 to 3 mCi of thallium.
- The patient exercises an additional 45 to 60 seconds to permit circulation and uptake of the isotope.
- Stop the stress imaging immediately if the patient develops chest pain, dyspnea, fatigue, syncope, hypotension, ischemic ECG changes, significant arrhythmias, or other critical signs or symptoms (confusion, staggering, or pale, clammy skin).
- Disconnect the patient from monitoring equipment as long as he's clinically stable, and position him on his back under the nuclear medicine camera.
- Additional scans may be taken after the patient rests and occasionally after 24 hours.
- Scanning after rest is helpful in differentiating between an ischemic area and an infarcted or scarred area of the myocardium.
- Resting imaging: Give the patient an injection of thallium I.V. or Cardiolyte.
- Scanning is performed as in stress imaging.

Patient care

- If further scanning is required, have the patient rest and restrict foods and beverages other than water.
- Monitor vital signs and ECGs.
- Watch for cardiac arrhythmias and anginal symptoms.

Complications

- Cardiac arrhythmias
- Myocardial ischemia, MI
- Respiratory distress
- Cardiac arrest
- Hypotension or hypertension

Interpretation

Normal results

- Normal distribution of the isotope throughout the left ventricle without defects (cold spots)
- After coronary artery bypass surgery, improved regional perfusion, suggesting graft patency
- Improved perfusion after nonsurgical revascularization interventions, suggesting increased coronary flow

Abnormal results

- Persistent defects suggest MI.
- Transient defects (those that disappear after a 3- to 6-hour rest) suggest myocardial ischemia caused by CAD.

Interfering factors

- Improper ECG electrode placement

Thoracentesis

Overview

- Obtains specimens of pleural fluid for analysis, or therapeutically relieves respiratory symptoms caused by the accumulation of excess pleural fluid.
- Examines specimens for color, consistency, pH, glucose and protein content, cellular composition, and the enzymes lactate dehydrogenase (LD) and amylase; also examined cytologically for malignant cells and cultured for pathogens.
- Contraindicated in patients with uncorrected bleeding disorders or anticoagulant therapy.
- Also known as *pleural fluid aspiration*.

Purpose

- To provide pleural fluid specimens to determine the cause and nature of pleural effusion
- To provide symptomatic relief with large pleural effusion

Procedure

Preparation

- Make sure the patient has signed a consent form.
- Note and report all allergies.
- Record the patient's baseline vital signs.
- If the patient will receive sedation, restrict food and fluids.
- Explain to the patient that pleural fluid may be located by chest X-ray or ultrasound study.
- Tell the patient that he'll receive a local anesthetic.
- Instruct the patient to avoid coughing, deep breathing, or moving during the test.

Implementation

- Position the patient to widen the intercostal spaces and allow easier access to the pleural cavity.
- If the patient can't sit up, position him on his unaffected side with the arm on the affected side elevated.
- After the patient is in the proper position, prepare and drape the site.
- Inject a local anesthetic into the subcutaneous tissue; the thoracentesis needle is then inserted.
- When the needle reaches the pocket of fluid, it's attached to a 50-ml syringe or a vacuum bottle and the fluid is removed.
- During aspiration, the patient is monitored for signs of respiratory distress and hypotension.
- Pleural fluid characteristics and total volume are noted.
- After the needle is withdrawn, apply pressure until hemostasis is obtained and a small dressing is applied.
- Place specimens in proper containers, label appropriately, and send to the laboratory immediately.

- Pleural fluid for pH determination must be collected anaerobically, heparinized, kept on ice, and analyzed promptly.

Patient care

- Elevate the head of the bed to facilitate breathing.
- Obtain a chest X-ray.
- Tell the patient to immediately report difficulty breathing.
- Immediately report signs and symptoms of pneumothorax, tension pneumothorax, and pleural fluid reaccumulation.
- Monitor the patient for reexpansion pulmonary edema (RPE), a rare but serious complication of thoracentesis. Thoracentesis should be halted if the patient has sudden chest tightness or coughing.
- Monitor vital signs, pulse oximetry, and breath sounds.
- Observe the puncture site and dressings.
- Watch for subcutaneous emphysema.
- Monitor pleural pressure.

Complications

- Laceration of intercostal vessels
- Pneumothorax
- Mediastinal shift
- RPE
- Bleeding and infection

Interpretation

Normal results

- Negative pressure in the pleural cavity with less than 50 ml serous fluid.

Abnormal results

- Bloody fluid suggests possible hemothorax, malignancy, or traumatic tap.
- Milky fluid suggests chylothorax.
- Fluid with pus suggests empyema.
- Transudative effusion suggests heart failure, hepatic cirrhosis, or renal disease.
- Exudative effusion suggests lymphatic drainage abstraction, infections, pulmonary infarctions, and neoplasms.
- Positive cultures suggest infection.
- Predominating lymphocytes suggest tuberculosis or fungal or viral effusions.
- Elevated LD levels in a nonpurulent, nonhemolyzed, nonbloody effusion suggest possible malignant tumor.
- Pleural fluid glucose levels that are 30 to 40 mg/dl lower than blood glucose levels may indicate cancer, bacterial infection, or metastasis.
- Increased amylase suggests pleural effusions associated with pancreatitis.

Interfering factors

- Improper collection of the specimen

Thoracoscopy

Overview

- Insertion of an endoscope directly into the chest wall allowing visualization of the pleural space
- Used for both diagnostic and therapeutic purposes; can sometimes replace traditional thoracotomy
- Reduces morbidity (by avoiding open-chest surgery) and postoperative pain, decreases surgical and anesthesia time, and allows faster recovery

Purpose

- To diagnose pleural disease
- To obtain biopsy specimens from the mediastinum, lung, or pericardium
- To facilitate treatment of pleural conditions, such as cysts, blebs, and effusions
- To allow resection such as wedge biopsy

Procedure

Preparation

- Make sure the patient has signed an appropriate consent form.
- Note and report all allergies.
- Make sure appropriate preoperative tests (such as pulmonary function and coagulation tests, electrocardiogram, and chest X-ray) are complete; report abnormal results to the physician.
- Explain to the patient that it's common to use general anesthesia for this test.
- Instruct him to restrict food and fluids for 10 to 12 hours before the procedure.

Implementation

- The patient is anesthetized and a double-lumen endobronchial tube is inserted.
- The lung on the operative side is collapsed and a small intercostal incision is made, through which a trocar is inserted.
- A lens is inserted to view the area and assess thoracoscopy access.
- Two or three more small incisions are made, and trocars are placed for insertion of suctioning and dissection instruments.
- The camera lens and instruments are moved from site to site as needed.
- After thoracoscopy, the lung is reexpanded, and a chest tube is placed through one incision site.
- The other incisions are closed with adhesive strips and dressed.
- A water-seal drainage system is attached to the chest tube.

Patient care

- Give the patient analgesics.
- Tell the patient to resume his normal diet and activity.
- Monitor vital signs and respiratory status.
- Monitor the patient's intake and output.
- Observe patency of the chest tube and drainage system.
- Monitor the patient for bleeding and infection.

Complications

- Hemorrhage
- Nerve injury
- Perforation of the diaphragm
- Air emboli
- Tension pneumothorax

Interpretation

Normal results

- The pleural cavity contains a small amount of lubricating fluid that facilitates movement of the lung and chest wall.
- The parietal and visceral layers are lesion-free and able to separate from each other.

Abnormal results

- Lesions adjacent to or involving the pleura or mediastinum suggest possible malignancy; will be biopsied for diagnosis and determination of treatment.
- Blebs suggest possible presence of chronic lung disease; can be removed by wedge resection to reduce the risk of spontaneous pneumothorax.
- The presence of increased pleural fluid indicates pleural effusion; specimens can be obtained for analysis and diagnosis of the cause.

Interfering factors

- Excessive bleeding during the procedure (may necessitate open thoracotomy)
- Extensive or inaccessible pathology

Throat culture

Overview

- Requires swabbing the throat, streaking a culture plate, and allowing organisms to grow for isolation and identification of pathogens.
- Obtains preliminary identification through a Gram-stained smear, which guides clinical management and determines the need for further tests.
- Rapid nonculture antigen-testing methods detect group A streptococcal antigen in as few as 5 minutes; all negative specimens should be cultured.

Purpose

- To isolate and identify pathogens, especially group A beta-hemolytic streptococci
- To screen asymptomatic carriers of pathogens, especially *Neisseria meningitides*

Procedure

Preparation

- Make sure the patient has signed an appropriate consent form.
- Note and report all allergies.
- Maintain asepsis throughout all procedures.
- Wear personal protective equipment throughout the procedure.
- Check the patient's history for recent antimicrobial therapy.
- Determine immunization history if pertinent to the preliminary diagnosis.
- Tell the patient that he need not restrict food and fluids before the test.
- Warn the patient that he may gag during the swabbing.
- Obtain a specimen before beginning antimicrobial therapy.

Implementation

- Ask the patient to tilt his head back and close his eyes.
- With the throat well illuminated, check for inflamed areas, using a tongue blade.
- Swab the tonsillar areas from side to side; include any inflamed or purulent sites. Don't touch the tongue, cheeks, or teeth with the swab.
- Immediately place the swab in the culture tube. If a commercial sterile collection and transport system is used, crush the ampule and force the swab into the medium to keep it moist.
- Note recent antimicrobial therapy on the laboratory request.
- Label the specimen with the patient's name, physician's name, date and time of collection, and origin of the specimen. Also indicate the suspected organism, especially *Corynebacterium diphtheriae* (re-quires two swabs and a special growth medium) and *N. meningitidis* (requires enriched selective media).

Patient care

- Answer the patient's questions about the test.

Complications

None known

Interpretation

Normal results

- The presence of usual or normal flora: nonhemolytic and alpha-hemolytic streptococci, *Neisseria* species, staphylococci, diphtheroids, some *Haemophilus* species, pneumococci, yeasts, enteric gram-negative organisms, spirochetes, *Veillonella* species, and *Micrococcus* species

Abnormal results

- Group A beta-hemolytic streptococci *(Streptococcus pyogenes)* suggest possible scarlet fever or pharyngitis.
- *Candida albicans* suggests possible thrush.
- *C. diphtheriae* suggests possible diphtheria.
- *Bordetella pertussis* suggests possible whooping cough.
- *Legionella* species and *Mycoplasma pneumoniae* suggest bacterial pneumonia.
- *Histoplasma capsulatum, Coccidioides immitis,* and *Blastomyces dermatitidis* suggest fungal infections.
- Adenovirus, enterovirus, herpesvirus, rhinovirus, influenza virus, and parainfluenza virus suggest viral infections.

Interfering factors

- Improper collection of the sample

Thyroid biopsy

Overview

○ The excision of a thyroid tissue specimen for histologic examination
○ May be indicated for patients with thyroid enlargement or nodules; breathing and swallowing difficulties; vocal cord paralysis, weight loss, hemoptysis, or a sensation of fullness in the neck
○ Commonly performed when noninvasive tests, such as thyroid ultrasonography and scans, are abnormal or inconclusive
○ Specimens obtained with hollow needle under local anesthesia or during open (surgical) biopsy under general anesthesia

Purpose

○ To differentiate between benign and malignant thyroid disease
○ To diagnose Hashimoto's disease, hyperthyroidism, and nontoxic nodular goiter

Procedure

Preparation

○ Make sure the patient has signed an appropriate consent form.
○ Note and report all allergies.
○ Give the patient a sedative.
○ Obtain results of coagulation studies and report abnormal results to the physician.
○ Tell the patient that he need not restrict food and fluids unless he'll be receiving a general anesthetic.
○ Explain the use of a local anesthetic.
○ Warn the patient that he might experience some pressure when the tissue specimen is obtained.
○ Explain that results should be available in 48 to 72 hours.

Implementation

○ For needle biopsy, assist the patient into a supine position with a pillow under his shoulder blades. This position pushes the trachea and thyroid forward and allows the jugular veins to fall backward.
○ The biopsy site is prepared.
○ The patient is given a local anesthetic.
○ The carotid artery is palpated, and the biopsy needle is inserted parallel to and about 1″ (2.5 cm) from the thyroid cartilage to prevent damage to the deep structures and the larynx.
○ After the specimen is obtained, the needle is removed and the specimen is immediately placed in formalin.
○ Apply pressure to the biopsy site until hemostasis is obtained.
○ Clean and dress the biopsy site.

Patient care

○ Place the patient in semi-Fowler's position.
○ Explain that a sore throat is possible the day after the test.
○ Teach the patient to avoid undue strain on the biopsy site by putting both hands behind his neck when he sits up.
○ Keep the biopsy site clean and dry.
○ Monitor the patient's vital signs and voice quality.
○ Measure neck circumference.
○ Monitor the patient's swallowing ability.
○ Watch for signs of infection.
○ Observe for difficulty breathing associated with edema or hematoma, with resultant tracheal compression. Also check the back of the patient's neck and his pillow for bleeding every hour for 8 hours. Report bleeding immediately.
○ Bleeding may persist in a patient with abnormal prothrombin time or abnormal activated partial thromboplastin time or in a patient with a large, vascular thyroid and distended jugular veins.

Complications

○ Bleeding
○ Infection
○ Respiratory compromise

Interpretation

Normal results

○ Fibrous networks divide the gland into pseudolobules that consist of follicles and capillaries.
○ Cuboidal epithelium lines the follicle walls and contains the protein thyroglobulin, which stores triiodothyronine and thyroxine.

Abnormal results

○ Well-encapsulated, solitary nodules of uniform but abnormal structure suggest possible malignant tumors.
○ Hypertrophy, hyperplasia, and hypervascularity suggest possible benign conditions such as nontoxic nodular goiter.
○ Characteristic histologic patterns suggest possible subacute granulomatous thyroiditis, Hashimoto's disease, and hyperthyroidism.

Interfering factors

○ Failure to properly preserve the specimen in formalin

Thyroid-stimulating hormone, neonatal

Overview

- An immunoassay that confirms congenital hypothyroidism after a screening test detects low thyroxine (T_4) levels.
- Thyroid-stimulating hormone (TSH) levels should surge after birth, triggering a rise in thyroid hormone that's essential for neurologic development.
- In congenital hypothyroidism, the thyroid gland doesn't respond to TSH stimulation, resulting in diminished thyroid hormone levels and elevated TSH levels.
- Early detection and treatment of congenital hypothyroidism is critical to prevent mental retardation and cretinism.

Purpose

- To confirm diagnosis of congenital hypothyroidism

Procedure

Preparation

- Explain to the infant's parents that this test helps confirm the diagnosis of congenital hypothyroidism.
- Emphasize the importance of detecting the disorder early so that prompt therapy can prevent irreversible brain damage.

Implementation

Filter paper sample
- Assemble the necessary equipment, wash your hands thoroughly, and put on gloves.
- Wipe the infant's heel with an alcohol or povidone-iodine swab, and then dry it thoroughly with a gauze pad.
- Perform a heelstick. Squeezing the infant's heel gently, fill the circles on the filter paper with blood. Make sure the blood saturates the paper.
- Allow the filter paper to dry, label it appropriately, and send it to the laboratory.

Serum sample
- Perform a venipuncture and collect the sample in a 3-ml clot-activator tube.
- Label the sample and send it to the laboratory immediately.

Patient care

- Apply direct pressure to the venipuncture or heelstick site until bleeding stops.

Complications

- Hematoma at the venipuncture site

Interpretation

Normal results

- TSH level at age 1 to 2 days, 25 to 30 µIU/ml (SI, 25 to 30 mU/L)
- TSH level after age 1 to 2 days, < 25 µIU/ml (SI, < 25 mU/L)

Abnormal results

- Neonatal TSH levels must be interpreted in light of the T_4 level.
- Increased TSH levels with decreased T_4 levels indicate primary congenital hypothyroidism (thyroid gland dysfunction).
- Decreased TSH and T_4 levels may indicate secondary congenital hypothyroidism (pituitary or hypothalamic dysfunction).
- Normal TSH levels with decreased T_4 levels may indicate hypothyroidism caused by a congenital defect in T_4-binding globulin or transient congenital hypothyroidism caused by prematurity or prenatal hypoxia. A complete thyroid workup must be done to confirm the cause of hypothyroidism before treatment can begin.

Interfering factors

- Failure to let a filter paper sample dry completely
- Hemolysis from rough handling of the sample
- Corticosteroids, triiodothyronine, and T_4 (decrease)
- Lithium carbonate, potassium iodide, excessive topical resorcinol, and TSH injection (increase)

Thyroid-stimulating hormone, serum

Overview

- Measures serum thyroid-stimulating hormone (TSH) levels by radioimmunoassay.
- Detects primary hypothyroidism and determines whether the hypothyroidism results from thyroid gland failure or from pituitary or hypothalamic dysfunction.
- TSH, or thyrotropin, promotes increases in the size, number, and activity of thyroid cells and stimulates the release of triiodothyronine and thyroxine; these hormones affect total body metabolism and are essential for normal growth and development.
- Normal serum TSH levels rule out primary hypothyroidism.
- May not distinguish between low-normal and subnormal levels, especially in secondary hypothyroidism.

Purpose

- To confirm or rule out primary hypothyroidism and distinguish it from secondary hypothyroidism
- To monitor drug therapy in the patient with primary hypothyroidism

Procedure

Preparation

- Explain to the patient that this test helps assess thyroid gland function.
- Tell the patient that the test requires a blood sample. Explain who will perform the venipuncture and when.
- Explain to the patient that he may experience slight discomfort from the tourniquet and the needle puncture.
- Withhold steroids, thyroid hormones, aspirin, and other drugs that may influence test results. If the patient must continue taking them, note this on the laboratory request.
- Keep the patient relaxed and recumbent for 30 minutes before the test.

Implementation

- Between 6 a.m. and 8 a.m., perform a venipuncture and collect the sample in a 5-ml clot-activator tube.

Patient care

- Apply direct pressure to the venipuncture site until bleeding stops.
- Instruct the patient that he may resume medications stopped before the test, as ordered.

Complications

- Hematoma at the venipuncture site

Interpretation

Normal results

- Undetectable to 15 µIU/ml (SI, 15 mU/L)

Abnormal results

- TSH levels may be slightly increased in euthyroid patients with thyroid cancer.
- Levels > 20 µIU/ml (SI, 20 mU/L) suggest primary hypothyroidism or, possibly, endemic goiter.
- Decreased or undetectable TSH levels may be normal but occasionally indicate secondary hypothyroidism (with inadequate secretion of TSH or thyrotropin-releasing hormone [TRH]).
- Decreased TSH levels may also result from hyperthyroidism (Graves' disease) and thyroiditis; both are marked by hypersecretion of thyroid hormones, which suppresses TSH release. Provocative testing with TRH is necessary to confirm the diagnosis.

Interfering factors

- Failure to observe pretest restrictions
- Hemolysis from rough handling of the sample

Thyroid-stimulating immunoglobulin

Overview

- Detects thyroid-stimulating immunoglobulin (TSI), formerly called *long-acting thyroid stimulator*, which appears in the blood of most patients with Graves' disease.
- TSI reacts with the cell-surface receptors that usually combine with thyroid-stimulating hormone (TSH), activates intracellular enzymes, and promotes epithelial cell activity that functions outside the normal feedback regulation mechanism for TSH.
- TSI stimulates the thyroid gland to produce and excrete excessive amounts of thyroid hormone.
- Reportedly, 90% of people with Graves' disease have elevated TSI levels; positive results of this test strongly suggest Graves' disease, despite normal routine thyroid tests in patients still suspected of having Graves' disease or progressive exophthalmos.

Purpose

- To aid in the evaluation of suspected thyroid disease
- To aid in the diagnosis of suspected thyrotoxicosis, especially in patients with exophthalmos
- To monitor treatment of thyrotoxicosis

Procedure

Preparation

- Explain to the patient that this test evaluates thyroid function, as appropriate.
- Tell the patient that the test requires a blood sample. Explain who will perform the venipuncture and when.
- Explain to the patient that he may experience slight discomfort from the tourniquet and the needle puncture.

Implementation

- Perform a venipuncture and collect the sample in a 5-ml clot-activator tube.
- Handle the sample gently to prevent hemolysis and send it to the laboratory immediately.
- If the patient had a radioactive iodine scan within 48 hours of the test, note this on the laboratory request.

Patient care

- Apply direct pressure to the venipuncture site until bleeding stops.

Complications

- Hematoma at the venipuncture site

Interpretation

Normal results

- TSI doesn't normally appear in serum, but it's considered normal at < 130% of basal activity.

Abnormal results

- Increased TSI levels are linked to exophthalmos, Graves' disease (thyrotoxicosis), and recurrence of hyperthyroidism.

Interfering factors

- Hemolysis from rough handling of the sample
- Administration of radioactive iodine within 48 hours of the test

Thyroxine, serum

Overview

○ Immunoassay to measure the total circulating thyroxine (T_4) level when thyroxine-binding globulin (TBG) is normal; one of the most common thyroid diagnostic tools.
○ T_4 is an amine secreted by the thyroid gland in response to thyroid-stimulating hormone (TSH) and, indirectly, thyrotropin-releasing hormone.
○ The rate of secretion is normally regulated by a complex system of negative and positive feedback involving the thyroid, anterior pituitary, and hypothalamus.
○ The suspected precursor, or prohormone, of triiodothyronine (T_3), T_4 is believed to convert to T_3 by monodeiodination, which occurs mainly in the liver and kidneys.
○ Only a fraction of T_4 (about 0.05%) circulates freely in the blood; the rest binds strongly to plasma proteins, primarily TBG.
○ This minute fraction is responsible for the clinical effects of thyroid hormone.
○ TBG binds so tenaciously that T_4 survives in the plasma for a relatively long time, with a half-life of about 6 days.

Purpose

○ To evaluate thyroid function
○ To aid in the diagnosis of hyperthyroidism and hypothyroidism
○ To monitor the patient's response to antithyroid medication in hyperthyroidism or to thyroid replacement therapy in hypothyroidism (TSH estimates needed to confirm hypothyroidism)

Procedure

Preparation

○ Explain to the patient that this test helps evaluate thyroid gland function.
○ Inform the patient that he need not fast or restrict activity.
○ Tell the patient that the test requires a blood sample. Explain who will perform the venipuncture and when.
○ Withhold drugs that may interfere with test results. If they must be continued, note this on the laboratory request.
○ If this test is to monitor thyroid therapy, the patient should continue to receive daily thyroid supplements.

Implementation

○ Perform a venipuncture and collect the sample in a 7-ml clot-activator tube.
○ Handle the sample gently to prevent hemolysis.
○ Send the sample to the laboratory immediately so that the serum can be separated.

Patient care

○ Apply direct pressure to the venipuncture site until bleeding stops.
○ Instruct the patient that he may resume medications stopped before the test.

Complications

○ Hematoma at the venipuncture site

Interpretation

Normal results

○ Total T_4 levels, 5 to 13.5 µg/dl (SI, 60 to 165 mmol/L)

Abnormal results

○ Increased T_4 levels are consistent with primary and secondary hyperthyroidism, including excessive T_4 (levothyroxine) replacement therapy (factitious or iatrogenic hyperthyroidism).
○ Subnormal levels suggest primary or secondary hypothyroidism or may be caused by T_4 suppression by normal, elevated, or replacement T_3 levels.
○ When hypothyroidism can't be confirmed, it may be necessary to measure TSH levels.
○ Normal T_4 levels don't guarantee euthyroidism; for example, normal readings occur in T_3 toxicosis.
○ Overt signs of hyperthyroidism require further testing.

Interfering factors

○ Hemolysis from rough handling of the sample
○ Hereditary factors and hepatic disease (possible increase or decrease in TBG)
○ Protein-wasting disease (such as nephrotic syndrome) and androgens (possible decrease in TBG)
○ Estrogens, progestins, levothyroxine, and methadone (increase)
○ Free fatty acids, heparin, iodides, liothyronine sodium, lithium, methylthiouracil, phenylbutazone, phenytoin, propylthiouracil, salicylates (high doses), steroids, sulfonamides, and sulfonylureas (decrease)
○ Clofibrate (possible increase or decrease)

Thyroxine-binding globulin, serum

Overview

- Measures serum thyroxine-binding globulin (TBG) level, the predominant protein carrier for circulating thyroxine (T_4) and triiodothyronine (T_3).
- TBG values are identified by saturating the sample for TBG determination with radioactive T_4, then subjecting this to electrophoresis and measuring the amount of TBG by the amount of radioactive T_4 by radioimmunoassay.
- Any condition that affects TBG levels and subsequent binding capacity also affects the amount of free T_4 (FT_4) in circulation.
- An underlying TBG abnormality renders tests for total T_3 and T_4 inaccurate but doesn't affect the accuracy of tests for free T_3 (FT_3) and FT_4.

Purpose

- To evaluate abnormal thyrometabolic states that don't correlate with thyroid hormone (T_3 or T_4) values (for example, a patient with overt signs of hypothyroidism and a low FT_4 level with a high total T_4 level caused by a marked increase of TBG secondary to hormonal contraceptives)
- To identify TBG abnormalities

Procedure

Preparation

- Explain to the patient that this test helps evaluate thyroid function.
- Tell the patient that the test requires a blood sample.
- Explain to the patient that he may experience slight discomfort from the tourniquet and the needle puncture.
- Withhold drugs that may affect the accuracy of test results, such as estrogens, anabolic steroids, phenytoin, salicylates, or thyroid preparations. If the patient must continue taking them, note this on the laboratory request.
- Drugs may be continued to determine if prescribed drugs are affecting TBG levels.

Implementation

- Perform a venipuncture and collect the sample in a 7-ml clot-activator tube.
- Handle the sample gently to prevent hemolysis.

Patient care

- Apply direct pressure to the venipuncture site until bleeding stops.
- Instruct the patient that he may resume medications stopped before the test.

Complications

- Hematoma at the venipuncture site

Interpretation

Normal results

- TBG by immunoassay, 16 to 32 µg/dl (SI, 120 to 180 mg/ml)

Abnormal results

- Elevated TBG levels may indicate hypothyroidism or congenital (genetic) excess, some forms of hepatic disease, or acute intermittent porphyria.
- TBG levels rise during pregnancy and are high in neonates.
- Suppressed levels may indicate hyperthyroidism or congenital deficiency and can occur in active acromegaly, nephrotic syndrome, and malnutrition associated with hypoproteinemia, acute illness, or surgical stress.
- Patients with TBG abnormalities require additional testing, such as the serum FT_3 and T_4 tests, to evaluate thyroid function more precisely.

Interfering factors

- Hemolysis from rough handling of the sample
- Estrogens, including hormonal contraceptives, and phenothiazines such as perphenazine (increase)
- Androgens, prednisone, phenytoin, and high doses of salicylates (decrease)

Tonometry

Overview

- Indirectly measures intraocular pressure (IOP) to screen for glaucoma, which occurs in 2% of people over age 40 and is a common cause of blindness, using one of two procedures.
- *Indentation tonometry* measures IOP by observing how deeply a known weight depresses the cornea; *applanation tonometry* measures IOP by observing how much force is required to flatten an area of the cornea.
- The patient's cornea must be anesthetized, and careful examination technique followed for each procedure.
- If indentation tonometry shows that the IOP is elevated, confirm the diagnosis with other tests, such as applanation tonometry, visual field testing, and ophthalmoscopy.
- Tonometry should never be performed on a patient with a corneal ulcer or infection, except by a skilled examiner and only in an emergency such as suspected acute angle-closure glaucoma.
- Patients with increased IOP can monitor themselves at home using a portable tonometer.

Purpose

- To measure IOP
- To aid in the diagnosis and follow-up evaluation of glaucoma

Procedure

Preparation

- Explain to the patient that tonometry measures the pressure within his eyes.
- Tell the patient that the test takes only a few minutes and requires that his eyes be anesthetized; reassure him that the procedure is painless.
- If the patient wears contact lenses, tell him to remove them before the test and not to reinsert them until the anesthetic wears off completely.
- Ask the patient to lie supine. Make sure he's relaxed, and have him loosen restrictive clothing around his neck.
- Instruct him not to cough or squeeze his eyelids together.

Implementation

- Ask the patient to look down. Raise his superior eyelid with your thumb, place one drop of the topical anesthetic at the top of the sclera, and have the patient blink.
- Check the tonometer for a zero reading on the steel test block that comes with the instrument. Make sure the plunger moves freely. The first measurement on each eye is obtained with the 5.5-g weight.

- Have the patient look up and stare at a spot on the ceiling. Then ask him to open his mouth, take a deep breath, and exhale slowly for distraction.
- With the thumb and forefinger of one hand, hold the lids of his right eye open against the orbital rim.
- Hold the tonometer vertically with the thumb and forefinger of the other hand, and rest the footplate on the apex of the cornea.
- With the footplate in place, check the indicator needle for a rhythmic transmission caused by the ocular pulse, and then record the calibrated scale reading that converts to a measurement of IOP.
- If the reading doesn't exceed 4, add an additional weight (7.5, 10, or 15 g) to obtain a reliable result.
- Repeat the procedure on the left eye and record the time the test is performed.

Patient care

- Tell the patient not to rub his eyes for at least 20 minutes after the test to prevent corneal abrasion.
- If the patient wears contact lenses, tell him not to reinsert them for at least 2 hours.
- If the tonometer moved across the cornea during the test, tell the patient he may feel a slight scratching sensation in the eye when the anesthetic wears off. This sensation should disappear within 24 hours because most abrasions resulting from tonometry affect only the epithelium, which regenerates in 24 hours.

Complications

- Resting your fingers on the cornea or pressing on the cornea (increases IOP)
- Touching the patient's lashes (may trigger a blink response or Bell's phenomenon: upward movement of the eyes with forced closure of the lids, which can cause the footplate to move and scratch the cornea)

Interpretation

Normal results

- IOP is 12 to 20 mm Hg, with diurnal variations: the highest point is upon waking; the lowest point, in the evening.

Abnormal results

- Increased IOP requires further testing for glaucoma.
- Because IOP varies diurnally, findings must be supplemented with serial measurements obtained at different times on different days.

Interfering factors

- Poor patient cooperation
- Deformed corneal curvature that prevents proper placement of the footplate
- Corneoscleral rigidity or flaccidity, as determined by an ophthalmologist (falsely elevated or depressed readings)

TORCH test

Overview

- Detects exposure to pathogens from *to*xoplasmosis, *r*ubella, *c*ytomegalovirus, and *h*erpes simplex antibodies (TORCH).
- TORCH pathogens often linked to asymptomatic congenital and neonatal infections that may severely impair the central nervous system.
- Detects specific immunoglobulin M-associated antibodies in infant blood.

Purpose

- To aid in the diagnosis of acute, congenital, and intrapartum infections

Procedure

Preparation

- Explain to the infant's parents the purpose of the test; tell them that the test requires a blood sample. Explain who will perform the venipuncture and when.
- Explain that the infant may experience slight discomfort from the tourniquet and the needle puncture.

Implementation

- Obtain a 3-ml sample of venous or cord blood.
- Handle the sample gently to prevent hemolysis.
- Don't freeze the sample.
- Send the sample to the laboratory immediately.

Patient care

- Apply direct pressure to the venipuncture site until bleeding stops.

Complications

- Hematoma at the venipuncture site

Interpretation

Normal results

- Negative for TORCH pathogens

Abnormal results

- Toxoplasmosis is diagnosed by sequential examination that shows rising antibody titers, changing titers, and serologic conversion from negative to positive; a titer of 1:256 suggests recent *Toxoplasma* infection.
- In infants less than 6 months old, rubella infection is linked to a marked and persistent rise in complement-fixing antibody titer over time.
- Persistence of rubella antibody in an infant after age 6 months strongly suggests congenital infection, which may lead to cardiac anomalies, neurosensory deafness, growth retardation, and encephalitic symptoms.

- In infants, a screen for congenital infections may show the presence of antibodies, which may indicate diseases such as cytomegalovirus and syphilis.
- Detection of herpes antibodies in cerebrospinal fluid with signs of herpetic encephalitis and persistent herpes simplex virus type 2 antibody levels confirms herpes simplex infection in a neonate without obvious herpetic lesions.

Interfering factors

- Hemolysis from rough handling of the sample

Total carbon dioxide content

Overview

- When carbon dioxide (CO_2) pressure in red blood cells exceeds 40 mm Hg, CO_2 spills out of the cells and dissolves in plasma. There it may combine with water to form carbonic acid, which in turn may dissociate into hydrogen and bicarbonate ions.
- The total CO_2 content test measures the total concentration of all forms of CO_2 in serum, plasma, or whole blood samples.
- The test is commonly ordered for patients with respiratory insufficiency and is usually included in an assessment of electrolyte balance.
- Test results are most significant when considered with pH and arterial blood gas values.
- Since about 90% of CO_2 in serum is in the form of bicarbonate, this test closely assesses bicarbonate levels.
- Total CO_2 content reflects the adequacy of gas exchange in the lungs and the efficiency of the carbonic acid–bicarbonate buffer system, which maintains acid-base balance and normal pH.

Purpose

- To help evaluate acid-base balance

Procedure

Preparation

- Explain to the patient that the total CO_2 content test measures the amount of CO_2 in his blood.
- Tell the patient that the test requires a blood sample.
- Explain to the patient that he may experience discomfort from the tourniquet and the needle puncture.
- Inform the patient that he need not restrict food and fluids.
- Notify the laboratory and physician of drugs the patient is taking that may affect test results; it may be necessary to restrict them.

Implementation

- Perform a venipuncture.
- When CO_2 content is measured along with electrolytes, use a 3- or 4-ml clot-activator tube.
- When this test is performed alone, use a heparinized tube.
- Fill the tube completely to prevent diffusion of CO_2 into the vacuum.

Patient care

- Apply direct pressure to the venipuncture site until bleeding stops.
- Instruct the patient that he may resume medications stopped before the test.

Complications

- Hematoma at the venipuncture site

Interpretation

Normal results

- Total CO_2 levels, 22 to 26 mEq/L (SI, 22 to 26 mmol/L)
- Varying levels, depending on the patient's sex and age

Abnormal results

- High CO_2 levels may occur in metabolic alkalosis, respiratory acidosis, primary aldosteronism, and Cushing's syndrome.
- CO_2 levels may also increase after excessive loss of acids, such as severe vomiting and continuous gastric drainage.
- Decreased CO_2 levels are common in metabolic acidosis.
- Decreased total CO_2 levels in metabolic acidosis also result from loss of bicarbonate.
- Levels may decrease in respiratory alkalosis.

Interfering factors

- Underfilling the collection tube, letting CO_2 escape (inaccurate levels)
- Excessive use of corticotropin, cortisone, or thiazide diuretics; excessive ingestion of alkali or licorice (increase)
- Salicylates, paraldehyde, methicillin, dimercaprol, ammonium chloride, and acetazolamide; ingestion of ethylene glycol or methyl alcohol (decrease)

Total cholesterol

Overview

- The total cholesterol test, the quantitative analysis of serum cholesterol, measures the circulating levels of free cholesterol and cholesterol esters; it reflects the level of the two forms in which this biochemical compound appears in the body.
- High serum cholesterol levels may be linked to an increased risk of coronary artery disease (CAD).
- A 3-minute skin test is now available for use in physician offices. (See *Skin test for cholesterol*.)

Purpose

- To assess the risk of CAD
- To evaluate fat metabolism
- To aid in the diagnosis of nephrotic syndrome, pancreatitis, hepatic disease, hypothyroidism, and hyperthyroidism
- To assess the efficacy of lipid-lowering drug therapy

Procedure

Preparation

- Explain to the patient that the total cholesterol test assesses the body's fat metabolism.
- Tell the patient that the test requires a blood sample. Explain who will perform the venipuncture and when.
- Explain to the patient that he may experience slight discomfort from the tourniquet and the needle puncture.
- Instruct the patient not to eat or drink for 12 hours before the test, with the exception of water.

Skin test for cholesterol

A new 3-minute test that measures the amount of cholesterol in the skin rather than in the blood is the first noninvasive test of its kind. It measures how much cholesterol is present in other tissues in the body and provides additional data about a person's risk of heart disease.

The test, which doesn't require patients to fast, involves placing a bandagelike applicator pad on the palm of the hand. Drops of a special solution that reacts to skin cholesterol are then added to the pad; 3 minutes later, a hand-held computer translates the information into a skin cholesterol reading.

Because the test measures the amount of cholesterol that has accumulated in the tissues over time, results don't correlate with blood cholesterol levels, so the test isn't meant to be a substitute or surrogate for a blood cholesterol test. In addition, the Food and Drug Administration cautions that the test isn't intended for use as a screening tool for heart disease in the general population. Instead, it has been approved for use among adults with severe heart disease — those with at least a 50% blockage of two or more heart arteries.

- Notify the laboratory and physician of drugs the patient is taking that may affect test results; it may be necessary to restrict them.

Implementation

- The patient should be in a sitting position for 5 minutes before the blood is drawn.
- Perform a venipuncture and collect the sample in a 4-ml ethylenediaminetetraacetic acid tube.
- Fingersticks may also be used for initial screening when using an automated analyzer.

Patient care

- Apply direct pressure to the venipuncture site until bleeding stops.
- Instruct the patient that he may resume his usual diet and medications stopped before the test.

Complications

- Hematoma at the venipuncture site

Interpretation

Normal results

- Varying levels, depending on age and sex
- In men, < 205 mg/dl (SI, < 5.3 mmol/L)
- In women, < 190 mg/dl (SI, < 4.9 mmol/L)
- In children ages 12 to 18, < 170 mg/dl (SI, < 4.4 mmol/L)

Abnormal results

- Increased serum cholesterol levels (hypercholesterolemia) may indicate a risk of CAD, incipient hepatitis, lipid disorders, bile duct blockage, nephrotic syndrome, obstructive jaundice, pancreatitis, and hypothyroidism.
- Decreased serum cholesterol levels (hypocholesterolemia) are usually linked to malnutrition, cellular necrosis of the liver, and hyperthyroidism.
- Abnormal cholesterol levels usually require further testing to find the cause.

Interfering factors

- Failure to observe pretest restrictions
- Failure to send the sample to the laboratory immediately
- Cholestyramine, clofibrate, colestipol, dextrothyroxine, haloperidol, neomycin, niacin, and chlortetracycline (decrease)
- Epinephrine, chlorpromazine, trifluoperazine, hormonal contraceptives, and trimethadione (increase)
- Androgens (possible variable effect)

Total iron-binding capacity

Overview

- Measures the amount of iron that would appear in plasma if all the transferrin were saturated with iron (iron is essential to the formation and function of hemoglobin and other heme and nonheme compounds).
- After iron is absorbed by the intestine, it's distributed to various body compartments for synthesis, storage, and transport.
- The sample should be drawn in the morning because serum iron level is highest in the morning and declines progressively during the day.
- Serum iron level and total iron-binding capacity (TIBC) are more useful when performed with the serum ferritin assay, but together these tests may not accurately reflect the state of other iron compartments, such as myoglobin iron and the labile iron pool.
- Bone marrow or liver biopsy and iron absorption or excretion studies may yield more information.

Purpose

- To estimate total iron storage
- To aid in the diagnosis of hemochromatosis
- To help distinguish iron deficiency anemia from anemia of chronic disease
- To help evaluate nutritional status

Procedure

Preparation

- Explain to the patient that this test evaluates the body's capacity to store iron.
- Tell the patient that the test requires a blood sample.
- Inform the patient that he need not restrict food and fluids.
- Notify the laboratory and physician of drugs the patient is taking that may affect test results; it may be necessary to restrict them.
- Explain to the patient that he may feel slight discomfort from the tourniquet and the needle puncture.

Implementation

- Perform a venipuncture and collect the sample in a 4.5-ml clot-activator tube.
- Handle the sample gently to prevent hemolysis.
- Send the sample to the laboratory immediately.

Patient care

- Make sure subdermal bleeding has stopped before removing pressure.
- Instruct the patient that he may resume medications stopped before the test.
- If a large hematoma develops at the venipuncture site, monitor pulses distal to the site.

Complications

- Hematoma at the venipuncture site

Interpretation

Normal results

- In males and females, 300 to 360 µg/dl (SI, 54 to 64 µmol/L)
- Saturation in males and females, 20% to 50% (SI, 0.2 to 0.5)

Abnormal results

- In iron deficiency, TIBC increases, decreasing saturation.
- In patients with chronic inflammation (such as in rheumatoid arthritis), TIBC may remain unchanged or may decrease to preserve normal saturation.
- Iron overload may not alter serum levels until relatively late, but serum iron usually increases and TIBC remains the same, which increases the saturation.

Interfering factors

- Hemolysis from rough handling of the sample or failure to send the sample to the laboratory immediately
- Iron supplements (possible false-positive serum iron values but false-negative TIBC)

Total serum protein

Overview

○ Protein electrophoresis measures serum albumin and globulin, the major blood proteins, by separating the proteins into five distinct fractions: albumin, alpha$_1$, alpha$_2$, beta, and gamma globulin proteins.

Purpose

○ To aid in the diagnosis of hepatic disease, protein deficiency, renal disorders, and GI and neoplastic diseases

Procedure

Preparation

○ Explain to the patient that protein electrophoresis determines the protein content of blood.

○ Tell the patient that the test requires a blood sample. Explain who will perform the venipuncture and when.

○ Inform the patient that he need not restrict food and fluids.

○ Notify the laboratory and physician of drugs the patient is taking that may affect test results; it may be necessary to restrict them.

○ Explain to the patient that he may experience slight discomfort from the tourniquet and the needle puncture.

Implementation

○ Perform a venipuncture and collect the sample in a 7-ml clot-activator tube.

○ This test must be performed on a serum sample to avoid measuring the fibrinogen fraction.

Patient care

○ Apply direct pressure to the venipuncture site until bleeding stops.

○ Inform the patient that he may resume his usual medications stopped before the test.

Clinical implications of abnormal protein levels

	TOTAL PROTEINS	ALBUMIN	GLOBULINS
INCREASED LEVELS	• Chronic inflammatory disease (such as rheumatoid arthritis or early-stage Laënnec's cirrhosis) • Dehydration • Diabetic ketoacidosis • Fulminating and chronic infections • Multiple myeloma • Monocytic leukemia • Vomiting, diarrhea	• Multiple myeloma	• Chronic syphilis • Collagen diseases • Diabetes mellitus • Hodgkin's disease • Multiple myeloma • Rheumatoid arthritis • Subacute bacterial endocarditis • Systemic lupus erythematosus (SLE) • Tuberculosis
DECREASED LEVELS	• Benzene and carbon tetrachloride poisoning • Blood dyscrasias • Essential hypertension • GI disease • Heart failure • Hepatic dysfunction • Hemorrhage • Hodgkin's disease • Hyperthyroidism • Malabsorption • Malnutrition • Nephrosis • Severe burns • Surgical and traumatic shock • Toxemia of pregnancy • Uncontrolled diabetes mellitus	• Acute cholecystitis • Collagen diseases • Diarrhea • Essential hypertension • Hepatic disease • Hodgkin's disease • Hyperthyroidism • Hypogammaglobulinemia • Malnutrition • Metastatic carcinoma • Nephritis, nephrosis • Peptic ulcer • Plasma loss from burns • Rheumatoid arthritis • Sarcoidosis • SLE	• Benzene and carbon tetrachloride poisoning • Blood dyscrasias • Essential hypertension • GI disease • Heart failure • Hepatic dysfunction • Hemorrhage • Hodgkin's disease • Hyperthyroidism • Malabsorption • Malnutrition • Nephrosis • Severe burns • Surgical and traumatic shock • Toxemia of pregnancy • Uncontrolled diabetes mellitus

Complications

○ Hematoma at the venipuncture site

Interpretation

Normal results

○ Total serum protein levels, 6.4 to 8.3 g/dl (SI, 64 to 83 g/L)
○ Albumin fraction, 3.5 to 5 g/dl (SI, 35 to 50 g/L)
○ Alpha$_1$ globulin fraction, 0.1 to 0.3 g/dl (SI, 1 to 3 g/L)
○ Alpha$_2$ globulin, 0.6 to 1 g/dl (SI, 6 to 10 g/L)
○ Beta globulin, 0.7 to 1.1 g/dl (SI, 7 to 11 g/L)
○ Gamma globulin, 0.8 to 1.6 g/dl (SI, 8 to 16 g/L)

Abnormal results

(See *Clinical implications of abnormal protein levels.*)

Interfering factors

○ Pretest administration of a contrast agent, such as sulfobromophthalein (false-high total protein)
○ Pregnancy or cytotoxic drugs (possible decrease in serum albumin)
○ Use of plasma instead of serum

Transcranial Doppler studies

Overview

- Transcranial Doppler studies provide information about the presence, quality, and changing nature of circulation to an area of the brain by measuring the velocity of blood flow through cerebral arteries.
- Commonly, these studies aren't definitive but are advantageous because they provide diagnostic information in a noninvasive manner.
- After transcranial Doppler studies and before surgery, the patient may undergo cerebral angiography to further define cerebral blood flow patterns and to locate the exact vascular abnormality.

Purpose

- To measure the velocity of blood flow through certain cerebral vessels
- To detect and monitor the progression of cerebral vasospasm
- To determine the presence of collateral blood flow before surgical ligation or radiologic occlusion of diseased blood vessels

Procedure

Preparation

- Tell the patient that fasting before the test isn't necessary.
- Explain that the test typically takes less than 1 hour, depending on the number of vessels to be examined and any interfering factors.

Implementation

- The patient reclines in a chair or on a stretcher or bed.
- A small amount of gel is applied to the transcranial "window" (temporal, transorbital, and through the foramen magnum), where bone is thin enough to allow the Doppler signal to enter and be detected.
- The technician directs the signal toward the artery being studied and then records the velocities detected.
- In a complete study, the middle cerebral arteries, anterior cerebral arteries, ophthalmic arteries, carotid siphon, vertebral arteries, and basilar artery are studied.
- The Doppler signal can be transmitted to varying depths.
- Waveforms may be printed for later analysis.

Patient care

- Remove any remaining gel from the patient's skin.

Complications

None known

Interpretation

Normal results

- Normal waveforms and velocities

Abnormal results

- High velocities suggest that blood flow is too turbulent or the vessel is too narrow; or possible stenosis, vasospasm, or arteriovenous malformation.

Interfering factors

- Dressings over the test site

Transesophageal echocardiography

Overview

- Combines ultrasonography with endoscopy to provide a better view of the heart's structures
- Involves a small transducer attached to the end of a gastroscope and inserted into the esophagus, allowing images to be taken from the posterior aspect of the heart
- Causes less tissue penetration and interference from chest wall structures and produces high-quality images of the thoracic aorta, except for the superior ascending aorta, which is shadowed by the trachea

Purpose

- To visualize and evaluate thoracic and aortic disorders, such as dissection and aneurysm; valvular disease (especially of the mitral valve); endocarditis; and congenital heart disease
- To visualize and evaluate intracardiac thrombi, cardiac tumors, cardiac tamponade, and ventricular dysfunction

Procedure

Preparation

- Make sure the patient has signed an appropriate consent form.
- Note and report all allergies.
- Review the patient's medical history and report possible contraindications to the test, such as esophageal obstruction or varices, GI bleeding, previous mediastinal radiation therapy, or severe cervical arthritis.
- Note and report loose teeth.
- Tell the patient that he must fast for 6 hours before the procedure.
- Instruct the patient to remove dentures or oral prostheses.
- Explain the use of a topical anesthetic throat spray.
- Warn the patient that he may gag when the tube is inserted.
- Explain the need for I.V. sedation and continuous monitoring during the study.
- Explain that the study takes about 2 hours, including preparation and recovery.

Implementation

- Connect the patient to monitors for continual blood pressure, heart rate, and pulse oximetry assessment.
- Assist the patient into a supine position on his left side and give him a sedative.
- Spray the back of his throat with a topical anesthetic.
- Place a bite block in the patient's mouth and instruct him to close his lips around it.
- The endoscope is inserted and advanced 12" to 14" (30 to 36 cm) to the level of the right atrium.
- To visualize the left ventricle, the scope is advanced 16" to 18" (41 to 46 cm).
- Ultrasound images are obtained and reviewed.

Patient care

- Ensure the patient's safety and a patent airway until the sedative wears off.
- Withhold food and water until his gag reflex returns.
- If the procedure is done on an outpatient basis, advise the patient to have someone drive him home.
- Monitor the patient's level of consciousness and vital signs.
- Monitor the patient's respiratory status and cardiac arrhythmias.
- Watch for bleeding.
- Observe for gag reflex.
- Observe closely for a vasovagal response, which may occur with gagging.
- Keep resuscitation and suction equipment immediately available.
- Use pulse oximetry to detect hypoxia.
- If bleeding occurs, stop the procedure immediately.

Complications

- Laryngospasm
- Cardiac arrhythmias
- Bleeding
- Adverse reaction to sedation

Interpretation

Normal results

- The heart is without structural abnormalities.
- No vegetations or thrombi are visible.
- No tumors are visible.

Abnormal results

- Structural thoracic and aortic abnormalities suggest possible endocarditis, congenital heart disease, intracardiac thrombi, or tumors.
- Congenital defects suggest possible patent ductus arteriosus.

Interfering factors

- Laryngospasm, arrhythmias, or bleeding increases the risk of complications. If either of these occurs, postpone the test.

Transferrin

Overview

- The transferrin test, a quantitative analysis of serum transferrin (siderophilin) levels, evaluates iron metabolism.
- Transferrin is a glycoprotein formed in the liver.
- It transports circulating iron obtained from dietary sources or the breakdown of red blood cells by reticuloendothelial cells to bone marrow for use in hemoglobin synthesis or to the liver, spleen, and bone marrow for storage.
- A serum iron level is typically obtained simultaneously.

Purpose

- To determine the iron-transporting capacity of the blood
- To evaluate iron metabolism in iron deficiency anemia

Procedure

Preparation

- Explain to the patient that the transferrin test determines the cause of anemia.
- Tell the patient that the test requires a blood sample. Explain who will perform the venipuncture and when.
- Explain to the patient that he may experience slight discomfort from the tourniquet and the needle puncture.
- Inform the patient that he need not restrict food and fluids.
- Notify the laboratory and physician of drugs the patient is taking that may affect test results; it may be necessary to restrict them.

Implementation

- Perform a venipuncture and collect the sample in a 4-ml clot-activator tube.
- Handle the sample gently to prevent hemolysis.
- Send the sample to the laboratory immediately.

Patient care

- Apply direct pressure to the venipuncture site until bleeding stops.
- Inform the patient that he may resume his usual medications stopped before the test.

Complications

- Hematoma at the venipuncture site

Interpretation

Normal results

- 200 to 400 mg/dl (SI, 2 to 4 g/L)

Abnormal results

- Inadequate transferrin levels may lead to impaired hemoglobin synthesis and, possibly, anemia.
- Low serum levels may indicate inadequate transferrin production caused by hepatic damage or excessive protein loss from renal disease.
- Decreased transferrin levels may also result from acute or chronic infection and cancer.
- Increased serum transferrin levels may indicate severe iron deficiency.

Interfering factors

- Hemolysis from rough handling of the sample
- Hormonal contraceptives and late pregnancy (possible increase)

Transvaginal ultrasound

Overview

- Imaging technique using high-frequency sound waves to produce images of the pelvic structures
- Allows evaluation of pelvic anatomy and diagnosis of pregnancy at an earlier gestational age
- Eliminates the need for a full bladder and circumvents difficulties encountered with obese patients
- Also known as *endovaginal ultrasound*

Purpose

- To establish early pregnancy with fetal heart motion as early as the 5th to 6th week of gestation
- To identify ectopic pregnancy
- To monitor follicular growth during infertility treatment
- To evaluate abnormal pregnancy (such as blighted ovum, missed or incomplete abortion, or molar pregnancy)
- To visualize retained products of conception
- To diagnose fetal abnormalities, placental location, and cervical length
- To evaluate adnexal pathology, such as tubo-ovarian abscess, hydrosalpinx, and ovarian masses
- To evaluate the uterine lining (in patients with dysfunctional uterine bleeding and postmenopausal bleeding)

Procedure

Preparation

- Make sure the patient has signed an appropriate consent form.
- Note and report all allergies.
- Explain to the patient that the test requires insertion of a vaginal probe and that self-insertion may be possible.
- If the sonographer is a man, assure the patient that a female assistant will be present during the examination.

Implementation

- Assist the patient into the lithotomy position.
- Water-soluble gel is placed on the transducer tip to allow better sound transmission, and a protective sheath is placed over the transducer.
- Additional lubricant is placed on the sheathed transducer tip, which is gently inserted into the vagina by the patient or the sonographer.
- The pelvic structures are observed by rotating the probe 90 degrees to one side and then the other.

Patient care

- Help the patient remove any residual gel.

Complications

None known

Interpretation

Normal results

- The uterus and ovaries are normal in size and shape.
- The body of the uterus lies on the superior surface of the bladder; the uterine tubes are attached laterally.
- The ovaries are located on the lateral pelvic walls with the external iliac vessels above and the ureters posteroinferior, and are covered by the fimbria of the uterine tubes medially.
- In pregnancy, the gestational sac and fetus are of normal size for the gestational period.

Abnormal results

- Free peritoneal fluid in the pelvic cavity suggests possible peritonitis.
- A tubal mass suggests possible ectopic pregnancy.
- Structural abnormalities in a nonpregnant woman may indicate cancer of the uterus, ovaries, vagina, and other pelvic structures; noncancerous growths of the uterus and ovaries; ovarian torsion; areas of infection, including pelvic inflammatory disease; and congenital malformations.
- Structural abnormalities in a pregnant woman may suggest threatened abortion; multiple pregnancies; fetal death; placental abnormalities, including placenta previa and placental abruption; tumors of pregnancy, including gestational trophoblastic disease.

Interfering factors

None known

Triglycerides

Overview

- Provides quantitative analysis of triglycerides — the main storage form of lipids — which constitute about 95% of fatty tissue
- Allows early identification of hyperlipidemia and the risk of coronary artery disease (CAD)

Purpose

- To screen for hyperlipidemia or pancreatitis
- To help identify nephrotic syndrome and the individual with poorly controlled diabetes mellitus
- To assess the risk of CAD
- To calculate the low-density lipoprotein cholesterol level using the Friedewald equation

Procedure

Preparation

- Explain to the patient that the triglyceride test is used to detect fat metabolism disorders.
- Tell the patient that the test requires a blood sample. Explain who will perform the venipuncture and when.
- Notify the laboratory and physician of drugs the patient is taking that may affect test results; it may be necessary to restrict them.
- Instruct the patient to fast for at least 12 hours before the test and to abstain from alcohol for 24 hours. Tell him that he may drink water.
- Explain to the patient that he may experience slight discomfort from the tourniquet and the needle puncture.

Implementation

- Perform a venipuncture and collect the sample in a 4-ml ethylenediaminetetraacetic acid tube.
- Send the sample to the laboratory immediately.
- Avoid prolonged venous occlusion; remove the tourniquet within 1 minute of application.

Patient care

- Apply direct pressure to the venipuncture site until bleeding stops.
- Instruct the patient that he may resume his usual diet and medications stopped before the test.

Complications

- Hematoma at the venipuncture site

Interpretation

Normal results

- Varying levels, depending on age and sex
- In men, 44 to 180 mg/dl (SI, 0.44 to 2.01 mmol/L)
- In women, 10 to 190 mg/dl (SI, 0.11 to 2.21 mmol/L)

Abnormal results

- An increased or decreased serum triglyceride level is abnormal; additional tests are required for a definitive diagnosis.
- A mild to moderate increase in serum triglyceride levels indicates biliary obstruction, diabetes mellitus, nephrotic syndrome, endocrinopathies, or overconsumption of alcohol.
- Markedly increased levels without an identifiable cause reflect congenital hyperlipoproteinemia and necessitate lipoprotein phenotyping to confirm the diagnosis.
- Decreased serum triglyceride levels are rare and occur mainly in malnutrition and abetalipoproteinemia.

Interfering factors

- Failure to observe pretest restrictions
- Use of a glycol-lubricated collection tube
- Failure to send the sample to the laboratory immediately
- Antilipemics (decreased serum lipid levels)
- Cholestyramine and colestipol (decreased cholesterol levels but increased or unaffected triglyceride levels)
- Corticosteroids (long-term use), hormonal contraceptives, estrogen, ethyl alcohol, furosemide, and miconazole (increase)
- Clofibrate, dextrothyroxine, gemfibrozil, and niacin (decreased cholesterol and triglyceride levels)
- Probucol (decreased cholesterol levels but variable effect on triglyceride levels)

Triiodothyronine uptake

Overview

○ Indirectly measures free thyroxine (FT_4) levels by demonstrating the availability of serum protein-binding sites for thyroxine (T_4).
○ Results are often combined with a T_4 radioimmunoassay or $T_4(D)$ (competitive protein-binding test) to calculate the FT_4 index, which reflects FT_4 levels by correcting for thyroxine-binding globulin (TBG) abnormalities.
○ Has become less popular recently because rapid tests for T_3, T_4, and thyroid-stimulating hormone are readily available.
○ Also called the *T_3 uptake* test.

Purpose

○ To aid in the diagnosis of hypothyroidism and hyperthyroidism when TBG is normal
○ To aid in the diagnosis of primary disorders of TBG levels

Procedure

Preparation

○ Explain to the patient that this test helps evaluate thyroid function.
○ Tell the patient that the test requires a blood sample. Explain who will perform the venipuncture and when.
○ Withhold drugs that may interfere with test results, such as estrogens, androgens, phenytoin, salicylates, and thyroid preparations. If the patient must continue them, note this on the laboratory request.
○ Explain to the patient that he may experience slight discomfort from the tourniquet and the needle puncture.
○ Tell the patient that the laboratory requires several days to complete the analysis.

Implementation

○ Perform a venipuncture and collect the sample in a 7-ml clot-activator tube.

Patient care

○ Apply direct pressure to the venipuncture site until bleeding stops.
○ Instruct the patient that he may resume medications stopped before the test.

Complications

○ Hematoma at the venipuncture site

Interpretation

Normal results

○ 25% to 35%

Abnormal results

○ A high T_3 uptake percentage with increased T_4 levels indicates hyperthyroidism (implying few TBG free binding sites and high FT_4 levels).
○ A low T_3 uptake percentage with decreased T_4 levels indicates hypothyroidism (implying more TBG free binding sites and low FT_4 levels).
○ A high T_3 uptake percentage with a decreased or normal FT_4 level suggests decreased TBG levels. Such decreased levels may be caused by protein loss (as in nephrotic syndrome), decreased production (caused by androgen excess or genetic or idiopathic causes), or competition for T_4 binding sites by certain drugs (salicylates, phenylbutazone, and phenytoin).
○ A low T_3 uptake percentage and an increased or normal FT_4 level suggests increased TBG levels. Such increased levels may result from exogenous or endogenous estrogen levels (pregnancy) or from idiopathic causes.
○ In primary disorders of TBG levels, measured T_4 and free sites change in the same direction.
○ In primary thyroid disease, T_4 and T_3 uptake vary in the same direction; availability of binding sites varies inversely.
○ Discordant variance in T_4 and T_3 uptake suggests a TBG abnormality.

Interfering factors

○ Radioisotope scans performed before sample collection
○ Anabolic steroids, heparin, phenytoin, salicylates (high dose), thyroid preparations, and warfarin (possible increase in TBG and thyroxine-binding protein electrophoresis)
○ Antithyroid agents, clofibrate, estrogen, hormonal contraceptives, and thiazide diuretics (decreased uptake)

Triiodothyronine, serum

Overview

○ Highly specific radioimmunoassay that measures total (bound and free) serum content of triiodothyronine(T_3) to investigate clinical indications of thyroid dysfunction. T_3, the more potent thyroid hormone, is an amine derived primarily from thyroxine (T_4) through the process of mono-deiodination.
○ From 50% to 90% of T_3 may be derived from T_4 as a result of this pivotal transformation, during which T_4 loses one of its iodine atoms to become T_3.
○ The remaining 10% or more of T_3 is secreted directly by the thyroid gland, in response to thyroid-stimulating hormone (TSH) and thyrotropin-releasing hormone.
○ Although minute amounts of T_3 are in the bloodstream and T_3 is metabolically active for only a short time, its impact on body metabolism dominates that of T_4. Another significant difference between the two major thyroid hormones is that T_3 binds less firmly to thyroxine-binding globulin (TBG).
○ Half of T_3 disappears from the bloodstream in about 1 day; half of T_4 disappears in 6 days.

Purpose

○ To aid in the diagnosis of T_3 toxicosis
○ To aid in the diagnosis of hypothyroidism and hyperthyroidism
○ To monitor the patient's response to thyroid replacement therapy in hypothyroidism

Procedure

Preparation

○ Explain to the patient that this test helps evaluate thyroid gland function and determine the cause of his symptoms.
○ Tell the patient that the test requires a blood sample. Explain who will perform the venipuncture and when.
○ Withhold drugs, such as steroids, propranolol, and cholestyramine, which may influence thyroid function. If the patient must continue them, record this information on the laboratory request.
○ Explain to the patient that he may experience slight discomfort from the tourniquet and the needle puncture.
○ If the patient must receive thyroid preparations, note the administration time on the laboratory request.

Implementation

○ Perform a venipuncture and collect the sample in a 7-ml clot-activator tube.

○ Send the sample to the laboratory as soon as possible to avoid stasis and to allow early separation of serum from the clotted blood.

Patient care

○ Apply direct pressure to the venipuncture site until bleeding stops.
○ Instruct the patient that he may resume medications stopped before the test.

Complications

○ Hematoma at the venipuncture site

Interpretation

Normal results

○ 80 to 200 nanograms/dl (SI, 1.2 to 3 nmol/L)
○ In pregnant patients, increased serum T_3 levels
○ Serum T_3 and T_4 levels that rise and fall in tandem

Abnormal results

○ T_3 levels are usually a more accurate diagnostic indicator of hyperthyroidism than T_4 levels.
○ In T_3 toxicosis, T_3 levels rise, while total and free T_4 levels remain normal. T_3 toxicosis occurs in the patient with Graves' disease, toxic adenoma, or toxic nodular goiter.
○ T_3 levels also surpass T_4 levels in the patient receiving thyroid replacement therapy containing more T_3 than T_4.
○ In iodine-deficient areas, the thyroid may produce larger amounts of T_3 than of T_4 to try to maintain the euthyroid state.
○ Although T_3 and T_4 levels are increased in about 90% of patients with hyperthyroidism, there's a disproportionate increase in T_3.
○ In some patients with hypothyroidism, T_3 levels may fall within the normal range and not be diagnostically significant.
○ Low T_3 levels may appear in the euthyroid patient with systemic illness (especially hepatic or renal disease), during severe acute illness, and after trauma or major surgery; in such cases, TSH levels are within normal limits.
○ Low T_3 levels are sometimes found in the euthyroid patient with malnutrition.

Interfering factors

○ Hemolysis from rough handling of the sample
○ Markedly increased or decreased TBG levels, regardless of cause
○ Failure to take into account drugs that affect T_3 levels, such as steroids, clofibrate, cholestyramine, and propranolol

Troponin

Overview

○ Detects cardiac troponin I (cTnI) and cardiac troponin T (cTnT), proteins in the striated cells that are extremely specific markers of cardiac damage.
○ When injury occurs to the myocardial tissue, these proteins are released into the bloodstream.
○ Elevations in troponin levels can be seen within 1 hour of myocardial infarction (MI) and will persist for 1 week or longer.

Purpose

○ To detect and diagnose acute MI and reinfarction
○ To evaluate the possible causes of chest pain

Procedure

Preparation

○ Explain to the patient that this test helps assess myocardial injury and that multiple samples may be drawn to detect fluctuations in serum levels.
○ Tell the patient that the test requires a blood sample. Explain who will perform the venipuncture and when.
○ Inform the patient he need not restrict foods and fluids.
○ Explain to the patient that he may feel slight discomfort from the tourniquet and the needle puncture.

Implementation

○ Perform a venipuncture and collect the specimen in a 7-ml clot-activator tube.
○ Obtain each specimen on schedule and note the date and collection time on each.

Patient care

○ Apply direct pressure to venipuncture site until bleeding stops.

Complications

○ Hematoma at the venipuncture site

Interpretation

Normal results

○ cTnI levels, < 0.35 µg/L (SI, > 0.35 µg/L)
○ cTnT levels, < 0.1 µg/L (SI, < 0.1 µg/L)

Abnormal results

○ Some laboratories may call a test positive if it shows any detectable levels, and others may give a range for abnormal results.

○ cTnI levels > 2.0 µg/L (SI, > 2.0 µg/L) and cTnT rapid immunoassay results > 0.1 µg/L (SI, > 0.1 µg/L) suggest cardiac injury. As long as tissue injury continues, the troponin levels will remain high.
○ Troponin levels rise rapidly and are detectable within 1 hour of myocardial cell injury.

Interfering factors

○ Sustained vigorous exercise (increase in absence of significant cardiac damage)
○ Cardiotoxic drugs such as doxorubicin (increase)
○ Renal disease and certain surgical procedures (possible increase)

Tuberculin skin tests

Overview

- Screen for previous infection by the tubercle bacillus.
- Performed in children, young adults, and patients with radiographic findings that suggest tuberculosis (TB)
- In the old tuberculin (OT) and purified protein derivative (PPD) tests, intradermal injection of the tuberculin antigen causes a delayed hypersensitivity reaction in patients with active or dormant TB.
- The Mantoux test uses a single-needle intradermal injection of PPD, permitting precise dose measurement.
- Multipuncture tests, such as the tine test, Mono-Vacc tests, and Aplitest — usually used for screening — intradermally injectioned with tines impregnated with OT or PPD.
- Because they require less skill and are more rapidly given, multipuncture tests are generally used for screening.
- A positive multipuncture test usually requires a Mantoux test for confirmation.

Purpose

- To distinguish TB from blastomycosis, coccidioidomycosis, and histoplasmosis
- To identify people who need diagnostic investigation for TB because of possible exposure

Procedure

Preparation

- Explain to the patient that this test helps detect TB.
- Tell the patient that the test requires an intradermal injection, which may cause him discomfort.
- Check the patient's history for active TB, the results of previous skin tests, and hypersensitivities.
- If the patient has had TB, don't perform a skin test.
- If the patient has had a positive reaction to previous skin tests, consult the physician or follow facility policy.
- If the patient has had an allergic reaction to acacia, don't perform an OT test which contains it.
- If you're performing a tuberculin test on an outpatient, instruct him to return at the specified time so that test results can be read.
- Inform the patient that a positive reaction to a skin test appears as a red, hard, raised area at the injection site. Although the area may itch, instruct him not to scratch it.
- Stress that a positive reaction doesn't always indicate active TB.

Implementation

- Ask the patient to sit and support his extended arm on a flat surface.
- Clean the volar surface of the upper forearm with alcohol and allow the area to dry completely.
- Mantoux test: Perform an intradermal injection.
- Multipuncture test: Remove the protective cap on the injection device to expose the four tines.
- Hold the patient's forearm in one hand, stretching the skin of the forearm tightly. Then, with your other hand, firmly depress the device into the patient's skin without twisting it.
- Hold the device in place for at least 1 second before removing it.
- If you've applied sufficient pressure, you'll see four puncture sites and a circular depression made by the device on the patient's skin.

Patient care

- Both tests: Record where the test was given, the date and time, and when the results are to be read. Tuberculin skin tests are generally read 48 to 72 hours after injection; the Mono-Vacc tests can be read 48 to 96 hours after the test.
- If an ulceration or necrosis develops at the injection site, apply cold soaks or a topical steroid.
- Have epinephrine available to treat a possible anaphylactic or acute hypersensitivity reaction.

Complications

- Ulceration or necrosis at the injection site

 ALERT *Anaphylactic or acute hypersensitivity reaction*

Interpretation

Normal results

- In tuberculin skin tests, negative or minimal reactions
- In the Mantoux test, no induration or induration < 5 mm in diameter.
- In the tine test and Aplitest, no vesiculation or induration or induration < 2 mm in diameter.
- In the Mono-Vacc tests, no induration.

Abnormal results

- A positive tuberculin reaction indicates previous infection by tubercle bacilli. It doesn't distinguish between an active and a dormant infection or provide a definitive diagnosis.
- If a positive reaction occurs, sputum smear and culture and chest radiography are necessary for further information.
- In the Mantoux test, induration 5 to 9 mm in diameter indicates a borderline reaction; larger induration, a positive reaction.
- Because patients infected with atypical mycobacteria other than tubercle bacilli may have borderline reactions, repeat testing is necessary.
- In the tine test or Aplitest, vesiculation indicates a positive reaction; induration 2 mm in diameter without vesiculation requires confirmation by the Man-

toux test. Any induration in the Mono-Vacc tests indicates a positive reaction, but this reaction should be confirmed by the Mantoux test.

Interfering factors

○ Subcutaneous injection, usually indicated by erythema diameter > 10 mm without induration
○ Corticosteroids, other immunosuppressants, and live vaccine viruses, such as measles, mumps, rubella, and polio, within 4 to 6 weeks before the test (possible suppression of skin reaction)
○ In elderly people and patients with viral infection, malnutrition, febrile illness, uremia, immunosuppressive disorders, or miliary TB (possible suppression of skin reaction)
○ Less than 10-week period since infection (possible suppression of skin reaction)
○ Improper dilution, dosage, or storage of the tuberculin

Tubular reabsorption of phosphate

Overview

○ Indirectly measures parathyroid hormone (PTH) levels by measuring urine and serum phosphate and creatinine levels; the results allow the tubular reabsorption of phosphate to be calculated.
○ PTH maintains optimum blood levels of ionized calcium, controls renal excretion of calcium and phosphate, stimulates reabsorption of calcium, and inhibits reabsorption of phosphate from the glomerular filtrate.
○ PTH secretion decreases as ionized calcium levels return to normal.
○ In primary hyperparathyroidism, excessive secretion of PTH disrupts this calcium-phosphate balance.

Purpose

○ To evaluate parathyroid gland function
○ To aid in the diagnosis of primary hyperparathyroidism
○ To aid in the differential diagnosis of hypercalcemia

Procedure

Preparation

○ Explain to the patient that this test evaluates parathyroid gland function.
○ Advise the patient that the test requires a blood sample and urine collection over a 24-hour period.
○ Tell the patient who will perform the venipuncture and when.
○ Notify the laboratory and physician of drugs the patient is taking that may affect test results; it may be necessary to restrict them. If the patient must continue taking them, note this on the laboratory request.
○ Instruct the patient to maintain a normal-phosphate diet for 3 days before the test because a low-phosphate diet (< 500 mg/day) may elevate tubular reabsorption values and a high-phosphate diet (3,000 mg/day) may lower them. Common nutritional sources of phosphorus include legumes, nuts, milk, egg yolks, meat, poultry, fish, cereals, and cheese. These foods should be eaten in moderate amounts.
○ Instruct the patient to fast after midnight the night before the test.
○ Advise the patient that he may experience slight discomfort from the tourniquet and the needle puncture.

Implementation

○ Perform a venipuncture and collect the blood sample in a 10-ml clot-activator tube.

○ Instruct the patient to empty his bladder and discard the urine; record this as "time 0."
○ Collect the patient's urine over a 24-hour period with the first sample discarded and the last sample retained; occasionally, a 4-hour collection or a random collection is performed instead.
○ Tell the patient to avoid contaminating the specimen with toilet paper or feces.
○ Handle the blood collection tube gently to prevent hemolysis.
○ Keep the urine specimen container refrigerated or on ice during the collection period.
○ Label the specimen and send it to the laboratory as soon as the collection period has ended.

Patient care

○ Allow the patient to eat and encourage fluid intake to maintain adequate urine flow after the venipuncture.
○ Apply direct pressure to the venipuncture site until bleeding stops.
○ Inform the patient that he may resume his usual diet and medications.

Complications

○ Hematoma at the venipuncture site

Interpretation

Normal results

○ Renal tubules reabsorb 80% or more of phosphate.

Abnormal results

○ Renal tubules that reabsorb < 74% of phosphate strongly suggest primary hyperparathyroidism.
○ Hypercalcemia is the most common symptom of primary hyperparathyroidism, but a patient with hypercalcemia may require additional testing to verify that primary hyperparathyroidism is the cause.

Interfering factors

○ Uremia, renal tubular disease, osteomalacia, myeloma, and sarcoidosis (possible increase)
○ Furosemide and gentamicin (possible increase)
○ Renal calculi in the patient without a parathyroid tumor, amphotericin B, and thiazide diuretics (possible decrease)
○ Contamination of the specimen with toilet tissue or feces
○ Hemolysis from rough handling of the sample
○ Failure to keep the specimen on ice or to send it to the laboratory immediately after the collection is complete
○ Failure to follow dietary restrictions

Tumor markers

Overview

○ Detects tumor markers (CA 15-3 [27, 29]; CA 19-9; CA-125; and CA-50), substances produced and secreted by tumor cells that help determine tumor activity, found in serum of patients with cancer.
○ Specific test depends on the type of cancer the patient has.
○ The CA 15-3 antigen (breast-cystic fluid protein [BCFP]) may be used with carcinoembryonic antigen and is helpful particularly in the breast cancer patient (CA 27, metastatic breast cancer, breast-cystic fluid protein 29, BCFP).
○ CA 19-9 carbohydrate antigen may be performed in the patient with pancreas, hepatobiliary, or lung cancer.
○ The CA-125 glycoprotein antigen and serum carbohydrate antigen are usually used in patients with ovarian cancer.
○ The CA-50 may be performed in the patient with GI or pancreatic cancer.
○ A combination of markers may be used because of low sensitivity and specificity of the markers.
○ Few tumor markers meet Food and Drug Administration approval because of their controversial role in cancer diagnosis and treatment.

Purpose

○ To assist tumor staging and identify possible metastasis
○ To monitor and detect disease recurrence
○ To assess the patient's response to therapy

Procedure

Preparation

○ Explain the purpose of the particular test and its helpfulness in the patient's disorder, as appropriate.
○ Tell the patient that the test requires a blood sample. Explain who will perform the venipuncture and when.
○ Explain that it may be necessary for the patient to fast.
○ Identify factors that may interfere with test results and note them on the appropriate laboratory requests.
○ Follow specific directions from the laboratory or cancer center for the particular test.
○ Explain to the patient that he may experience slight discomfort from the tourniquet and the needle puncture.

Implementation

○ Obtain a 10-ml venous sample in the tube specified by the laboratory or cancer center and transport the sample as directed.

Patient care

○ Apply direct pressure to the venipuncture site until bleeding stops.

Complications

○ Hematoma at the venipuncture site

Interpretation

Normal results

○ CA 15-3 (27, 29): < 30 units/ml
○ CA 19-9: < 70 units/ml
○ CA-125: < 34 units/ml
○ CA-50: < 17 units/ml

Abnormal results

○ CA 15-3 (27, 29) is greatly increased in metastatic breast cancer; it's also increased in pancreas, lung, colorectal, ovarian, and liver cancers. It decreases with therapy; an increase after therapy suggests progressive disease.
○ CA 19-9 is increased in pancreas, hepatobiliary, and lung cancers. It may be mildly increased in gastric and colorectal cancers.
○ CA-125 is increased in epithelial ovary, fallopian tube, endometrium, endocervix, pancreas, and liver cancers. It's less increased in colon, breast, lung, and GI cancers.
○ CA-50 is increased in GI and pancreatic cancers.

Interfering factors

○ CA 15-3 (27, 29) increased in benign breast or ovarian disease
○ CA 19-9 increased in pancreatitis, cholecystitis, cirrhosis, gallstones, and cystic fibrosis (minimal elevations)
○ CA-125 increased in pregnancy, endometriosis, pelvic inflammatory disease, menstruation, acute and chronic hepatitis, ascites, peritonitis, pancreatitis, GI disease, Meig's syndrome, pleural effusion, and pulmonary disease

Tuning fork test

Overview

- Screens for hearing loss and obtains preliminary information about the type of hearing loss.
- Use low frequency for most reliable test results.
- Weber's test determines whether a patient lateralizes the tone of the tuning fork to one ear.
- The Rinne test compares air and bone conduction in both ears.
- Schwabach's test compares the patient's bone conduction response with that of the examiner, who's assumed to have normal hearing.
- Results of Weber's test may be misleading, and the Rinne test commonly doesn't detect a mild conductive hearing loss (10 to 35 dB) because testing relies on subjective factors, such as the examiner's ability to strike the fork with equal force each time and the patient's ability to report audible tones correctly. Abnormal results require confirmation by pure tone audiometry.

Purpose

- To screen for or confirm hearing loss
- To help distinguish conductive from sensorineural hearing loss

Procedure

Preparation

- Explain to the patient that concentration and prompt responses are essential for accurate testing.
- Have him use hand signals to indicate whether a tone is louder in his right ear or left ear and to indicate when he stops hearing the tone.

Implementation

- Using a low-frequency tuning fork (256 or 512 Hz), practice achieving a consistent tone by gently striking a prong against your elbow or the heel of your hand, by stroking the prongs upward, or by pinching them together.
- When performing each test, be careful to strike the tuning fork with equal force. Hold the fork at its base to allow the prongs to vibrate freely. Record the name of the test, the result, and the vibrating frequency of the tuning fork.

Weber's test
- Vibrate the fork, and place its base on the midline of the patient's skull at the forehead.
- Ask the patient whether the tone is louder in his left ear or his right ear or is equally loud in both.
- Record the results as "Weber left," "Weber right," or "Weber midline," according to his response.

Rinne test
- Test bone conduction by holding the tuning fork between your thumb and index finger and placing the base of the vibrating fork against the patient's mastoid process.
- Test air conduction by moving the vibrating prongs next to (but not touching) the external ear. Ask the patient which location has the louder or longer sound. Repeat the procedure for the other ear.
- Record the results as "Rinne-positive," if the air-conducted sound is heard louder or longer, or "Rinne-negative," if the bone-conducted sound is heard louder or longer.

Schwabach's test
- Holding the tuning fork between your thumb and index finger, place the base of the vibrating tuning fork against the patient's left mastoid process, and ask whether he hears the tone. If he does, immediately place the tuning fork on your left mastoid process and listen for the tone.
- Alternate the tuning fork between the patient's left mastoid process and your own until one of you stops hearing the sound.
- Record the length of time the patient continues to hear it.
- Repeat the procedure on the right mastoid process.

Patient care

- Refer the patient for further audiologic testing if the tuning fork test suggests hearing loss.

Complications

None known

Interpretation

Normal results

- In Weber's test, the patient hears the same tone equally loudly in both ears (Weber midline result).
- In the Rinne test, the patient hears the air-conducted tone louder or longer than the bone-conducted tone (Rinne-positive result).
- In Schwabach's test, the patient hears the tone for the same duration as the examiner.

Abnormal results

- In Weber's test, lateralization of the tone to one ear suggests a conductive loss on that side or a sensorineural loss on the other side.
- Lateralization results if the tone is louder in one ear (Stenger effect) or reaches one ear sooner (phase effect).
- If one ear has a sensorineural loss, the Stenger effect causes lateralization to the unaffected ear; if one ear has a conductive loss, either the Stenger or the phase effect produces lateralization to that ear.
- In the Rinne test, hearing the bone-conducted tone louder or longer than the air-conducted tone indicates a conductive loss.
- In unilateral hearing loss, the tone may be heard louder when conducted by bone, but in the opposite ear; this is a false-negative Rinne test result.

○ A sensorineural loss is indicated when the sound is heard louder by air conduction.

○ In Schwabach's test, hearing the tone longer than the examiner hears it suggests a conductive loss; conversely, a shorter duration indicates a sensorineural loss.

○ A conductive loss attenuates (decreases the energy of) air-conducted sound in a room with ambient noise, enabling the patient with this type of loss to hear bone-conducted sound longer than the examiner can hear it.

Interfering factors

○ Failure to strike the tuning fork with equal force or to hold it correctly during the procedure

○ Striking the tuning fork on a hard surface rather than on the elbow or knee

○ Failure to use the 512-Hz frequency tuning fork or the more sensitive 256-Hz tuning fork

○ Inaccurate patient response because of poor understanding of his task

○ Undetected hearing loss in the examiner

Two-hour postprandial plasma glucose

Overview

- Screens for diabetes mellitus
- Performed when the patient shows symptoms of diabetes (polydipsia and polyuria) or when results of the fasting plasma glucose test suggest diabetes
- Also called the 2-*hour postprandial blood sugar test*

Purpose

- To aid in the diagnosis of diabetes mellitus
- To monitor drug or diet therapy in the patient with diabetes mellitus

Procedure

Preparation

- Explain to the patient that the 2-hour postprandial plasma glucose test evaluates glucose metabolism and detects diabetes.
- Tell the patient that the test requires a blood sample. Explain who will perform the venipuncture and when.
- Notify the laboratory and physician of drugs the patient is taking that may affect test results; it may be necessary to restrict them.
- Tell the patient to eat a balanced meal or one containing 100 g of carbohydrates before the test and then fast for 2 hours. Instruct him to avoid smoking and exercising strenuously after the meal.
- Explain to the patient that he may experience slight discomfort from the tourniquet and the needle puncture.

Implementation

- Perform a venipuncture and collect the sample in a 5-ml clot-activator tube.
- Send the sample to the laboratory immediately or refrigerate it.
- Specify on the laboratory request when the patient last ate, the time of the sample collection, and when the last pretest dose of insulin or oral antidiabetic drug was given.

Patient care

- Apply direct pressure to the venipuncture site until bleeding stops.
- Instruct the patient that he may resume his usual diet, medications, and activity stopped before the test.

Complications

- Hematoma at the venipuncture site

Two-hour postprandial plasma glucose levels by age

The greatest difference in normal and diabetic insulin responses, and thus in plasma glucose concentration, occurs about 2 hours after a glucose challenge. Test values can fluctuate according to the patient's age. After age 50, for example, normal levels rise markedly and steadily, sometimes reaching 160 mg/dl (SI, 8.82 mmol/L) or higher. In a younger patient, a glucose concentration of more than 145 mg/dl (SI > 8 mmol/L) suggests incipient diabetes and requires further evaluation.

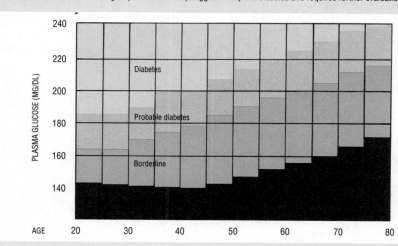

Interpretation

Normal results

○ In patients who don't have diabetes, postprandial glucose values are < 145 mg/dl (SI, < 8 mmol/L) by the glucose oxidase or hexokinase method.

○ Levels are slightly higher in patients older than age 50. (See *Two-hour postprandial plasma glucose levels by age*.)

Abnormal results

○ Two-hour postprandial blood glucose values of 200 mg/dl (SI, 11.1 mmol/L) or above indicate diabetes mellitus.

○ High glucose levels (hyperglycemia) occur with pancreatitis, Cushing's syndrome, acromegaly, pheochromocytoma, hyperlipoproteinemia (especially type III, IV, or V), chronic hepatic disease, nephrotic syndrome, brain tumor, sepsis, gastrectomy with dumping syndrome, eclampsia, anoxia, and seizure disorders.

○ Low glucose levels (hypoglycemia) occur in hyperinsulinism, insulinoma, von Gierke's disease, functional and reactive hypoglycemia, myxedema, adrenal insufficiency, congenital adrenal hyperplasia, hypopituitarism, malabsorption syndrome, and hepatic insufficiency.

Interfering factors

○ Recent illness, infection, or pregnancy (possible increase)

○ Acetaminophen, if using the glucose oxidase or hexokinase method (possible false-positive)

○ Chlorthalidone, thiazide diuretics, furosemide, triamterene, hormonal contraceptives, benzodiazepines, phenytoin, phenothiazines, lithium, epinephrine, arginine, phenolphthalein, dextrothyroxine, diazoxide, large doses of nicotinic acid, corticosteroids, and recent I.V. glucose infusions (increase)

○ Ethacrynic acid (possible increase); large doses in patients with uremia (possible decrease)

○ Beta-adrenergic blockers, amphetamines, ethanol, clofibrate, insulin, oral antidiabetic drugs, and monoamine oxidase inhibitors (possible decrease)

○ Strenuous exercise or stress (possible decrease)

○ Glycolysis caused by failure to refrigerate the sample or to send it to the laboratory immediately (possible decrease)

Ultrasonography

Overview

- Transmits high-frequency sound waves into the targeted tissue; resultant echoes are converted to electrical impulses, amplified by a transducer, and displayed on a monitor.
- Sound waves travel at varying speeds, depending on the density of tissue they're passing through; images on the display screen reflect this difference.

Purpose

- To measure organ size and evaluate structure
- To detect foreign bodies and differentiate between a cyst and solid tumor
- To monitor tissue response to radiation or chemotherapy

Procedure

Preparation

- Make sure the patient has signed an appropriate consent form.
- Note and report all allergies.
- Explain that the procedure is painless and safe and that no radiation exposure is involved.
- Stress the importance of remaining still during scanning to prevent a distorted image.

Implementation

- Assist the patient into a supine position; use pillows to support the area to be examined.
- Coat the target area with a water-soluble jelly. The transducer is used to scan the area, projecting the images on the oscilloscope screen. The image on the screen is photographed for subsequent examination.
- It may be necessary to assist the patient into right or left lateral positions for subsequent views.

Patient care

- After the procedure, remove the contact jelly from the patient's skin.

Complications

None known

Interpretation

Normal results

- See "Normal results" for a specific type of ultrasonography (abdominal aorta, gallbladder and biliary system, kidney and perirenal, liver, pancreas, pelvis, spleen, and thyroid).

Abnormal results

- See "Abnormal results" for a specific type of ultrasonography (abdominal aorta, gallbladder and biliary system, kidney and perirenal, liver, pancreas, pelvis, spleen, and thyroid).

Interfering factors

- Refer to "Interfering factors" for a specific type of ultrasonography (abdominal aorta, gallbladder and biliary system, kidney and perirenal, liver, pancreas, pelvis, spleen, and thyroid).

Ultrasonography, abdominal aorta

Overview

○ Confirms a suspected aortic aneurysm.
○ Method of choice in measuring diameter of aortic aneurysm.
○ A transducer directs a focused beam of high-frequency sound waves into the abdomen over a wide area from the xiphoid process to the umbilical region, creating echoes that vary with changes in tissue density.
○ The sound waves are transmitted as electrical impulses and displayed on a monitor to show the size and course of the abdominal aorta and other major vessels.
○ Performed every 6 months to monitor changes in a patient's status.

Purpose

○ To detect and measure a suspected abdominal aortic aneurysm
○ To monitor expansion of a known abdominal aortic aneurysm

Procedure

Preparation

○ Make sure the patient has signed an appropriate consent form.
○ Note and report all allergies.
○ Tell the patient that he must fast for 12 hours before the test to minimize bowel gas and motility.
○ Give the patient simethicone to reduce bowel gas if necessary.
○ Inform the patient that he will feel slight pressure in the area being tested.
○ Instruct the patient to remain still during scanning and to hold his breath when requested.
○ Explain that the test takes 30 to 45 minutes.

Implementation

○ Assist the patient into a supine position.
○ Apply acoustic coupling gel or mineral oil to the abdomen.
○ Longitudinal scans are then made at 0.5- to 1-cm intervals to the left and right of midline until the entire abdominal aorta is outlined.
○ Transverse scans are made at 1- to 2-cm intervals from the xiphoid process to the bifurcation at the common iliac arteries.
○ It may be necessary to place the patient in right and left lateral positions.
○ Appropriate views are photographed or videotaped.

Patient care

○ Remove residual gel from the patient's skin.
○ Have the patient resume his usual diet and medications.

▽ ALERT *Remember that sudden onset of constant abdominal or back pain accompanies rapid expansion of the aneurysm; sudden, excruciating pain with weakness, sweating, tachycardia, and hypotension signals rupture.*

Complications

None known

Interpretation

Normal results

○ The abdominal aorta tapers from about ½″ to 1″ (1 to 2.5 cm) in diameter along its length from the diaphragm to the bifurcation.
○ The abdominal aorta descends through the retroperitoneal space, anterior to the vertebral column and slightly left of the midline.
○ Four of the abdominal aorta's major branches are usually well visualized: the celiac trunk, the renal arteries, the superior mesenteric artery, and the common iliac arteries.

Abnormal results

○ Luminal diameter of the abdominal aorta > 4 cm indicates an aneurysm.
○ Luminal diameter of the abdominal aorta > 7 cm indicates an aneurysm with a high risk of rupture.

Interfering factors

○ Bowel gas and motility, excessive body movement, surgical wounds, and severe dyspnea
○ Residual barium from GI contrast studies within the past 24 hours
○ Mesenteric fat in the obese patient

Ultrasonography, gallbladder and biliary system

Overview

○ Reveals the size, shape, structure, and position of the gallbladder and biliary system.
○ Procedure of choice for evaluating jaundice and emergency diagnosing of patients with signs of acute cholecystitis.
○ A transducer directs a focused beam of high-frequency sound waves into the right upper quadrant of the abdomen, creating echoes that vary with changes in tissue density.
○ The sound waves are transmitted as electrical impulses and displayed on a monitor.

Purpose

○ To confirm the diagnosis of cholelithiasis
○ To diagnose acute cholecystitis
○ To distinguish between obstructive and nonobstructive jaundice

Procedure

Preparation

○ Make sure the patient or responsible party has signed a consent form.
○ Note and report all allergies.
○ Provide a fat-free meal in the evening before the study.
○ Tell the patient that he must fast for 8 to 12 hours before the procedure, if possible.
○ Instruct the patient to remain as still as possible during the procedure and to hold his breath when requested.

Implementation

○ Assist the patient into a supine position.
○ A water-soluble lubricant is applied to the face of the transducer, and transverse scans of the gallbladder are taken at ½" (1-cm) intervals, starting at the level of the xiphoid and moving laterally to the right subcostal area.
○ Longitudinal oblique scans are taken at ⅛" (5-mm) intervals parallel to the long axis of the gallbladder marked on the patient's skin, beginning medial to the gallbladder and continuing through to its lateral border.
○ During each scan the patient is asked to exhale deeply and hold his breath.
○ If the gallbladder is positioned deeply under the right costal margin, a scan may be taken through the intercostal spaces, while the patient inhales deeply and holds his breath.

○ Assist the patient into a left lateral decubitus position; he's then scanned beneath the right costal margin. This allows for displacing stones lodged in the cystic duct region, which escape detection in the supine position.
○ Oscilloscopic views are obtained and photographed for later study.

Patient care

○ Remove the lubricating jelly from the patient's skin.
○ Have the patient resume his normal diet.

Complications

None known

Interpretation

Normal results

○ The gallbladder is sonolucent; it's circular on transverse scans and pear-shaped on longitudinal scans.
○ Although the gallbladder's size varies, its outer walls normally appear sharp and smooth.
○ Intrahepatic radicles seldom appear.
○ The cystic duct may be indistinct.
○ The cystic duct is serpentine.
○ The common bile duct has a linear appearance but is sometimes obscured by overlying bowel gas.

Abnormal results

○ Mobile, echogenic areas, usually linked to an acoustic shadow, suggest gallstones within the gallbladder lumen or the biliary system.
○ When the gallbladder is shrunken or filled with gallstones, inadequate bile may make gallstone detection difficult, and the gallbladder itself may not be visible.
○ An acoustic shadow in the cystic and common bile ducts suggests possible choledocholithiasis.
○ Fixed echogenic areas within the gallbladder lumen suggest possible polyps or tumors; polyps usually appear as sharply defined, echogenic areas; carcinoma appears as a poorly defined mass commonly linked to a thickened gallbladder wall.
○ A fine layer of echoes that slowly gravitates to the dependent portion of the gallbladder as the patient changes position, suggests biliary sludge within the gallbladder lumen.
○ An enlarged gallbladder with thickened, double-rimmed walls, usually accompanied by gallstones within the lumen, suggests acute cholecystitis.
○ A contracted gallbladder with thickened walls suggests chronic cholecystitis.
○ A dilated biliary system and, usually, a dilated gallbladder suggest obstructive jaundice.

Interfering factors

○ Failure to observe pretest dietary restrictions
○ Overlying bowel gas or retained barium from previous testing
○ Deficiency of body fluids in a dehydrated patient

Ultrasonography, kidney and perirenal

Overview

○ A transducer directs a focused beam of high-frequency sound waves through the kidneys and perirenal structures, creating echoes that vary with changes in tissue density.
○ The echoes are converted into electrical impulses and displayed on a screen as images.
○ Especially valuable when excretory urography is ruled out — for example, because of hypersensitivity to the contrast medium or the need for serial examinations.
○ Useful in patients with renal failure because test doesn't require adequate renal function (unlike excretory urography).
○ Evaluation of urologic disorders may also include ultrasonography of the ureter, bladder, and gonads.

Purpose

○ To determine the size, shape, and position of the kidneys, their internal structures, and perirenal tissues
○ To evaluate and localize urinary obstruction and abnormal accumulation of fluid
○ To assess and diagnose complications after kidney transplantation
○ To detect renal or perirenal masses
○ To differentiate between renal cysts and solid masses
○ To verify placement of a nephrostomy tube

Procedure

Preparation

○ Explain to the patient that this test detects abnormalities in the kidneys.
○ Tell the patient that he need not restrict food and fluids before the test.
○ Explain that the test is safe and painless and takes about 30 minutes.

Implementation

○ Assist the patient into a prone position and expose the area to be scanned.
○ Apply ultrasound jelly to the area before the scanning begins.
○ The longitudinal axis of the kidneys is located using measurements from excretory urography or by performing transverse scans through the upper and lower renal poles.
○ These points are marked on the skin and connected with straight lines.
○ Sectional images ½″ to 1″ (1 to 2.5 cm apart) can then be obtained by moving the transducer longitudinally and transversely or at any other angle required.

○ During the test the patient may be asked to breathe deeply to reveal upper portions of the kidney.

Patient care

○ Remove the conduction jelly from the patient's skin.
○ If bladder abnormalities are found, prepare the patient for further testing.
○ If rejection of a transplanted kidney is suspected or diagnosed, monitor intake and output, blood pressure, blood urea nitrogen and creatinine levels, and vital signs.
○ If an adrenal tumor is detected, monitor for adrenal dysfunction (hypotension, decreased urine output, and electrolyte imbalances).
○ If a nephrostomy tube has been placed, monitor the amount and characteristics of drainage and tube patency.

Complications

None known

Interpretation

Normal results

○ The kidneys are between the superior iliac crests and the diaphragm.
○ The renal capsules are outlined sharply; the cortex produces more echoes than the medulla.
○ In the center of each kidney, the renal collecting systems appear as irregular areas of higher density than surrounding tissue.

Abnormal results

○ Fluid-filled, circular structures that don't reflect sound waves suggest cysts.
○ Multiple echoes appearing as irregular shapes suggest tumors.
○ Fluid-filled structures with slightly irregular boundaries that don't reflect sound waves well suggest abscesses.
○ A renal capsule that appears irregular and a kidney that appears smaller than normal and is associated with an increased number of echoes arising from the parenchyma because of fibrosis may suggest acute pyelonephritis and glomerulonephritis.
○ A large, echo-free, central mass that compresses the renal cortex may indicate hydronephrosis.
○ After kidney transplantation, compensatory hypertrophy of the transplanted kidney is normal, but an acute increase in size indicates rejection of the transplant.
○ Abnormal accumulations of fluid within or around the kidneys may suggest an obstruction.
○ Increased urine volume or residual urine postvoiding may indicate bladder dysfunction.

Interfering factors

None known

Ultrasonography, liver

Overview

- Transmits high-frequency sound waves into the right upper quadrant of the abdomen; the resultant echoes are converted to electrical energy, amplified by a transducer, and displayed on a monitor.
- Depicts various tissue densities by different shades of gray.
- Shows intrahepatic structures as well as organ size, shape, and position.
- Performed in patients with jaundice of unknown etiology, unexplained hepatomegaly and abnormal biochemical test results, suspected metastatic tumors and elevated serum alkaline phosphatase levels, and recent abdominal trauma.
- When used to complement liver-spleen scanning, ultrasonography can define cold spots (focal defects that fail to pick up the radionuclide) as tumors, abscesses, or cysts; it also provides better views of the periportal and perihepatic spaces than does liver-spleen scanning.

Purpose

- To distinguish between obstructive and nonobstructive jaundice
- To screen for hepatocellular disease
- To detect hepatic metastases and hematoma
- To define cold spots as tumors, abscesses, or cysts

Procedure

Preparation

- Make sure the patient has signed a consent form.
- Note and report all allergies.
- Tell the patient to fast for 8 to 12 hours before the test.
- Warn the patient that he may feel mild pressure as the transducer presses against the skin.
- Stress the need for the patient to remain as still as possible during the procedure and to hold his breath when requested.

Implementation

- Assist the patient into a supine position.
- A water-soluble lubricant is applied to the face of the transducer, and transverse scans are taken at ½" (1-cm) intervals, using a single-sweep technique between the costal margins.
- Sector scans are taken through the intercostal spaces to view the remainder of the right lobe.
- Scans are taken longitudinally, from the right border of the liver to the left.
- Oblique cephalad-angled scans may be taken beneath the right costal margin for better demonstration of the right lateral dome.
- Scans are then taken parallel to the hepatic portal, at a 45-degree angle toward the superior right lateral dome, to examine the peripheral anatomy, portal venous system, common bile duct, and biliary tree.
- During each scan, the patient should hold his breath briefly in deep inspiration.
- Clear images are photographed for later study.

Patient care

- Remove lubricating jelly from the patient's skin.
- Have the patient resume his usual diet.

Complications

None known

Interpretation

Normal results

- The liver demonstrates a homogeneous, low-level echo pattern, interrupted only by the different echo patterns of its vascular channels.
- Intrahepatic biliary radicles and hepatic arteries aren't apparent, but portal and hepatic veins, the aorta, and the inferior vena cava appear.
- Hepatic veins appear completely sonolucent; portal veins have margins that are highly echogenic.

Abnormal results

- Dilated intrahepatic biliary radicles and extrahepatic ducts suggest obstructive jaundice.
- Variable liver size, dilated, tortuous portal branches associated with portal hypertension, and an irregular echo pattern with increased echo amplitude, suggest possible cirrhosis.
- Hepatomegaly and a regular echo pattern that, although greater in echo amplitude than that of normal parenchyma, don't alter attenuation suggest possible fatty infiltration of the liver.
- Hypoechoic or echogenic and either poorly defined or well-defined areas suggest possible metastasis in the liver.
- Sonolucent masses with ill-defined, slightly thickened borders and an accentuated posterior wall transmission suggest possible abscesses.
- The presence of fluid lacking internal echoes with a more regular border suggests possible ascitic fluid.
- Spherical, sonolucent areas with well-defined borders and an accentuated posterior wall transmission suggest possible cysts.
- Poorly defined, relatively sonolucent masses, with possible scattered internal echoes caused by clotting, suggest possible intrahepatic hematomas.
- A focal, sonolucent mass on the periphery of the liver or a diffuse, sonolucent area surrounding part of the liver suggests possible subcapsular hematoma.

Interfering factors

- Overlying ribs and gas or residual barium in the stomach or colon
- Deficiency of body fluids in a dehydrated patient.

Ultrasonography, pancreas

Overview

○ Transmits high-frequency sound waves into the epigastric region; resultant echoes are converted to electrical impulses, amplified by a transducer, and displayed on a monitor.
○ The display pattern varies with tissue density and represents the size, shape, and position of the pancreas and surrounding viscera.
○ Can't provide a sensitive measure of pancreatic function but is useful in detecting anatomic abnormalities, such as pancreatic carcinoma and pseudocysts, and in guiding the insertion of biopsy needles.
○ Has largely replaced hypotonic duodenography, endoscopic retrograde cholangiopancreatography, radioisotope studies, and arteriography.

Purpose

○ To aid in the diagnosis of pancreatitis, pseudocysts, and pancreatic carcinoma

Procedure

Preparation

○ Make sure the patient has signed an appropriate consent form.
○ Note and report all allergies.
○ Tell the patient to fast for 8 to 12 hours before the test to reduce bowel gas, which hinders transmission of ultrasound.
○ Instruct the patient to abstain from smoking before the test to eliminate the risk of swallowing air while inhaling, which interferes with test results.
○ Provide reassurance that this study isn't harmful or painful, although the patient may experience mild pressure.
○ Instruct the patient to inhale deeply during scanning, when requested.
○ Stress the need for the patient to remain as still as possible during imaging.

Implementation

○ Assist the patient into a supine position.
○ Apply a water-soluble lubricant or mineral oil to the abdomen. With the patient at full inspiration, transverse scans are taken at ½" (1-cm) intervals, starting from the xiphoid and moving caudally.
○ Other techniques include the longitudinal scan to view the head, body, and tail of the pancreas in sequence; the right anterior oblique view for the head and body of the pancreas; the oblique sagittal view for the portal vein; and the sagittal view for the vena cava.

○ Good oscilloscopic views are photographed for later study.

Patient care

○ Remove the lubricating jelly from the patient's skin.
○ Have the patient resume his usual diet.

Complications

None known

Interpretation

Normal results

○ The pancreas demonstrates a coarse, uniform echo pattern (reflecting tissue density) and is usually more echogenic than the adjacent liver.

Abnormal results

○ Alterations in the size, contour, and parenchymal texture of the pancreas suggest possible pancreatic disease.
○ An enlarged pancreas with decreased echogenicity and distinct borders suggests pancreatitis.
○ A well-defined mass with an essentially echo-free interior suggests a pseudocyst.
○ An ill-defined mass with scattered internal echoes, or a mass in the head of the pancreas (obstructing the common bile duct) and a large noncontracting gallbladder suggest pancreatic carcinoma.

Interfering factors

○ Failure of patient to fast before test
○ Bowel gas
○ Dehydration
○ Barium from previous diagnostic tests
○ Obesity

Ultrasonography, pelvis

Overview

- Transmits high-frequency sound waves into the interior pelvic region; resultant echoes are converted to electrical impulses, amplified by a transducer, and displayed on a monitor.
- A-mode technique records only distances between interfaces.
- B-mode (brightness modulation) technique creates a two-dimensional or cross-sectional image.
- Gray-scale technique represents organ texture in shades of gray on a screen.
- Real-time imaging creates instant images of the tissues in motion, similar to fluoroscopic examination.
- Selected views may be photographed for later examination and kept as a permanent record of the test.
- Often used to evaluate symptoms that suggest pelvic disease, to confirm a tentative diagnosis, and to determine fetal growth during pregnancy.
- Often needed in pregnant women with a history or signs of fetal anomalies or multiple pregnancies, a history of bleeding, inconsistency of fetal size and conception date, or indications for amniocentesis.

Purpose

- To detect foreign bodies and distinguish between cysts and solid masses (tumors)
- To measure organ size
- To evaluate fetal viability, position, gestational age, and growth rate
- To detect multiple pregnancy
- To confirm fetal abnormalities (such as molar pregnancy, and abnormalities of the arms and legs, spine, heart, head, kidneys, and abdomen)
- To confirm maternal abnormalities (such as posterior placenta and placenta previa)
- To guide amniocentesis by determining placental location and fetal position

Procedure

Preparation

- Make sure the patient has signed an appropriate consent form.
- Note and report all allergies.
- Instruct the patient to drink fluids and avoid urination before the test because pelvic ultrasonography requires a full bladder as a landmark to define pelvic organs.
- Explain that the test won't harm the fetus.

Implementation

- With the patient in a supine position, coat the lower abdomen with mineral oil or water-soluble jelly to increase sound wave conduction.

- The transducer crystal is guided over the area, images are observed on the oscilloscope screen, and good images are photographed.

Patient care

- Allow the patient to empty her bladder immediately after the test.
- Remove ultrasound gel from the patient's skin.

Complications

None known

Interpretation

Normal results

- The uterus is normal in size and shape.
- The ovaries are normal in size, shape, and sonographic density.
- The body of the uterus lies on the superior surface of the bladder; the uterine tubes are attached laterally.
- The ovaries are located on the lateral pelvic walls, with the external iliac vessels above and the ureters posteroinferior, and are covered by the fimbria of the uterine tubes medially.
- No other masses are visible.
- If the patient is pregnant, the gestational sac and fetus are of normal size for date; the placenta is located in the fundus of the uterus.

Abnormal results

- Homogeneous densities suggest both cysts and solid masses; however, solid masses (such as fibroids) appear more dense on ultrasonography.
- Inappropriate fetal size suggests possible miscalculation of conception or delivery date.
- Abnormal echo patterns suggest possible foreign bodies (such as an intrauterine device), multiple pregnancy, placenta previa or abruptio placentae, or fetal abnormalities (such as molar pregnancy or abnormalities of the arms and legs, spine, heart, head, kidneys, and abdomen).
- Fetal abnormalities suggest possible malpresentation (such as breech or shoulder presentation) and cephalopelvic disproportion.

Interfering factors

- When the bladder is empty, the uterus is more difficult to see because it's farther down inside the pelvis.
- Bones disrupt ultrasound signals.
- Failure to keep the bladder full will interfere with the study results, making interpretation difficult.

Ultrasonography, spleen

Overview

○ Transmits high-frequency sound waves into the left upper quadrant of the abdomen, creating echoes that vary with changes in tissue density
○ Echoes converted to electrical energy, amplified by transducer, and displayed on a monitor
○ Indicated for patients with a left upper quadrant mass of unknown origin, with known splenomegaly to evaluate changes in the spleen's size, with left upper quadrant pain and local tenderness, and with recent abdominal trauma
○ Can show splenomegaly, but usually doesn't identify the cause
○ As a supplementary diagnostic procedure after liver-spleen scanning, can clarify the nature of cold spots or detect focal defects not infiltrated by tracer radioisotopes

Purpose

○ To demonstrate splenomegaly
○ To monitor progression of primary and secondary splenic disease
○ To evaluate the effectiveness of therapy
○ To evaluate the spleen after abdominal trauma
○ To detect splenic cysts and subphrenic abscess

Procedure

Preparation

○ Make sure the patient has signed an appropriate consent form.
○ Note and report all allergies.
○ Tell the patient to fast for 8 to 12 hours before the procedure.
○ Inform the patient that he will feel only mild pressure during the procedure.
○ Instruct the patient to remain as still as possible during the procedure and to hold his breath when requested.

Implementation

○ Because the procedure for ultrasonography varies, depending on the size of the spleen or the patient's body habitus, it's usually necessary to reposition the patient several times.
○ A water-soluble lubricant is applied to the face of the transducer, and transverse scans of the spleen are taken at ½″ to 1″ (1- to 2.5-cm) intervals, beginning at the level of the diaphragm and moving posteriorly while the transducer is angled anteromedially.
○ After the patient is placed in right lateral decubitus position, additional transverse scans are taken through the intercostal spaces using a sectoring motion.

○ For longitudinal scans, the patient remains in the right lateral decubitus position, and scans are taken from the axilla toward the iliac crest.
○ To prevent rib artifacts, oblique scans are taken by passing the transducer face along the intercostal spaces; this scan provides the best view of the splenic parenchyma.
○ During each scan, the patient may be asked to hold his breath briefly at varying stages of inspiration.

Patient care

○ Remove the lubricating jelly from the patient's skin.
○ Have the patient resume his usual diet.

Complications

None known

Interpretation

Normal results

○ The splenic parenchyma demonstrates a homogeneous, low-level echo pattern.
○ The superior and lateral splenic borders are clearly defined, each having a convex margin.
○ The undersurface and medial borders, in contrast, show indentations from surrounding organs.
○ The hilar region, where the vascular pedicle enters the spleen, commonly produces an area of highly reflected echoes.
○ The medial surface is usually concave, a characteristic particularly useful when differentiating between left upper quadrant masses and an enlarged spleen.
○ Even when splenomegaly is present, the spleen usually remains concave medially, unless a space-occupying lesion distorts this contour.

Abnormal results

○ Increased echogenicity and enlarged vascular channels, especially in the hilar region, suggest splenomegaly.
○ Splenomegaly and an irregular, sonolucent area (the presence of free intraperitoneal fluid) suggest splenic rupture.
○ Splenomegaly as well as the presence of a double contour (blood accumulation between the splenic parenchyma and the intact splenic capsule), altered splenic position, and a relatively sonolucent area on the periphery of the spleen suggest subcapsular hematoma.
○ A sonolucent area beneath the diaphragm suggests possible subphrenic abscess.
○ Spherical, sonolucent areas with well-defined, regular margins with acoustic enhancement behind them suggest cysts.

Interfering factors

○ Overlying ribs, failure to fast, bowel gas, dehydration, and barium from previous diagnostic tests
○ Patients with a splenic injury may be unable to tolerate the procedure because of pain

Ultrasonography, thyroid

Overview

- Emits pulses from a piezoelectric crystal in a transducer, directed at the thyroid gland, and reflected back to the transducer; these pulses are converted electronically to produce structural visualization on an oscilloscope screen.
- Differentiates between a cyst and a tumor larger than ½" (1 cm) with about 85% accuracy when the mass is located by palpation or by thyroid imaging
- Especially useful in evaluating thyroid nodules during pregnancy because it doesn't expose the fetus to radioactive iodine used in other diagnostic procedures.
- Can also be performed on parathyroid glands

Purpose

- To evaluate the thyroid structure
- To differentiate between a cyst and a solid tumor
- To monitor the size of the thyroid gland during suppressive therapy
- To allow accurate measurement of a nodule
- To aid in the performance of thyroid needle biopsy

Procedure

Preparation

- Make sure the patient has signed an appropriate consent form.
- Note and report all allergies.
- Tell the patient that he need not restrict food and fluids before the test.
- Explain that the study is painless and safe.

Implementation

- Assist the patient into a supine position with a pillow under his shoulder blades to hyperextend his neck.
- Coat the patient's neck with water-soluble gel.
- The transducer scans the thyroid, projecting its echographic image on the oscilloscope screen.
- The image on the screen is photographed for subsequent examination.

Patient care

- Thoroughly clean the patient's neck to remove the contact solution.

Complications

None known

Interpretation

Normal results

- A uniform echo pattern throughout the gland

Abnormal results

- Smooth-bordered, echo-free areas with enhanced sound transmission suggest cysts.
- Solid and well-demarcated areas with identical echo patterns suggest adenomas and carcinomas.

Interfering factors

None known

Unstable hemoglobin

Overview

○ Detects presence of unstable hemoglobin (Hb), a rare, congenital defect caused by amino acid substitutions in the structure of Hb, causing Hb to decompose easily
○ Best detected by precipitation tests (using heat stability or isopropanol solubility)
○ Unstable Hb may lead to the formation of small masses called *Heinz bodies,* which may accumulate on red blood cell membranes and may cause mild to severe hemolysis. (See *Signs and symptoms of unstable hemoglobin.*)

Purpose

○ To detect unstable Hb

Procedure

Preparation

○ Explain to the patient that the unstable Hb test detects abnormal Hb in the blood.
○ Tell the patient that the test requires a blood sample. Explain who will perform the venipuncture and when.
○ Notify the laboratory and physician of drugs the patient is taking that may affect test results; it may be necessary to restrict them.
○ Inform the patient that he need not restrict food and fluids.
○ Explain to the patient that he may feel slight discomfort from the tourniquet and the needle puncture.

Implementation

○ Perform a venipuncture and collect the sample in a 3- or 4.5-ml ethylenediaminetetraacetic acid tube.
○ Completely fill the collection tube and invert it gently several times to mix the sample and the anticoagulant thoroughly.
○ To avoid hemolysis, don't shake the tube vigorously.

Patient care

○ Make sure that subdermal bleeding has stopped before removing pressure.
○ Instruct the patient that he may resume medications stopped before the test.
○ If a large hematoma develops at the venipuncture site, monitor pulses distal to the site.

Complications

○ Hematoma at the venipuncture site

Signs and symptoms of unstable hemoglobin

More than 60 varieties of unstable hemoglobin (Hb) exist, each named after the city in which it was discovered. Their effects vary according to their number, the degree of instability, the condition of the spleen, and the oxygen-binding abilities of the unstable Hb.

Patients with unstable Hb typically exhibit pallor, jaundice, splenomegaly, and—with severely unstable Hb—cyanosis, pigmenturia, and hemoglobinuria. Thalassemia commonly causes similar signs and symptoms, but the molecular bases of the two diseases differ greatly.

Interpretation

Normal results

○ Heat stability test result is negative; isopropanol solubility test result is stable.

Abnormal results

○ A positive heat stability test result or unstable solubility test result, especially with hemolysis, strongly suggests the presence of unstable Hb.

Interfering factors

○ Failure to fill the tube completely, to use the proper anticoagulant, or to adequately mix the sample and the anticoagulant
○ Hemoconcentration from prolonged tourniquet constriction
○ Hemolysis from rough handling of the sample
○ Hemolysis from antimalarials, furazolidone (in infants), nitrofurantoin, phenacetin, procarbazine, and sulfonamides (possible false-positive or unstable results)
○ High levels of fetal Hb (possible false-positive isopropanol)
○ Recent blood transfusion

Upper GI and small-bowel series

Overview

- Fluoroscopically examines the esophagus, stomach, and small intestine after ingestion of barium sulfate, a contrast agent.
- As barium passes through the digestive tract, fluoroscopy shows peristalsis and the mucosal contours of organs; spot films record significant findings.
- Indicated for patients with upper GI symptoms (difficulty swallowing, regurgitation, burning or gnawing epigastric pain), signs of small-bowel disease (diarrhea, weight loss), or signs of GI bleeding (hematemesis, melena).
- Detects mucosal abnormalities; many patients need a biopsy afterward to rule out cancer or distinguish specific inflammatory diseases.
- Contraindicated in patients with obstruction or GI tract perforation because barium may intensify the obstruction or seep into the abdominal cavity; also contraindicated in pregnant patients because of the possible teratogenic effects of radiation.
- For suspected GI tract perforation, use Gastrografin (a water-soluble contrast medium) instead of barium.

Purpose

- To detect hiatal hernia, diverticula, and varices
- To aid in the diagnosis of strictures, ulcers, tumors, regional enteritis, and malabsorption syndrome
- To detect motility disorders

Procedure

Preparation

- Make sure the patient has signed an appropriate consent form.
- Note and report all allergies.
- Withhold oral medications after midnight and anticholinergics and opioids for 24 hours because these drugs affect small intestine motility.
- Withhold antacids, histamine-2 receptor antagonists, and proton pump inhibitors if gastric reflux is suspected.
- Instruct the patient to maintain a low-residue diet for 2 or 3 days before the test and to fast and avoid smoking after midnight before the test.
- Instruct the patient to remove all jewelry and metal objects.
- Inform the patient that the barium mixture has a milkshake consistency and chalky taste; although flavored, the patient may find the taste unpleasant. Tell him that he will need 16 to 20 oz (475 to 600 ml) for a complete examination.

- Warn the patient that the abdomen may be compressed to ensure proper coating of the stomach or intestinal walls with barium or to separate overlapping bowel loops.
- Explain that the test may take up to 6 hours to complete, so the patient should bring something to read or otherwise pass the time.

Implementation

- After securing the patient in a supine position on the X-ray table, the table is tilted until the patient is erect, and the heart, lungs, and abdomen are examined fluoroscopically.
- The patient is then instructed to take several swallows of the barium suspension; its passage through the esophagus is observed.
- Occasionally, the patient is given a thick barium suspension, especially when esophageal pathology is strongly suspected.
- During fluoroscopic examination, spot films of the esophagus are taken from lateral angles and from right and left posteroanterior angles.
- When barium enters the stomach, the patient's abdomen is palpated or compressed to ensure adequate coating of the gastric mucosa with barium.
- To perform a double-contrast examination, the patient is instructed to sip the barium through a perforated straw. As he does so, a small amount of air is also introduced into the stomach to allow detailed examination of the gastric rugae, and spot films of significant findings are taken.
- The patient is instructed to ingest the remaining barium suspension, and the filling of the stomach and emptying into the duodenum are observed fluoroscopically.
- Two series of spot films of the stomach and duodenum are taken from posteroanterior, anteroposterior, oblique, and lateral angles, with the patient erect and then in a supine position.
- The passage of barium into the remainder of the small intestine is then observed fluoroscopically, and spot films are taken at 30- to 60-minute intervals until the barium reaches the ileocecal valve and the region around it.
- If abnormalities in the small intestine are detected, the area is palpated and compressed to help clarify the defect, and a spot film is taken.
- When barium enters the cecum, the examination is complete.

Patient care

- Make sure additional X-rays aren't needed before allowing the patient food, fluids, and oral drugs.
- Instruct the patient to drink plenty of fluid (unless contraindicated) to help eliminate the barium.
- Give a cathartic or enema.
- Inform him that his feces will be light-colored for 24 to 72 hours.
- Because barium retention in the intestine may cause obstruction or fecal impaction, notify the physician if the patient doesn't pass barium within 2 to 3 days.

- Tell the patient to notify the physician if he experiences abdominal fullness or pain or a delay in return to brown feces.
- Monitor the patient's vital signs, intake and output, and bowel movements.
- Watch for abdominal distention.
- Monitor bowel sounds.

Complications

- Bowel obstruction
- Fecal impaction

Interpretation

Normal results

- After the patient swallows the barium suspension, it pours over the base of the tongue into the pharynx and is propelled by a peristaltic wave through the entire length of the esophagus in about 2 seconds.
- The bolus evenly fills and distends the lumen of the pharynx and esophagus, and the mucosa appears smooth and regular.
- When the peristaltic wave reaches the base of the esophagus, the cardiac sphincter opens, allowing the bolus to enter the stomach; this is followed by closing of the cardiac sphincter.
- As barium enters the stomach, it outlines the characteristic longitudinal folds called *rugae*, which are best observed using the double-contrast technique.
- When the stomach is completely filled with barium, its outer contour appears smooth and regular without evidence of flattened, rigid areas suggesting intrinsic or extrinsic lesions.
- After barium enters the stomach, it quickly empties into the duodenal bulb through relaxation of the pyloric sphincter.
- Although the mucosa of the duodenal bulb is relatively smooth, circular folds become apparent as barium enters the duodenal loop; these folds deepen and become more numerous in the jejunum.
- Barium temporarily lodges between these folds, producing a speckled pattern on the X-ray film.
- As barium enters the ileum, the circular folds become less prominent and, except for their broadness, resemble those in the duodenum.
- The diameter of the small intestine tapers gradually from the duodenum to the ileum.

Abnormal results

- Structural abnormalities of the esophagus suggest possible strictures, tumors, hiatal hernia, diverticula, varices, and ulcers.
- Dilatation of the esophagus suggests possible benign strictures.
- Erosive changes in the esophageal mucosa suggest possible malignant strictures.
- Filling defects in the column of barium suggest possible esophageal tumors; malignant esophageal tumors change the mucosal contour.

- Narrowing of the distal esophagus strongly suggests achalasia (cardiospasm).
- Backflow of barium from the stomach into the esophagus suggests gastric reflux.
- Filling defects in the stomach, which usually disrupt peristalsis, suggest malignant tumors, usually adenocarcinomas.
- Outpouchings of the gastric mucosa that usually don't affect peristalsis suggest benign tumors, such as adenomatous polyps and leiomyomas.
- Evidence of partial or complete healing, characterized by radiating folds extending to the edge of the ulcer crater, suggests benign ulcers.
- Radiating folds that extend beyond the ulcer crater to the edge of the mass suggest malignant ulcers.
- Edematous changes in the mucosa of the antrum or duodenal loop, or dilation of the duodenal loop suggests possible pancreatitis or pancreatic carcinoma.
- Edematous changes, segmentation of the barium column, and flocculation in the small intestine suggest possible malabsorption syndrome.
- Filling defects of the small intestine suggest possible Hodgkin's disease and lymphosarcoma.

Interfering factors

- Failure to observe restrictions on diet, smoking, and medication (may invalidate results)
- Excess air in the small bowel (possible poor imaging)
- Failure to remove metallic objects in the X-ray field (possible poor imaging)

Uric acid, serum

Overview

- Measures serum levels of uric acid, the major end metabolite of purine
- Helps detect disorders of purine metabolism, rapid destruction of nucleic acids, and conditions marked by impaired renal excretion, which typically raise serum uric acid levels

Purpose

- To confirm the diagnosis of gout
- To help detect renal dysfunction

Procedure

Preparation

- Explain to the patient that the uric acid test detects gout and kidney dysfunction.
- Tell the patient that the test requires a blood sample. Explain who will perform the venipuncture and when.
- Notify the laboratory and physician of drugs the patient is taking that may affect test results; it may be necessary to restrict them.
- Instruct the patient to fast for 8 hours before the test.
- Explain to the patient that he may experience slight discomfort from the tourniquet and the needle puncture.

Implementation

- Perform a venipuncture and collect the sample in a 3- or 4-ml clot-activator tube.

Patient care

- Apply direct pressure to the venipuncture site until bleeding stops.
- Inform the patient that he may resume his usual diet and medications stopped before the test.

Complications

- Hematoma at the venipuncture site

Interpretation

Normal results

- In men, 3.4 to 7 mg/dl (SI, 202 to 416 µmol/L)
- In women, 2.3 to 6 mg/dl (SI, 143 to 357 µmol/L)

Abnormal results

- Increased uric acid levels may indicate gout or impaired kidney function.
- Levels may also rise in heart failure, glycogen storage disease (type I, von Gierke's disease), infections, hemolytic and sickle cell anemia, polycythemia, neoplasms, and psoriasis.
- Low uric acid levels may indicate defective tubular absorption (such as Fanconi's syndrome) or acute hepatic atrophy.

Interfering factors

- Failure to observe pretest restrictions
- Loop diuretics, ethambutol, vincristine, pyrazinamide, thiazides, and low doses of aspirin (possible increase)
- Acetaminophen, ascorbic acid, and levodopa (possible false-high if using colorimetric method)
- Aspirin in high doses (possible decrease)
- Starvation, high-purine diet, stress, and alcohol abuse (possible increase)

Uric acid, urine

Overview

○ A quantitative analysis of urine uric acid levels that may supplement serum uric acid testing to identify disorders that alter production or excretion of uric acid (such as leukemia, gout, and renal dysfunction).
○ The most specific laboratory method is spectrophotometric absorption after treatment of the specimen with the enzyme uricase.

Purpose

○ To detect enzyme deficiencies and metabolic disturbances (such as gout) that affect uric acid production
○ To help measure the efficiency of renal clearance and to determine the risk of stone formation

Procedure

Preparation

○ Explain to the patient that this test measures the body's production and excretion of a waste product known as *uric acid*.
○ Notify the laboratory and physician of drugs the patient is taking that may affect test results; it may be necessary to restrict them.
○ It may be necessary to change the patient's diet to one that is low or high in purines before or during urine collection.
○ Tell the patient that the test requires urine collection over a 24-hour period, and teach him the proper collection technique.

Implementation

○ Collect the patient's urine over a 24-hour period, discarding the first specimen and retaining the last.
○ Send the specimen to the laboratory immediately after the collection is complete.

Patient care

○ Instruct the patient that he may resume his usual diet and medications.

Complications

None known

Interpretation

Normal results

○ 250 to 750 mg/24 hours (SI, 1.48 to 4.43 mmol/d), depending on patient's diet

Abnormal results

○ Increased levels may result from chronic myeloid leukemia, polycythemia vera, multiple myeloma, early remission in pernicious anemia, lymphosarcoma and lymphatic leukemia during radiotherapy, or tubular reabsorption defects, such as Fanconi's syndrome and hepatolenticular degeneration (Wilson's disease).
○ Decreased levels occur in gout (when uric acid production is normal but excretion inadequate) and in severe renal damage such as that resulting from chronic glomerulonephritis, diabetic glomerulosclerosis, and collagen disorders.

Interfering factors

○ Diuretics, such as benzthiazide, furosemide, and ethacrynic acid (decrease); pyrazinamide, salicylates, phenylbutazone, probenecid, and allopurinol (increase)
○ High-purine diet (increase)
○ Low-purine diet (decrease)
○ Failure to send the sample to the laboratory immediately after the collection is completed

Urinalysis

Overview

○ Evaluates physical characteristics of urine; determines specific gravity and pH; detects and measures protein, glucose, and ketone bodies; examines sediment for blood cells, casts, and crystals
○ Includes visual examination, reagent strip screening, refractometry for specific gravity, and microscopic inspection of centrifuged sediment

Purpose

○ To screen the patient's urine for renal or urinary tract disease
○ To help detect metabolic or systemic disease unrelated to renal disorders
○ To detect substances (drugs)

Procedure

Preparation

○ Explain that this analysis helps to diagnose renal or urinary tract disease and to evaluate overall body function.
○ Inform the patient that he need not restrict food and fluids.
○ Notify the laboratory and physician of drugs the patient is taking that may affect laboratory results.

Implementation

○ Collect a random urine specimen of at least 15 ml. Obtain a first-voided morning specimen if possible.
○ Strain the specimen to catch calculi or calculus fragments if the patient is being evaluated for renal colic. Carefully pour the urine through an unfolded 4″ × 4″ gauze pad or a fine-mesh sieve placed over the specimen container.

Patient care

○ Inform the patient that he may resume his usual diet and medications.

Complications

None known

Interpretation

Normal results

○ Color, straw to dark yellow
○ Odor, slightly aromatic
○ Appearance, clear
○ Specific gravity, 1.005 to 1.035
○ pH, 4.5 to 8
○ Red blood cells (RBCs), 0 to 2 per high-power field
○ White blood cells (WBCs) or epithelial cells, 0 to 5 per high-power field
○ Casts, none except 1 to 2 hyaline casts/low-power field
○ Crystals, present

Abnormal results

○ Nonpathologic variations in normal values may result from diet, nonpathologic conditions, specimen collection time, and other factors.
○ An alkaline pH (above 7.0) — characteristic of a vegetarian diet — causes turbidity and the formation of phosphate, carbonate, and amorphous crystals.
○ An acid pH (below 7.0) — typical of a high-protein diet — produces turbidity and the formation of oxalate, cystine, leucine, tyrosine, amorphous urate, and uric acid crystals.
○ Protein may be present in a benign condition known as *orthostatic (postural) proteinuria.*
○ Most common in patients ages 10 to 20, proteinuria is intermittent, appears after prolonged standing, and disappears after recumbency.
○ Transient benign proteinuria may also occur with fever, exposure to cold, emotional stress, or strenuous exercise.
○ Systemic diseases that may cause proteinuria include lymphoma, hepatitis, diabetes mellitus, toxemia, hypertension, lupus erythematosus, and febrile illnesses.
○ Proteinuria suggests renal failure or disease or multiple myeloma.
○ Sugars may appear under normal conditions; most common sugar in urine is glucose.
○ Transient nonpathologic glycosuria may result from emotional stress or pregnancy and may follow ingestion of a high-carbohydrate meal.
○ Centrifuged urine sediment contains cells, casts, crystals, bacteria, yeast, and parasites. RBCs commonly don't appear in urine without pathologic significance; however, strenuous exercise can cause hematuria.
○ Color change can result from diet, drugs, and many diseases.
○ In diabetes mellitus, starvation, and dehydration, a fruity odor accompanies formation of ketone bodies.
○ In urinary tract infections (UTIs), a fetid odor commonly is associated with *Escherichia coli.*
○ Maple syrup urine disease and phenylketonuria also cause distinctive odors.
○ Other abnormal odors include those similar to a brewery, sweaty feet, cabbage, fish, and sulfur.
○ Turbid urine may contain RBCs or WBCs, bacteria, fat, or chyle and may reflect renal infection.
○ Low-specific gravity (< 1.005) is characteristic of diabetes insipidus, nephrogenic diabetes insipidus, acute tubular necrosis, and pyelonephritis.
○ Fixed-specific gravity, in which values remain 1.010 regardless of fluid intake, occurs in chronic glomerulonephritis with severe renal damage.
○ High-specific gravity (> 1.035) occurs in nephrotic syndrome, dehydration, acute glomerulonephritis, heart failure, liver failure, and shock.

○ Alkaline urine pH may result from Fanconi's syndrome, UTI caused by urea-splitting bacteria (*Proteus* and *Pseudomonas*), and metabolic or respiratory alkalosis.

○ Acid urine pH is associated with renal tuberculosis, pyrexia, phenylketonuria, alkaptonuria, and acidosis.

○ Glycosuria usually indicates diabetes mellitus, but may result from pheochromocytoma, Cushing's syndrome, impaired tubular reabsorption, advanced renal disease, and increased intracranial pressure.

○ Ketonuria occurs in diabetes mellitus when cellular energy needs exceed available cellular glucose. In the absence of glucose, cells metabolize fat for energy. Ketone bodies — the end products of incomplete fat metabolism — accumulate in plasma and are excreted in the urine.

○ Ketonuria may also occur in starvation states, low- or no-carbohydrate diets, and following diarrhea or vomiting.

○ Bilirubin in urine may occur in liver disease resulting from obstructive jaundice or hepatotoxic drugs or toxins or from fibrosis of the biliary canaliculi (which may occur in cirrhosis).

○ Increased urobilinogen in the urine may indicate liver damage, hemolytic disease, or severe infection.

○ Decreased levels may occur with biliary obstruction, inflammatory disease, antimicrobial therapy, severe diarrhea, or renal insufficiency.

○ Hematuria indicates bleeding within the genitourinary tract and may result from infection, obstruction, inflammation, trauma, tumors, glomerulonephritis, renal hypertension, lupus nephritis, renal tuberculosis, renal vein thrombosis, renal calculi, hydronephrosis, pyelonephritis, scurvy, malaria, parasitic infection of the bladder, subacute bacterial endocarditis, polyarteritis nodosa, and hemorrhagic disorders.

○ Strenuous exercise or exposure to toxic chemicals may also cause hematuria.

○ An excess of WBCs in urine usually implies urinary tract inflammation, especially cystitis or pyelonephritis.

○ WBC and WBC casts in urine suggest renal infection or noninfective inflammatory disease.

○ Numerous epithelial cells suggest renal tubular degeneration, such as heavy metal poisoning, eclampsia, and kidney transplant rejection.

○ Casts form in the renal tubules and collecting ducts by agglutination of protein cells or cellular debris and are flushed loose by urine flow.

○ Excessive numbers of casts indicate renal disease.

○ Hyaline casts are associated with renal parenchymal disease, inflammation, trauma to the glomerular capillary membrane, and some physiologic states (such as the one following exercise); epithelial casts, with renal tubular damage, nephrosis, eclampsia, amyloidosis, and heavy metal poisoning; coarse and fine granular casts, with acute or chronic renal failure, pyelonephritis, and chronic lead intoxication; fatty and waxy casts, with nephrotic syndrome, chronic renal disease, and diabetes mellitus; RBC casts, with

renal parenchymal disease (especially glomerulonephritis), renal infarction, subacute bacterial endocarditis, vascular disorders, sickle cell anemia, scurvy, blood dyscrasias, malignant hypertension, collagen disease, and acute inflammation; and WBC casts, with acute pyelonephritis and glomerulonephritis, nephrotic syndrome, pyogenic infection, and lupus nephritis.

○ Numerous calcium oxalate crystals suggest hypercalcemia or ethylene glycol ingestion. Cystine crystals (cystinuria) reflect an inborn error of metabolism.

○ Bacteria, yeast cells, and parasites in urine sediment reflect genitourinary tract infection or contamination of external genitalia.

○ The most common parasite in sediment is *Trichomonas vaginalis,* which causes vaginitis, urethritis, and prostatovesiculitis.

Interfering factors

○ Strenuous exercise before routine urinalysis (may cause transient myoglobulinuria)

○ Insufficient urinary volume, < 2 ml (may limit the range of procedures)

○ Failure to send the specimen to the laboratory immediately after collection is complete or failure to refrigerate the specimen (false-low urobilinogen)

○ Foods such as beets, berries, and rhubarb (false change in color)

○ Certain drugs

○ Highly dilute urine such as in diabetes insipidus

Urinary calculi

Overview

○ Strains urine to remove any urinary calculi, so they can be chemically analyzed to reveal their cause.
○ Urinary calculi (urolithiasis or, more commonly, *urinary stones*) are insoluble substances formed when mineral salts — calcium oxalate, calcium phosphate, magnesium ammonium phosphate, urate, or cystine — accumulate around the nuclei of bacteria, fibrin, blood clots, or epithelial cells.
○ Calculi commonly form in the kidney, pass into the ureter, and are excreted in the urine, ranging in size from microscopic to several centimeters. Calculi that don't pass spontaneously may require surgical extraction or pulverization.
○ Urinary calculi can result from reduced urinary volume, increased excretion of mineral salts, urinary stasis, pH changes, and decreased protective substances.
○ Symptoms may include hematuria, severe flank pain, dysuria, and urinary retention, frequency, and urgency.

Purpose

○ To detect and analyze calculi in the urine

Procedure

Preparation

○ Tell the patient that this test detects urinary calculi; explain that laboratory analysis will reveal their composition.
○ Tell the patient that his urine will be collected and strained.
○ Advise the patient that he need not restrict food and fluids.
○ Inform the patient that he will receive medication to control pain.

Implementation

○ Have the patient void into the strainer.
○ Inspect the strainer carefully because calculi may be minute, appearing like gravel or sand.
○ Document the appearance of the calculi and the number, if possible.
○ Place the calculi in a properly labeled container.
○ Send the container to the laboratory immediately for analysis.

Patient care

○ Observe the patient for severe flank pain, dysuria, and urinary retention, frequency, or urgency. Hematuria should subside.
○ Keep the strainer and urinal or bedpan within the patient's reach if he has received analgesics because he may be drowsy and unable to get out of bed to void.

Complications

None known

Interpretation

Normal results

○ No calculi present

Abnormal results

○ More than one-half of all calculi in urine are of mixed composition, containing two or more mineral salts; calcium oxalate is the most common component.
○ Determining the composition of calculi helps identify various metabolic disorders. This guides proper treatment and prevention measures.

Interfering factors

○ Improper collection technique

Urine amino acid screening

Overview

○ Screens for elevated urine amino acid levels (aminoaciduria), which may result from inborn errors of metabolism caused by the absence of specific enzymatic activities.
○ Best used to indicate secondary (renal) aminoaciduria; the plasma amino acid test is best used to indicate primary (overflow) aminoaciduria. To screen for congenital aminoaciduria, plasma or urine test may be used.
○ Chromatography is the preferred technique. Positive results can be elaborated by fractionation, showing specific amino acid levels.
○ Testing for specific amino acid levels is necessary for infants or young children with acidosis, severe vomiting and diarrhea, and abnormal urine odor.
○ Because aminoaciduria can cause mental retardation if not diagnosed early in neonates, testing for specific amino acid levels is especially important in this age-group.
○ More specific defects, such as cystinuria, may also cause aminoaciduria.

Purpose

○ To screen for renal aminoaciduria
○ To follow up on plasma test findings when results of these tests suggest overflow aminoaciduria

Procedure

Preparation

○ Explain to the patient (or the parents if the patient is an infant or a child) that the urine amino acid screening test helps detect amino acid disorders. Advise him that additional tests may be necessary.
○ Tell the patient that the test requires a urine specimen.
○ Notify the laboratory and physician of drugs the patient is taking that may affect test results; it may be necessary to restrict them. If the patient must continue taking them, note this on the laboratory request.
○ If the patient is a breast-fed infant, record any drugs the mother is receiving.
○ Inform the patient that he need not restrict food and fluids.

Implementation

○ If the patient is an infant, clean and dry the genital area, attach the collection device, and observe for voiding. Transfer at least 20 ml of urine to a specimen container.
○ If the patient is an adult or a child, collect a fresh random specimen.
○ Send the specimen to the laboratory immediately after collection.

Patient care

○ Remove the infant collection device carefully to prevent skin irritation, and make sure to remove all adhesive residues.

Complications

None known

Interpretation

Normal results

○ Depending on the patient's age, patterns on thin-layer chromatography are reported as normal

Abnormal results

○ If thin-layer chromatography shows gross changes or abnormal patterns, blood and 24-hour urine quantitative column chromatography are performed to identify specific amino acid abnormalities and to differentiate overflow and renal aminoaciduria.

Interfering factors

○ Failure to send the urine specimen to the laboratory immediately after collection
○ In the neonate, failure to ingest dietary protein during the 48 hours preceding the test

Urine Bence Jones protein

Overview

- Detects presence of Bence Jones proteins, abnormal low-molecular-weight, light-chain immunoglobulins derived from the clone of a single plasma cell.
- Appears in the urine of 50% to 80% of patients with multiple myeloma and in most patients with Waldenström's macroglobulinemia.
- Thermal coagulation and Bradshaw's tests screen for presence of Bence Jones proteins, but urine immunoelectrophoresis is preferred for quantitative studies. (Serum immunoelectrophoresis is less sensitive than other tests.)
- Urine and serum studies are usually used together when multiple myeloma is suspected.

Purpose

- To confirm the presence of multiple myeloma in the patient with symptoms such as bone pain (especially in the back and the thorax) and persistent anemia and fatigue

Procedure

Preparation

- Tell the patient that the test detects an abnormal protein in the urine.
- Explain to the patient that the test requires an early-morning urine specimen; teach him how to collect a midstream clean-catch specimen.

Implementation

- Collect an early-morning urine specimen of at least 50 ml.
- Instruct the patient not to contaminate the urine specimen with toilet tissue or feces.
- Send the specimen to the laboratory immediately after collection, or refrigerate it if transport is delayed.
- A refrigerated specimen must be analyzed within 24 hours, or it should be discarded.

Patient care

- Answer the patient's questions about the test.

Complications

None known

Interpretation

Normal results

- No Bence Jones proteins found

Abnormal results

- The presence of Bence Jones proteins in urine suggests multiple myeloma or Waldenström's macroglobulinemia.
- A low level of Bence Jones proteins in asymptomatic patients may result from benign monoclonal gammopathy.

Interfering factors

- Connective tissue disease, renal insufficiency, and certain cancers (possible false-positive)
- Contamination of the specimen with menstrual blood, prostatic secretions, or semen (possible false-positive)
- Contamination of the specimen with toilet tissue or feces
- Failure to store the specimen properly during the collection period or to send the sample to the laboratory immediately after the collection is complete (possible false-positive from protein deterioration)

Urine culture

Overview

○ Evaluates urinary tract infection (UTI), usually bladder infection.
○ Identifies pathogenic fungi such as *Coccidioides immitis*.
○ May use quick urine screen to determine if urine contains high bacteria or white blood cell (WBC) counts; only urine with bacteria or WBCs is processed for culture.
○ Clean-voided midstream collection, rather than suprapubic aspiration or catheterization, is the method of choice for obtaining a urine specimen.
○ To distinguish between true bacteriuria and contamination, it's necessary to know the number of organisms in a milliliter of urine, estimated by a culture technique known as a *colony count*; an additional quick centrifugation test determines where a UTI originates.
○ Specimen collection may be required on three consecutive mornings for a patient with suspected urogenital tuberculosis.

Purpose
○ To diagnose UTI
○ To monitor microorganism colonization after urinary catheter insertion

Procedure

Preparation
○ Make sure the patient has signed an appropriate consent form.
○ Note and report all allergies.
○ Check the patient's history for current use of antimicrobial drugs.
○ Explain that the test requires a urine specimen. Obtain the urine specimen before beginning antibiotic therapy.
○ Maintain asepsis throughout the procedure as indicated.
○ Instruct the patient to collect a clean-voided midstream specimen. Stress the importance of cleaning the external genitalia thoroughly.
○ Warn of possible discomfort during specimen collection in catheterization.

Implementation
○ Collect the first-voided urine specimen.
○ Collect at least 3 ml of urine, but don't fill the specimen cup more than halfway.
○ Record the suspected diagnosis, the collection time and method, current antimicrobial therapy, and fluid- or drug-induced diuresis on the laboratory request.

○ Seal the cup with a sterile lid and send it to the laboratory at once.
○ If transport is delayed for more than 30 minutes, store the specimen at 39.2° F (4° C) or place it on ice unless the urine transport tube contains a preservative.

Patient care
○ Answer the patient's questions about the test.

Complications
○ Possible infection when specimens are obtained by catheterization

Interpretation

Normal results
○ Sterile urine with no bacterial growth

Abnormal results
○ Bacterial count of 100,000 or more organisms of a single microbe species per milliliter suggest UTI; < 100,000/ml may be significant, depending on the patient's age, sex, history, and other individual factors.
○ Bacterial count of < 10,000/ml usually suggest that the organisms are contaminants, except in symptomatic patients or those with urologic disorders.
○ Isolation of *Mycobacterium tuberculosis* in a special test for acid-fast bacteria suggests tuberculosis of the urinary tract.
○ Isolation of more than two species of organisms or of vaginal or skin organisms usually suggests contamination and requires a repeat culture.

Interfering factors
○ Antibiotics and diuretics

Urine delta-aminolevulinic acid

Overview

○ Using the colorimetric technique for quantitative analysis, determines urine delta-aminolevulinic acid (ALA) levels, to help diagnose porphyrias, hepatic disease, and lead poisoning.
○ In an emergency, performed by a simple qualitative screening test.
○ ALA, the basic precursor of the porphyrins, normally converts to porphobilinogen during heme synthesis. Impaired conversion, which occurs in porphyrias and lead poisoning, causes urine ALA levels to rise before other chemical or hematologic changes occur.

Purpose

○ To screen for lead poisoning
○ To help diagnose porphyrias and certain hepatic disorders, such as hepatitis and hepatic carcinoma

Procedure

Preparation

○ Explain to the patient that the urine ALA test detects the amount of delta-ALA in the urine.
○ If lead poisoning is suspected, tell the patient (or parents, because the patient is usually a child) that the test helps detect the presence of too much lead in the body.
○ Notify the laboratory and physician of drugs the patient is taking that may affect test results; it may be necessary to restrict them.
○ Inform the patient or his parents that he need not restrict food and fluids.
○ Tell the patient that the test requires urine collection over a 24-hour period, and teach him or his parents the proper collection technique.

Implementation

○ Collect the patient's urine over a 24-hour period, discarding the first specimen and retaining the last.
○ Use a light-resistant bottle containing a preservative (usually glacial acetic acid) to prevent ALA degradation.
○ Refrigerate the specimen or keep it on ice during the collection period.
○ Insert the drainage bag in a dark plastic bag if the patient has an indwelling urinary catheter in place.
○ Send the specimen to the laboratory as soon as the collection is complete.

Patient care

○ Instruct the patient that he may resume his usual medications.

Complications

None known

Interpretation

Normal results

○ 1.3 to 7.0 mg/24 hours (SI, 10 to 53 μmol/d)

Abnormal results

○ Increased levels may occur in lead poisoning, hereditary tyrosinemia, acute porphyria, hepatic carcinoma, or hepatitis.

Interfering factors

○ Failure to collect all urine during the test period, to store the specimen properly and protect it from light, or to send the specimen to the laboratory immediately after the collection is complete
○ Barbiturates and griseofulvin (increase caused by accumulation of porphyrins in the liver)
○ Vitamin E in pharmacologic doses (possible decrease)

Urine 17-hydroxycorticosteroids

Overview

○ Measures urine levels of 17-hydroxycorticosteroid (17-OHCS) — metabolites of the hormones that regulate glyconeogenesis (more than 80% are metabolites of cortisol, the primary adrenocortical steroid)
○ Reflects cortisol secretion and, indirectly, adrenocortical function
○ Most accurately determined from a 24-hour specimen because cortisol secretion varies diurnally and in response to stress and many other factors
○ Uses column chromatography and spectrophotofluorometry with the Porter-Silber reagent
○ Measure plasma cortisol; urine-free cortisol; and urine 17-ketosteroid levels, and test corticotropin stimulation and suppression to confirm test results.

Purpose

○ To assess adrenocortical function

Procedure

Preparation

○ Explain to the patient that this test evaluates how his adrenal glands are functioning.
○ Inform the patient that he should restrict food and fluids that will alter test results (coffee, tea) and avoid excessive physical exercise and stressful situations during the collection period.
○ Tell the patient that the test requires collection of urine over a 24-hour period, and instruct him in the proper collection technique.
○ Notify the laboratory and physician of drugs the patient is taking that may affect test results; it may be necessary to restrict them.

Implementation

○ Collect the patient's urine over a 24-hour period, discarding the first specimen and retaining the last.
○ Use a bottle containing a preservative to prevent deterioration of the specimen.
○ Label the specimen appropriately, including the patient's gender, on the request forms.
○ Refrigerate the specimen or place it on ice during the collection period.

Patient care

○ Instruct the patient that he may resume his usual activities, diet, and medications.

Complications

None known

Interpretation

Normal results

○ In men, 4.5 to 12 mg/24 hours (SI, 12.4 to 33.1 µmol/d)
○ In women, 2.5 to 10 mg/24 hours (SI, 6.9 to 27.6 µmol/d)
○ In children ages 8 to 12, < 4.5 mg/24 hours (SI, < 12.4 µmol/d)
○ In children younger than age 8, < 1.5 mg/24 hours (SI, < 4.14 µmol/d)

Abnormal results

○ Increased levels may occur in Cushing's syndrome, adrenal carcinoma or adenoma, pituitary tumor, virilism, hyperthyroidism, severe hypertension, and extreme stress induced by such conditions as acute pancreatitis and eclampsia.
○ Decreased levels may indicate Addison's disease, hypopituitarism, or myxedema.

Interfering factors

○ Failure to observe restrictions, to collect all urine during the test period, or to store the specimen properly
○ Meprobamate, phenothiazines, spironolactone, ascorbic acid, chloral hydrate, glutethimide, chlordiazepoxide, penicillin G, hydroxyzine, quinidine, quinine, iodides, and methenamine (possible increase)
○ Hydralazine, phenytoin, thiazide diuretics, estrogens, hormonal contraceptives, phenothiazines, nalidixic acid, and reserpine (possible decrease)

Urine hydroxyproline

Overview

○ Determines hydroxyproline levels colorimetrically on a timed urine sample or by ion-exchange or gas-liquid chromatography.
○ Total urine levels of hydroxyproline, an amino acid found mainly in collagen (a component of skin and bone), are a good index of bone matrix turnover because levels increase when collagen breaks down during bone resorption.
○ Bone matrix turnover and hydroxyproline levels normally rise in children during periods of rapid skeletal growth. However, they also rise in disorders that increase bone resorption, such as Paget's disease, metastatic bone tumors, and certain endocrine disorders.
○ A collagen-restricted diet is essential for this test because hydroxyproline levels reflect collagen intake.
○ Free hydroxyproline, a small component of total hydroxyproline and a sensitive indicator of dietary collagen intake, may be measured to validate results.

Purpose

○ To monitor treatment for disorders characterized by bone resorption, including Paget's disease, metastatic bone tumors, certain endocrine disorders (hyperthyroidism), rheumatoid arthritis, and osteoporosis
○ To aid in the diagnosis of disorders characterized by bone resorption

Procedure

Preparation

○ Explain to the patient that the urine hydroxyproline test helps monitor treatment or detect an amino acid disorder related to bone formation.
○ Notify the laboratory and physician of drugs the patient is taking that may affect test results; it may be necessary to restrict them.
○ Inform the patient that he must follow a collagen-free diet and avoid eating ice cream, candy, meat, fish, poultry, jelly, and any foods containing gelatin for 24 hours before the test and during the test period itself.
○ Tell the patient that the test requires urine collection over a 2-hour or 24-hour period, and teach him the correct collection technique.
○ Note the patient's age and sex on the laboratory request.

Implementation

○ Collect the patient's urine over a 2- or 24-hour period. In a 24-hour collection, discard the first sample and retain the last.
○ Use a container that has a preservative to prevent hydroxyproline degradation.
○ Refrigerate the specimen or keep it on ice during the collection period.
○ Send the specimen to the laboratory immediately after the collection is complete.

Patient care

○ Instruct the patient that he may resume his usual diet and medications.

Complications

None known

Interpretation

Normal results

○ 1 to 9 mg/24 hours (SI, 1.0 to 3.4 IU/d)

Abnormal results

○ Decreased levels may occur during therapy for bone resorption disorders.
○ Increased levels may indicate bone disease, metastatic bone tumors, or endocrine disorders that stimulate hormonal secretion.

Interfering factors

○ Failure to observe restrictions, to collect all urine during the collection period, to store the specimen properly, or to send the specimen to the laboratory immediately after the collection is complete
○ Ascorbic acid, vitamin D, aspirin, glucocorticoids, antineoplastic agents, calcium gluconate, corticosteroids, estradiol, propranolol, calcitonin, and mithramycin — used to treat Paget's disease (possible decrease)
○ Psoriasis and burns (possible increase caused by collagen turnover)
○ Growth hormone, parathyroid hormone, phenobarbital, and sulfonylureas (increase)

Urine 17-ketogenic steroids

Overview

- Determines urine levels of the 17-ketogenic steroids (17-KGS), using spectrophotofluorometry; 17-KGS consists of the 17-hydroxycorticosteroids (cortisol and its metabolites, for example) and other adrenocortical steroids, such as pregnanetriol, that can be oxidized in the laboratory to 17-ketosteroids.
- Provides an excellent overall assessment of adrenocortical function.
- For accurate diagnosis of a specific disease, results must be compared with those of other tests, including plasma corticotropin, plasma cortisol, corticotropin stimulation, single-dose metyrapone, and dexamethasone suppression.

Purpose

- To evaluate adrenocortical and testicular function
- To aid in the diagnosis of Cushing's syndrome and Addison's disease

Procedure

Preparation

- Explain to the patient that the urine 17-KGS test evaluates adrenal function.
- Notify the laboratory and physician of drugs the patient is taking that may affect test results; it may be necessary to restrict them.
- Inform the patient that he need not restrict food and fluids but should avoid excessive physical exercise and stressful situations during the collection period.
- Tell the patient that the test requires urine collection over a 24-hour period, and teach him how to collect the specimen correctly.

Implementation

- Collect the patient's urine over a 24-hour period, discarding the first specimen and retaining the last.
- Use a bottle containing a preservative to keep the specimen at a pH of 4.0 to 4.5.
- Appropriately label the specimen and laboratory requests with the patient's name and gender.
- Refrigerate the specimen or keep it on ice during the collection period.
- Send the specimen to the laboratory as soon as the collection is complete.

Patient care

- Instruct the patient that he may resume his usual activities and medications.

Complications

None known

Interpretation

Normal results

- In men, 4 to 14 mg/24 hours (SI, 13 to 49 μmol/d)
- In women, 2 to 12 mg/24 hours (SI, 7 to 42 μmol/d)
- In children ages 11 to 14, 2 to 9 mg/24 hours (SI, 7 to 31 μmol/d)
- In children younger than 11 and infants, 0.1 to 4 mg/24 hours (SI, 0.3 to 14 μmol/d)

Abnormal results

- Increased levels may be caused by hyperadrenalism, from Cushing's syndrome, adrenogenital syndrome (congenital adrenal hyperplasia), or adrenal carcinoma or adenoma; or by severe physical stress (such as that caused by burns, infections, or surgery) or emotional stress.
- Decreased levels may reflect hypoadrenalism, caused by Addison's disease, panhypopituitarism, cretinism, or cachexia.

Interfering factors

- Failure to observe restrictions, to collect all urine during the collection period, to store the specimen properly, or to send it to the laboratory immediately after the collection is complete
- Corticotropin, meprobamate, phenothiazines, spironolactone, penicillin, oleandomycin, and hydralazine (possible increase)
- Estrogens, quinine, reserpine, thiazide diuretics, and long-term corticosteroid therapy (possible decrease)
- Nalidixic acid, dexamethasone, carbamazepine, cephalothin, and tiaprofenic acid (possible increase or decrease)

Urine melanin

Overview

○ Measures urine levels of melanin, the brown-black pigment produced by specialized cells and melanocytes that covers the skin, hair, and eyes.
○ Cutaneous malignant melanomas, which produce excessive amounts of melanin, develop most commonly around the head and neck but may also originate in mucous membranes (as in the rectum), the retinas, or the central nervous system. Patients may excrete melanin precursors—melanogen—in their urine. If the urine is left standing, exposure to air converts the melanogen to melanin in about 24 hours.
○ In Thormählen's test, sodium nitroprusside (nitroferricyanide) detects melanin in urine, based on characteristic color changes.
○ A more specific test, such as chromatography, isolates and measures the pigment.

Purpose

○ To aid in the diagnosis of malignant melanomas

Procedure

Preparation

○ Explain to the patient what melanin is, and tell him the urine melanin test detects its presence in urine.
○ Inform the patient that he need not restrict food and fluids.
○ Tell the patient that the test requires a random urine specimen, and teach him the correct collection technique.

Implementation

○ Collect a random urine specimen.
○ Send the specimen to the laboratory immediately.

Patient care

○ Answer the patient's questions about the test.

Complications

None known

Interpretation

Normal results

○ No melanogen or melanin found

Abnormal results

○ In a patient with a visible skin tumor, the presence of melanin or melanogen in urine indicates advanced internal metastasis.
○ In a patient without a visible skin tumor, because malignant melanomas may also develop in internal organs, the presence of melanin or melanogen in urine indicates an internal melanoma.

Interfering factors

○ Failure to send the urine specimen to the laboratory immediately after collection

Urine osmolality

Overview

- Evaluates the concentrating ability of the kidneys in acute and chronic renal failure by measuring the number of osmotically active ions or particles present per kilogram of water.
- Osmolality is high in concentrated urine and low in dilute urine. It's determined by the effect of solute particles on the freezing point of the fluid.
- Normal kidneys concentrate or dilute urine according to fluid intake.
- When intake is excessive, the kidneys excrete more water in the urine; when intake is limited, they excrete less. To make such variation possible, the distal segment of the tubule varies its permeability to water in response to antidiuretic hormone.
- Osmolality is a more sensitive indicator of renal function than dilution techniques that measure specific gravity.

Purpose

- To evaluate renal tubular function
- To detect renal impairment

Procedure

Preparation

- Explain to the patient that this test evaluates kidney function.
- Tell the patient that the test requires a urine specimen and collection of blood within 1 hour before or after the urine is collected.
- Withhold diuretics.
- Emphasize to the patient that his cooperation is necessary to obtain accurate results.

Implementation

- Collect a random urine specimen and draw a blood sample within 1 hour of urine collection.
- If a 24-hour urine collection is necessary, record the total urine volume on the laboratory request. (Preservatives aren't required for a 24-hour container.)
- If the patient can't urinate into the specimen containers, give him a clean bedpan, urinal, or toilet specimen pan.
- Rinse the collection device after each use.
- If the patient is catheterized, empty the drainage bag before the test. Obtain the specimen from the catheter.
- Send each specimen to the laboratory immediately after collection.

Patient care

- After collecting the final specimen, provide the patient with a balanced meal or snack.

- Make sure the patient voids within 8 to 10 hours after the catheter has been removed.

Complications

None known

Interpretation

Normal results

- In a random specimen, 50 to 1,400 mOsm/kg
- In a 24-hour urine specimen, 300 to 900 mOsm/kg

Abnormal results

- Decreased renal capacity to concentrate urine in response to fluid deprivation, or to dilute urine in response to fluid overload, may indicate tubular epithelial damage, decreased renal blood flow, loss of functional nephrons, or pituitary or cardiac dysfunction.

Interfering factors

- Diuretics (increase urine volume and dilution, thereby lowering specific gravity)
- Nephrotoxic drugs (cause tubular epithelial damage, thereby decreasing renal concentrating ability)
- Patients who have been markedly overhydrated for several days before the test (may have depressed concentration values)
- Patients who are dehydrated or have electrolyte imbalances (may retain fluids, leading to inaccurate results)

Urine porphyrins

Overview

○ Quantitatively analyzes uroporphyrins and coproporphyrins and their precursors (porphyrinogens such as porphobilinogen).
○ Porphyrins are red-orange fluorescent compounds produced during heme biosynthesis; normally found in protoplasm and excreted in urine in small amounts.
○ Increased urine levels of porphyrins or porphyrinogens may be caused by impaired heme biosynthesis, resulting from inherited enzyme deficiencies (congenital porphyrias) or from hemolytic anemia or hepatic disease (acquired porphyrias).
○ Determination of the specific porphyrins and porphyrinogens found in a urine specimen can help identify the impaired metabolic step in heme biosynthesis.
○ For correct diagnosis of a specific porphyria, urine porphyrin levels should be correlated with plasma and fecal porphyrin levels.
○ Sometimes a preliminary qualitative screening test is performed on a random specimen. A positive screening test result must be confirmed by the quantitative analysis of a 24-hour specimen.

Purpose

○ To aid in the diagnosis of congenital or acquired porphyria

Procedure

Preparation

○ Explain to the patient that the urine porphyrin test detects abnormal heme formation.
○ Tell the patient that the test requires urine collection over a 24-hour period, and teach him the proper collection technique.
○ Notify the laboratory and physician of drugs the patient is taking that may affect test results; it may be necessary to restrict them.
○ Inform the patient that he need not restrict food and fluids.

Implementation

○ Collect the patient's urine over a 24-hour period, discarding the first specimen and retaining the last.
○ Use a light-resistant specimen bottle containing a preservative to prevent degradation of the light-sensitive porphyrins and their precursors.
○ Put the collection bag in a dark plastic bag if an indwelling urinary catheter is in place.
○ Refrigerate the specimen or keep it on ice during the collection period.
○ Send the specimen to the laboratory immediately.

Patient care

○ Instruct the patient that he may resume his usual medications.

Complications

None known

Interpretation

Normal results

○ Uroporphyrins, 27 to 52 µg/24 hours (SI, 32 to 63 nmol/d)
○ Coproporphyrins, 34 to 230 µg/24 hours (SI, 52 to 351 nmol/d)

Abnormal results

○ Increased urine levels of porphyrins and porphyrin precursors may indicate porphyria, infectious hepatitis, Hodgkin's disease, central nervous system disorders, cirrhosis, or heavy metal, benzene, or carbon tetrachloride toxicity.

Interfering factors

○ Failure to store the specimen properly during the collection period, to protect it from exposure to light, or to send the specimen to the laboratory immediately after the collection is complete
○ Barbiturates, chloral hydrate, chlorpropamide, sulfonamides, meprobamate, and chlordiazepoxide (induce porphyria or porphyrinuria): stop 12 days before the test if possible (possible increase or decrease)
○ Hormonal contraceptives and griseofulvin (increase)
○ Pregnancy or menstruation (possible increase or decrease)
○ Rifampin (elevated urine urobilinogen)

Urine urobilinogen

Overview

○ Detects impaired liver function by measuring urine levels of urobilinogen, the colorless, water-soluble product that results from the reduction of bilirubin by intestinal bacteria.
○ Quantitative analysis of urine urobilinogen involves the addition of a reagent to a 2-hour urine specimen.
○ The resulting color reaction is read promptly by spectrophotometry.

Purpose

○ To aid in the diagnosis of extrahepatic obstruction such as blockage of the common bile duct
○ To aid in the differential diagnosis of hepatic and hematologic disorders

Procedure

Preparation

○ Explain to the patient that the urine urobilinogen test assesses liver and biliary tract function.
○ Tell the patient that the test requires a 2-hour urine specimen, and teach him the proper collection technique.
○ Notify the laboratory and physician of drugs the patient is taking that may affect test results; it may be necessary to restrict them.
○ Inform the patient that he need not restrict food and fluids, except for bananas, which he should avoid for 48 hours before the test.

Implementation

○ Most laboratories request a random urine specimen; others prefer a 2-hour specimen, usually during the afternoon (ideally, between 1 p.m. and 3 p.m.), when urobilinogen levels peak.
○ Send the specimen to the laboratory immediately after collection.
○ This test must be performed within 30 minutes of collection because urobilinogen quickly oxidizes into an orange compound called urobilin.

Patient care

○ Instruct the patient that he may resume his usual diet and medications.

Complications

None known

Interpretation

Normal results

○ 0.1 to 0.8 EU/2 hours (SI, 0.1 to 0.8 EU/2 hours) or 0.5 to 4.0 EU/24 hours (SI, 0.5 to 4.0 EU/d)

Abnormal results

○ Absence of urine urobilinogen may result from hepatic damage or dysfunction, complete obstructive jaundice, or treatment with broad-spectrum antibiotics.
○ Decreased levels may result from congenital enzymatic jaundice (hyperbilirubinemia syndromes) or treatment with drugs that acidify urine, such as ammonium chloride or ascorbic acid.
○ Increased levels may indicate hemolysis of red blood cells, hemolytic jaundice, hepatitis, or cirrhosis.

Interfering factors

○ Failure to observe pretest restrictions or to send the specimen to the laboratory immediately after collection
○ Para-aminosalicylic acid, phenazopyridine, procaine, phenothiazines, and sulfonamides (possible decrease)
○ Acetazolamide and sodium bicarbonate (increase)
○ Bananas eaten up to 48 hours before the test (increase)

Urine vanillylmandelic acid

Overview

- Determines urine levels of vanillylmandelic acid (VMA), a phenolic acid, using spectrophotofluorometry; helps to detect pheochromocytoma and to evaluate adrenal medulla function.
- VMA, the product of hepatic conversion of epinephrine and norepinephrine, is the catecholamine metabolite that's normally most prevalent in the urine; urine VMA levels reflect endogenous production of these major catecholamines.
- Should be performed on a 24-hour urine specimen (not a random specimen) to overcome the effects of diurnal variations in catecholamine secretion.
- Other catecholamine metabolites — metanephrine, normetanephrine, and homovanillic acid (HVA) — may be measured at the same time.
- If evaluating hypertension, specimen collection may be of greatest value during the hypertensive episode.

Purpose

- To help detect pheochromocytoma, neuroblastoma, and ganglioneuroma
- To evaluate the function of the adrenal medulla

Procedure

Preparation

- Explain to the patient that the urine VMA test evaluates hormonal secretion.
- Tell the patient that the test requires collection of urine over a 24-hour period, and teach him the proper collection technique.
- Notify the laboratory and physician of drugs the patient is taking that may affect test results; it may be necessary to restrict them.
- Instruct the patient to restrict foods and beverages containing phenolic acid, such as coffee, tea, bananas, citrus fruits, chocolate, and vanilla, and carbonated beverages for 3 days before the test.
- Advise the patient to avoid stressful situations and excessive physical activity during the urine collection period.

Implementation

- Collect the patient's urine over a 24-hour period, discarding the first specimen and retaining the last. Use a bottle containing a preservative to keep the specimen at a pH of 3.
- Refrigerate the specimen or keep it on ice during the collection period.
- Send the specimen to the laboratory immediately after the collection is completed.

Patient care

- Instruct the patient that he may resume his usual activities, diet, and medications.
- Tell family members of a patient with confirmed pheochromocytoma that they, too, should receive a careful evaluation for multiple endocrine neoplasia.

Interpretation

Normal results

- 1.4 to 6.5 mg/24 hours (SI, 7 to 33 μmol/d)

Abnormal results

- Increased levels may result from a catecholamine-secreting tumor. Further testing, such as measurement of urine HVA levels to rule out pheochromocytoma, is necessary for precise diagnosis.
- If pheochromocytoma is confirmed, it may be necessary to test the patient for multiple endocrine neoplasia, an inherited condition commonly associated with pheochromocytoma.

Interfering factors

- Excessive exercise or emotional stress (increase)
- Failure to observe restrictions, to store the specimen properly during the collection period, or to send the sample to the laboratory immediately after the collection is complete
- Epinephrine, norepinephrine, lithium carbonate, and methocarbamol (increase); chlorpromazine, guanethidine, reserpine, monoamine oxidase inhibitors, and clonidine (decrease); levodopa and salicylates (increase or decrease)

Urobilinogen, fecal

Overview

○ Measures fecal urobilinogen, the end product of bilirubin metabolism, a brown pigment formed by bacterial enzymes in the small intestine. It's excreted in feces or reabsorbed into portal blood, where it's returned to the liver and excreted in bile. A small amount is excreted in urine.

○ May be a useful indicator of hepatobiliary and hemolytic disorders, but rarely performed because it's easier to measure serum bilirubin and urine urobilinogen.

○ Proper bilirubin metabolism depends on normal hepatobiliary system functioning and a normal erythrocyte life span.

Purpose

○ To aid in the diagnosis of hepatobiliary and hemolytic disorders

Procedure

Preparation

○ Explain to the patient that the fecal urobilinogen test evaluates liver and bile duct function or detects red blood cell disorders.

○ Tell the patient that the test requires collection of a random feces specimen.

○ Notify the laboratory and physician of drugs the patient is taking that may affect test results; it may be necessary to restrict them.

○ Inform the patient that he need not restrict food and fluids.

Implementation

○ Collect a random feces specimen.

○ Tell the patient not to contaminate the feces specimen with toilet tissue or urine.

○ Use a light-resistant collection container because urobilinogen breaks down to urobilin when exposed to light.

○ Send the specimen to the laboratory immediately after collection.

○ Refrigerate the specimen if transport or testing is delayed more than 30 minutes; freeze the specimen if the test is to be performed by an outside laboratory.

Patient care

○ Tell the patient that he may resume his usual medications.

Complications

None known

Interpretation

Normal results

○ 50 to 300 mg/24 hours (SI, 100 to 400 EU/100 g)

Abnormal results

○ Absent or low levels of urobilinogen in the feces indicate obstructed bile flow, the result of intrahepatic disorders (such as hepatocellular jaundice caused by cirrhosis or hepatitis) or extrahepatic disorders (such as choledocholithiasis or tumor of the head of the pancreas, ampulla of Vater, or bile duct); or depressed erythropoiesis (such as in aplastic anemia).

Interfering factors

○ Contamination of the specimen or failure to use a light-resistant collection container

○ Broad-spectrum antibiotics (possible decrease caused by inhibition of bacterial growth in the colon)

○ Sulfonamides, which react with the reagent used by the laboratory in this test, and large doses of salicylates (possible increase)

Uroflowmetry

Overview

- Detects and evaluates dysfunctional voiding patterns by a simple, noninvasive test.
- The patient voids into a funnel containing a uroflowmeter, which measures flow rate (volume of urine voided per second), continuous flow (time of measurable flow), and intermittent flow (total voiding time, including interruptions).
- The gravimetric system weighs urine as it's voided and plots the weight against time; it's the simplest to use and widely available.
- Other types of uroflowmeters are the rotary disc, electromagnetic, and spectrophotometric systems.

Purpose

- To evaluate lower urinary tract function
- To demonstrate bladder outlet obstruction

Procedure

Preparation

- Make sure the patient has signed an appropriate consent form.
- Note and report all allergies.
- Stop drugs that may affect bladder and sphincter tone.
- Instruct the patient not to urinate for several hours before the test and to increase fluid intake so he'll have a full bladder and a strong urge to void.
- Instruct the patient to remain still while voiding during the test to help ensure accurate results.
- Provide complete privacy during the test.

Implementation

- The test procedure is the same with all types of equipment.
- Ask a male patient to void while standing.
- Ask a female patient to void while sitting.
- Instruct the patient to avoid straining to empty the bladder.
- Check cable connections, and leave the patient.
- The patient pushes the start button on the commode chair, counts for 5 seconds, and voids.
- When finished, he counts for 5 seconds and pushes the button again.
- The volume of urine voided is then recorded and plotted as a curve over the time of voiding.
- Note the patient's position and the route of fluid intake (oral or I.V.).

Patient care

- Have the patient resume his medications.
- Teach self-catheterization if indicated.
- Provide bladder training as needed.
- Monitor the patient for urine retention and bladder distension.
- Monitor intake and output.

Complications

None known

Interpretation

Normal results

- Vary by age, sex, and the volume of urine voided

Abnormal results

- An increased flow rate suggests reduced urethral resistance, which may be associated with external sphincter dysfunction.
- A high peak on the curve plotted over the voiding time suggests decreased outflow resistance, which may be associated with stress incontinence.
- A decreased flow rate suggests outflow obstruction or hypotonia of the detrusor muscle.
- More than one distinct peak in a normal curve suggests abdominal straining, which may result from pushing against an obstruction to empty the bladder.

Interfering factors

- A transducer that isn't level or a beaker that isn't centered beneath the funnel
- A beaker not large enough to hold all urine
- Anticholinergics and spasmolytics
- Straining to urinate, toilet tissue in the beaker, and moving while seated on the toilet

Uroporphyrinogen I synthase

Overview

- Measures blood levels of uroporphyrinogen I synthase, an enzyme involved in heme biosynthesis; able to detect acute intermittent porphyria (AIP) during its latent phase, identifying an affected individual before an acute episode occurs.
- Differentiates hereditary deficiency AIP from other types of porphyria.
- Uroporphyrinogen I synthase is normally present in erythrocytes, fibroblasts, lymphocytes, hepatic cells, and amniotic fluid cells.
- AIP can be latent until certain factors (some sex hormones and drugs, a low-carbohydrate diet, or an infection) precipitate active disease.
- Enzyme activity is determined by fluorometrically measuring the conversion rate of porphobilinogen to uroporphyrinogen.
- If levels are indeterminate, urine and feces tests for aminolevulinic acid (ALA) and porphobilinogen may be necessary to support the diagnosis because excretion of these porphyrin precursors increases substantially during an acute episode of AIP and may increase slightly during the latent phase.

Purpose

- To aid in the diagnosis of latent or active AIP
- To differentiate AIP from other types of porphyria

Procedure

Preparation

- Explain to the patient that this test detects a red blood cell disorder.
- Tell the patient that the test requires a blood sample. Explain who will perform the venipuncture and when.
- Notify the laboratory and physician of drugs the patient is taking that may affect test results; it may be necessary to restrict them.
- Inform the patient that he'll need to fast for 12 to 14 hours before the test and to abstain from alcohol for 24 hours, but that he may drink water.
- Explain to the patient that he may experience slight discomfort from the tourniquet and the needle puncture.
- If the patient's hematocrit is available, note it on the laboratory request.

Implementation

- Perform a venipuncture and collect the sample in a 10-ml heparinized tube.

Patient care

- Apply direct pressure to the venipuncture site until bleeding stops.
- Instruct the patient that he may resume his usual diet and medications.
- If AIP is present, refer the patient for nutrition and genetic counseling. Advise him to avoid low-carbohydrate diets, alcohol, and medications that may trigger an acute episode and to seek prompt care for all infections.

Complications

- Hematoma at the venipuncture site

Interpretation

Normal results

- 7 nmol/sec/L

Abnormal results

- Decreased uroporphyrinogen I synthase levels usually indicate latent or active AIP; symptoms differentiate these phases.
- Levels that are < 6 nmol/sec/L confirm AIP.
- Levels between 6 and 6.9 nmol/sec/L are indeterminate, in which case urine and feces tests for the porphyrin precursors ALA and porphobilinogen may be necessary to support the diagnosis.

Interfering factors

- Failure to observe pretest restrictions or to freeze the sample (false-positive)
- Hemolysis from rough handling of the sample
- Hemolytic and hepatic diseases (possible increase)
- Alcohol and use of drugs, such as steroid hormones, estrogens, barbiturates, sulfonamides, phenytoin, griseofulvin, chlordiazepoxide, meprobamate, glutethimide, and ergot alkaloids (possible decrease)

Venography of the leg

Overview

○ Radiographically examines veins in the leg to assess the condition of the deep leg veins after injection of a contrast medium; used in patients whose duplex ultrasound findings are equivocal
○ Not used for routine screening because it exposes the patient to relatively high doses of radiation and can cause phlebitis, local tissue damage, and, occasionally, deep vein thrombosis (DVT)
○ Also known as *ascending contrast phlebography*

Purpose

○ To confirm a diagnosis of DVT
○ To distinguish clot formation from venous obstruction (such as a large tumor of the pelvis impinging on the venous system)
○ To evaluate congenital venous abnormalities
○ To assess deep vein valvular competence (helpful in identifying underlying causes of leg edema)
○ To locate a suitable vein for arterial bypass grafting
○ To evaluate chronic venous disease

Procedure

Preparation

○ Make sure the patient has signed a consent form.
○ Tell the patient that this test evaluates deep leg veins.
○ Note and report all allergies.
○ Report hypersensitivity to iodine, iodine-containing foods, or contrast media.
○ Stop anticoagulant therapy.
○ Instruct the patient to restrict food and drink only clear liquids for 4 hours before the test.
○ Reassure the patient that contrast media complications are rare, but tell him to report nausea, severe burning or itching, constriction in the throat or chest, or dyspnea at once.
○ Give the patient a sedative.
○ Warn the patient that he might experience a burning sensation in the leg when the contrast medium is injected and some discomfort during the procedure.
○ Explain that the test takes 30 to 45 minutes.

Implementation

○ Position the patient on a tilting X-ray table so that the leg being tested doesn't bear any weight.
○ Tie a tourniquet around the ankle to expedite venous filling.
○ Normal saline solution is injected into a superficial vein in the dorsum of the patient's foot, and a contrast medium is injected after placement has been confirmed.
○ Using a fluoroscope, the distribution of the contrast medium is monitored, and spot films of the thigh and femoroiliac regions are taken from the anteroposterior and oblique views.
○ Overhead films are taken of the calf, knee, thigh, and femoral area.
○ After filming, reposition the patient horizontally, quickly elevate the leg being tested, and infuse normal saline solution to flush the contrast medium from the veins.
○ The fluoroscope is checked to confirm complete emptying.
○ After the needle is removed, apply a dressing to the injection site.

Patient care

○ Give the patient analgesics.
○ Tell the patient to resume usual diet and medications.
○ Encourage the patient's oral fluid intake.
○ If DVT is documented, initiate therapy (heparin infusion, bed rest, leg elevation or support).
○ Monitor vital signs and fluid intake and output.
○ Because of the high volume of contrast used, especially if bilateral venography is necessary, monitor renal function and hydration status very carefully.
○ Because most allergic reactions to the contrast medium occur within 30 minutes of injection, carefully observe the patient for signs and symptoms of anaphylaxis, such as flushing, urticaria, and laryngeal stridor.
○ Monitor the injection site for bleeding, infection, hematoma, and erythema.

Complications

○ Adverse reactions to contrast media or drugs
○ Thrombophlebitis
○ Local tissue damage
○ Renal insufficiency or failure
○ Small extravasations of contrast media (less than 10 ml) don't usually pose a problem, but tissue necrosis and ulceration may occur, especially with larger extravasations and in patients with arterial insufficiency.

Interpretation

Normal results

○ Steady opacification of the superficial and deep vasculature with no filling defects

Abnormal results

○ Consistent filling defects, abrupt termination of a column of contrast material, unfilled major deep veins, or diversion of flow (through collaterals, for example) suggest DVT.
○ Improper needle placement in a superficial vein, weight bearing or muscle contraction, or use of tourniquets can produce artifacts of poor filling.
○ Diagnosis errors often result from incomplete filling.
○ Fluoroscopy is essential for establishing that the contrast medium has reached the vessels being filmed and that opacification is adequate.

Vertebral radiography

Overview

○ Radiographically shows all or part of the vertebral column, to determine bone density, texture, erosion, and changes in bone relationships.
○ X-rays of bone cortex reveal any widening or narrowing and signs of irregularity.
○ Joint X-rays may reveal fluid, spur formation, narrowing or widening of the cortex, and changes in joint structure.
○ The type and extent of vertebral radiography depend on the patient's condition; for example, a patient with lower back pain requires a study of only the lumbar and sacral segments.

Purpose

○ To detect vertebral fractures, dislocations, subluxations, and deformities
○ To detect vertebral degeneration, infection, and congenital disorders
○ To detect disorders of the intervertebral disks
○ To determine the vertebral effects of arthritic and metabolic disorders
○ To follow the progression of certain disorders (such as scoliosis in children)

Procedure

Preparation

○ Make sure the patient has signed an appropriate consent form.
○ Explain to the patient that this test evaluates bone structure in the vertebral column.
○ Note and report all allergies.
○ Tell the patient that he need not restrict food and fluids.
○ Inform the patient that positioning for the radiographic films may cause slight discomfort and that cooperation helps to ensure accurate results.
○ Stress to the patient the importance of remaining still and holding his breath for film exposure during the procedure.
○ Explain that the test usually takes 15 to 30 minutes.

Implementation

○ The procedure varies considerably, depending on which vertebral segment is being examined.
○ Assist the patient into a supine position on the X-ray table for an anteroposterior view.
○ Reposition him for lateral or right and left oblique views; specific positioning depends on the vertebral segment or adjacent structures of interest.
○ X-rays are obtained as required.

Patient care

○ Answer the patient's questions about the test.

○ Exercise extreme caution when handling trauma patients with suspected spinal injuries, especially of the cervical area. Such patients should be filmed while on the stretcher to avoid further injury during transfer to the X-ray table.

Complications

 ALERT Potential for spinal injury in a trauma patient

Interpretation

Normal results

○ Vertebrae are without fractures, subluxations, dislocations, abnormal curvatures, or other abnormalities.
○ Specific positions and spacing of the vertebrae vary with the patient's age. In the lateral view, adult vertebrae are aligned to form four alternately concave and convex curves.
○ The cervical and lumbar curves are convex anteriorly; the thoracic and sacral curves are concave anteriorly.
○ Although the structure of the coccyx varies, it usually points forward and downward.
○ Neonatal vertebrae form only one curve, which is concave anteriorly.

Abnormal results

○ Spondylolisthesis, fractures, subluxations, dislocations, wedging
○ Deformities of the spine, such as kyphosis, scoliosis, and lordosis
○ Absence of sacral or lumbar vertebrae (congenital abnormalities)
○ Hypertrophic spurs and osteoarthritis (degenerative processes)
○ Thinning of the bone (osteoporosis)
○ Intervertebral discs and adjacent surfaces of vertebral bodies destroyed by lesions (tuberculosis)
○ Benign or malignant intraspinal tumors visible on X-ray

Interfering factors

○ Improper positioning

Visual acuity

Overview

- Evaluates a patient's ability to distinguish the form and detail of an object.
- The patient is asked to read letters on a standardized visual chart, called the *Snellen chart,* from a distance of 20′ (6.1 m). This test should be performed on all patients with eye complaints.
- Charts showing the letter "E" in various positions and sizes are used for young children and other people who can't read.
- The smaller the symbol the patient can identify, the sharper his visual acuity.
- A patient's near (reading) vision may be tested as well, using a standardized chart such as the *Jaeger card* (a card with print in graded sizes).
- The near-vision test is routine for those complaining of eyestrain or reading difficulty and for everyone over age 40.
- Results serve as a baseline for treatments, follow-up examinations, and referrals.

Purpose

- To test distance and near visual acuity
- To identify refractive errors in vision

Procedure

Preparation

- Tell the patient that these tests evaluate distance and near vision.
- Tell the patient that the tests take only a few minutes. If he wears glasses, tell him to bring them to the examination.

Implementation

Distance visual acuity

- Have the patient sit 20′ (6.1 m) away from the eye chart. If he's wearing glasses, tell him to remove them so his uncorrected vision can be tested first.
- Begin with the right eye unless vision in the left eye is known to be more acute.
- Have the patient occlude the left eye; then ask him to read the smallest line of letters he can see on the chart.
- Encourage him to try to read lines he can't see clearly because intelligent guesses usually indicate that the patient can recognize some details of the symbols.

※ *AGE AWARE If using the "E" chart with preschool children, have the child compare the letter to a table with three legs. Then ask the child to point to the direction in which the legs of the table are pointing.*

- Record the number of the smallest line the patient can read. This number is expressed as a fraction. The numerator is the distance between the patient and the chart; the denominator is the distance from which a patient with normal vision can read the line. The greater the denominator, the poorer the vision.
- If the patient makes an error on a line, record the results with a minus number. For example, if the patient reads the 20/40 line but makes one error, record his vision as 20/40 −1. If the patient reads the 20/40 line and one symbol on the next line, record his vision as 20/40 +1.
- Have the patient occlude the right eye; then repeat the test for the left eye. To minimize recall, use a different set of symbols or have the patient read the lines backward.
- If the patient wears glasses, test his corrected vision using the same procedure. If he normally wears glasses but doesn't have them with him, note this on the test results.
- In recording the patient's responses, indicate which eye was tested and whether it was tested with or without corrective lenses.

Near visual acuity

- Have the patient remove his glasses and occlude the left eye. Ask him to read the Jaeger card at his customary reading distance.
- Test both eyes, with and without corrective lenses.
- In reporting near visual acuity, specify the size of the smallest print legible to the patient and the nearest distance at which reading is possible.

Patient care

- If the patient can't read the largest letter on the chart, further testing is necessary.

Complications

None known

Interpretation

Normal results

- Distance visual acuity, 20/20 (the smallest symbol the patient can identify at 20′ [6.1 m] is the same symbol a patient with normal vision can identify from the same distance)
- Near visual acuity, 14/14 (a person can read at 14″ [36 cm] what a person with normal vision can read from the same distance)

Abnormal results

- If the denominator is more than 20 (for example, 40), his visual acuity is less than normal. In this case, it means he reads at 20′ what a person with normal vision can read at 40′ (12.2 m).
- A person with visual acuity of 20/200 in the better eye is considered legally blind. Similarly, if the denominator is less than 20, the patient's distance visual acuity is better than normal. For example, 20/15 vision means that the patient can read at 20′ (6.1 m) what a person with normal visual acuity can see at 15′ (4.6 m).

○ Decreased near visual acuity is indicated by a larger denominator. For example, 14/20 near vision means that the patient can read at 14″ (36 cm) what a person with normal vision can read at 20″ (50.8 cm).

○ Normal or better-than-normal visual acuity doesn't necessarily indicate normal vision. For example, a visual field defect may be present if the patient consistently misses the letters on one side of all the lines.

○ A field defect is present if the patient states that one or more of the letters disappear or become illegible when he's looking at a nearby letter. Such findings indicate the need for further visual field testing, such as Amsler's grid test or the tangent screen examination.

○ Patients with less-than-normal visual acuity require further testing, including refraction and complete ophthalmologic examination, to determine whether visual loss is from injury, disease, or a need for corrective lenses.

Interfering factors

○ The patient's failure to bring glasses to the examination

○ Glasses improperly prescribed or outdated in their degree of correction (possible to have better visual acuity without them)

○ The patient's inability to cooperate

Vitamin A and carotene

Overview

○ Measures serum levels of vitamin A (retinol) and its precursor, carotene; the color reactions produced by vitamin A and related compounds with various reagents provide quantitative and qualitative information.
○ A fat-soluble vitamin normally supplied by diet, vitamin A is important for reproduction, vision (especially night vision), and epithelial tissue and bone growth. Vitamin A is found mostly in fruits, vegetables, eggs, poultry, meat, and fish. Carotene is present in leafy green vegetables and in yellow fruits and vegetables.

Purpose

○ To investigate suspected vitamin A deficiency or toxicity
○ To aid in the diagnosis of visual disturbances, especially night blindness and xerophthalmia
○ To aid in the diagnosis of skin diseases, such as keratosis follicularis or ichthyosis
○ To screen for malabsorption

Procedure

Preparation

○ Explain to the patient that this test measures the vitamin A level in blood.
○ Tell the patient that the test requires a blood sample. Explain who will perform the venipuncture and when.
○ Instruct the patient to fast overnight, but tell him that he need not restrict water intake.
○ Explain to the patient that he may experience slight discomfort from the tourniquet and the needle puncture.

Implementation

○ Perform a venipuncture and collect the sample in a chilled 7-ml siliconized tube.
○ Protect the sample from light because vitamin A characteristically absorbs light.
○ Keep the specimen on ice.
○ Handle the sample gently and send it to the laboratory immediately.

Patient care

○ Apply direct pressure to the venipuncture site until bleeding stops.
○ Instruct the patient that he may resume his usual diet.

Complications

○ Hematoma at the venipuncture site

Interpretation

Normal results

○ Vitamin A, 30 to 80 µg/dl (SI, 1.05 to 2.8 µmol/L)
○ Carotene, 10 to 85 µg/dl (SI, 0.19 to 1.58 µmol/L)

Abnormal results

○ Decreased vitamin A levels (hypovitaminosis A) may indicate impaired fat absorption, as in celiac disease, infectious hepatitis, cystic fibrosis of the pancreas, or obstructive jaundice; chronic nephritis; or protein-calorie malnutrition (marasmic kwashiorkor).
○ Increased vitamin A levels (hypervitaminosis A) usually indicate chronically excessive intake of vitamin A supplements or of foods high in vitamin A; other causes are hyperlipemia and hypercholesterolemia of uncontrolled diabetes mellitus.
○ Decreased serum carotene levels may result from pregnancy or from impaired fat absorption or, rarely, insufficient dietary intake of carotene.
○ Increased carotene levels indicate grossly excessive dietary intake.

Interfering factors

○ Failure to observe overnight fast
○ Hemolysis from rough handling of the sample
○ Mineral oil, neomycin, and cholestyramine (possible decrease)
○ Glucocorticoids and hormonal contraceptives (possible increase)

Vitamin B$_2$, serum

Overview

- Evaluates serum levels of vitamin B$_2$ (riboflavin), a vitamin essential for growth and tissue function.
- Considered more reliable than the urine test, which can produce artificially high values in patients after surgery or prolonged fasting.

Purpose

- To detect vitamin B$_2$ deficiency

Procedure

Preparation

- Explain to the patient that this test evaluates vitamin B$_2$ levels.
- Tell the patient that the test requires a blood sample. Explain who will perform the venipuncture and when.
- Instruct the patient to maintain a normal diet before the test.
- Explain to the patient that he may experience slight discomfort from the tourniquet and the needle puncture.

Implementation

- Perform a venipuncture and collect the sample in a 4.5-ml siliconized tube.
- Handle the sample gently to prevent hemolysis.
- Don't refrigerate or freeze the sample.
- Send the sample to the laboratory immediately.

Patient care

- Apply direct pressure to the venipuncture site until bleeding stops.
- Inform the patient with vitamin B$_2$ deficiency that good dietary sources of vitamin B$_2$ are milk products, organ meats (liver and kidneys), fish, green leafy vegetables, legumes, and fortified breads and cereals.

Complications

- Hematoma at the venipuncture site

Interpretation

Normal results

- 3 to 15 µg/dl

Abnormal results

- Less than 2 µg/dl indicates vitamin B$_2$ deficiency, from insufficient dietary intake of vitamin B$_2$, malabsorption syndrome, or conditions that increase metabolic demands such as stress.

Interfering factors

- Hemolysis from rough handling of the sample

Vitamin B$_{12}$, serum

Overview

- A radioisotope assay of competitive binding to quantitatively analyze serum levels of vitamin B$_{12}$ (also called *cyanocobalamin*, *antipernicious anemia factor*, or extrinsic factor); usually performed concurrently with measurement of serum folic acid levels.
- A water-soluble vitamin containing cobalt, vitamin B$_{12}$ is essential to hematopoiesis, deoxyribonucleic acid synthesis and growth, myelin synthesis, and central nervous system (CNS) integrity.
- This vitamin is found almost exclusively in animal products, such as meat, shellfish, milk, and eggs.

Purpose

- To aid in the differential diagnosis of megaloblastic anemia, which may be caused by a vitamin B$_{12}$ or folic acid deficiency
- To aid in the differential diagnosis of CNS disorders that are affecting peripheral and spinal myelinated nerves

Procedure

Preparation

- Explain to the patient that this test determines the amount of vitamin B$_{12}$ in blood.
- Tell the patient that the test requires a blood sample. Explain who will perform the venipuncture and when.
- Instruct the patient to fast overnight before the test.
- Check the patient's history for drugs that may alter test results, and note these on the laboratory request.
- Explain to the patient that he may experience slight discomfort from the tourniquet and the needle puncture.

Implementation

- Perform a venipuncture and collect the sample in a 4.5-ml siliconized tube.
- Handle the sample gently to prevent hemolysis.
- Send the sample to the laboratory immediately.

Patient care

- Apply direct pressure to the venipuncture site until bleeding stops.
- Tell the patient that he may resume his usual diet.

Complications

- Hematoma at the venipuncture site

Interpretation

Normal results

- 200 to 900 pg/ml (SI, 148 to 664 pmol/L)

Abnormal results

- Decreased serum vitamin B$_{12}$ levels may indicate inadequate dietary intake, especially if the patient is a strict vegetarian; malabsorption syndromes such as celiac disease; isolated malabsorption of vitamin B$_{12}$; hypermetabolic states such as hyperthyroidism; pregnancy; and CNS damage (for example, posterolateral sclerosis or funicular degeneration).
- Increased serum vitamin B$_{12}$ levels may result from excessive dietary intake; hepatic disease, such as cirrhosis or acute or chronic hepatitis; and myeloproliferative disorders such as myelocytic leukemia.

Interfering factors

- Failure to fast overnight and administration of substances that decrease vitamin B$_{12}$ absorption
- Neomycin, metformin, anticonvulsants, and ethanol (possible decrease)
- Hormonal contraceptives (increase)

Vitamin C, serum

Overview

○ Chemical assay to measure plasma levels of vitamin C (ascorbic acid), a water-soluble vitamin required for collagen synthesis and cartilage and bone maintenance; for promoting iron absorption and influencing folic acid metabolism; for withstanding stresses of injury and infection.
○ This vitamin is present in generous amounts in citrus fruits, berries, tomatoes, raw cabbage, green peppers, green leafy vegetables, and fortified juices.
○ Severe vitamin C deficiency, or scurvy, causes capillary fragility, joint abnormalities, and multisystemic symptoms.

Purpose

○ To aid in the diagnosis of scurvy, scurvylike conditions, and metabolic disorders, such as malnutrition and malabsorption syndromes

Procedure

Preparation

○ Explain to the patient that this test detects the amount of vitamin C in his blood.
○ Tell the patient that the test requires a blood sample. Explain who will perform the venipuncture and when.
○ Instruct the patient to fast overnight before the test.
○ Explain to the patient that he may experience slight discomfort from the tourniquet and the needle puncture.

Implementation

○ Perform a venipuncture and collect the sample in a 4.5-ml heparinized tube.
○ Avoid rough handling or excessive agitation of the sample to prevent hemolysis.
○ Send the sample to the laboratory immediately.

Patient care

○ Apply direct pressure to the venipuncture site until bleeding stops.
○ Instruct the patient that he may resume his usual diet.

Complications

○ Hematoma at the venipuncture site

Interpretation

Normal results

○ 0.2 to 2 mg/dl (SI, 11 to 114 µmol/L)

Abnormal results

○ Decreased levels may be caused by pregnancy, infection, fever, or anemia and may result in scurvy.
○ Increased levels may indicate increased ingestion of vitamin C. This is significant because excess vitamin C is converted to oxalate, which is excreted in the urine and excessive oxalate levels can produce urinary calculi.

Interfering factors

○ Failure to observe pretest restrictions
○ Hemolysis from rough handling of the sample
○ Failure to send the sample to the laboratory promptly

Vitamin D₃, serum

Overview

○ A competitive protein-binding assay that determines serum levels of 25-hydroxycholecalciferol after chromatography has separated it from other vitamin D metabolites and contaminants; usually combined with a measurement of serum calcium and alkaline phosphatase levels.
○ Vitamin D_3 (cholecalciferol), the major form of vitamin D, is endogenously produced in the skin from the sun's ultraviolet rays and occurs naturally in fish liver oils, egg yolks, liver, and butter.

Purpose

○ To evaluate skeletal disease, such as rickets and osteomalacia
○ To aid in the diagnosis of hypercalcemia
○ To detect vitamin D toxicity
○ To monitor therapy with vitamin D_3

Procedure

Preparation

○ Explain to the patient that this test measures vitamin D in the body.
○ Tell the patient that the test requires a blood sample. Explain who will perform the venipuncture and when.
○ Instruct the patient to restrict food and fluids for 8 to 12 hours before the test.
○ Check for drugs that alter test results (corticosteroids or anticonvulsants); it may be necessary to restrict them. If the patient must continue them, note this on the laboratory request.
○ Explain to the patient that he may experience slight discomfort from the tourniquet and the needle puncture.

Implementation

○ Perform a venipuncture and collect the sample in a 4.5-ml siliconized tube.
○ Handle the sample carefully to prevent hemolysis.

Patient care

○ Apply direct pressure to the venipuncture site until bleeding stops.
○ Inform the patient that he may resume his usual medications after the test.

Complications

○ Hematoma at the venipuncture site

Interpretation

Normal results

○ 10 to 60 nanograms/ml (SI, 25 to 150 nmol/L)

Abnormal results

○ Low or undetectable levels may result from poor diet, decreased exposure to the sun, or impaired absorption of vitamin D (from hepatobiliary disease, pancreatitis, celiac disease, cystic fibrosis, or gastric or small-bowel resection); or from various hepatic, parathyroid, and renal diseases. This deficiency can cause rickets or osteomalacia.
○ Levels > 100 nanograms/ml (SI, > 250 nmol/L) may indicate toxicity caused by excessive self-medication or prolonged therapy; increased levels linked to hypercalcemia may be from hypersensitivity to vitamin D, as in sarcoidosis.

Interfering factors

○ Hemolysis from rough handling of the sample
○ Anticonvulsants, isoniazid, mineral oil, corticosteroids, aluminum hydroxide, cholestyramine, and colestipol (possible decrease)

Voiding cystourethrography

Overview

- Involves use of contrast medium instilled by gentle syringe or gravity into the bladder through a urethral catheter
- Fluoroscopic films or overhead X-rays: demonstrate bladder filling and excretion of the contrast as the patient voids
- May be performed to investigate possible causes of chronic urinary tract infection
- Other indications: suspected congenital anomaly of the lower urinary tract, abnormal bladder emptying, and incontinence
- In men or boys, used to assess hypertrophy of the prostatic lobes, urethral stricture, and the degree of compromise of a stenotic prostatic urethra

Purpose

- To detect abnormalities of the bladder and urethra, such as vesicoureteral reflux, neurogenic bladder, prostatic hyperplasia, urethral strictures, or diverticula

Procedure

Preparation

- Make sure the patient has signed an appropriate consent form.
- Note and report all allergies.
- Check the patient's history for hypersensitivity to contrast media or iodine-containing foods such as shellfish; mark the chart and notify the physician of sensitivities.
- Tell the patient that he need not restrict food and fluids before the test.
- Give the patient a sedative.
- Explain that the test requires a catheter to be inserted into the patient's bladder.
- Warn of a possible feeling of fullness and an urge to void when the contrast agent is instilled.
- Explain that the test takes 45 to 60 minutes.

Implementation

- Assist the patient into a supine position and insert an indwelling urinary catheter into the bladder.
- Contrast medium is instilled through the catheter until the bladder is full. The catheter is clamped and radiographic films are obtained with the patient in supine, oblique, and lateral positions.
- The catheter is removed, and the patient assumes the right oblique position — right leg flexed to 90 degrees, left leg extended, and in men or boys, penis parallel to the right leg — and begins to void.

- High-speed exposures of the bladder and urethra, coned down to reduce radiation exposure, are obtained during voiding.
- If the right oblique view doesn't delineate both ureters, the patient is asked to stop urinating and to begin again in the left oblique position.
- The most reliable voiding cystourethrograms are obtained with the patient recumbent.
- Patients who can't urinate in the recumbent position may do so standing (not sitting).
- Young children who can't void on command may need to undergo expression cystourethrography under general anesthesia.

Patient care

- Encourage the patient's oral fluid intake.
- Prepare the patient for surgery if indicated.
- Instruct the patient to report any fever, chills, or lower abdominal pain.
- Monitor the patient's vital signs and intake and output.
- Watch for bleeding and infection.
- Observe and record the time, color, and volume of the patient's voiding. If hematuria is present after the third voiding, notify the physician.

Complications

- Bleeding
- Infection
- Adverse reaction to contrast media

Interpretation

Normal results

- Delineation of the bladder and urethra shows normal structure and function, with no reflux of contrast medium into the ureters.

Abnormal results

- Structural and anatomical abnormalities suggest possible urethral stricture, vesical or urethral diverticula, ureterocele, prostatic enlargement, vesicoureteral reflux, or neurogenic bladder.

Interfering factors

- Embarrassment at voiding in the presence of others
- Painful urination that may cause an interrupted or less vigorous stream, muscle spasm, or incomplete sphincter relaxation
- Previous X-ray study using dye
- Presence of feces or gas in the bowel
- Difficulties encountered in bladder catheterization, especially in children (may prevent completion of the study)

Whitaker test

Overview

○ Correlates radiographic findings with measurements of pressure and flow in the kidneys and ureters and helps assess the upper urinary tract's efficiency in emptying.
○ Urethral catheterization, I.V. administration of a contrast medium, percutaneous cannulation of the kidney, and renal perfusion of the contrast medium are performed.
○ X-rays are taken; then intrarenal and bladder pressures are measured.
○ Also called a *pressure* or *flow study*.

Purpose

○ To identify and evaluate renal obstruction

Procedure

Preparation

○ Check the patient's history for hypersensitivity reactions to iodine, iodine-containing foods such as shellfish, and contrast media.
○ Instruct the patient to avoid food and fluids for at least 4 hours before the test.
○ Warn the patient that the X-ray machine makes loud clacking sounds as films are exposed.
○ Instruct the patient to void; give prescribed sedatives just before the procedure.
○ Give prophylactic antimicrobials to prevent infection from the instrumentation.

Implementation

○ Assist the patient into a supine position on the X-ray table. The table must be horizontal and must remain at the same height throughout the test.
○ To prepare for measurement of bladder pressure, a urethral catheter is placed in the bladder.
○ If an obstruction is suspected, ask the patient to void before the test. If a condition such as a bladder hypertonia is the suspected cause of insufficient emptying, he shouldn't void.
○ A plain film of the urinary tract is taken to obtain anatomic landmarks.
○ The catheter is connected to a three-way stopcock on a manometer line linked to the transducer and recorder. The line is then filled with sterile water.
○ Contrast medium is injected intravenously.
○ Assist the patient into a prone position, and make him comfortable with pillows.
○ When urography demonstrates contrast medium in the kidney, clean and drape the skin.
○ Pressure recording equipment is calibrated. The renal perfusion tubing is filled with sterile water or normal saline solution and held at the level of the kidney.

○ Local anesthetic is injected, and an incision is made through the flank for cannulation of the kidney.
○ Ask the patient to hold his breath while the needle is inserted into the renal pelvis. Aspiration of urine confirms that the needle is in position.
○ The cannula is then connected by a four-way stopcock to the perfusion tubing and the manometer line.
○ Perfusion of the contrast medium is begun, serial X-rays are taken, and intrarenal pressure is measured. Bladder pressure is then measured.
○ Perfusion continues at a steady rate of 10 ml/minute until bladder pressure is constant.
○ When pressure holds steady for a few minutes and adequate films have been taken, perfusion is stopped.
○ Residual fluid is aspirated from the kidney, the cannula is removed, and the wound is dressed.

Patient care

○ Keep the patient supine for 12 hours after the test.
○ Check vital signs every 15 minutes for the first hour, every 30 minutes for the next hour, and then every 2 hours for 24 hours.
○ Check the puncture site for bleeding, hematoma, or urine leakage each time you check the vital signs.
○ Monitor fluid intake and urine output for 24 hours. Report hematuria that persists after the third voiding.
○ Watch the patient for signs of sepsis or similar signs of contrast medium extravasation.
○ Inform the patient that colicky pains are transient.
○ Give analgesics.
○ Give antimicrobials for several days after the test to prevent infection.
○ If an obstruction is present, prepare the patient for surgery.

Complications

○ Bleeding
○ Hematoma
○ Urine leakage

Interpretation

Normal results

○ Renal pelvis and calyces are outlined normally.
○ The ureter fills uniformly and appears normal in size and course; intrarenal pressure is 15 cm H_2O and bladder pressure is 5 to 10 cm H_2O.

Abnormal results

○ Enlargement of the renal pelvis, calyces, or ureteropelvic junction may indicate obstruction.
○ Subtraction of bladder pressure from intrarenal pressure results in a differential that aids diagnosis.
○ A differential of 12 to 15 cm H_2O indicates obstruction; a differential of < 10 cm H_2O indicates an abnormality, such as hypertonia or neurogenic bladder.

Interfering factors

○ Recent barium studies or feces or gas in the bowel
○ Patient movement

White blood cell count

Overview

- Part of a complete blood count that indicates the number of white blood cells (WBCs) in a microliter (μl, or cubic millimeter) of whole blood
- May vary by as much as 2,000 cells/μl (SI, 2 × 10⁹/L) on any given day because of strenuous exercise, stress, or digestion
- May increase or decrease significantly in certain diseases but is diagnostically useful when the patient's WBC differential and condition are considered.
- Also called a *leukocyte count*

Purpose

- To determine infection or inflammation
- To determine the need for further tests, such as the WBC differential or bone marrow biopsy
- To monitor response to chemotherapy or radiation therapy

Procedure

Preparation

- Explain to the patient that the WBC test detects an infection or inflammation.
- Tell the patient that the test requires a blood sample. Explain who will perform the venipuncture and when.
- Notify the laboratory and physician of drugs the patient is taking that may affect test results; it may be necessary to restrict them.
- Inform the patient that he should avoid strenuous exercise for 24 hours before the test. Also tell him that he should avoid eating a heavy meal before the test.
- Explain to the patient that he may feel slight discomfort from the needle puncture and the tourniquet.
- If the patient is being treated for an infection, advise him that this test will be repeated to monitor his progress.

Implementation

- Perform a venipuncture and collect the sample in a 3- or 4.5-ml ethylenediaminetetraacetic acid tube.
- Completely fill the sample collection tube.
- Invert the sample gently several times to mix it with the anticoagulant.

Patient care

- Make sure subdermal bleeding has stopped before removing pressure.
- Instruct the patient that he may resume his usual diet, activity, and medications stopped before the test.
- A patient with severe leukopenia may have little or no resistance to infection and requires protective isolation.
- If a large hematoma develops at the venipuncture site, monitor pulses distal to the site.

Complications

- Hematoma at the venipuncture site

Interpretation

Normal results

- 4,000 to 10,000/μl (SI, 4 to 10 × 10⁹/L)

Abnormal results

- An increased count (leukocytosis) commonly signals infection, such as an abscess, meningitis, appendicitis, or tonsillitis; or may result from leukemia and tissue necrosis caused by burns, myocardial infarction, or gangrene.
- A decreased count (leukopenia) indicates bone marrow depression that may result from viral infections or from toxic reactions, such as those following treatment with antineoplastics, ingestion of mercury or other heavy metals, or exposure to benzene or arsenicals; may also indicate influenza, typhoid fever, measles, infectious hepatitis, mononucleosis, and rubella.

Interfering factors

- Hemolysis from rough handling of the sample
- Exercise, stress, or digestion
- Most antineoplastics; anti-infectives, such as metronidazole and flucytosine; anticonvulsants such as phenytoin derivatives; thyroid hormone antagonists; and nonsteroidal anti-inflammatory drugs such as indomethacin (decrease)

Wound culture

Overview

○ Microscopic analysis of a specimen from a lesion to confirm infection
○ May be aerobic (for detection of organisms that usually require oxygen to grow and typically appear in a superficial wound) or anaerobic (for organisms that need little or no oxygen and appear in areas of poor tissue perfusion, such as postoperative wounds, ulcers, or compound fractures)

Purpose

○ To identify an infectious microbe in a wound

Procedure

Preparation

○ Make sure the patient has signed an appropriate consent form.
○ Tell the patient that this test confirms the presence of an infection.
○ Note and report all allergies.

Anaerobic specimen collector

Some anaerobes die when exposed to oxygen. To facilitate anaerobic collection and culturing, tubes filled with carbon dioxide (CO_2) or nitrogen are used for oxygen-free transport.

The anaerobic specimen collector shown here consists of a rubber-stopper tube filled with CO_2, a small inner tube, and a swab attached to a plastic plunger. The drawing (below, left) shows the tube before specimen collection. The small inner tube containing the swab is held in place by the rubber stopper.

After specimen collection (below, right), the swab is quickly replaced in the inner tube, and the plunger is depressed. This separates the inner tube from the stopper, forcing it into the larger tube and exposing the specimen to the CO_2-rich environment.

The tube should be kept upright.

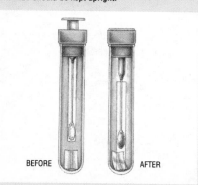

BEFORE   AFTER

Implementation

○ Maintain aseptic technique throughout the procedure.
○ Wear personal protective equipment throughout the procedure.
○ Prepare a sterile field.
○ Clean the area around the wound with antiseptic solution.
○ *For an aerobic culture:* Express the wound and swab as much exudate as possible, or insert the swab deep into the wound and gently rotate. Immediately place the swab in the aerobic culture tube.
○ *For an anaerobic culture:* Insert the swab deep into the wound, gently rotate it, and immediately place it in the anaerobic culture tub. (See *Anaerobic specimen collector.*)
○ Record recent antimicrobial therapy, the source of the specimen, and the suspected organism on the laboratory request.
○ Label the specimen container appropriately with the patient's name, physician's name, hospital number, wound site, and time of specimen collection.
○ Because some anaerobes die in the presence of oxygen, place the specimen in the culture tube quickly; take care that no air enters the tube, and check that the double stoppers are secure.
○ Keep the specimen container upright and send it to the laboratory within 15 minutes to prevent growth or deterioration of microbes.

Patient care

○ Clean the area around the wound thoroughly to limit contamination of the culture by normal skin flora.
○ Make sure no antiseptic enters the wound.
○ Re-dress the wound.

Complications

○ Spread of any existing infection

Interpretation

Normal results

○ No pathogenic organisms found

Abnormal results

○ The presence of *Staphylococcus aureus,* group A beta-hemolytic streptococci, *Proteus* species, *Escherichia coli* and other Enterobacteriaceae, and some *Pseudomonas* species suggests an aerobic wound infection.
○ The presence of *Clostridium, Bacteroides, Peptococcus,* and *Streptococcus* species suggests an anaerobic wound infection.

Interfering factors

○ Failure to report recent or current antimicrobial therapy (possible false-negative)
○ Failure to use the proper collection technique
○ Failure to use the proper transport medium, allowing the specimen to dry and the bacteria to deteriorate

Zinc

Overview

○ Measures serum zinc levels through analysis by atomic absorption spectroscopy; its deficiency can seriously impair body metabolism, growth, and development.
○ Zinc is an integral component of more than 80 enzymes and proteins and plays a critical role in enzyme catalytic reactions.
○ An important trace element, zinc occurs naturally in water and in most foods; high levels are found in meat, seafood, dairy products, whole grains, nuts, and legumes.

Purpose

○ To detect zinc deficiency or toxicity

Procedure

Preparation

○ Explain to the patient that this test determines the level of zinc in blood.
○ Tell the patient that the test requires a blood sample. Explain who will perform the venipuncture and when.
○ Inform the patient that he need not restrict food and fluids.
○ Explain to the patient that he may experience slight discomfort from the tourniquet and the needle puncture.

Implementation

○ Perform a venipuncture and collect a 7- to 10-ml sample in a zinc-free collection tube.
○ Handle the sample gently to prevent hemolysis.
○ Send the sample to the laboratory immediately. Reliable analysis must begin before platelet disintegration can alter test results.

Patient care

○ Apply direct pressure to the venipuncture site until bleeding stops.

Complications

○ Hematoma at the venipuncture site

Interpretation

Normal results

○ 70 to 120 µg/dl (SI, 10.7 to 18.4 µmol/L)

Abnormal results

○ A decreased serum zinc level may result from an acquired deficiency (from insufficient dietary intake or from an underlying disease) or a hereditary deficiency; and from alcoholic cirrhosis of the liver, myocardial infarction, ileitis, chronic renal failure, rheumatoid arthritis, or hemolytic or sickle cell anemia.
○ An extremely decreased zinc level may result from leukemia because of impaired zinc-dependent enzyme systems.
○ An increased or potentially toxic zinc level may result from accidental ingestion or industrial exposure.

Interfering factors

○ Failure to use a metal-free collection tube
○ Hemolysis from rough handling of the sample
○ Delayed transport to the laboratory
○ Time of day and time of last meal (possible increase or decrease)
○ Zinc-chelating agents, such as penicillinase, and corticosteroids (decrease)
○ Estrogens; penicillamine; antineoplastics, such as cisplatin; antimetabolites; and diuretics (possible decrease)

Normal and abnormal serum drug levels

Drug name and therapeutic level for adults	Purpose of test	Significance of abnormal level
Acetaminophen 10 to 20 mcg/ml (SI, 66.2 to 132.4 µmol/L)	Monitoring for overdose	• > 200 mcg/ml (SI, > 1,324 µmol/L) 4 hours after ingestion or > 50 mcg/ml (SI, > 331 µmol/L) 12 hours after ingestion signifies toxicity and potential for liver damage.
Amikacin *Peak:* 20 to 30 mcg/ml (SI, 34.2 to 51.3 µmol/L) *Trough:* 1 to 8 mcg/ml (SI, 1.71 to 13.68 µmol/L)	Monitoring drug therapy	• Adjust time or amount of dose or both.
Digoxin 0.8 to 2 nanograms/ml (SI, 1.024 to 2.56 nmol/L)	Monitoring drug therapy	• ≥ 3 nanograms/ml (SI, ≥ 3.8 nmol/L) may signify toxicity. • Decreased level shows that drug may have decreased therapeutic effect.
Ethosuximide 40 to 100 mcg/ml (SI, 283.2 to 708 µmol/L)	Monitoring drug therapy	• ≥ 100 mcg/ml (SI, ≥ 708 µmol/L) may signify toxicity. • Decreased level shows that drug may have decreased therapeutic effect.
Gentamicin *Peak:* 4 to 12 mcg/ml (SI, 8.36 to 25.08 µmol/L) *Trough:* < 2 mcg/ml (SI, 4.18 µmol/L)	Monitoring drug therapy	• Adjust time or amount of dose or both.
Lidocaine 2 to 5 mcg/ml (SI, 8.54 to 21.35 µmol/L)	Monitoring drug therapy	• ≥ 6 mcg/ml (SI, ≥ 25.62 µmol/L) may signify toxicity. • Decreased level shows that drug may have decreased therapeutic effect.
Lithium Therapeutic range:0.6 to 1.2 mEq/L (SI, 0.6 to 1.2 nmol/L)	Monitoring drug therapy and evaluating toxicity	• Levels > 1.2 mEq/L (SI, > 1.2 nmol/L) may signify toxicity. • Decreased level shows that drug may have decreased therapeutic effect.
Nitroprusside **(thiocyanate level)** 4 to 20 mcg/ml	Evaluating toxicity	• > 100 mcg/ml may signify toxicity. • Decreased level shows that drug may have decreased therapeutic effect.
Phenobarbital 15 to 40 mcg/ml (SI, 64.65 to 172.4 µmol/L)	Monitoring drug therapy, evaluating toxicity, and evaluating for possible abuse	• Decreased level shows that drug may have decreased therapeutic effect.

Drug name and therapeutic level for adults	Purpose of test	Significance of abnormal level
Phenytoin *Plasma:* 10 to 20 mcg/ml (SI, 39.6 to 79.2 µmol/L)	Monitoring drug therapy and evaluating toxicity	• > 20 mcg/ml (SI, > 79.2 µmol/L) may signify toxicity. • Decreased level shows that drug may have decreased therapeutic effect.
Procainamide 3 to 10 mcg/ml (SI, 12.69 to 42.3 µmol/L)	Monitoring drug therapy and evaluating toxicity	• > 14 mcg/ml (SI, > 60 µmol/L). • Decreased level shows that drug may have decreased therapeutic effect.
Quinidine 2 to 6 mcg/ml (SI, 6.16 to 18.48 µmol/L)	Monitoring drug therapy and evaluating toxicity	• ≥ 7 mcg/ml (SI, ≥ 21.56 µmol/L) may signify toxicity. • Decreased level shows that drug may have decreased therapeutic effect.
Theophylline 10 to 20 mcg/ml (SI, 55.5 to 111 µmol/L)	Monitoring drug therapy and evaluating toxicity	• ≥ 20 mcg/ml (SI, ≥ 111 µmol/L) may signify toxicity. • Decreased level shows that drug may have decreased therapeutic effect.
Tobramycin *Peak:* 4 to 8 mcg/ml (SI, 4 to 16.7 µmol/L) *Trough:* < 2 mcg/ml (SI, < 4.28 µmol/L)	Monitoring drug therapy	• Adjust time or amount of dose or both.
Valproic acid 50 to 100 mcg/ml (SI, > 346.5 to 693 µmol/L)	Monitoring drug therapy	• Decreased level shows that drug may have decreased therapeutic effect.
Vancomycin *Peak:* 20 to 40 mcg/ml (SI, 20 to 40 mg/L) *Trough:* 5 to 15 mcg/ml (SI, 5 to 15 mg/L)	Monitoring drug therapy	• Decreased level shows that drug may have decreased therapeutic effect.

Key diagnostic findings in major disorders

Abbreviations used in key diagnostic findings

ABG	arterial blood gas		HCO_3^-	bicarbonate
AFP	alpha-fetoprotein		HCT	hematocrit
ALT	alanine aminotransferase		hGH	human growth hormone
ANA	antinuclear antibody		HIV	human immunodeficiency virus
ASO	antistreptolysin-O		HLA	human leukocyte antigen
AST	aspartate aminotransferase		Ig	immunoglobulin
BUN	blood urea nitrogen		kat	katal
CBC	complete blood count		kPa	kilopascal
CEA	carcinoembryonic antigen		KS	ketosteroids
CK	creatine kinase		KUB	kidney-ureter-bladder
CO_2	carbon dioxide		LD	lactate dehydrogenase
CSF	cerebrospinal fluid		LH	luteinizing hormone
CT	computed tomography		MRI	magnetic resonance imaging
CXR	chest X-ray		$Paco_2$	partial pressure of arterial carbon dioxide
D&C	dilatation and curettage		Pao_2	partial pressure of arterial oxygen
DNA	deoxyribonucleic acid		Pap	Papanicolaou
ECG	electrocardiogram		PAWP	pulmonary artery wedge pressure
EEG	electroencephalogram		PET	positron emission tomography
ELISA	enzyme-linked immunosorbent assay		PFT	pulmonary function test
EMG	electromyography		PT	prothrombin time
ESR	erythrocyte sedimentation rate		PTT	partial thromboplastin time
FEV_1	forced expiratory volume		RBC	red blood cell
FSH	follicle-stimulating hormone		RF	rheumatoid factor
FVC	forced vital capacity		T_4	thyroxine
GFR	glomerular filtration rate		TSH	thyroid-stimulating hormone
Hb	hemoglobin		T_3	triiodothyronine
hCG	human chorionic gonadotropin		WBC	white blood cell

Abdominal aortic aneurysm
○ CT scan, MRI, or ultrasonography reveals the size, shape, and location of the aneurysm.
○ Anteroposterior and lateral abdominal X-rays may detect aortic calcification, which outlines the mass.
○ Aortography shows the condition of vessels proximal and distal to the aneurysm and the extent of the aneurysm but may underestimate the aneurysm diameter because it shows only the blood flow channel and not the surrounding clot.

Abruptio placentae
○ History includes mild to moderate vaginal bleeding (usually during second half of pregnancy).
○ Amniocentesis reveals "port wine" fluid.

○ Coagulation tests reveal a rise in fibrin split product levels.
○ CBC reveals decreased Hb level and platelet counts.
○ Pelvic ultrasonography reveals abnormal echo patterns.

Acceleration-deceleration cervical injuries
○ Full cervical spine CT scans or X-rays indicate absence of cervical fracture.
○ If the X-rays find no obvious cervical fracture, examination emphasizes motor ability and sensation below the cervical spine to detect signs of nerve root compression.

Acquired immunodeficiency syndrome
○ ELISA identifies the HIV-1 antibody.

- Western blot test should be performed after a positive ELISA result to confirm the diagnosis (antibody may not be detected in late stages because of the inability to mount an antibody response).
- CD4+ T-lymphocyte assay reveals a decreased lymphocyte count in an HIV-infected individual.

Actinomycosis
- Culture of tissue or exudate identifies *Actinomyces israelii*.
- Gram staining of excised tissue or exudates reveals branching gram-positive rods.
- CXR reveals lesions in unusual locations such as the shaft of a rib.

Acute leukemia
- Bone marrow aspiration indicates a proliferation of immature WBCs.
- Bone marrow biopsy reveals cancerous cells.
- CBC indicates pancytopenia with circulating blasts.

Acute poststreptococcal glomerulonephritis
- History includes recent streptococcal infection.
- Serum electrolyte studies show elevated calcium, chloride, phosphate, potassium, and sodium levels.
- BUN and serum creatinine levels are elevated.
- Urinalysis reveals RBCs, WBCs, mixed cell casts, and protein.
- ASO test reveals elevated streptozyme titers, indicating a recent streptococcal infection (in 80% of patients).
- Anti-DNase B titers are elevated, indicating a recent streptococcal infection.
- Serum complement assay level is low, indicating recent streptococcal infection.
- Throat culture may show group A beta-hemolytic streptococci.
- KUB X-rays show bilateral kidney enlargement.
- Renal biopsy reveals histologic changes indicating glomerulonephritis.

Acute pyelonephritis
- Urinalysis reveals sediment containing leukocytes singly, in clumps, and in casts and, possibly, a few RBCs as well as low-specific gravity and osmolality and a slight alkaline urine pH.
- Urine culture reveals more than 100,000 organisms/ml of urine.
- KUB X-rays may reveal calculi, tumors, or cysts in the kidneys and the urinary tract.
- Excretory urography may show asymmetrical kidneys.

Acute renal failure
- History includes renal disease.
- BUN and serum creatinine levels are elevated.
- ABG analysis indicates a blood pH < 7.35 and HCO_3^- level < 22 mEq/L (SI, < 22 mmol/L).

Acute respiratory failure in chronic obstructive pulmonary disease
- ABG measurements show progressive deterioration when compared with normal values for the patient; an increased HCO_3^- level may indicate metabolic alkalosis or metabolic compensation for chronic respiratory acidosis.
- CXR reveals such pulmonary pathology as emphysema, atelectasis, lesions, pneumothorax, infiltrates, or effusions.
- Hb level and HCT are decreased.
- Serum electrolyte studies reveal hypokalemia.
- WBC count is elevated if bacterial infection is present.
- ECG indicates arrhythmias that suggest cor pulmonale and myocardial hypoxia.

Acute tubular necrosis
- Urinalysis reveals urinary sediment containing RBCs and casts, specific gravity of 1.010 or less, and osmolality < 400 mOsm/kg (SI, < 400 mmol/kg).
- BUN and serum creatinine levels are elevated.
- Serum electrolyte studies reveal hyperkalemia.

Adrenal hypofunction
- Plasma cortisol level is decreased.
- Fasting blood glucose and serum sodium levels are decreased (in Addison's disease).
- Serum potassium and BUN levels are increased.
- CBC reveals increased HCT and elevated lymphocyte and eosinophil counts.
- X-rays reveal a small heart.
- Corticotropin level is increased.
- Rapid corticotropin test reveals low cortisol levels.
- Urine 17-hydroxycorticosteroid and urine 17-KS levels are decreased.

Age-related macular degeneration
- Indirect ophthalmoscopy reveals gross macular changes.
- I.V. fluorescein angiography reveals leaking vessels.
- Amsler's grid reveals visual field loss.

Alcoholism
- History includes chronic and excessive ingestion of alcohol.
- Liver function studies reveal increased levels of serum cholesterol, LD, ALT, AST, and CK in patients with liver damage.
- Serum amylase and lipase levels are elevated (in pancreatitis).

Allergic rhinitis
- Personal or family history includes allergies.
- Sputum and nasal smears reveal a large numbers of eosinophils.
- Skin test for specific allergen is positive, supported by tested response to environmental stimuli.

Alport's syndrome
- Family history includes recurrent hematuria, deafness, and renal failure (especially in men).
- Urinalysis indicates presence of RBCs.
- Renal biopsy reveals histologic changes characteristic of Alport's syndrome.
- Blood tests reveal Ig and complement components.
- Eye examination may reveal cataracts and, less commonly, keratoconus, micro spherophakia, myopia, nystagmus, and retinitis pigmentosa.

Alzheimer's disease

○ History includes progressive personality, mental status, and neurologic changes.
○ PET scan reveals alteration in the metabolic activity of the cerebral cortex.
○ Elevated Tau proteins with low levels of soluble amyloid beta-protein precursor in CSF correlate with Alzheimer's disease.
○ EEG and CT scan may help diagnose later stages of illness.
○ Autopsy reveals neurofibrillary tangles, neuritic plaques, and granulovascular degeneration.

Amputation, traumatic

○ History and examination reveal trauma to an extremity.
○ CBC reveals decreased Hb level and HCT, indicating hemorrhage.

Amyloidosis

○ Histologic examination of tissue specimen (rectal mucosa, gingiva, skin, or nerve biopsy) or abdominal fat pad aspiration using a polarizing or electron microscope and appropriate tissue staining reveals amyloid deposits.
○ Liver function study results are usually normal, except for slightly elevated serum alkaline phosphatase levels.
○ ECG shows low voltage and conduction or rhythm abnormalities resembling those characteristic of myocardial infarction (with cardiac amyloidosis).
○ Echocardiography (M-mode and two-dimensional) may detect myocardial infiltration.

Anaphylaxis

○ Diagnosis is based on the patient's history, physical examination, and signs and symptoms, which may include a rapid onset of severe respiratory or cardiovascular symptoms after ingesting or injecting a drug, vaccine, diagnostic agent, food, or food additive or after being stung by an insect.

Ankylosing spondylitis

○ Family history includes the disorder.
○ X-rays reveal blurring of the bony margins of joints (in early stage), bilateral sacroiliac involvement, patchy sclerosis with superficial bony erosions, squaring of vertebral bodies, and "bamboo spine" (with complete ankylosis).
○ Serum HLA-B27 is present in about 95% of patients with primary disease and 80% of patients with secondary disease.
○ CBC reveals slightly elevated ESR and alkaline phosphatase and creatine phosphatase levels in active disease.
○ Serum IgA levels may be elevated.

Anorexia nervosa

○ History includes weight loss of at least 25% with no organic basis; compulsive dieting; bulimic episodes, or gorging and purging; and laxative or diuretic abuse.
○ Emaciated appearance is accompanied by maintenance of physical vigor.
○ CBC reveals decreased Hb level, platelet count, WBC count, and ESR.

○ Bleeding time is prolonged (because of thrombocytopenia).
○ Serum creatinine, BUN, uric acid, cholesterol, total protein, albumin, sodium, potassium, chloride, and calcium levels are decreased.
○ Fasting blood glucose level is decreased.
○ ECG reveals nonspecific ST interval, T-wave changes, prolonged PR interval, and ventricular arrhythmias.
○ Additional diagnostic testing may be performed to rule out other disorders that may cause wasting.

Anthrax

○ History includes exposure to wool, hides, or other animal products.
○ Inspection reveals a large, pruritic, painless skin lesion.
○ Tissue culture with Gram stain reveals large gram-positive rods.
○ Drainage cultures reveal *Bacillus anthracis*.
○ Indirect hemagglutination reveals a fourfold rise in titer.

Aortic insufficiency

○ Cardiac catheterization shows reduced arterial diastolic pressure, aortic insufficiency, and valvular abnormalities.
○ Echocardiography reveals left ventricular enlargement and changes in left ventricular function; it may show a dilated aortic root, a flail leaflet, thickening of the cusps, or valve prolapse.
○ Doppler echocardiography readily detects mild degrees of aortic insufficiency that may be inaudible. It also shows a rapid, high-frequency, diastolic fluttering of the anterior mitral leaflet that results from aortic insufficiency.
○ ECG may show left ventricular hypertrophy, ST-segment depression, and T-wave inversion.
○ Radionuclide angiography helps to determine the degree of regurgitant blood flow and to assess left ventricular function.

Aortic stenosis

○ Cardiac catheterization reveals the pressure gradient across the aortic valve (indicating the severity of obstruction), increased left ventricular end-diastolic pressures (indicating left ventricular dysfunction), and the number of cusps.
○ CXR shows valvular calcification, left ventricular enlargement, dilation of the ascending aorta, pulmonary venous congestion, and — in later stages — left atrial, pulmonary artery, right atrial, and right ventricular enlargement.
○ Echocardiography demonstrates a thickened aortic valve and left ventricular wall and possible coexistent mitral valve stenosis.
○ Doppler echocardiography allows calculation of the aortic pressure gradient.
○ ECG reveals left ventricular hypertrophy and ST-segment and T-wave abnormalities. As hypertrophy progresses in severe aortic stenosis, left atrial enlargement is noted. Up to 10% of patients have atrioventricular and intraventricular conduction defects.

Aplastic or hypoplastic anemia
○ CBC reveals normochromic and normocytic RBCs with a total count of 1 million or less, as well as decreased platelet, neutrophil, and WBC counts.
○ Serum iron is elevated. (Hemosiderin is present and tissue iron storage is visible microscopically.)
○ Bleeding time is prolonged.
○ Bone marrow biopsy yields a "dry tap" or shows severely hypocellular or aplastic marrow, with a varying amount of fat, fibrous tissue, or gelatinous replacement; absence of tagged iron and megakaryocytes; and depression of erythroid elements.

Appendicitis
○ History includes right upper quadrant abdominal pain that eventually localizes in lower right quadrant, plus patient complaints of nausea and vomiting, diarrhea, anorexia, and constipation.
○ Temperature is elevated.
○ WBC count is elevated, with increased numbers of immature cells.

Arm and leg fractures
○ History includes trauma to an arm or leg.
○ Physical examination reveals pain and difficulty moving parts distal to the injury.
○ Anteroposterior and lateral X-rays of arm or leg reveal fracture.

Arterial occlusive disease
○ Arteriography demonstrates the type (thrombus or embolus), location, and degree of obstruction, and the collateral circulation.
○ Doppler ultrasonography and plethysmography show decreased blood flow distal to the occlusion.
○ Ophthalmodynamometry helps determine degree of obstruction in the internal carotid artery by comparing ophthalmic artery pressure to brachial artery pressure on the affected side. More than a 20% difference between pressures suggests insufficiency.

Asbestosis
○ History includes occupational, family, or neighborhood exposure to asbestos fibers.
○ CXR reveals fine, irregular, and linear diffuse infiltrates; extensive fibrosis results in "honeycomb" or "ground glass" appearance. X-rays also show pleural thickening and calcification, with bilateral oblation of costophrenic angles.
○ PFTs reveal decreased vital capacity, FVC, and total lung capacity; decreased or normal FEV_1 in 1 second; a normal ratio of FEV_1 to FVC; and reduced diffusing capacity for CO_2.
○ ABG analysis may reveal decreased Pao_2 and $Paco_2$.

Aspergillosis
○ History includes ocular trauma or surgery.
○ CXR reveals crescent-shaped radiolucency surrounding a circular mass.
○ Culture of exudate identifies *Aspergillus*.

Asphyxia
○ History includes change in mental status and alteration of respiratory pattern.

○ ABG analysis reveals Pao_2 < 60 mm Hg (SI, < 8.02 kPa) and $Paco_2$ > 50 mm Hg (SI, > 6.64 kPa).
○ CXR may reveal presence of foreign body, pulmonary edema, or atelectasis.
○ Toxicology screening may reveal abnormal Hb level or ingestion of drugs or chemicals.
○ PFTs may indicate respiratory muscle weakness.

Asthma
○ PFTs may reveal decreased peak expiratory flow and FEV_1
○ ABG analysis may demonstrate Pao_2 < 75 mm Hg (SI, < 10.03 kPa) and $Paco_2$ > 45 mm Hg (SI, > 5.3 kPa), indicating severe bronchial obstruction.
○ CBC reveals eosinophil count > 7%.
○ CXR shows hyperinflation.

Asystole
○ ECG reveals a waveform that's almost a flat line.
○ Atrial rhythm is usually indiscernible; no ventricular rhythm is present.
○ Atrial rate is usually indiscernible; no ventricular rate is present.
○ P wave may be present.
○ PR interval isn't measurable.
○ QRS complex is absent, or occasional escape beats are present.
○ T wave is absent.
○ QT interval isn't measurable.

Atelectasis
○ Chest auscultation reveals decreased or absent breath sounds.
○ CXR reveals characteristic horizontal lines in the lower lung zones (in widespread atelectasis) and dense shadows (with segmental or lobar collapse) with hyperinflation of neighboring lung.

Atrial fibrillation
○ ECG findings include:
 – Atrial and ventricular rhythms are grossly irregular.
 – The atrial rate, almost indiscernible, usually exceeds 400 beats/minute. The ventricular rate usually varies from 100 to 150 beats/minute but can be < 100 beats/minute.
 – P wave is absent. Erratic baseline fibrillatory (f) waves appear instead. These chaotic f waves represent atrial tetanization from rapid atrial depolarizations. When f waves are pronounced, the arrhythmia is called *coarse atrial fibrillation*. When they aren't pronounced, the arrhythmia is called *fine atrial fibrillation*.
 – PR interval is indiscernible.
 – Duration and configuration of QRS complex are usually normal. If ventricular conduction is aberrant, the QRS complex may be wide and abnormally shaped.
 – T wave is indiscernible.
 – QT interval isn't measurable.
 – *Atrial fib-flutter*, a rhythm that frequently varies between a fibrillatory line and flutter waves, may appear.

Atrial flutter
○ ECG findings include:

– Atrial rhythm is regular. Ventricular rhythm depends on the atrioventricular (AV) conduction pattern; it's often regular, although cycles may alternate. An irregular pattern may herald atrial fibrillation or indicate a block.
– Atrial rate is 250 to 400 beats/minute. Ventricular rate depends on the degree of AV block; usually, it's 60 to 100 beats/minute, but it may accelerate to 125 to 150 beats/minute.
– P wave is saw-toothed, referred to as flutter (F) waves.
– PR interval isn't measurable.
– Usually, duration of QRS complex is within normal limits, but the complex may be widened if F waves are buried within.
– T wave isn't identifiable.
– QT interval isn't measurable because T wave can't be identified.
– The patient may develop an atrial rhythm that frequently varies between a fibrillatory line and F waves. This is called *atrial fib-flutter;* the ventricular response is irregular.

Atrial septal defect

○ Echocardiography measures right ventricular enlargement, may locate the defect, and shows volume overload in the right heart.
○ ECG reveals incomplete or complete right bundle-branch block in nearly all cases.
○ Cardiac catheterization reveals a left-to-right shunt, determines the extent of shunting and pulmonary vascular disease, detects the size and location of pulmonary venous drainage, and competence of the atrioventricular valves.

Atrial tachycardia

○ ECG findings include:
– Atrial and ventricular rhythms are regular.
– Atrial rate is characterized by three or more consecutive ectopic atrial beats occurring at a rate between 160 and 250 beats/minute; the rate rarely exceeds 250 beats/minute. The ventricular rate depends on the atrioventricular conduction ratio.
– Usually positive, the P wave may be aberrant, invisible, or hidden in the previous T wave. If visible, it precedes each QRS complex.
– PR interval may be immeasurable if the P wave is indistinguishable from the preceding T wave.
– Duration and configuration of QRS complex are usually normal.
– T wave usually is indistinguishable.
– QT interval is usually within normal limits but may be shorter because of the rapid rate.

Atrioventricular (AV) block, third-degree

○ ECG findings include:
– Atrial and ventricular rhythms are regular.
– Atrial rate, which is usually within normal limits, exceeds the ventricular rate. The slow ventricular rate ranges from 40 to 60 beats/minute, but this rate is determined by the block's location and the origin of the subsidiary impulse.
– P wave has normal size and configuration.

– PR interval isn't measurable because the atria and ventricles beat independently.
– Configuration of the QRS complex depends on where the ventricular beat originates. A high AV junctional pacemaker produces a narrow QRS complex; a pacemaker in the bundle of His produces a wide QRS complex; a ventricular pacemaker produces a wide, bizarre QRS complex.
– T wave has normal size and configuration.
– QT interval may or may not be within normal limits.

Basal cell carcinoma

○ Inspection reveals skin lesions.
○ Tissue biopsy reveals basal cell carcinoma.

Bell's palsy

○ Inspection reveals facial paresthesia with an inability to raise the eyebrow, close the eyelid, smile, show the teeth, or puff the cheek.
○ EEG distinguishes temporary conduction defect from pathologic interruption of nerve fibers (after 10 days).

Benign prostatic hyperplasia

○ History includes problems with urination.
○ Rectal examination reveals enlarged prostate gland.
○ Prostate biopsy reveals histologic changes characteristic of benign prostatic hyperplasia.
○ Excretory urography may indicate urinary tract obstruction, hydronephrosis, calculi, or tumors, and filling and emptying defects in the bladder.
○ Elevated BUN and creatinine levels suggest impaired renal function.
○ Urinalysis and urine culture show hematuria, pyuria, and, when bacterial count is elevated, infection.
○ Cystourethroscopy indicates prostate enlargement (usually performed immediately before surgery to help determine the best operative procedure).

Bladder cancer

○ Cystoscopy with biopsy reveals the presence of malignant cells and may reveal that the bladder is fixed to the pelvic wall or prostate.
○ Arylsulfatase A level is elevated.
○ Retrograde cystography evaluates bladder structure and integrity and confirms the diagnosis.
○ Excretory urography reveals an early-stage or infiltrating tumor, ureteral obstruction, or a rigid deformity of the bladder wall. This test may also delineate functional problems in the upper urinary tract and help assess the degree of hydronephrosis.
○ Urinalysis indicates presence of blood and malignant cytology.
○ Ultrasonography may detect metastases in tissue beyond the bladder and can distinguish a bladder cyst from a bladder tumor.
○ Pelvic arteriography reveals tumor invasion of the bladder wall.
○ CT scan reveals the thickness of the involved bladder wall and detects enlarged retroperitoneal lymph nodes.

Blood transfusion reaction

○ Crossmatching reveals conflicting blood types.
○ Urinalysis reveals hemoglobinuria.

- Antibody screening reveals anti-A or anti-B antibodies in the blood.
- Serum haptoglobin level falls below pretransfusion level after 24 hours.
- Blood cultures may indicate bacterial contamination.

Blunt and penetrating abdominal injuries

- History includes trauma to abdomen or chest area.
- CXR or abdominal X-ray indicates presence of free air.
- Peritoneal lavage reveals blood, urine, bile, stool, or pus.
- Elevated serum amylase level indicates pancreatic injury.
- Hb level and HCT show a serial decrease.
- Excretory urography and retrograde cystography indicate renal and urinary tract damage.
- CT scan indicates abdominal organ rupture.
- Exploratory laparotomy reveals specific injuries when other clinical evidence is incomplete.

Blunt chest injuries

- History includes trauma to chest area.
- With hemothorax, percussion reveals dullness.
- With tension pneumothorax, percussion reveals tympany.
- CXR may indicate rib and sternal injuries, pneumothorax, flail chest, pulmonary contusion, lacerated or ruptured aorta, diaphragmatic rupture, lung compression, or hemothorax.
- CT scan reveals aortic laceration or rupture, or diaphragmatic rupture.
- CK-MB level shows mild elevation.

Bone tumor, primary malignant

- Physical examination detects palpable mass over bony area.
- Biopsy reveals malignant cells.
- Bone X-ray and radioisotope bone scan reveal tumor location and size.
- CT scan reveals tumor location and size.
- MRI reveals tumor.
- Serum alkaline phosphatase level is elevated (in patients with sarcomas).

Botulism

- Offending toxin is detected in the patient's serum, stool, gastric content, or the suspected food.
- EMG shows diminished muscle action potential after a single supramaximal nerve stimulus.

Brain abscess

- History includes congenital heart disease or infection, especially of the middle ear, mastoid, nasal sinuses, heart, or lungs.
- CT scan or MRI reveals site of abscess.
- Arteriography highlights the abscess with a halo.
- Culture of drainage reveals causative organism, such as *Staphylococcus aureus, Streptococcus viridans,* or *Streptococcus hemolyticus.*

Breast cancer

- Breast examination is abnormal.
- Mammography, ultrasonography, or thermography indicates presence of mass.

- Surgical biopsy reveals malignant cells.
- CEA level is elevated in metastatic disease.

Bronchiectasis

- History includes recurrent bronchial infections, pneumonia, and hemoptysis.
- CXR show pleural thickening, areas of atelectasis, and scattered cystic changes.

Bronchitis, chronic

- CXRs may show hyperinflation and increased bronchovascular markings.
- PFTs demonstrate increased residual volume, decreased vital capacity and forced expiratory flow, and normal static compliance and diffusing capacity.
- ABG analysis reveals decreased Pao_2 and normal or increased $Paco_2$.
- Sputum culture reveals the presence of microorganisms and neutrophils.
- ECG may detect atrial arrhythmias; peaked P waves in leads II, III, and aV_F; and, occasionally, right ventricular hypertrophy.
- Bronchography reveals location and extent of disease.

Burns

- History includes exposure to heat, electricity, or chemicals.
- Examination reveals depth of skin and tissue damage and area affected.
- Urinalysis may reveal myoglobinuria and hemoglobinuria.
- ABG analysis reveals reduced respiratory function.
- Fiber-optic bronchoscopy may reveal epithelial damage to the trachea and bronchi.
- Serum protein studies show increased albumin levels.
- BUN level is increased because of increased protein catabolism.
- Fibrin split products are increased.
- Serum magnesium level is suppressed.
- Osmotic fragility is high (increased tendency to hemolysis).
- Changes are noted in serum electrolyte levels, including elevated potassium and decreased sodium levels.
- WBC count reveals leukocytosis.

Calcium imbalance

- In hypocalcemia, serum calcium level is decreased.
- In hypercalcemia, serum calcium level is increased and urinalysis reveals increased calcium precipitation.
- Because about one-half of serum calcium is bound to albumin, changes in serum protein must be considered when interpreting serum calcium levels.

Candidiasis

- Culture of skin, vaginal scrapings, pus, sputum, blood, or tissue reveals *Candida albicans.*

Cardiac tamponade

- CXR reveals slightly widened mediastinum and cardiomegaly.
- Echocardiography reveals pericardial effusion with signs of right ventricular and atrial compression.

○ Pulmonary artery monitoring reveals increased right atrial pressure, right ventricular diastolic pressure, and central venous pressure.

Cardiogenic shock

○ Auscultation detects gallop rhythm, faint heart sounds, and a holosystolic murmur (with ruptured ventricular septum or papillary muscles).
○ Pulmonary artery pressure monitoring reveals:
  – increased pulmonary artery pressure
  – increased PAWP
  – increased systemic vascular resistance
  – increased peripheral vascular resistance
  – decreased cardiac output.
○ Invasive arterial pressure monitoring reveals hypotension.
○ CK level is increased.
○ ABG analysis may show metabolic acidosis and hypoxia.
○ ECG shows acute myocardial infarction, ischemia, or ventricular aneurysm.

Carpal tunnel syndrome

○ Physical examination reveals decreased sensation to light touch or pinpricks in the affected fingers.
○ Tinel's sign is positive.
○ Wrist-flexion test reveals positive Phalen's sign.
○ Compression test provokes pain and paresthesia along the distribution of the median nerve.
○ EMG detects a median nerve motor conduction delay of more than 5 milliseconds.

Cataract

○ Eye examination reveals the white area behind the pupil (unnoticeable until the cataract is advanced).
○ Ophthalmoscopy or slit-lamp examination reveals a dark area in the normally homogeneous red reflex.

Celiac disease

○ Tissue biopsy of the small bowel reveals a mosaic pattern of alternating flat and bumpy areas on the bowel surface (because of an almost total absence of villi) and an irregular, blunt, and disorganized network of blood vessels (usually prominent in the jejunum).
○ Stool samples (after 72-hour collection) reveal excess fat.
○ HLA test reveals presence of HLA-B8 antigen.
○ D-xylose absorption test reveals depressed blood and urine D-xylose levels.
○ Upper GI series followed by a small-bowel series demonstrates protracted barium passage: Barium shows up in a segmented, coarse, scattered, and clumped pattern; the jejunum shows generalized dilation.
○ Glucose tolerance test indicates poor glucose absorption.
○ Low serum carotene levels, indicating malabsorption.
○ CBC indicates decreased Hb level and HCT as well as decreased WBC and platelet counts.
○ Decreased serum albumin, sodium, potassium, cholesterol, and phospholipid levels.
○ PT may be shortened.

Cerebral aneurysm

○ History includes headache and change in mental status (usually with rupture or leakage).
○ Angiography shows location and size of unruptured aneurysm.
○ CT scan reveals location of clot, hydrocephalus, areas of infarction, and extent of blood spillage within the cisterns around the brain.

Cerebral contusion

○ History includes head trauma.
○ CT scan reveals ischemic tissue and hematoma.
○ Skull X-ray indicates fracture is absent.

Cerebral palsy

○ Infant displays:
  – difficulty sucking or keeping food in his mouth
  – infrequent voluntary movement
  – arm or leg tremors with movement
  – crossing legs when lifted from behind rather than pulling them up or "bicycling"
  – legs difficult to separate to change diapers
  – persistent use of one hand or ability to use hands well but not legs.

Cervical cancer

○ Pap test reveals abnormal cells.
○ Cone biopsy of cervical tissue reveals malignant cells.
○ Colposcopy determines the source of the abnormal cells seen on the Pap test.

Chancroid

○ History includes sexual contact with a partner with chancroid.
○ Tissue culture of ulcer exudate, bubo aspirate, or blood reveals *Haemophilus ducreyi.*

Chlamydial infections

○ History includes sexual contact with a partner with chlamydial infection.
○ Culture of site indicates *Chlamydia trachomatis* (findings may reveal urethritis, cervicitis, salpingitis, endometritis, or proctitis).
○ Culture of blood, pus, or CSF reveals *C. trachomatis* (findings may reveal epididymitis, prostatitis, or lymphogranuloma venereum).

Cholelithiasis and related disorders

○ Ultrasonography of the gallbladder indicates presence of stones.
○ Percutaneous transhepatic cholangiography reveals gallbladder disease.
○ Endoscopic retrograde cholangiopancreatography shows the biliary tree.
○ Hida scan of the gallbladder reveals obstruction of the cystic duct.
○ Oral cholecystography shows stones in the gallbladder and biliary duct obstruction.
○ Technetium-labeled iminodiacetic acid scan of the gallbladder indicates cystic duct obstruction and acute or chronic cholecystitis if the gallbladder isn't visible.
○ Blood studies may reveal elevated serum alkaline phosphatase, LD, AST, and total bilirubin levels and icteric index.

○ WBC count is slightly elevated during a cholecystitis attack.

Cholera
○ Patient reports voluminous, gray-tinged diarrhea.
○ Stool or vomitus culture reveals presence of *Vibrio cholerae*.
○ Agglutination and other clear reactions to group — and type-specific antisera provide definitive diagnosis.
○ Dark-field microscopic examination of fresh stool shows rapidly moving bacilli.
○ Immunofluorescence allows for rapid diagnosis.

Chronic glomerulonephritis
○ Urinalysis reveals proteinuria, hematuria, cylindruria, and RBC casts.
○ BUN level is elevated.
○ Serum creatinine level is elevated.
○ Kidney X-rays or ultrasonography reveals small kidneys.
○ Renal biopsy indicates presence of underlying disease.

Chronic lymphocytic leukemia
○ CBC reveals numerous abnormal lymphocytes.
○ WBC count is mildly but persistently elevated in early stages.
○ Granulocytopenia is present.
○ Bone marrow aspiration and biopsy reveal lymphocytic invasion.

Chronic renal failure
○ History includes chronic progressive debilitation.
○ BUN level is elevated.
○ Serum creatinine level is elevated.
○ Serum potassium level may be elevated.
○ Urinalysis may show proteinuria, glycosuria, erythrocytes, leukocytes, and casts.
○ Kidney biopsy identifies underlying pathology.

Cirrhosis and fibrosis
○ Liver biopsy reveals destruction and fibrosis of hepatic tissue.
○ Abdominal X-rays show liver size and cysts or gas within the biliary tract or liver, liver calcification, and massive ascites.
○ CT and liver scans determine the liver size, identify liver masses, and reveal hepatic blood flow and obstruction.
○ Esophagogastroduodenoscopy reveals bleeding esophageal varices, stomach irritation or ulceration, or duodenal bleeding and irritation.
○ ALT, AST, total serum bilirubin, and indirect bilirubin levels are elevated.
○ Serum albumin and protein levels are decreased.
○ PT is prolonged.
○ HCT, Hb, and serum electrolyte levels are decreased.

Coarctation of the aorta
○ Physical examination reveals resting systolic hypertension, absent or diminished femoral pulses, and wide pulse pressure.
○ CXR reveals notching of the undersurfaces of the ribs because of collateral circulation.

○ Echocardiography reveals left ventricular muscle thickening, coexisting aortic valve abnormalities, and the coarctation site.
○ Aortography locates the site and extent of coarctation.
○ ECG may reveal left ventricular hypertrophy.

Colorectal cancer
○ Hemoccult test (guaiac) reveals blood in stool.
○ Proctoscopy or sigmoidoscopy reveals presence of mass.
○ Colonoscopy reveals lesion.
○ Tissue biopsy reveals malignant cells.
○ Barium X-ray reveals lesion.
○ CEA level is > 5 nanograms/ml (SI, > 5 µg/L).

Concussion
○ History includes head trauma, with or without loss of consciousness.
○ Patient demonstrates amnesia with regard to traumatic event.
○ Patient reports headache.
○ Neurologic examination results are normal for patient.
○ Skull X-ray and CT scan results may be negative.

Congenital hip dysplasia
○ Ortolani or Trendelenburg's sign is positive.
○ Inspection reveals extra thigh fold on affected side, higher buttock fold on the affected side, and restricted abduction of the affected hip.
○ X-ray reveals the location of the femur head and a shallow acetabulum.

Conjunctivitis
○ Inspection reveals inflammation of the conjunctiva.
○ Stained smear of conjunctival scrapings reveals monocytes (viral conjunctivitis), polymorphonuclear cells (bacterial conjunctivitis), or eosinophils (allergic conjunctivitis).
○ Conjunctival culture reveals causative organism.

Corneal abrasion
○ History includes eye trauma or prolonged wearing of contact lenses.
○ Fluorescein stain of the cornea turns the injured area green during flashlight examination.
○ Slit-lamp examination discloses the depth of the abrasion.

Coronary artery disease
○ History includes angina and risk factors for coronary artery disease.
○ ECG reveals ischemia and, possibly, arrhythmias during an anginal attack. ECG returns to normal when pain ceases.
○ Coronary angiography reveals coronary artery stenosis or obstruction, collateral circulation, and condition of the arteries beyond the narrowing.
○ Myocardial perfusion imaging with thallium-201 during treadmill exercise detects ischemic areas.

Cor pulmonale
○ Pulmonary artery pressure measurements reveal increased right ventricular and pulmonary artery pressures as well as elevated right ventricular systolic, pul-

monary artery systolic, and pulmonary artery diastolic pressures.
○ CXR reveals large central pulmonary arteries and rightward enlargement of cardiac silhouette.
○ Echocardiography reveals right ventricular enlargement.

Crohn's disease
○ History includes diarrhea and abdominal cramping.
○ Barium enema reveals the string sign (segments of stricture separated by normal bowel).
○ Sigmoidoscopy and colonoscopy reveal patchy areas of inflammation.
○ Biopsy of bowel tissue reveals histologic changes indicative of Crohn's disease.

Cryptococcosis
○ Inspection may reveal signs of meningeal irritation.
○ Sputum, urine, prostatic secretion culture; bone marrow aspirate or biopsy; or pleural biopsy reveals *Cryptococcus neoformans*.
○ Blood culture reveals *C. neoformans* (with severe infection).
○ CXR reveals pulmonary lesion.
○ Cryptococcal antigen and positive cryptococcal culture occur in 90% of tests.

Cushing's syndrome
○ Serum cortisol level is consistently elevated.
○ A 24-hour urine sample demonstrates elevated free cortisol levels.
○ Dexamethasone suppression test reveals an elevated cortisol level (failure to suppress).
○ Urine 17-hydroxycorticosteroid level is elevated.
○ Urine 17-KS level is elevated.
○ Ultrasonography, CT scan, or angiography localizes adrenal tumors.
○ CT scan of the head identifies pituitary tumors.

Cystic fibrosis
○ Family history includes the disorder.
○ Pulmonary disease or pancreatic insufficiency (absence of trypsin) is present.
○ Sweat test reveals elevated sodium and chloride levels.
○ DNA testing may locate the Delta 508 deletion and help to confirm the diagnosis.
○ PFTs evaluate lung function.
○ Sputum culture allows the detection of concurrent infectious disease.
○ ABG analysis helps determine pulmonary status.
○ CXR helps diagnose respiratory obstruction and monitor its progress.

Cystinuria
○ Family history includes renal disease or renal calculi.
○ Chemical analysis of calculi shows cystine crystals, with a variable amount of calcium.
○ Clearance of cystine, lysine, arginine, and ornithine is elevated.
○ Urinalysis with amino acid chromatography indicates aminoaciduria, as evidenced by the presence of cystine, lysine, arginine, and ornithine.
○ Urine pH is usually < 5.0.

○ Microscopic examination of urine shows hexagonal, flat cystine crystals.
○ Cyanide-nitroprusside test result is positive.
○ Excretory urography or KUB X-rays reveal size and location of calculi.

Cytomegalovirus infection
○ Culture of urine, saliva, throat, or blood, or biopsy specimens reveal virus.
○ Indirect immunofluorescent test reveals IgM antibody.

Dermatitis
○ Family history includes allergy and chronic inflammation.
○ Patient demonstrates characteristic distribution of skin lesions.
○ Serum IgE level is elevated.

Dermatophytosis
○ Inspection reveals skin lesions.
○ Microscopic examination or culture of lesion scrapings reveals infective organism.
○ Wood's light examination may reveal types of tinea capitis.

Diabetes insipidus
○ History includes head trauma or neurologic surgery.
○ Urinalysis reveals almost colorless urine of low osmolality and low-specific gravity.

Diabetes mellitus
○ In nonpregnant adults, findings include:
   – symptoms of uncontrolled diabetes and a random blood glucose level ≥ 200 mg/dl (SI, ≥ 10.6 mmol/L)
   – fasting plasma glucose level ≥ 126 mg/dl (SI, ≥ 7 mmol/L) on at least two occasions
○ Ophthalmologic examination may show diabetic retinopathy.
○ Urinalysis reveals presence of acetone.

Dilated cardiomyopathy
○ CXR reveals cardiomegaly, usually affecting all heart chambers, and may also show pulmonary congestion, pleural or pericardial effusion, or pulmonary venous hypertension.
○ ECG may reveal ST-segment and T-wave changes.
○ Echocardiography reveals left ventricular thrombi, global hypokinesia, and degree of left ventricular dilation.

Diphtheria
○ Inspection reveals characteristic thick, patchy, grayish-green membrane over the mucous membranes of the pharynx, larynx, tonsils, soft palate, and nose.
○ Throat culture or culture of other suspect lesions reveals *Corynebacterium diphtheriae*.

Dislocated or fractured jaw
○ History includes trauma to jaw or face.
○ Maxillary or mandibular mobility is abnormal.
○ X-ray of the jaw shows fracture.

Dislocations and subluxations
○ Inspection confirms joint deformity.

- X-ray is negative for fracture but may reveal dislocation or subluxation.
- Arthroscopy reveals dislocation or subluxation.

Disseminated intravascular coagulation
- Patient displays abnormal bleeding in the absence of a known hematologic disorder.
- Platelet count is decreased.
- Fibrinogen is decreased.
- PT is prolonged.
- PTT is prolonged.
- Fibrin split products reveal increased fibrin degradation products.
- D-dimer test (a specific fibrinogen test for disseminated intravascular coagulation) is positive.

Diverticular disease
- Upper GI series reveals barium-filled pouches in the esophagus and upper bowel.
- Barium enema reveals barium-filled pouches in the lower bowel; barium outlines diverticula filled with stool.

Down syndrome
- History includes hypotonia at birth.
- Karyotype reveals chromosome abnormality.
- Prenatal ultrasonography may suggest Down syndrome if a duodenal obstruction or an atrioventricular canal defect is present.
- Maternal serum AFP levels are reduced.
- Amniocentesis reveals the translocated chromosome.

Dysmenorrhea
- History includes abdominal pain related to menstruation.
- Pelvic examination may reveal the physical cause.
- Laparoscopy may reveal an underlying cause such as endometriosis or uterine leiomyoma.
- D&C may reveal an underlying cause such as cervical stenosis or pelvic inflammatory disease.

Dyspareunia
- History includes discomfort during sexual intercourse.
- Pelvic examination may reveal a physical disorder as underlying cause of discomfort.

Ectopic pregnancy
- Serum pregnancy test shows presence of hCG.
- Real-time ultrasonography (performed if serum pregnancy test result is positive) reveals no intrauterine pregnancy.
- Culdocentesis (performed if ultrasonography detects the absence of a gestational sac in the uterus) reveals free blood in the peritoneum.
- Laparoscopy (performed if culdocentesis is positive) reveals pregnancy outside the uterus.

Electric shock
- History includes electrical contact, voltage, and length of contact.
- Physical examination reveals electrical burn.
- ECG reveals ventricular fibrillation or other arrhythmias that progress to fibrillation or myocardial infarction.

- Urine myoglobin test result is positive.

Emphysema
- Examination reveals barrel chest, pursed-lip breathing, and use of accessory muscles of respiration; palpation may reveal decreased tactile fremitus and decreased chest expansion; percussion may reveal hyperresonance; auscultation may reveal decreased breath sounds, crackles and wheezing on inspiration, prolonged expiratory phase with grunting respirations, and distant heart sounds.
- In advanced disease, CXR may show a flattened diaphragm, reduced vascular markings at the lung periphery, overaeration of the lungs, a vertical heart, enlarged anteroposterior chest diameter, and large retrosternal air space.
- PFTs indicate increased residual volume and total lung capacity, reduced diffusing capacity, and increased inspiratory flow.
- ABG analysis usually shows reduced Pao_2 and normal $Paco_2$ until late in the disease when $Paco_2$ increases.
- ECG may reveal tall, symmetrical P waves in leads II, III, and aV_F; a vertical QRS axis; and signs of right ventricular hypertrophy late in the disease.
- RBC count usually demonstrates an increased Hb level late in the disease, when the patient has persistent severe hypoxia.

Encephalitis
- Lumbar puncture reveals elevated CSF pressure and clear CSF, with slightly elevated WBC and protein levels.
- CSF or blood culture reveals virus.
- Serologic studies (in herpes encephalitis) may show rising titers of complement-fixing antibodies.
- EEG reveals abnormalities such as generalized slowing of waveforms.

Endocarditis
- Auscultation reveals a loud, regurgitant murmur.
- Blood cultures (three or more during a 24- to 48-hour period) reveal infecting organism.
- WBC count is elevated.
- ESR is elevated.
- Serum creatinine level is elevated.
- Echocardiography or transesophageal echocardiography reveals valvular damage and endocardial vegetation.

Endometriosis
- Pelvic examination reveals multiple tender nodules on uterosacral ligaments or in the rectovaginal septum, which enlarge and become more tender during menses.
- Palpation may uncover ovarian enlargement in patients with endometrial cysts on the ovaries or thickened, nodular adnexa (as in pelvic inflammatory disease).
- Laparoscopy shows small, blue powder burns on the peritoneum or the serosa of any pelvic or abdominal structure.
- Barium enema rules out malignant or inflammatory bowel disease.

Enterocolitis

- Stool Gram stain reveals numerous gram-positive cocci and polymorphonuclear leukocytes with few gram-negative rods.
- Stool culture identifies *Staphylococcus aureus* as the causative organism.
- Blood studies reveal leukocytosis, moderately increased BUN level, and decreased serum albumin level.

Epicondylitis

- History includes traumatic injury or strain from athletic activity.
- Examination reveals pain with wrist extension and supination with lateral involvement, or with flexion and pronation with epicondyle involvement.
- X-rays are normal at first, but later bony fragments, osteophyte sclerosis, or calcium deposits appear.
- Arthrography is normal with some minor irregularities on the tendon undersurface.
- Arthrocentesis identifies causative organism if joint infection is suspected.

Epididymitis

- History includes unilateral, dull aching pain radiating to the spermatic cord, lower abdomen, and flank.
- Physical examination shows characteristic waddle, as an attempt to protect the groin and scrotum when walking.
- WBC count in urine is increased.
- Urine culture and sensitivity tests reveal causative organism.
- Elevated serum WBC count indicates infection.

Epiglottiditis

- History reveals acute onset with sore throat, fever, hoarseness, dysphagia and respiratory distress characterized by stridor, drooling, inspiratory retractions and nostril flaring.
- Direct laryngoscopy reveals swollen, beefy-red epiglottis (not done if significant obstruction is suspected or immediate intubation isn't possible).
- Lateral neck X-rays show an enlarged epiglottis and distended hypopharynx.

Epilepsy

- CT scan provides brain density readings indicating abnormalities in internal structures.
- EEG may show paroxysmal abnormalities and help classify the disorder.
- MRI helps identify the cause of the seizure by providing clear images of the brain in regions where bone normally hampers visualization.

Epistaxis

- History includes trauma to the nose, chemical irritation, sinus infection, or coagulopathy.
- Inspection with a bright light and nasal speculum locates the site of bleeding.

Erythroblastosis fetalis

- Maternal history reveals risk factors for incompatibility of fetal and maternal blood, such as erythroblastotic stillbirths, abortions, previously affected children, previous anti-Rh titers, and blood transfusions.
- Maternal blood typing indicates mother is Rh-negative (titers determine changes in the degree of maternal immunization).
- Amniocentesis reveals an increase in bilirubin levels (indicating possible hemolysis) and elevations in anti-Rh titers.
- Radiologic studies may show edema and, in hydrops fetalis, the halo sign (edematous, elevated, subcutaneous fat layers) and the Buddha position (fetus's legs are crossed).
- Direct Coombs' test of umbilical cord blood confirms maternal-neonate Rh incompatibility.
- A decreased umbilical cord Hb count signals severe disease.
- Stained RBC examination reveals many nucleated peripheral RBCs.

Esophageal cancer

- X-rays of the esophagus, with barium swallow and motility studies, reveal structural and filling defects and reduced peristalsis.
- CXR or esophagography reveals pneumonitis.
- Esophagoscopy, punch-and-brush biopsies, and exfoliative cytologic tests confirm esophageal tumors.
- Bronchoscopy may reveal tumor growth in the tracheobronchial tree.
- Endoscopic ultrasonography (combined with endoscopy and ultrasonography) identifies depth of tumor penetration.
- Mediastinoscopy reveals lesion and extent of disease.
- Esophageal biopsy reveals malignant cells.

Esophageal diverticula

- Barium swallow reveals characteristic outpouching in esophagus.
- Esophagoscopy rules out other lesions as cause.

Exophthalmos

- Physical examination reveals forward displacement of the eyeballs.
- Exophthalmometer readings reveal the degree of anterior projection and asymmetry between the eyes to be > 12 mm.
- X-rays show orbital fracture or bony erosion by an orbital tumor.
- CT scan identifies lesions in optic nerve, orbit, or ocular muscle within the orbit.

Extrapulmonary tuberculosis

- Acid-fast smear reveals *Mycobacterium tuberculosis*.
- Tuberculin skin test result is positive.
- CXR reveals primary pulmonary nodular infiltrates and cavitations (often, however, CXR is negative in extrapulmonary tuberculosis).
- Fluid specimen culture (urine, synovial fluid) reveals *M. tuberculosis*.

Fallopian tube cancer

- History includes unexplained postmenopausal bleeding.
- Pap test reveals abnormal cells.
- Ultrasonography defines tumor mass.
- Barium enema rules out intestinal obstruction.
- Laparotomy and biopsy reveal malignant cells.

Fatty liver

○ Examination reveals large, tender liver.
○ Liver function studies reveal low albumin, elevated globulin, elevated total bilirubin, low aminotransferase, and — commonly — elevated cholesterol levels.
○ PT is prolonged.
○ Liver biopsy reveals excessive fat.

Femoral and popliteal aneurysms

○ Palpation reveals a pulsating mass above or below the inguinal ligament (in femoral aneurysm) or in the popliteal space (in popliteal aneurysm).
○ Arteriography or ultrasonography reveals location and size of aneurysm.

Folic acid deficiency anemia

○ Serum folate level is decreased.
○ Reticulocyte count is decreased.
○ Schilling test result is positive.
○ Serum blood studies show macrocytosis, increased mean corpuscular volume, and abnormal platelets.

Galactosemia

○ Deficiency of the enzyme galactose-1-phosphate uridyl transferase in RBCs indicates classic galactosemia; decreased galactokinase level in RBCs indicates galactokinase deficiency.
○ Serum and urine galactose level is increased.
○ Ophthalmoscopy reveals punctate lesions in the fetal lens nucleus.
○ Liver biopsy reveals acinar formation.
○ AST and ALT levels are elevated.
○ Urinalysis reveals presence of albumin.
○ Amniocentesis provides prenatal diagnosis (recommended for heterozygous and homozygous parents).

Gallbladder and bile duct carcinoma

○ Liver function test may show elevated urobilirubin levels and may show elevated levels of bile and bilirubin.
○ Patient may be jaundiced.
○ PT is prolonged.
○ Serum alkaline phosphatase level is consistently elevated.
○ Liver-spleen scan identifies abnormality.
○ Cholecystography shows stones or calcifications.
○ MRI may show areas of tumor growth.
○ Cholangiography outlines common bile duct obstruction.
○ Ultrasonography of the gallbladder shows a mass.
○ Endoscopic retrograde cholangiopancreatography identifies tumor site.
○ Biopsy reveals malignant cells.

Gas gangrene

○ History includes recent surgery or a deep puncture wound with rapid onset of pain and crepitation around the wound.
○ Anaerobic cultures of wound drainage reveal *Clostridium perfringens*.
○ Gram stain of wound drainage reveals large, gram-positive, rod-shaped bacteria.
○ X-rays reveal gas in tissues.
○ Blood studies reveal leukocytosis and, later, hemolysis.

Gastric carcinoma

○ Barium X-rays with fluoroscopy reveal tumor or filling defect in the outline of the stomach, loss of flexibility and distensibility, and abnormal gastric mucosa with or without ulceration.
○ Gastroscopy with fiber-optic endoscope shows mucosal lesions and allows gastroscopic biopsy (biopsy reveals malignant cells).
○ Photography with fiber-optic endoscope provides a permanent record of gastric lesions that may help determine disease progression and effect of treatment.
○ CT scans, CXR, liver and bone scans, and liver biopsy may rule out specific organ metastasis.

Gastritis

○ History includes gastric discomfort or bleeding.
○ Gastroscopy demonstrates inflammation of mucosa and confirms diagnosis.
○ Stool or vomitus may contain occult blood.
○ Hb level and HCT are decreased if bleeding has occurred.

Gastroenteritis

○ History includes acute onset of diarrhea accompanied by abdominal pain and discomfort.
○ Stool or blood culture reveals causative bacteria, parasites, or amoebae.
○ Barium enema reveals inflammation.

Gastroesophageal reflux

○ Barium swallow with fluoroscopy may be normal except in patients with advanced disease; in children, barium esophagography under fluoroscope reveals reflux.
○ Esophageal acidity test reveals pH of 1.5 to 2.0.
○ Acid perfusion test elicits pain or burning.
○ Gastroesophageal reflux scanning detects radioactivity in the esophagus.
○ Endoscopy and biopsy identify pathologic mucosal changes.

Genital herpes

○ History includes oral, vaginal, or anal sexual contact with an infected person or other direct contact with lesions.
○ Examination reveals vesicles on the genitalia, mouth, or anus.
○ Tissue culture and histologic biopsy of vesicular fluid reveals herpes simplex virus type 2.

Genital warts

○ Dark-field examination of scrapings from wart cells shows marked vascularization of epidermal cells, which helps to differentiate genital warts from condylomata lata.
○ Applying 5% acetic acid (white vinegar) to the warts turns them white, indicating papillomas.

Giardiasis

○ History includes such risk factors as recent travel to an endemic area, participation in sexual activity involving oral-anal contact, ingestion of suspect water, or institutionalization.
○ Stool specimen shows cysts.

○ Duodenal aspirate or biopsy shows trophozoites.
○ Small-bowel biopsy shows parasitic infection.

Glaucoma

○ History includes gradual loss of peripheral vision.
○ Tonometry reveals increased intraocular pressure.
○ Gonioscopy determines the angle of the anterior chamber of the eye, differentiating between chronic open-angle glaucoma and acute angle-closure glaucoma.
○ Ophthalmoscopy reveals cupping and atrophy of the optic disk.
○ Slit-lamp examination shows anterior structures of the eye, demonstrating effects of glaucoma.
○ Perimetry or visual field tests evaluate the extent of visual field loss of open-angle deterioration.
○ Fundus photography reveals changes in the optic disk.

Glycogen storage diseases

○ In type Ia:
  – Liver biopsy reveals normal glycogen synthetase and phosphorylase enzyme activities but reduced or absent glucose-6-phosphatase activity.
  – Liver biopsy reveals normal glycogen structure but elevated amounts.
  – Serum glucose level is low.
  – Plasma studies reveal high levels of free fatty acids, triglycerides, cholesterol, and uric acid.
  – Injection of glucagon or epinephrine increases pyruvic and lactic acid levels but doesn't increase blood glucose levels.
  – Glucose tolerance test curve reveals depletional hypoglycemia and reduced insulin output.
○ In type II (Pompe's):
  – Muscle biopsy reveals increased level of glycogen with normal structure and decreased alpha-1,4-glucosidase level.
  – ECG (in infants) shows large QRS complexes in all leads, inverted T waves, and a shortened PR interval.
  – EMG (in adults) demonstrates muscle fiber irritability and myotonic discharges.
  – Amniocentesis reveals a deficiency in alpha-1,4-glucosidase level.
  – Placenta or umbilical cord examination shows an alpha-1,4-glucosidase deficiency.
  – Liver biopsy shows deficient debranching activity and increased glycogen level.
○ In type III (Cori's):
  – Laboratory tests (in children only) may reveal elevated AST or ALT levels and an increase in erythrocyte glycogen.
○ In type IV (Andersen's):
  – Liver biopsy demonstrates deficient branching enzyme activity and longer outer branches of the glycogen molecule.
○ In type V (McArdle's):
  – Serum studies indicate no increase in venous levels of lactate in sample drawn from extremity after ischemic exercise.
  – Muscle biopsy reveals a lack of phosphorylase activity and increased glycogen content.
○ In type VI (Hers'):
  – Liver biopsy shows decreased phosphorylase beta activity and increased glycogen level.
○ In type VII:

– Serum studies indicate no increase in venous levels of lactate in sample drawn from extremity after ischemic exercise.
– Blood studies reveal low erythrocyte phosphofructokinase activity and reduced half-life of RBCs.
– Muscle biopsy shows deficient phosphofructokinase with a marked rise in glycogen level with normal structure.
○ In type VIII:
  – Liver biopsy shows deficient phosphorylase beta activity and increased liver glycogen levels.
  – Blood studies show deficient phosphorylase beta kinase in leukocytes.

Goiter, simple

○ History includes residence in an area known for nutritionally related risk factors (such as iodine-depleted soil or malnutrition) or ingestion of goitrogenic medications or foods.
○ Serum TSH or T_3 level is high to normal.
○ T_4 level is low to normal.
○ Uptake of ^{131}I is normal to increased.
○ Protein-bound iodine is low to normal.
○ Urinary excretion of iodine is low.

Gonorrhea

○ History includes sexual contact with a partner with gonorrhea.
○ Culture from site of infection (urethra, cervix, rectum, pharynx) reveals *Neisseria gonorrhoeae*.
○ Culture of joint fluid and skin lesions reveals gram-negative diplococci (gonococcal arthritis).
○ Culture of conjunctival scrapings confirms gonococcal conjunctivitis.
○ Complement fixation and immunofluorescent assays of serum reveal antibody titers four times the normal rate.

Goodpasture's syndrome

○ Immunofluorescence of alveolar basement membrane shows linear deposition of Ig as well as complement 3 and fibrinogen.
○ Immunofluorescence of glomerular basement membrane (GBM) shows linear deposition of Ig combined with detection of circulating anti-GBM antibody.
○ Lung biopsy shows interstitial and intra-alveolar hemorrhage with hemosiderin-laden macrophages.
○ CXR reveals pulmonary infiltrates in a diffuse, nodular pattern.
○ Renal biopsy reveals focal necrotic lesions and cellular crescents.
○ Serum creatinine and BUN levels typically increase two to three times normal.
○ Urinalysis may reveal RBCs and cellular casts, granular casts, and proteinuria.

Gout

○ Microscopic analysis of synovial fluid obtained by needle aspiration reveals needlelike intracellular crystals of sodium urate; presence of monosodium urate monohydrate crystals confirms diagnosis.
○ Serum uric acid level is usually normal but may be increased; the higher the level, the more likely a gout attack will occur.

- Urine uric acid level is increased (in about 20% of patients).
- X-rays reveal damage to the articular cartilage and subchondral bone (in chronic gout).

Granulocytopenia
- Patient demonstrates marked neutropenia.
- WBC count is markedly decreased.
- CBC reveals few observable granulocytes.
- Bone marrow aspiration reveals a scarcity of granulocytic precursor cells beyond the most immature forms.

Guillain-Barré syndrome
- History includes minor febrile illness 1 to 4 weeks before current symptoms.
- Examination reveals progressive muscle weakness.
- CSF analysis reveals normal WBC count, rising protein levels (peaks in 4 to 6 weeks), and increasing pressure.
- EMG reveals repeated firing of the same motor unit instead of widespread sectional stimulation.
- Electrophysiologic studies may reveal marked slowing of nerve conduction velocities.

Haemophilus influenzae infection
- Blood culture reveals *H. influenzae* infection.
- CBC reveals polymorphonuclear leukocytosis and, in young children with severe infection, leukopenia.

Hearing loss
- Audiometry identifies and quantifies hearing loss.
- The Weber, the Rinne, and Schwabach tests differentiate between conductive and sensorineural hearing loss.
- Auditory brain stem response and behavioral tests may help to identify neonatal or infant hearing loss.
- CT scan evaluates vestibular and auditory pathways.
- Pure tone audiometry identifies the presence and degree of hearing loss.
- MRI detects acoustic tumors and lesions.

Heart failure
- Auscultation reveals dyspnea or crackles.
- CXR reveals increased pulmonary vascular markings, interstitial edema, or pleural effusion and cardiomegaly.
- Pulmonary artery monitoring reveals elevated pulmonary artery and capillary wedge pressures and elevated left ventricular end-diastolic pressure in left-sided heart failure, and elevated right atrial pressure or central venous pressure in right-sided heart failure.

Hemochromatosis
- Serum or plasma iron level is elevated.
- Transferrin level is increased to 70% to 100% saturation.
- A 24-hour urine collection shows excretion of iron after administration of deferoxamine, an iron-chelating agent.
- Liver biopsy may also confirm diagnosis.

Hemophilia
- History suggests disorder runs in family.

- History includes prolonged bleeding after surgery or trauma or of episodes of spontaneous bleeding into muscles or joints.
- Hemophilia A:
  - Factor VIII assay is 0% to 55% of normal.
  - PTT is prolonged.
  - Platelet count and function, bleeding time, and PT are normal.
- Hemophilia B:
  - Factor IX assay is deficient.
  - PTT is prolonged.
- Hemophilia C:
  - Assay testing reveals deficient factor XI but normal factors VIII and IX levels (rules out hemophilias A and B).
  - PTT is prolonged.
- Hb levels may be decreased depending on the degree of blood loss.

Hepatic encephalopathy
- History includes liver disease, with symptoms beginning with slight personality changes progressing to mental confusion and coma.
- Serum ammonia level is elevated.
- EEG shows slowing waves as the disease progresses.

Hepatitis, nonviral
- History includes exposure to hepatotoxic chemicals or drugs.
- Serum ALT level is elevated.
- Serum AST level is elevated.
- Serum total and direct bilirubin levels are elevated (with cholestasis).
- Serum alkaline phosphatase level is elevated.
- Differential WBC count reveals elevated eosinophils.

Hepatitis, viral
- Hepatitis profile identifies serum antigens and antibodies (serum markers) specific to the causative virus, establishing the type of hepatitis (types A, B, C, D, and E).
- PT is prolonged (more than 3 seconds longer than normal indicates liver damage).
- AST and ALT levels are elevated.
- Serum alkaline phosphatase level is elevated.
- Serum and urine bilirubin levels are elevated (with jaundice).
- Serum albumin is decreased and serum globulin is increased.
- Liver biopsy and liver scan show patchy necrosis.

Hereditary hemorrhagic telangiectasia
- History includes an established family pattern of bleeding disorders.
- Examination reveals localized aggregations of dilated capillaries on the skin of the face, ears, scalp, hands, arms, and feet, and under the nails; characteristic telangiectases are raised or flat, nonpulsatile, violet in color, blanch under pressure, and bleed easily.
- Bone marrow aspiration shows depleted iron stores, which confirms secondary iron deficiency anemia.
- Platelet count may be abnormal.

Herniated disk

○ History includes unilateral low back pain radiating to the buttocks, legs, and feet, often associated with a previous traumatic injury or back strain.
○ X-rays show degenerative changes and rule out other abnormalities.
○ MRI also rules out spinal compression.
○ Lasègue's test causes resistance and pain, as well as loss of ankle or knee-jerk reflex.
○ Myelography pinpoints the level of herniation and reveals spinal canal compression by herniated disk material.
○ CT scan identifies soft tissue and bone abnormalities.
○ EMG confirms nerve involvement.
○ Neuromuscular tests identify motor and sensory loss and leg muscle weakness.

Herpangina

○ Examination reveals vesicular lesions on the mucous membranes of the soft palate, tonsillar pillars, and throat.
○ Cultures of mouth washings or stool reveal the coxsackieviruses.
○ Antibody titers are elevated.

Herpes simplex

○ Examination reveals edema with small vesicles on an erythematous base that rupture, leaving a painful ulcer followed by yellow crusting.
○ Isolation of virus from local lesions and biopsy reveal *Herpesvirus hominis*.

Herpes zoster

○ Examination reveals small red, nodular skin lesions that spread unilaterally around the thorax or vertically over the arms or legs, and vesicles filled with clear fluid or pus.
○ Examination of vesicular fluid and infected tissue reveals eosinophilic intranuclear inclusions and varicella virus.
○ Lumbar puncture shows increased CSF pressure; CSF analysis shows increased protein levels and, possibly, pleocytosis (with CNS involvement).

Hiatal hernia

○ CXR reveals air shadow behind the heart (with large hernia).
○ Barium swallow with fluoroscopy reveals outpouching at lower end of the esophagus and identifies diaphragmatic abnormalities.
○ Serum Hb level and HCT may be decreased (with paraesophageal hernia).
○ Endoscopy and biopsy rule out varices and other small gastroesophageal lesions.
○ Esophageal motility studies reveal esophageal motor or lower esophageal pressure abnormalities.
○ pH studies reveal reflux of gastric contents.
○ Acid perfusion test reveals heartburn resulting from esophageal reflux.

Hirschsprung's disease

○ Rectal biopsy reveals absence of ganglion cells.
○ Barium enema studies reveal a narrowed segment of distal colon with a sawtooth appearance and a funnel-shaped segment above it; barium is retained longer than the usual 12 to 24 hours.
○ Rectal manometry detects failure of the internal anal sphincter to relax and contract.
○ Upright films of the abdomen show marked colonic distention.

Histoplasmosis

○ History includes an immunocompromised condition or exposure to contaminated soil in an endemic area.
○ Tissue biopsy and sputum culture reveal *Histoplasma capsulatum* (in acute primary and chronic pulmonary histoplasmosis).
○ Histoplasmosis skin test result is positive.
○ Complement fixation test results and agglutination titers are increased.

Hodgkin's disease

○ Lymph node biopsy reveals Reed-Sternberg's abnormal histiocyte proliferation and nodular fibrosis and necrosis.
○ CT scan shows lymph node abnormality.
○ Lymphangiography shows lymph node abnormality.
○ Bone marrow, liver, mediastinal, and spleen biopsies; abdominal CT scan; and lung and bone scans identify organ involvement.
○ Blood studies show normochromic anemia (in 50% of patients) and elevated, normal, or reduced WBC count and differential showing any combination of neutrophilia, lymphocytopenia, monocytosis, and eosinophilia.
○ Serum alkaline phosphatase level is increased.

Huntington's disease

○ History includes family inheritance pattern along with progressive chorea and dementia, with usual onset between age 35 and 40.
○ PET scan identifies disease.
○ DNA analysis identifies marker for gene linked to the disease.
○ Evoked potential studies reveal bilateral abnormal P100 latencies.
○ Pneumoencephalography reveals the characteristic butterfly dilation of the brain's lateral ventricles.
○ CT scan reveals brain atrophy.

Hydatidiform mole

○ History includes vaginal bleeding, ranging from brownish red spotting to bright red hemorrhage.
○ Examination reveals an abnormally enlarged uterus; pelvic examination reveals grapelike vesicles.
○ Histologic identification of hydatid vesicles after passage helps confirm diagnosis.
○ Ultrasonography shows grapelike structures rather than a fetus; use of a Doppler ultrasonic flowmeter demonstrates the absence of fetal heart tones.
○ Amniography reveals the absence of a fetus.
○ WBC count and ESR are increased.
○ Hb level, HCT, RBC count, PT, PTT, fibrinogen levels, and hepatic and renal function studies are abnormal.
○ Serum hCG level is elevated 100 days or more after the last menstrual period.
○ Serum human placental lactogen level is subnormal.

Hydrocephalus

○ Examination reveals an abnormally large head size for age.
○ Skull X-rays reveal thinning of the skull with separation of sutures and widening of the fontanels.
○ Ventriculography reveals enlargement of the brain's ventricles.
○ Angiography, CT scan, or MRI of the brain reveals areas of altered density and rules out intracranial lesions.

Hydronephrosis

○ KUB X-rays reveal bilateral kidney enlargement.
○ Renal ultrasonography reveals large, echo-free, central mass that compromises the renal cortex.
○ Excretory urography reveals abnormal kidneys.
○ Urine studies reveal the inability to concentrate urine, a decreased GFR, and, if infection exists, pyuria.

Hyperaldosteronism

○ Serum potassium level is persistently low (in the absence of edema, diuretic use, GI loss, or abnormal sodium intake).
○ Low plasma renin level after volume depletion by diuretic administration and upright posture and a high plasma aldosterone level after volume expansion by salt loading confirms primary hyperaldosteronism in a hypertensive patient without edema.
○ Serum HCO_3^- level is elevated, with ensuing alkalosis resulting from the loss of hydrogen and potassium in the distal tubules.
○ Serum and urine aldosterone levels are increased.
○ Plasma volume level is increased.
○ Adrenal angiography or CT scan reveals adrenal tumor.
○ Suppression testing reveals decreased plasma aldosterone and urine metabolites (secondary hyperaldosteronism) or normal plasma aldosterone and urine metabolites (primary hyperaldosteronism).
○ ECG reveals ST-segment depression and the presence of U waves, indicating hypokalemia.
○ CXR shows left ventricular hypertrophy from chronic hypertension.
○ CT scan, ultrasonography, or MRI identifies tumor location.

Hyperbilirubinemia

○ Examination reveals jaundice.
○ Serum bilirubin level is elevated.

Hyperemesis gravidarum

○ History includes uncontrolled nausea and vomiting that persist beyond the first trimester of pregnancy.
○ Examination reveals substantial weight loss.
○ Serum sodium, chloride, potassium, and protein levels are decreased.
○ BUN level is elevated.
○ Urinalysis reveals ketonuria and proteinuria.

Hyperlipoproteinemia

○ In type I (Fredrickson's hyperlipoproteinemia, fat-induced hyperlipemia, idiopathic familial):
 – Chylomicrons (very-low-density lipoproteins [VLDL], low-density lipoproteins [LDL], high-density lipoproteins [HDL]) are present in plasma 14 hours or more after last meal.
 – Serum chylomicron and triglyceride levels show high elevation; serum cholesterol level is slightly elevated.
 – Serum lipoprotein lipase level is decreased.
 – Leukocytosis is present.
○ In type II (familial hyperbetalipoproteinemia, essential familial hypercholesterolemia):
 – Plasma levels of LDL are increased.
 – Serum LDL and cholesterol levels are elevated.
 – Increased LDL level is detected by amniocentesis.
○ In type III (familial broad-beta disease, xanthoma tuberosum):
 – Serum beta-lipoprotein level is abnormal.
 – Cholesterol and triglyceride levels are elevated.
 – Glucose level is slightly elevated.
○ In type IV (endogenous hypertriglyceridemia, hyperbetalipoproteinemia):
 – Plasma VLDL level is elevated.
 – Plasma triglyceride level is moderately increased.
 – Serum cholesterol level is normal or slightly elevated.
 – Glucose tolerance is mildly abnormal.
 – History includes early coronary artery disease.
○ In type V (mixed hypertriglyceridemia, mixed hyperlipidemia):
 – Chylomicrons are present in plasma.
 – Plasma VLDL level is elevated.
 – Serum cholesterol and triglyceride level are elevated.

Hyperparathyroidism

○ Serum parathyroid hormone level is increased.
○ Serum calcium level is increased.
○ Urine cyclic adenosine monophosphate test reveals failure to respond to parathyroid hormone.
○ X-rays show diffuse demineralization of bones, bone cysts, outer cortical bone absorption, and subperiosteal erosion of the radial aspect of the middle fingers.
○ X-ray spectrophotometry demonstrates increased bone turnover.
○ Radioimmunoassay shows increased level of parathyroid hormone with accompanying hypercalcemia.
○ Serum phosphorus level is increased.
○ Serum and urine chloride, uric acid, creatinine, and alkaline phosphatase levels are increased; basal acid secretion is present.
○ Serum immunoreactive gastrin level is increased.

Hyperpituitarism

○ Growth hormone (GH) immunoassay shows increased plasma GH levels.
○ Glucose suppression test shows failure to suppress GH level to below accepted norm of 5 nanograms/ml (SI, 5 µg/L).
○ Skull X-rays, CT scan, arteriography, and pneumoencephalography reveal the presence and extent of a pituitary lesion.
○ Bone X-rays reveal a thickening of the cranium (especially of frontal, occipital, and parietal bones) and of the long bones, as well as osteoarthritis in the spine.

Hypersplenism

○ I.V. infusion of chromium-labeled RBCs or platelets reveals high spleen-liver ratio of radioactivity, indicating splenic destruction or sequestration.

- CBC shows decreased Hb levels, WBC count, and platelet count, and elevated reticulocyte count.
- Examination reveals splenomegaly.

Hypertension

- Serial blood pressure measurements on a sphygmomanometer are more than 140/90 mm Hg.
- Urinalysis reveals presence of protein, RBCs, WBCs, or glucose.
- Excretory urography may reveal renal atrophy.
- BUN and serum creatinine levels are normal or elevated, suggesting renal disease.

Hyperthyroidism

- Radioimmunoassay shows increased serum T_4 and T_3 levels.
- Thyroid scan reveals increased uptake of ^{131}I.
- Thyroid-releasing hormone (TRH) stimulation test reveals failure of the TSH level to rise within 30 minutes after administration of TRH.
- Autoantibody tests reveal presence of thyroid-stimulating Ig.

Hypervitaminoses A and D

- History includes accidental or misguided use of supplemental vitamin preparations.
- Serum vitamin A level is elevated.
- Serum vitamin D level is elevated.
- Serum carotene level is elevated.
- X-rays show calcification of tendons, ligaments, and subperiosteal tissues in hypervitaminosis D.

Hypoglycemia

- Blood glucose is decreased.
- c-peptide assay identifies fasting hypoglycemia.

Hypogonadism

- Serum and urine gonadotropin levels are increased in primary (hypergonadotropic) hypogonadism and decreased in secondary (hypogonadotropic) hypogonadism.
- Chromosomal analysis identifies the cause.
- Testicular biopsy and semen analysis reveal impaired spermatogenesis and low testosterone levels.
- X-rays and bone scans show delayed closure of epiphyses and immature bone age.

Hypoparathyroidism

- Radioimmunoassay shows decreased serum parathyroid hormone levels.
- Urine and serum calcium levels are decreased.
- Serum phosphorus level is increased.
- Urine creatinine level is decreased.
- X-rays show increased bone density and malformation.
- Cyclic adenosine monophosphate test result shows a 10- to 20-fold increase.
- ECG shows increased QT and ST intervals because of hypercalcemia.

Hypopituitarism

- Radioimmunoassay shows decreased plasma levels of some or all pituitary hormones.
- Serum T_4 level is decreased (with thyroid dysfunction).

- Arginine test reveals failure of hGH levels to rise after arginine infusion (with pituitary dysfunction).
- Insulin tolerance test reveals failure of stimulation or a blunted response of hGH levels (with hypothalamic-pituitary-adrenal axis dysfunction).
- Urine 17-KS level is decreased (with hypoadrenalism).
- Levels of serum pituitary hormones (FSH, LH, and TSH) are decreased.
- CT scan, pneumoencephalography, or cerebral angiography confirms the presence of tumors inside or outside the sella turcica.

Hypothermic injuries

- History includes severe and prolonged exposure to cold.
- Core body temperature is $< 95°$ F ($35°$ C).
- Physical examination shows burning, tingling, numbness, swelling, pain, and mottled blue-gray skin in exposed areas.

Hypothyroidism, in adults

- Radioimmunoassay shows low serum levels of thyroid hormones.
- Serum TSH level may be increased (because of thyroid insufficiency) or decreased (because of hypothalamic or pituitary insufficiency).
- Radioactive iodine uptake test reveals below normal percentages of iodine uptake.
- Radionuclide thyroid imaging reveals "cold spots."
- Thyroid ultrasonography identifies cysts or tumors.
- Serum antithyroid antibodies are elevated (in autoimmune thyroiditis).

Hypothyroidism, in children

- An elevated serum TSH level is linked to low T_3 and T_4 levels.
- Thyroid scan (^{131}I uptake test) shows decreased uptake levels and confirms the absence of thyroid tissue in athyroid children.
- Gonadotropin level is increased and compatible with sexual precocity in older children.
- Hip, knee, and thigh X-rays reveal absence of the femoral or tibial epiphyseal line and delayed skeletal development that's markedly inappropriate for the child's chronological age.

Hypovolemic shock

- History includes recent loss of blood volume.
- Blood pressure auscultation reveals mean arterial pressure under 60 mm Hg in adults and a narrowing pulse pressure.
- Blood studies show low Hb level and HCT, low RBC count, and low platelet levels.
- Serum potassium, sodium, LD, creatinine, and BUN levels are elevated.
- Urine specific gravity is increased.
- Urine osmolality is elevated.
- Urine creatinine level is decreased.

Idiopathic thrombocytopenic purpura

- Platelet count is markedly decreased.
- Bleeding time is prolonged.

- Bone marrow studies show an abundance of mega-karyocytes (platelet precursors) and a shortened circulating platelet survival time.

Impetigo
- Inspection reveals characteristic lesions.
- Microscopic visualization, Gram stain, or culture of exudate identifies *Staphylococcus aureus* as causative organism.
- WBC count may be elevated.

Infectious mononucleosis
- WBC count is elevated during 2nd and 3rd week of illness, with lymphocytes and monocytes making up 50% to 70% of WBCs (10% of lymphocytes are abnormal).
- Heterophil agglutination tests indicate the presence of heterophil antibodies; testing at 3- to 4-week intervals reveals a rise to four times normal levels.
- Indirect immunofluorescence shows antibodies to Epstein-Barr virus and cellular antigens.
- Liver function studies are abnormal.

Infertility, female
- History includes inability to achieve pregnancy after having regular intercourse, without contraception, for at least 1 year.
- Progesterone blood levels reveal a luteal phase deficiency.
- FSH level is decreased.
- Hysterosalpingography reveals tubal obstruction or uterine abnormalities.
- Endoscopy shows tubal obstruction or uterine abnormalities.
- Laparoscopy of abdominal and pelvic areas may reveal peritubular adhesions or ureterotubal obstruction.
- Postcoital (Sims-Huhner) test shows inadequate motile sperm cells in cervical fluid after intercourse.
- Immunologic or antibody test detects spermicidal antibodies in the sera of the female.

Infertility, male
- History includes abnormal sexual development, delayed puberty, or infertility in previous relationships.
- Medical history also includes prolonged fever, mumps, impaired nutritional status, previous surgery, or trauma to genitalia.
- Semen analysis reveals subnormal sperm counts, decreased sperm motility, abnormal morphology, or absence of viable spermatozoa.
- Urine 17-KS level is decreased.
- Serum testosterone level is decreased.

Influenza
- Nose and throat culture identifies the causative virus.
- Cold agglutinin titers are elevated.
- Serum antibody titers are increased.
- WBC count is decreased and lymphocytes are increased (uncomplicated cases).

Inguinal hernia
- History includes sharp or "catching" pain when lifting, straining, or coughing excessively, or following a recent pregnancy.

- Examination reveals a swelling or lump in the inguinal area.
- Palpation of the inguinal area, while the patient is performing Valsalva's maneuver, reveals pressure against the fingertip (indirect hernia) or pressure against the side of the finger (direct hernia).
- Abdominal X-ray rules out obstruction.
- WBC count may be elevated.

Intestinal obstruction
- History includes progressive, colicky abdominal pain and distention.
- Abdominal X-ray reveals the presence and location of intestinal gas or fluid.
- In X-ray, small-bowel obstruction appears as a typical "stepladder" pattern of alternating gas and fluid levels.
- In X-ray, large-bowel obstruction reveals a distended, air-filled colon or a closed loop of sigmoid with extreme distention.
- Serum sodium, chloride, and potassium levels may decrease because of vomiting.
- WBC count may be normal or slightly elevated if necrosis, peritonitis, or strangulation occurs.
- Serum amylase level may increase.
- Sigmoidoscopy, colonoscopy, or barium enema may help identify the cause of obstruction.

Intussusception
- Barium enema reveals characteristic coiled spring sign and delineates the extent of intussusception.
- Upright abdominal X-rays may show a soft-tissue mass and signs of complete or partial obstruction, with dilated loops of bowel.
- Elevated WBC count may indicate obstruction, strangulation, or bowel infarction.

Iodine deficiency
- Serum T_4 level is low, with high ^{131}I uptake.
- A 24-hour urine collection reveals low iodine levels.
- Serum TSH level is high.
- Radioiodine uptake test traces ^{131}I in the thyroid 24 hours after administration.

Iron deficiency anemia
- Bone marrow studies reveal depleted or absent iron stores and normoblastic hyperplasia.
- Hb level is decreased.
- HCT is decreased.
- Serum iron level is low, with high iron-binding capacity.
- Serum ferritin level is low.
- RBC count is low, with microcytic and hypochromic cells.
- GI studies rule out or confirm the bleeding.

Irritable bowel syndrome
- History includes diarrhea alternating with constipation and bowel upset related to diet or psychological stress.
- Sigmoidoscopy may reveal spastic contraction.
- Barium enema may reveal colonic spasm and tubular appearance of descending colon.
- Colonoscopy, rectal examination, or rectal biopsy may rule out other disorders.

○ Fecal tests for occult blood, parasites, and pathogenic bacteria are negative.

Junctional tachycardia

ECG findings include:
○ Atrial and ventricular rhythms are usually regular. The atrial rhythm may be difficult to determine if the P wave is hidden in the QRS complex.
○ Atrial and ventricular rates exceed 100 beats/minute (usually between 100 and 200 beats/minute). The atrial rate may be difficult to determine if the P wave is hidden in the QRS complex.
○ P wave is usually inverted. It may occur before or after the QRS complex, or may be hidden in the QRS complex.
○ If the P wave precedes the QRS complex, the PR interval is shortened ($<$ 0.12 second). Otherwise, the PR interval can't be measured.
○ Duration of QRS complex is within normal limits. The configuration is usually normal.
○ T-wave configuration is usually normal but may be abnormal if the P wave is hidden in the T wave. Fast rate may make the T wave indiscernible.
○ QT interval is usually within normal limits.

Keratitis

○ History includes recent infection of the upper respiratory tract accompanied by cold sores.
○ Slit-lamp examination reveals one or more small branchlike (dendritic) lesions (caused by herpes simplex virus).
○ Touching the cornea with cotton reveals reduced corneal sensation.

Kidney cancer

○ Renal ultrasonography and CT scan identify renal tumor.
○ Excretory urography, nephrotomography, and KUB X-ray identify renal tumor.
○ Liver function studies show increased alkaline phosphatase, bilirubin, and transaminase levels.
○ PT is prolonged.
○ Blood studies show anemia, polycythemia, hypercalcemia, and increased ESR.
○ Urinalysis reveals hematuria.
○ Antegrade urography and cytologic studies reveal malignancy.
○ Renal biopsy reveals malignant cells.
○ Radionuclide renal imaging reveals malignant tumor.

Kyphosis

○ History includes severe pain.
○ Examination reveals curvature of the thoracic spine and bone destruction.
○ X-rays reveal vertebral wedging, Schmorl's nodes, irregular plates and, possibly, mild scoliosis of 10 to 20 degrees.

Labyrinthitis

○ History includes nausea and vomiting, hearing loss, and severe vertigo from any movement of the head.
○ Examination reveals spontaneous nystagmus with jerking movements of the eyes toward the unaffected ear.

○ Culture of drainage identifies infective organism.
○ Audiometry reveals sensorineural hearing loss.
○ CT scan rules out brain lesion.

Laryngeal cancer

○ History includes hoarseness that lasts longer than 2 weeks.
○ Laryngoscopy reveals lesion.
○ Laryngeal tomography, CT scan, or laryngography defines the borders of a lesion.
○ Laryngeal biopsy reveals malignant cells.
○ CXR identifies metastasis.

Laryngitis

○ History includes hoarseness, ranging from mild to complete loss of voice.
○ Indirect laryngoscopy reveals red, inflamed and, occasionally, hemorrhagic vocal cords, with rounded rather than sharp edges, and exudate; bilateral swelling may be present, which restricts movement but doesn't cause paralysis.

Legionnaires' disease

○ Cultures of respiratory tract secretions and tissue culture identify *Legionella pneumophila*.
○ Direct immunofluorescence testing reveals *L. pneumophila*.
○ Indirect fluorescent serum antibody testing shows convalescent serum with a fourfold or greater rise in antibody titer for *L. pneumophila*.
○ CXR reveals patchy, localized infiltration, which progresses to multilobar consolidation, pleural effusions, and, in fulminant disease, opacification of the entire lung.
○ Blood studies show leukocytosis, increased ESR, and increases in alkaline phosphatase, ALT, and AST levels.
○ ABG analysis shows decreased Pao_2 and, initially, decreased $Paco_2$.
○ Bronchial washings, blood and pleural fluid cultures, and transtracheal aspirate studies rule out pulmonary infections.

Leprosy

○ Examination reveals skin lesions and muscular and neurologic deficits.
○ Biopsy of skin lesions, peripheral nerves, or smear of skin or ulcerated mucous membranes allows identification of *Mycobacterium leprae*.

Liver abscess

○ Liver scan reveals filling defects at the area of the abscess longer than ¾″ (2 cm).
○ Hepatic ultrasonography reveals defects caused by abscess.
○ CT scan reveals a low-density, homogenous area with well-defined borders.
○ CXR reveals the diaphragm on the affected side to be raised and fixed.
○ Blood tests show elevated levels of AST, ALT, alkaline phosphatase, and bilirubin.
○ Serum albumin is decreased.
○ WBC count is elevated.
○ Blood cultures and percutaneous liver aspiration identify causative organism.

○ Stool cultures and serologic and hemagglutination tests isolate *Entamoeba histolytica* (in amoebic abscesses).

Liver cancer
○ Needle biopsy or open biopsy reveals malignant cells.
○ AFP level is elevated in 70% of patients with hepatocellular carcinoma.
○ Liver scan shows filling defects.
○ Liver function tests are abnormal.
○ CXR rules out metastasis to lungs.
○ Arteriography may define large tumors.
○ Serum electrolyte measurements show increased levels of sodium.
○ Serum glucose and cholesterol levels are decreased.

Lower urinary tract infection
○ Microscopic urinalysis reveals RBC and WBC counts > 10 per high-power field.
○ Clean-catch urinalysis reveals bacterial count of more than 100,000/ml.
○ Voiding cystoureterography or excretory urography shows congenital anomalies predisposing the patient to urinary tract infections.

Lung abscess
○ Auscultation of the chest may reveal crackles and decreased breath sounds.
○ CXR shows a localized infiltrate with one or more clear spaces, usually containing air or fluid.
○ Percutaneous aspiration of an abscess or bronchoscopy may be used to obtain cultures to identify the causative organism.
○ Blood and sputum cultures and Gram stain identify causative organism.
○ WBC count is elevated.

Lung cancer
○ CXR reveals lesion or mass.
○ Sputum cytology reveals malignant cells.
○ Bronchoscopy reveals site of mass.
○ Biopsy reveals malignant cells.
○ Tissue biopsy reveals evidence of metastasis.

Lupus erythematosus
○ Examination reveals classic butterfly rash occurring over the nose and cheeks.
○ ANA, anti-DNA, and lupus erythematosus cell tests are positive.
○ Urine studies may show RBCs, WBCs, urine casts, sediment, and protein loss.
○ CXR reveals pleurisy or lupus pneumonitis.
○ Blood studies may show decreased serum complement 3 and complement 4 levels, indicating active disease; ESR is usually elevated; leukopenia, mild thrombocytopenia, and anemia may also be evident.
○ ECG may show a conduction defect (with cardiac involvement or pericarditis).
○ Renal biopsy identifies progression and extent of renal involvement.

Lyme disease
○ History includes recent travel to endemic areas or exposure to ticks.
○ Examination reveals the classic skin lesion called *erythema chronicum migrans,* beginning as a red macule or papule at the tick bite site and growing up to 2″ (5 cm), described as hot and pruritic, with bright red outer rims and white centers.
○ Mild anemia and elevated ESR, leukocyte count, serum IgM level, and AST level support the diagnosis.
○ Antibody titers, ELISA, or blood culture may reveal *Borrelia burgdorferi;* lumbar puncture with CSF analysis allows for identification of antibodies to *B. burgdorferi* (if Lyme disease involves the central nervous system).

Lymphocytopenia
○ Lymphocyte count is markedly decreased.
○ Bone marrow aspiration and lymph node biopsies identify the cause.

Magnesium imbalance
○ Hypomagnesemia:
  – Serum magnesium level is decreased.
  – Serum potassium and calcium levels are decreased.
  – ECG shows tachyarrhythmias, slightly prolonged PR interval, prolonged QT interval, slightly prolonged QRS complex, ST-segment depression, prominent U waves, and broad flattened T waves.
○ Hypermagnesemia:
  – Serum magnesium level is elevated.
  – Serum potassium and calcium levels are elevated.
  – ECG shows prolonged PR interval, prolonged QRS complex, and elevated T wave.

Malaria
○ History includes travel to an endemic area, recent blood transfusion, or I.V. drug use.
○ Blood smears reveal parasites in RBCs.
○ Indirect immunofluorescent serum antibody tests reveal malaria (2 weeks after onset).
○ CBC shows decreased Hb level and a normal or decreased WBC count.
○ Urinalysis reveals protein and WBCs in urine sediment.
○ Serum blood studies show a reduced platelet count, prolonged PT, prolonged PTT, and decreased plasma fibrinogen levels (in falciparum malaria).

Malignant brain tumor
○ Skull X-ray, brain scan, CT scan, or MRI reveals lesion.
○ Biopsy of lesion reveals malignant cells.
○ Lumbar puncture shows increased protein levels and decreased glucose levels in CSF; increased CSF pressure, indicating increased intracranial pressure; and, occasionally, tumor cells in CSF.

Malignant lymphoma
○ Examination reveals enlarged lymph nodes.
○ Biopsy of lymph nodes, tonsils, bone marrow, liver, bowel, or skin reveals malignant cells.
○ CXR; lymphangiography; liver, bone, and spleen scans; CT scan of the abdomen; and excretory urography show disease progression.
○ Serum uric acid level is normal or elevated.
○ Serum calcium level may be elevated, indicating bone lesions.

Malignant melanoma

○ Examination reveals skin lesion or nevus with recent changes in appearance.
○ Excisional biopsy and full-depth punch biopsy reveal malignant cells.
○ Urine test reveals melanin.

Mallory-Weiss syndrome

○ History includes recent bout of forceful vomiting followed by vomiting blood or passing blood rectally (after a few hours to several days).
○ Endoscopy identifies esophageal tear.
○ Angiography reveals bleeding site.
○ Serum HCT is decreased. (Measurements help to quantify blood loss.)

Mastitis and breast engorgement

○ History includes breast discomfort or other symptoms of inflammation in a lactating woman.
○ Examination reveals redness, swelling, warmth, hardness, tenderness, cracks or fissures of the nipple, and enlarged lymph nodes.
○ Cultures of expressed milk identify infective organism (generalized mastitis).
○ Cultures of breast skin identify infective organism (localized mastitis).

Mastoiditis

○ X-rays of the mastoid area reveal hazy mastoid air cells, and the bony walls between the cells appear decalcified.
○ Otoscopy reveals a dull, thickened, and edematous tympanic membrane, if the membrane isn't concealed by obstruction.
○ Culture and sensitivity tests identify causative organism.
○ Audiometry shows a conductive hearing loss.

Ménière's disease

○ History includes vertigo, tinnitus, and hearing loss or distortion.
○ Audiometric studies indicate a sensorineural hearing loss and loss of discrimination and recruitment.
○ MRI rules out brain lesions or tumors.
○ Auditory brain stem response test rules out cochlear or retrocochlear lesion as the cause of hearing loss.

Meningitis

○ Lumbar puncture reveals cloudy CSF, elevated CSF pressure, high protein level, and depressed glucose level.
○ CSF culture and sensitivity tests reveal gram-positive or gram-negative organisms.
○ CXR shows pneumonitis or lung abscess, tubercular lesions, or granulomas (secondary to fungal infection).
○ Sinus and skull X-rays may help identify cranial osteomyelitis, paranasal sinusitis, or skull fracture.
○ WBC count shows leukocytosis.
○ CT scan rules out cerebral hematoma, hemorrhage, or tumor.
○ Brudzinski's and Kernig's signs are positive.

Meningococcal infection

○ Blood, CSF, or lesion culture reveals *Neisseria meningitidis*.

○ Platelet and clotting levels are decreased (with skin or adrenal hemorrhages).

Menopause

○ History includes menstrual cycle irregularities.
○ Pap test results show changes indicating the influence of estrogen deficiency on vaginal mucosa.
○ Radioimmunoassay blood studies show decreased estrogen levels and plasma estradiol level of 0 to 30 pg/ml (SI, 9 to 92 pmol/L).
○ Pelvic examination, endometrial biopsy, and D&C rule out suspected organic disease.
○ Serum FSH level is 30 to 100 mIU/ml (SI, 30 to 100 IU/L).
○ Plasma LH level is 20 to 100 mIU/ml (SI, 20 to 100 IU/ml).

Metabolic acidosis

○ ABG analysis reveals:
  – $pH < 7.35$
  – $Paco_2$ normal
  – HCO_3^- level decreased.
○ Serum potassium level is usually elevated.
○ Blood glucose and serum ketone body levels are elevated (in diabetes mellitus).
○ Plasma lactic acid level is elevated (in lactic acidosis).

Metabolic alkalosis

○ ABG analysis reveals:
  – $pH > 7.45$
  – $Paco_2$ normal
  – HCO_3^- level increased.
○ Serum potassium, calcium, and chloride levels are usually decreased.

Mitral insufficiency

○ Cardiac catheterization may indicate signs of mitral insufficiency, including increased left ventricular end-diastolic volume and pressure, increased PAWP and atrial pressure, and decreased cardiac output.
○ CXR may demonstrate left atrial and ventricular enlargement, pulmonary venous congestion, and calcification of the mitral leaflets.
○ Echocardiography may reveal abnormal motion of the valve leaflets, left atrial enlargement, and a hyperdynamic left ventricle.
○ ECG may show left atrial and ventricular hypertrophy, sinus tachycardia, or atrial fibrillation.

Mitral stenosis

○ Cardiac catheterization shows a diastolic pressure gradient across the mitral valve and elevated left atrial and pulmonary artery pressures as well as an elevated PAWP. Catheterization may also reveal elevated right ventricular pressure, decreased cardiac output, and abnormal contraction of the left ventricle. This test may not be indicated in patients who have isolated mitral stenosis with mild symptoms.
○ CXR shows left atrial and left ventricular enlargement (in severe mitral stenosis), straightening of the left border of the cardiac silhouette, enlarged pulmonary arteries, dilation of the pulmonary veins of the upper lobes of the lungs, and mitral valve calcification.

- Echocardiography may disclose thickened mitral valve leaflets and left atrial enlargement.
- ECG can reveal atrial fibrillation, right ventricular hypertrophy, left atrial enlargement (in sinus rhythm), and right-axis deviation.

Multiple myeloma

- CBC shows moderate to severe anemia; differential may show 40% to 50% lymphocytes but seldom more than 3% plasma cells.
- Rouleaux formation is visible on differential smear results.
- Analysis of urine proteins reveals Bence Jones protein, proteinuria, and hypercalciuria.
- Serum calcium level is elevated.
- Serum electrophoresis shows an elevated globulin spike, which is electrophoretically and immunologically abnormal.
- Excretion tests show phenolsulfonphthalein level > 25% in 15 minutes, > 80% in 2 hours.
- Bone marrow aspiration detects myelomatous cells.
- KUB X-rays reveal bilateral renal enlargement.
- X-rays reveal multiple, sharply circumscribed osteolytic lesions, especially on the skull, pelvis, and spine.

Multiple sclerosis

- History includes multiple neurologic attacks with characteristic remissions and exacerbations.
- EEG results are abnormal.
- CSF analysis reveals elevated gamma globulin fraction of IgG (with normal serum gamma globulin levels).
- MRI reveals multifocal white matter lesions resulting from demyelination.
- Evoked potential studies show slowed conduction of nerve impulses (in 80% of patients).
- CT scan may show lesions within the brain's white matter.

Mumps

- History includes inadequate immunization and exposure to person infected with mumps.
- Examination reveals swelling and tenderness of the parotid glands and one or more of the other salivary glands.
- Antibody titer increases fourfold 3 weeks after acute phase of illness.
- Serum amylase level may be elevated.

Muscular dystrophy

- History includes progressive muscle weakness and evidence of genetic transmission.
- Muscle biopsy reveals fat and connective tissue deposits, degeneration and necrosis of muscle fibers, and, in Duchenne's and Becker's dystrophies, a deficiency of the muscle protein dystrophin.
- EMG shows short, weak bursts of electrical activity in affected muscles.
- Genetic testing identifies the gene defect (in some patients).
- Urine creatinine, serum CK, LD, ALT, and AST levels are elevated.

Myasthenia gravis

- History includes progressive muscle weakness and muscle fatigability that improves with rest.
- Tensilon test result is positive, showing improved muscle function after an I.V. injection of edrophonium or neostigmine.
- Serum acetylcholine receptor antibodies test result is positive in symptomatic adults.
- EMG reveals motor unit potentials that are initially normal but progressively diminish in amplitude with continuing contractions.
- CXR or CT scan may show a thymoma.

Myelitis and acute transverse myelitis

- WBC count is normal or slightly elevated.
- CSF analysis may show normal or increased lymphocyte and protein levels and allows for isolation of the causative agent.
- Throat washings may reveal the causative virus (in poliomyelitis).
- CT scan or MRI may rule out spinal tumor.
- Examination may reveal focal neck and back pain with development of paresthesia and sensory loss.

Myocardial infarction

- History includes substernal chest pain, with radiation.
- Serial 12-lead ECG may be normal or inconclusive during the first hours after a myocardial infarction (MI); may reveal serial ST-segment depression (in subendocardial MI) and ST-segment elevation and Q waves (in transmural MI).
- Cardiac enzyme tests reveal elevated CK levels, with CK-MB isoenzyme > 5% of total CK over a 72-hour period.
- Cardiac protein tests reveal elevated troponin T and I levels. Elevations of troponin I are specific for myocardial injury.
- Echocardiography shows ventricular wall dyskinesia (with a transmural MI).
- Radioisotope scans using I.V. technetium 99m pertechnetate show "hot spots," indicating damaged muscle.
- Myocardial perfusion imaging with thallium-210 reveals a "cold spot" in most patients during the first few hours after a transmural MI.

Myocarditis

- History includes recent febrile upper respiratory tract infection, viral pharyngitis, or tonsillitis.
- Cardiac examination reveals supraventricular and ventricular arrhythmias, S_3 and S_4 gallops, a faint S_1, possibly a murmur of mitral insufficiency, and a pericardial friction rub (in patients with pericarditis).
- Endomyocardial biopsy reveals histologic changes consistent with myocarditis.
- Cardiac enzyme levels, including CK, CK-MB, serum AST, and LD, are elevated.
- WBC count and ESR are elevated.
- Antibody titers such as ASO are elevated.
- ECG shows diffuse ST-segment and T-wave abnormalities, conduction defects, and other ventricular and supraventricular arrhythmias.
- Cultures of stool, throat, pharyngeal washings, or other body fluids identify the causative bacteria or virus.

Necrotizing enterocolitis

- Anteroposterior and lateral abdominal X-rays reveal nonspecific intestinal dilation and, in later stages, gas or air in the intestinal wall.
- Platelet count is decreased.
- Serum sodium level is decreased.
- Serum bilirubin levels (indirect, direct, and total) may be elevated.
- Blood and stool cultures are positive for *Escherichia coli, Clostridia, Salmonella, Pseudomonas,* or *Klebsiella.*
- Hb level is decreased.
- PT and PTT are prolonged.
- Fibrin degradation products are increased.
- Guaiac test detects occult blood in stool.

Nephrotic syndrome

- Urinalysis shows marked proteinuria and reveals increased number of hyaline, granular, and waxy, fatty casts and oval fat bodies.
- Renal biopsy provides histologic identification of the lesion.
- T_3 resin uptake percentage is high with a low or normal free T_4 level.
- Serum protein electrophoresis reveals decreased albumin and gamma globulin levels and markedly increased alpha$_2$ and beta globulin levels.
- Serum triglyceride, phospholipid, and cholesterol levels are elevated.

Neurogenic bladder

- History includes neurologic disease or spinal cord injury.
- CSF analysis shows increased protein level indicating cord tumor; increased gamma globulin level may indicate multiple sclerosis.
- X-rays of the skull and vertebral column show fracture, dislocation, congenital anomalies, or metastasis.
- Myelography shows spinal cord compression.
- EMG confirms presence of peripheral neuropathy.
- Cystometry reveals abnormal micturition and vesical function.
- External sphincter EMG reveals detrusor-external sphincter dyssynergia.
- Voiding cystourethrography reveals neurogenic bladder.
- Whitaker test reveals bladder abnormality.

Obesity

- Observation and comparison of height and weight to a standardized table reveals weight exceeding ideal body weight by 20% or more. In morbid obesity, body weight > 200% of standard range.
- Measurement of the thickness of subcutaneous fat folds with calipers reveals excess body fat.

Optic atrophy

- Slit-lamp examination reveals a pupil that reacts sluggishly to direct light stimulation.
- Ophthalmoscopy shows pallor of the nerve head from loss of microvascular circulation in the disk and deposit of fibrous or glial tissue.
- Visual field testing reveals a scotoma and, possibly, major visual field impairment.

Orbital cellulitis

- Examination reveals eyelid edema and purulent discharge.
- Culture of eye discharge identifies *Streptococcus, Staphylococcus,* or *Pneumococcus* as the causative organism.

Osteoarthritis

- History includes deep, aching joint pain, particularly after exercise or weight bearing, usually relieved by rest; and morning stiffness that lasts less than 30 minutes.
- Examination may reveal nodes in the distal and proximal joints that become red, swollen, and tender.
- X-rays reveal narrowing of the joint space or margin, cystlike bony deposits in joint space and margins, sclerosis of the subchondral space, joint deformity because of degeneration or articular damage, bony growths at weight-bearing areas, and fusion of joints.

Osteomyelitis

- History includes sudden pain in the affected bone accompanied by tenderness, heat, swelling, and restricted movement.
- Blood cultures identify *Staphylococcus aureus, Streptococcus pyogenes, Pneumococcus, Pseudomonas aeruginosa, Escherichia coli,* or *Proteus vulgaris* as the causative organism.
- Bone scan shows infection site in early stages of illness.
- X-ray reveals abnormal areas of calcification (may not be evident until 2 to 3 weeks).
- ESR is elevated.
- WBC count reveals leukocytosis.

Osteoporosis

- X-rays may reveal typical degeneration in the lower thoracic and lumbar vertebrae; vertebral bodies may appear flattened and more dense than normal.
- Photon absorptiometry reveals deterioration of bone mass.
- Bone biopsy reveals thin, porous, but otherwise normal-looking bone.
- Bone densitometry reveals decreased bone density.

Otitis externa

- Examination reveals pain on palpation of the tragus or auricle.
- Otoscopy reveals a swollen external ear canal (sometimes to the point of complete closure), periauricular lymphadenopathy (tender nodes in front of the tragus, behind the ear, or in the upper neck), and, occasionally, regional cellulitis.
- In fungal otitis externa, examination reveals thick, red epithelium after removal of growth.
- Microscopic examination or culture and sensitivity tests identify *Aspergillus niger* or *Candida albicans* as the causative organism for fungal otitis externa; *Pseudomonas, Proteus vulgaris, Streptococcus,* or *Staphylococcus aureus* as the causative organism for bacterial otitis externa.
- In chronic otitis externa, examination of the ear canal reveals a thick red epithelium.

Otitis media

○ In acute suppurative otitis media:
    – Otoscopy reveals obscured or distorted bony landmarks of the tympanic membrane.
    – Pneumatoscopy may show decreased tympanic membrane mobility.
    – Examination shows that pulling on the auricle doesn't exacerbate the pain.
○ In acute secretory otitis media:
    – Otoscopy demonstrates tympanic membrane retraction, causing the bony landmarks to appear more prominent, with clear or amber fluid detected behind the tympanic membrane, possibly with a meniscus and bubbles.
    – If hemorrhage into the middle ear has occurred, the tympanic membrane appears blue-black.
○ In chronic otitis media:
    – History discloses recurrent or unresolved otitis media; otoscopy shows thickening and sometimes scarring, and decreased mobility of the tympanic membrane.
    – Pneumatoscopy reveals decreased or absent tympanic membrane movement.
○ History of recent air travel or scuba diving suggests barotitis media.

Ovarian cancer

○ Examination reveals abdominal mass.
○ CT scan shows the abdominal tumor.
○ Pelvic ultrasonography reveals mass.
○ Exploratory laparotomy with biopsy reveals malignant cells.
○ Transvaginal ultrasonography shows ovarian enlargement and growth.
○ Transvaginal Doppler color flow imaging reveals ovarian growth.
○ CEA level is elevated.
○ Serum hCG level is elevated in a nonpregnant woman.
○ Barium enema reveals obstruction and size of tumor.

Ovarian cysts

○ Pelvic ultrasonography reveals ovarian mass.
○ Laparoscopy reveals a bubble on the surface of the ovary, which may be clear, serous, or mucus-filled.
○ The hCG titers are highly elevated (with theca-lutein cysts).
○ Progesterone level is elevated.

Paget's disease

○ X-rays reveal increased bone expansion and density (before overt symptoms appear).
○ Bone scan reveals radioisotope concentrates in areas of active lesions (early pagetic lesions).
○ Bone biopsy reveals characteristic mosaic pattern.
○ Serum alkaline phosphatase level is highly elevated.
○ Urine hydroxyproline level is increased.

Pancreatic cancer

○ Ultrasonography, CT scan, or MRI reveals mass size and locations.
○ Laparotomy and biopsy reveal malignant cells.
○ Barium swallow shows neoplasm or changes in the duodenum or stomach indicating carcinoma of the head of the pancreas.
○ Endoscopic retrograde cholangiopancreatography shows mass and abnormalities of the pancreatic ducts.
○ Cholangiography shows obstructed bile ducts caused by carcinoma of the pancreas.
○ Secretin test reveals an abnormal volume of secretions, HCO_3^-, or enzymes.
○ Serum alkaline phosphatase and serum bilirubin levels are markedly elevated with biliary obstruction.
○ Plasma insulin immunoassay reveals measurable serum insulin (with islet cell tumors).
○ Stool guaiac testing shows presence of occult blood, suggesting ulceration in GI tract or ampulla of Vater.

Parkinson's disease

○ History and examination reveal muscle rigidity, akinesia, and pill-roll tremors, which increase during stress or anxiety.
○ Urinalysis reveals decreased dopamine levels.
○ Evoked potential studies reveal bilateral abnormal P100 latencies.

Pediculosis

○ In pediculosis capitis, examination reveals oval, grayish nits that can't be shaken loose.
○ In pediculosis corporis, examination reveals characteristic skin lesions and nits found on clothing.
○ In pediculosis pubis, examination reveals nits attached to pubic hairs, which feel coarse and grainy to the touch.

Pelvic inflammatory disease

○ History includes recent sexual intercourse, intrauterine device insertion, childbirth, or abortion.
○ Cultures and Gram stain of secretions from the endocervix or cul-de-sac identify *Neisseria gonorrhoeae* or *Chlamydia trachomatis* as the infective organism.
○ Ultrasonography reveals an adnexal or uterine mass.
○ Laparoscopy reveals infection or abscess.

Penetrating chest wounds

○ Examination reveals chest wound and a sucking sound during breathing.
○ Hb level and HCT are markedly decreased, indicating severe blood loss.
○ CXR reveals pneumothorax and possible lung laceration.

Penile cancer

○ Tissue biopsy reveals malignant cells.
○ Examination reveals small circumscribed lesion, pimple, or sore on the penis, which may be accompanied by pain, hemorrhage, dysuria, purulent discharge, and urinary meatal obstruction (in late stages).

Peptic ulcers

○ History includes heartburn, midepigastric pain, or gastric bleeding.
○ Endoscopy reveals ulcer.
○ Upper GI X-rays show abnormalities in the mucosa.
○ Gastric secretory studies show hyperchlorhydria.
○ Biopsy rules out malignancy.
○ Stool guaiac testing reveals presence of occult blood.

Perforated eardrum

○ History includes trauma to the ear accompanied by severe earache and bleeding from the ear.
○ Direct visual inspection of the tympanic membrane with an otoscope confirms perforation; flaccid, thin areas indicate previous perforation.
○ Audiometric testing reveals hearing loss.

Pericarditis

○ Chest auscultation reveals pericardial friction rub.
○ Pericardial fluid culture identifies infecting organism (in bacterial or fungal pericarditis).
○ ECG reveals ST-segment elevation in the standard limb leads and most precordial leads without the significant changes in QRS morphology that occur with myocardial infarction.
○ ECG may also reveal atrial ectopic rhythms and diminished QRS voltage (with pericardial effusion).
○ Echocardiography reveals an echo-free space between the ventricular wall and the pericardium (with pericardial effusion).

Peritonitis

○ Examination reveals severe abdominal pain with direct or rebound tenderness.
○ Abdominal X-rays reveal edematous and gaseous distention of the small and large bowel, or air in the abdominal cavity (with perforation of a visceral organ).
○ Paracentesis reveals bacteria in fluid, exudate, pus, blood, or urine.
○ CXR may show elevation of the diaphragm.
○ Elevated WBC count indicates leukocytosis.

Pernicious anemia

○ Hb level is markedly decreased.
○ RBC count is decreased.
○ Mean corpuscular volume is increased.
○ Serum vitamin B_{12} is decreased.
○ Schilling test reveals < 3% excretion of radioactive B_{12} in urine collected over 24 hours.
○ Bone marrow aspiration reveals erythroid hyperplasia with increased numbers of megaloblasts but few normally developing RBCs.
○ Gastric analysis reveals absence of free hydrochloric acid after histamine or pentagastrin injection.

Pharyngitis

○ Examination reveals generalized redness and inflammation of the posterior wall of the pharynx and red, edematous mucous membranes studded with white or yellow follicles.
○ Exudate is usually confined to the lymphoid areas of the throat, sparing the tonsillar pillars.
○ Throat culture identifies the infective organism, most commonly *Streptococcus*.

Phenylketonuria

○ Family history indicates presence of autosomal recessive gene.
○ Guthrie screening test reveals elevated serum phenylalanine levels.
○ Drops of 10% ferric chloride solution added to a wet diaper turn a deep, bluish-green color, indicating phenylpyruvic acid in the urine.

○ Low serum tyrosine level in neonates age 1 week or less.
○ Urine testing reveals presence of phenylpyruvic acid.

Pheochromocytoma

○ History includes acute episodes of hypertension, headache, sweating, and tachycardia, particularly in a patient with hyperglycemia, glycosuria, and hypermetabolism.
○ A 24-hour urine test reveals increased excretion of total free catecholamine and its metabolites, vanillylmandelic acid, and metanephrine.
○ Total plasma catecholamines may show levels 10 to 50 times higher than normal.
○ Angiography reveals an adrenal medullary tumor.
○ Excretory urography with nephrotomography, adrenal venography, or CT scan helps localize a tumor.

Phosphate imbalance

○ Hypophosphatemia: Serum phosphate level decreased.
○ Hyperphosphatemia: Serum phosphate level increased.

Pituitary tumors

○ Skull X-rays with tomography reveal enlargement of the sella turcica or erosion of its floor and enlargement of the paranasal sinuses and mandible, thickened cranial bones, and separated teeth (if growth hormone predominates).
○ Carotid angiography reveals displacement of the anterior cerebral and internal carotid arteries (with enlarging tumor mass).
○ Intracranial CT scan may confirm the existence of the adenoma and accurately depict its size.
○ Orbital radiography shows superior orbital fissure enlargement.
○ MRI of the brain differentiates healthy, benign, and malignant tissues and blood vessels.
○ Tangent screen examination reveals bitemporal hemianopsia.
○ hGH levels are elevated.
○ Urine 17-hydroxycorticosteroid levels are elevated.

Placenta previa

○ History includes painless bleeding during third trimester of pregnancy.
○ Pelvic ultrasonography reveals abnormal echo patterns.
○ Pelvic examination (performed only immediately before delivery) reveals only cervix and minimal descent of fetal presenting part.

Plague

○ History includes exposure to rodents (bubonic plague).
○ Culture of skin lesion reveals *Yersinia pestis*.
○ WBC count is elevated; WBC differential reveals increased polymorphonuclear leukocytes.
○ CXR reveals fulminating pneumonia (with pneumonic plague).

Platelet function disorders

○ History includes excessive bleeding or bruising.
○ Bleeding time is prolonged.
○ PT and PTT are normal.

- Platelet count is normal.
- Platelet function tests measure platelet release reaction and aggregation to identify defective mechanism.

Pleural effusion and empyema

- CXR reveals radiopaque fluid in dependent regions.
- Lung auscultation reveals decreased breath sounds.
- Percussion detects dullness over the effused area, which doesn't change with respiration.
- Pleural fluid analysis reveals:
  - transudative effusions with decreased specific gravity
  - empyema with acute inflammatory WBCs and microorganisms
  - empyema or rheumatoid arthritis with extremely decreased pleural fluid glucose levels.

Pleurisy

- Auscultation of the chest reveals characteristic pleural friction rub — a coarse, creaky sound heard during late inspiration and early expiration, directly over the area of pleural inflammation.
- Palpation may reveal coarse vibration.

Pneumocystis carinii pneumonia

- History includes an immunocompromising condition (such as HIV infection, leukemia, and lymphoma) or procedure (such as organ transplantation).
- Histologic studies of sputum specimen confirm presence of *P. carinii.*
- CXR shows slowly progressing, fluffy infiltrates and occasional nodular lesions or a spontaneous pneumothorax.
- Gallium scan of the chest shows increased uptake over the lungs even if the CXR appears relatively normal.

Pneumonia

- Percussion reveals dullness; auscultation discloses crackles, wheezing, or rhonchi over the affected lung area as well as decreased breath sounds and decreased vocal fremitus.
- CXR discloses infiltrates, confirming the diagnosis.
- Gram stain and culture of sputum show acute inflammatory cells.
- WBC count indicates leukocytosis in bacterial pneumonia and a normal or low count in viral or mycoplasmal pneumonia.
- Blood cultures reflect bacteremia and help determine the causative organism.

Pneumothorax

- History includes sudden, sharp pain on affected side and shortness of breath.
- CXR reveals air in the pleural space and, possibly, mediastinal shift.
- Examination reveals overexpansion and rigidity of the affected chest side; in tension pneumothorax, examination may reveal jugular vein distention.
- Palpation of chest reveals crackling beneath the skin and decreased vocal fremitus.
- Chest auscultation reveals decreased or absent breath sounds on the affected side.
- ABG analysis reveals pH < 7.35, decreased Pao_2, and increased $Paco_2$.

Poisoning

- History includes ingestion, inhalation, injection of, or skin contact with a poisonous substance.
- Toxicologic studies (including drug screens) reveal poison in the mouth, vomitus, urine, stool, blood, or on the victim's hands or clothing.
- CXR (with inhalation poisoning) reveals pulmonary infiltrates or edema, or aspiration pneumonia (with petroleum distillate inhalation).

Poliomyelitis

- Throat culture or stool examination reveals poliovirus.
- Convalescent serum antibody titers rise fourfold from acute titers.
- CSF pressure and protein levels may be slightly increased.
- WBC count may be elevated initially, mostly because of polymorphonuclear leukocytes, which constitute 50% to 90% of the total count; thereafter, the number of cells is diminished with mononuclear leukocytes accounting for most of them.

Polycystic kidney disease

- Family history includes polycystic kidney disease.
- Physical examination reveals large bilateral, irregular masses in the flanks.
- Excretory or retrograde urography reveals enlarged kidneys, with elongation of pelvis, flattening of the calyces, and indentations caused by cysts.
- Excretory urography of the neonate shows poor excretion of contrast agent.
- Ultrasonography, CT scan, and radioisotope scans of the kidney show kidney enlargement and presence of cysts. CT scan also demonstrates multiple areas of cystic damage.

Polycythemia, secondary

- RBC mass is increased.
- Hb level, HCT, mean corpuscular volume, and mean corpuscular Hb level are increased.
- Urine erythropoietin and blood histamine levels are elevated.
- Arterial oxygen saturation may be decreased.
- Bone marrow biopsies reveal hyperplasia confined to the erythroid series.

Polycythemia, spurious

- Hb level, HCT, and RBC count are elevated.
- RBC mass is normal.
- WBC count is normal.

Polycythemia vera

- Laboratory studies confirm polycythemia vera by showing increased RBC mass and normal arterial oxygen saturation in association with splenomegaly or two of the following:
  - elevated platelet count
  - elevated WBC count
  - elevated leukocyte alkaline phosphatase level
  - elevated serum B_{12} elevation or unbound B_{12}-binding capacity.
- Bone marrow biopsy reveals panmyelosis.
- Serum and urine uric acid levels are increased.

Polymyositis and dermatomyositis

○ Muscle biopsy reveals necrosis, degeneration, regeneration, and interstitial chronic lymphocytic infiltration.
○ Muscle enzyme levels (CK, aldolase, AST) are elevated and not attributable to hemolysis of RBCs or hepatic or other diseases.
○ Urine creatine level is markedly increased.
○ EMG reveals polyphasic short-duration potentials, fibrillation, and bizarre high-frequency repetitive changes.
○ ANA test result is positive.

Porphyrias

○ Screening tests reveal porphyrins or their precursors (such as aminolevulinic acid and porphobilinogen) in urine, stool, blood, or skin biopsy.
○ Urinary lead level is > 400 mg/24-hour collection.

Potassium imbalance

○ In hypokalemia:
  – Serum potassium level is decreased.
  – ECG shows flattened T waves, elevated U waves, and depressed ST segment.
○ In hyperkalemia:
  – Serum potassium level is increased.
  – ECG shows tall, tented T waves; widened QRS complex; prolonged PR interval; flattened or absent P waves; and depressed ST segment.

Precocious puberty, in girls

○ X-rays of hands, wrists, knees, and hips reveal advanced bone age and possible premature epiphyseal closure.
○ Androstenedione level is > 3 nanograms/ml.
○ Radioimmunoassays for estrogen and FSH levels are abnormally high for patient's age.
○ Vaginal smear for estrogen secretion reveals abnormally high levels.
○ Urinary test for gonadotropic activity and excretion of 17-KS show abnormally high levels.

Precocious puberty, in boys

○ Detailed patient history reveals recent growth pattern, behavior changes, family history of precocious puberty, or hormonal ingestion.
○ In true precocious puberty:
  – Serum levels of LH, FSH, and corticotropin are elevated.
  – Plasma tests for testosterone demonstrate elevated levels (equal to those of an adult male).
  – Evaluation of ejaculate indicates true precocity by revealing presence of live spermatozoa.
  – Skull and hand X-rays reveal advanced bone age.
○ In pseudoprecocious puberty:
  – Chromosome analysis may demonstrate an abnormal pattern of autosomes and sex chromosomes.
  – Steroid excretion levels, such as testosterone and 24-hour 17-KS levels, are elevated.

Pregnancy

○ Serum hCG level is elevated.
○ Urine hCG level is elevated.
○ Pelvic examination reveals changes to uterus consistent with pregnancy.

○ Ultrasonography reveals presence of fetus in the uterus.

Pregnancy-induced hypertension

○ In mild preeclampsia:
  – Systolic blood pressure is 140 mm Hg or shows a rise of 30 mm Hg or more above the patient's normal systolic pressure (measured on two occasions, 6 hours apart).
  – Diastolic blood pressure is 90 mm Hg or shows a rise of 15 mm Hg or more above the patient's normal diastolic pressure (measured on two occasions, 6 hours apart).
  – Proteinuria (urine protein level) is increased.
○ In severe preeclampsia:
  – Blood pressure measurements are 160/110 mm Hg or higher (measured on two occasions, 6 hours apart) on bed rest.
  – Proteinuria is increased.
  – Patient has oliguria (urine output ≤ 400 ml/24 hours).
  – Deep tendon reflexes are hyperactive.
○ In eclampsia:
  – History and examination reveal signs of severe preeclampsia and seizure activity.
  – Ophthalmoscope examination may reveal vascular spasm, papilledema, retinal edema or detachment, and arteriovenous nicking or hemorrhage.

Premature labor

○ Physical examination reveals rhythmic uterine contractions, cervical dilation and effacement, possible rupture of membranes, expulsion of cervical mucus plug, and bloody discharge occurring before expected date of delivery.
○ Vaginal examination reveals progressive cervical effacement and dilation.
○ Pelvic ultrasonography identifies fetus's position in the mother's pelvis.

Premature rupture of the membranes

○ History includes passage of amniotic fluid before the expected date of delivery.
○ Examination reveals amniotic fluid in the vagina.
○ Nitrazine paper test of fluid from posterior fornix turns deep blue.
○ Fluid from posterior fornix smeared on slide and allowed to dry takes on a fernlike pattern.

Premenstrual syndrome

○ History includes menstruation-related symptoms, including mild to severe personality changes, nervousness, irritability, fatigue, lethargy, depression, breast tenderness or bloating, joint pain, headache, diarrhea, and exacerbations of skin, respiratory, or neurologic problems recorded for 2 to 3 months.
○ Serum estrogen and progesterone levels are normal (ruling out hormonal imbalance).

Pressure ulcers

○ History includes immobility, malnutrition, or skin irritation.
○ Inspection reveals skin breakdown.

○ Wound culture and sensitivity identify the infecting organisms.

Proctitis
○ In acute proctitis, sigmoidoscopy reveals edematous, bright-red or pink rectal mucosa that's thick, shiny, friable, and possibly ulcerated.
○ In chronic proctitis, sigmoidoscopy reveals thickened mucosa, loss of vascular pattern, and stricture of the rectal lumen.
○ Biopsy reveals absence of malignant cells.

Prostatic cancer
○ Digital rectal examination reveals small, hard nodule in prostate area.
○ Serum prostate-specific antigen level is elevated.
○ Serum prostatic acid phosphatase is elevated.
○ Serum alkaline phosphatase level is elevated.
○ Biopsy reveals malignant cells.

Prostatitis
○ Examination reveals tender, indurated, swollen, and warm prostate.
○ Urine samples, taken at start of voiding, midstream, after a physician massages the prostate, and final specimen, reveal a significant increase in colony count of the prostatic specimens.

Protein-calorie malnutrition
○ History includes poor diet lacking in protein.
○ Examination reveals a small, gaunt, and emaciated appearance with no adipose tissue; dry and "baggy" skin; general weakness; sparse hair and dull brown or reddish yellow eyes; and slow pulse rate and respirations.
○ Anthropometry reveals height and weight less than 80% of standard for the patient's age and sex, and below standard arm circumference and triceps skinfolds.
○ Serum albumin and prealbumin levels are markedly decreased.

Pseudomembranous enterocolitis
○ History includes sudden onset of copious, watery, or bloody diarrhea; abdominal pain; and fever.
○ Rectal biopsy reveals characteristic histologic changes, such as plaquelike lesions on the colonic mucosal surface consisting of fibrinopurulent exudate and necrotic epithelial debris.
○ Stool cultures identify *Clostridium difficile*.

Pseudomonas infections
○ Culture of blood, spinal fluid, urine, exudate, or sputum identifies the *Pseudomonas* organism.
○ Gram stain reveals gram-negative bacillus.

Psoriasis
○ Examination reveals dry, cracked, encrusted lesions (erythematous plaques) accompanied by itching on the scalp, chest, elbows, knees, back, or buttocks.
○ Skin biopsy reveals psoriasis.
○ Serum uric acid level is elevated, without indications of gout.

Puerperal infection
○ History includes fever within 48 hours after delivery or abortion.
○ Culture of lochia, blood, incisional exudate (from cesarean incision or episiotomy), uterine tissue, or material collected from the vaginal cuff reveals *Streptococcus*, coagulase-negative staphylococci, *Clostridium perfringens, Bacteroides fragilis,* or *Escherichia coli* as the causative organism.
○ Elevated WBC count shows leukocytosis and an increased sedimentation rate.
○ Pelvic examination reveals induration without purulent discharge (parametritis).
○ Culdoscopy shows adnexal induration and thickening.

Pulmonary edema
○ Examination reveals respiratory distress.
○ Chest auscultation reveals crackles in the lung fields.
○ ABG analysis usually shows decreased Pao_2 (hypoxia) and variable $Paco_2$. Profound respiratory alkalosis and acidosis may occur; metabolic acidosis occurs when cardiac output is low.
○ CXR shows diffuse haziness of the lung fields and, often, cardiomegaly and pleural effusions.
○ Pulmonary artery catheterization reveals elevated PAWP.

Pulmonary embolism and infarction
○ Lung scan reveals perfusion defects in areas beyond occluded vessels.
○ Pulmonary angiography reveals emboli.
○ CXR shows areas of atelectasis, elevated diaphragm and pleural effusion, prominent pulmonary artery, and, occasionally, a wedge-shaped infiltrate suggesting pulmonary infarction.
○ ECG may show right-axis deviation; right bundle-branch block; tall, peaked P waves; ST-segment depression; T-wave inversion; and supraventricular tachycardia.
○ Auscultation reveals right ventricular gallop, increased intensity of the pulmonic component of S_2, crackles, and pleural rub at the site of the embolism.
○ ABG analysis may show decreased Pao_2 and $Paco_2$.

Pulmonary hypertension
○ Pulmonary artery catheterization reveals elevated pulmonary systolic pressure and PAWP.
○ Pulmonary angiography reveals filling defects in pulmonary vasculature.
○ PFTs may show decreased flow rates and increased residual volume (with underlying obstructive disease); total lung capacity may be decreased (with underlying restrictive disease).
○ ABG analysis reveals decreased Pao_2.
○ ECG shows right-axis deviation and tall or peaked P waves in inferior leads (with right ventricular hypertrophy).

Pulmonic insufficiency
○ Cardiac catheterization shows pulmonic insufficiency, increased right ventricular pressure, and associated cardiac defects.
○ CXR shows enlargement of the right ventricle and pulmonary artery.

- Echocardiography shows right ventricular or right atrial enlargement.
- ECG may be normal in mild cases or show right ventricular or right atrial hypertrophy.

Pulmonic stenosis

- Cardiac catheterization reveals increased right ventricular pressure, decreased pulmonary artery pressure, and an abnormal valve orifice.
- CXR usually reveals a normal heart size and normal lung vascularity, although the pulmonary arteries may be evident. With severe obstruction and right-sided heart failure, CXR may reveal right atrial and ventricular enlargement.
- Echocardiography reveals the abnormality in the pulmonic valve.
- ECG results may be normal in mild cases, or they may indicate right-axis deviation and right ventricular hypertrophy. High amplitude P waves in leads II, III, aV_F, and V_1 indicate right atrial enlargement.

Rabies

- History reveals recent animal bite.
- Throat and saliva culture identifies virus.
- Serum fluorescent rabies antibody test result is positive.
- WBC count is elevated, with increased polymorphonuclear and large mononuclear cells.
- Urine glucose, acetone, and protein levels are elevated.

Radiation exposure

- History includes exposure to radiation, along with nausea and vomiting.
- CBC reveals decreased Hb level and HCT, and decreased WBC, platelet, and lymphocyte counts.
- Bone marrow studies reveal blood dyscrasias.
- X-rays may show bone necrosis.
- Geiger counter measurement reveals the amount of radiation in an open wound.

Rape-trauma syndrome

- History includes being the victim of a rape or attempted rape, accompanied by feelings of anxiety, grief, anger, fear, or revenge.
- Examination shows signs of physical trauma.
- X-rays may reveal fractures.
- Vaginal specimen is positive for semen.
- Fingernail and pubic hair scrapings and semen analysis may help to identify alleged rapist.

Raynaud's disease

- History and examination reveal changes in skin color induced by cold or stress, bilateral involvement, minimal cutaneous gangrene or absence of gangrene, and clinical symptoms of 2 years' duration or more.
- Cold stimulation test demonstrates Raynaud's syndrome.
- Arteriography reveals no underlying secondary disease.

Rectal polyps

- Proctosigmoidoscopy or colonoscopy reveals type, size, and location of polyps.
- Biopsy reveals histologic changes consistent with polyps.

- Barium enema reveals polyps high in the colon.
- Stool guaiac testing reveals presence of occult blood.

Rectal prolapse

- In complete prolapse, visual examination reveals the full thickness of the bowel wall and, possibly, the sphincter muscle protruding and mucosa falling into bulky, concentric folds.
- In partial prolapse, visual examination reveals only partially protruding mucosa and a smaller mass of radial mucosal folds.

Reiter's syndrome

- History includes venereal or enteric infection.
- HLA testing reveals presence of HLA-B27.
- Analysis of urethral discharge and synovial fluid reveals numerous WBCs, mostly polymorphonuclear leukocytes.
- Synovial fluid analysis reveals increased complement and protein; fluid is grossly purulent.
- WBC count and ESR are elevated.

Renal calculi

- KUB X-rays reveal renal calculi.
- Excretory urography reveals size and location of calculi.
- Kidney ultrasonography reveals obstructive changes.
- Urine culture may reveal urinary tract infection.
- Urinalysis may be normal or may show increased specific gravity, acid or alkaline pH (depending on the type of stone), hematuria, crystals, casts, and pyuria (with or without WBCs).
- A 24-hour urine collection shows presence of calcium oxalate, phosphorus, or uric acid.

Renal infarction

- Urinalysis reveals proteinuria and microscopic hematuria.
- Urine enzyme levels, especially LD and alkaline phosphatase, are elevated.
- Serum ALT, AST, and LD levels are elevated.
- Excretory urography shows diminished or absent excretion of contrast dye (with vascular occlusion or urethral obstruction).
- Isotopic renal scan demonstrates absent or reduced blood flow to the kidneys.
- Renal arteriography reveals infarction.

Renal tubular acidosis

- Urine studies reveal pH > 6.0, low titratable acids and ammonia content, increased HCO_3^- and potassium levels, and low specific gravity.
- Blood pH is < 7.35.
- Serum HCO_3^- level is decreased.
- Serum potassium and phosphorus levels are decreased.

Renal vein thrombosis

- Excretory urography reveals enlarged kidneys and diminished excretory function (in acute thrombosis); urography contrast medium seems to "smudge" necrotic renal tissue.

- In chronic thrombosis, excretory urography may show ureteral indentations that result from collateral venous channels.
- Renal venography reveals filling defects.
- Renal biopsy reveals characteristic histologic changes.
- Urinalysis reveals gross or microscopic hematuria, proteinuria ($>$ 2 g/day in chronic disease), casts, and oliguria.
- Blood studies show leukocytosis, hypoalbuminemia, hyperlipemia, and thrombocytopenia.

Respiratory acidosis
- ABG analysis reveals:
  - pH $<$ 7.35
  - increased $Paco_2$
  - normal HCO_3^- level.

Respiratory alkalosis
- ABG analysis reveals:
  - pH $>$ 7.45
  - decreased $Paco_2$
  - normal HCO_3^- level.

Respiratory distress syndrome, adult
- ABG analysis reveals:
  - pH $<$ 7.35
  - decreased Pao_2 (despite oxygen therapy)
  - increased $Paco_2$.
- Serial CXRs initially show bilateral infiltrates; later X-rays reveal ground-glass appearance and eventually "whiteouts" of both lungs.

Respiratory distress syndrome, child
- CXR reveals fine reticulonodular pattern (may be normal for first 6 to 12 hours after birth).
- ABG measurements reveal pH $<$ 7.35 and Pao_2 $<$ 75 mm Hg (SI, $<$ 10.03 kPa).
- Chest auscultation reveals normal or diminished air entry and crackles (rare in early stages).
- Amniocentesis reveals lecithin-sphingomyelin ratio of $<$ 2 (used to assess risk of respiratory distress syndrome).

Respiratory syncytial virus infection
- Cultures of nasal and pharyngeal secretions identify respiratory syncytial virus infection (not always reliable).
- Serum antibody titers elevated (maternal antibodies may impair results before age 6 months).
- CXR may reveal pneumonia.
- Indirect immunofluorescence and ELISA tests are positive.

Restrictive cardiomyopathy
- CXR reveals massive cardiomegaly, affecting all four chambers of the heart, pericardial effusion, and pulmonary congestion (advanced stage).
- Echocardiography detects increased left ventricular muscle mass and differences in end-diastolic pressures between the ventricles.
- Carotid palpation reveals blunt carotid upstroke with small volume.
- Cardiac catheterization demonstrates increased left ventricular end-diastolic pressure.

- ECG may show low-voltage complexes, hypertrophy, atrioventricular conduction defects, or arrhythmias.

Retinal detachment
- Ophthalmoscopy reveals the usually transparent retina to be gray and opaque.
- In severe detachment, ophthalmoscopy reveals folds in the retina and a ballooning out of the area.
- Indirect ophthalmoscopy reveals retinal tears.
- Ocular ultrasonography shows a dense sheetlike echo on a B-scan.

Retinitis pigmentosa
- Family history indicates a possible predisposition to retinitis pigmentosa.
- Electroretinography shows a retinal response time slower than normal or absent.
- Visual field testing (using a tangent screen) detects ring scotomata.
- Fluorescein angiography shows white dots (areas of dyspigmentation) in the epithelium.
- Ophthalmoscopy may initially show normal fundi but later reveals characteristic black pigmentary disturbance.

Reye's syndrome
- History includes recent viral disorder with varying degrees of encephalopathy and cerebral edema.
- ALT level is elevated.
- AST level is elevated.
- Liver biopsy reveals fatty droplets uniformly distributed throughout cells.
- PT and PTT are prolonged.
- CSF analysis reveals decreased WBCs; in coma, CSF pressure is increased.
- Serum ammonia level is elevated.
- Serum fatty acid and lactate levels are elevated.
- Serum glucose level is normal or low.

Rheumatic fever and rheumatic heart disease
- History includes streptococcal infection.
- Examination reveals joint pain and swelling and one or more of the following symptoms: carditis, polyarthritis, chorea, erythema marginatum, or subcutaneous nodules.
- C-reactive protein is positive.
- ASO titer is elevated (within 2 months of onset).
- Echocardiography and cardiac catheterization reveal valvular damage.
- Cardiac enzymes may be elevated (in severe carditis).

Rheumatoid arthritis, adult
- Serum RF titer is above 1:80.
- X-rays reveal bone demineralization and soft-tissue swelling (in early stages), loss of cartilage and narrowing of joint spaces, and cartilage and bone destruction, erosion, subluxations, and deformities.
- Synovial fluid analysis reveals increased volume and turbidity but decreased viscosity and complement 3 and complement 4 levels, and elevated WBC count.
- ESR is increased.
- CBC shows moderate decrease in RBC count, Hb level, and HCT, and slight leukocytosis.

Rheumatoid arthritis, juvenile

○ History includes persistent joint stiffness and pain in the morning or after periods of inactivity.
○ ANA test may be positive in patients who have pauciarticular juvenile rheumatoid arthritis (JRA) with chronic iridocyclitis.
○ RF is present in 15% of patients with JRA, as compared with 85% of patients with rheumatoid arthritis.
○ Early changes seen on X-ray include soft-tissue swelling, effusion, and periostitis in affected joints.
○ In later X-ray studies, osteoporosis and accelerated bone growth may appear, followed by subchondral erosions, joint space narrowing, bone destruction, and fusion.
○ CBC usually shows decreased Hb levels, increased neutrophil count, increased platelet levels, and elevated ESR.
○ Blood studies reveal elevated C-reactive protein, serum haptoglobin, Ig, and complement 3 levels.
○ HLA testing reveals presence of HLA-B27, forecasting later development of ankylosing spondylitis.

Rocky Mountain spotted fever

○ History includes tick bite or travel to a tick-infested area.
○ Complement fixation test shows a fourfold rise in convalescent antibodies compared to acute titers.
○ Blood culture identifies *Rickettsia rickettsii*.
○ Decreased platelet count indicates thrombocytopenia during second week of illness.
○ WBC count is elevated during second week of illness.

Roseola infantum

○ History includes temperature of 103° to 105° F (39.4° to 40.4° C) followed by rash 48 hours after fever subsides.
○ Examination reveals maculopapular, nonpruritic rash that blanches on pressure.

Rubella

○ History includes exposure to infected person.
○ Examination reveals maculopapular rash, beginning on the face and spreading to the trunk and arms and legs.
○ Cell cultures of throat, blood, urine, and CSF reveal rubella virus.
○ Convalescent serum antibody titers rise fourfold from acute titers.

Rubeola

○ History includes exposure to person infected with the measles virus (patient may be unaware of contact).
○ Examination reveals the pathognomonic Koplik's spots.
○ Cultures of blood, nasopharyngeal secretions, and urine identify measles virus (during the febrile period).
○ Serum antibody titers appear within 3 days after onset of the rash and reach peak titers 2 to 4 weeks later.

Salmonellosis

○ Culture of blood, stool, urine, bone marrow, pus, or vomitus identifies gram-negative bacilli of the genus *Salmonella*.
○ Widal's test reveals a fourfold rise in titer.

Sarcoidosis

○ Kveim skin test confirms discrete epithelioid cell granuloma.
○ CXR reveals bilateral hilar and right paratracheal adenopathy with or without diffuse interstitial infiltrates; occasionally, large nodular lesions appear in lung parenchyma.
○ Lymph node, skin, or lung biopsy reveals noncaseating granulomas with negative cultures for mycobacteria and fungi.
○ PFTs show decreased total lung capacity and compliance and decreased diffusing capacity.
○ Tuberculin skin test results, fungal serologies, sputum cultures for mycobacteria and fungi, and biopsy cultures are negative.

Scabies

○ Visual examination of the contents of the scabietic burrow may reveal itch mite.
○ Mineral oil placed over the burrow, followed by superficial scraping and examination of expressed material, reveals ova or mite feces.
○ Pediculicide administration to affected area clears skin.

Scarlet fever

○ History includes recent streptococcal pharyngitis.
○ Examination reveals "strawberry tongue" and fine erythematous rash that blanches on pressure.
○ Pharyngeal culture identifies group A beta-hemolytic streptococci.
○ CBC reveals granulocytosis and, possibly, a reduced RBC count.

Scoliosis

○ Examination reveals unequal shoulder height, elbow levels, and heights of iliac crests, and asymmetry of the paraspinal muscles.
○ Scoliosometer (an apparatus for measuring curvature of the spinal column) reveals angle of trunk rotation to be abnormal.
○ Anterior, posterior, and lateral spinal X-rays reveal degree of curvature and flexibility of the spine.

Septal perforation and deviation

○ History and examination reveal whistle on inspiration, rhinitis, epistaxis, nasal crusting, and watery discharge.
○ Inspection of the nasal mucosa with bright light and a nasal speculum reveals perforation or deviation.

Septic arthritis

○ Synovial fluid Gram stain and culture or biopsy of synovial membrane reveals gram-positive cocci *(Staphylococcus aureus, Streptococcus pyogenes, Streptococcus pneumoniae,* or *Streptococcus viridans)*, gram-negative cocci *(Neisseria gonorrhoeae* or *Haemophilus influenzae)*, or gram-negative bacilli *(Escherichia coli, Salmonella,* or *Pseudomonas)* as the causative organism.
○ Joint fluid analysis reveals gross pus or watery, cloudy fluid of decreased viscosity, with markedly elevated WBCs/ml, containing primarily neutrophils.

- Culture of skin exudate, sputum, urethral discharge, feces, urine, blood, or nasopharyngeal secretions is positive for causative organism.
- Skeletal X-rays show distention of joint capsules, followed by narrowing of joint space (indicating cartilage damage) and erosions of bone (joint destruction).
- WBC count may be elevated with many polymorphonuclear cells; ESR is increased.

Septic shock
- History includes infection accompanied by fever, confusion, nausea, vomiting, and hyperventilation.
- Blood cultures identify gram-negative bacteria (*Escherichia coli, Klebsiella, Enterobacter, Pseudomonas, Proteus,* or *Bacteroides*) or gram-positive bacteria (*Streptococcus pneumoniae, S. pyogenes,* or *Actinomyces*) as the causative organism.
- WBC count is elevated.
- Pulmonary artery catheterization reveals decreased central venous pressure, pulmonary artery pressures, wedge pressure, cardiac output (may be initially elevated), and systemic vascular resistance.
- ABG analysis reveals decreased $Paco_2$, low or normal HCO_3^- level, and pH > 7.45 (in early stages); as shock progresses, decreasing $Paco_2$, Pao_2, HCO_3^- level, and pH indicate the development of metabolic acidosis with hypoxemia.
- Serum BUN and creatinine levels increase; creatinine clearance decreases.
- ECG reveals ST-segment depression, inverted T waves, and arrhythmias.

Shigellosis
- Microscopic examination of fresh feces may reveal mucus, RBCs, and polymorphonuclear leukocytes.
- Stool culture identifies *Shigella.*
- Hemagglutinating antibodies may be present, indicating severe infection.

Sickle cell anemia
- Family history includes homozygous inheritance.
- Stained blood smear reveals sickle cells.
- Hb electrophoresis reveals HbS.
- CBC may reveal decreased RBC count and elevated WBC and platelet counts.
- ESR is decreased.
- Serum iron level is increased.

Sideroblastic anemias
- Bone marrow aspirate reveals ringed sideroblasts.
- Microscopic examination reveals RBCs that are hypochromic or normochromic and slightly macrocytic; RBC precursors may be megaloblastic, with anisocytosis and poikilocytosis.
- Hb level is decreased.
- Serum iron and transferrin levels are increased.

Silicosis
- History includes occupational exposure to silica dust.
- Examination reveals decreased chest expansion, diminished intensity of breath sounds, areas of hyporesonance and hyperresonance, fine to medium crackles, and tachypnea (with chronic silicosis).
- CXR reveals:

– small, discrete, nodular lesions distributed throughout both lung fields but typically concentrated in the upper lung zones
– enlarged hilar lung nodes that exhibit "eggshell" calcification (in simple silicosis)
– one or more conglomerate masses of dense tissue (in complicated silicosis).
- PFTs reveal:
– reduced FVC (in complicated silicosis)
– reduced FEV_1 (in obstructed disease)
– reduced maximal voluntary ventilation (in restrictive and obstructive disease)
– reduced diffusing capacity for carbon monoxide when fibrosis destroys alveolar walls and oblates pulmonary capillaries, or when fibrosis thickens the alveolar capillary membrane.
- ABG measurements reveal:
– decreased or normal $Paco_2$ in the early stages; may increase as restrictive pattern develops
– significantly decreased Pao_2 in the late stages of chronic or complicated disease.

Sinus bradycardia
- ECG reveals:
– regular atrial and ventricular rhythm
– atrial and ventricular rates < 60 beats/minute
– P wave of normal size and configuration with a P wave preceding each QRS complex
– PR interval within normal limits and constant
– QRS complex of normal duration and configuration
– T wave of normal size and configuration
– QT interval within normal limits, but possibly prolonged.

Sinus tachycardia
- ECG reveals:
– regular atrial and ventricular rhythms
– atrial and ventricular rates > 100 beats/minute (usually between 100 and 160 beats/minute)
– P wave of normal size and configuration with a P wave preceding each QRS complex
– PR interval within normal limits and constant
– QRS complex of normal duration and configuration
– T wave of normal size and configuration
– QT interval within normal limits, but commonly shortened.

Sinusitis
- Nasal examination reveals inflammation and pus.
- Sinus X-rays reveal cloudiness in the affected sinus, air-fluid levels, or thickened mucosal lining.
- Transillumination allows inspection of the sinus cavities by passing a light through them; in sinusitis, purulent drainage prevents passage of light.

Sjögren's syndrome
- History and examination reveal two of the following three conditions: xerophthalmia, xerostomia (with salivary gland biopsy showing lymphocytic infiltration), and autoimmune or lymphoproliferative disorder.
- ESR is elevated.
- Hypergammaglobulinemia is present.
- RF test result is positive (75% to 90% of patients).
- ANA test result is positive (50% to 80% of patients).

- Schirmer's tearing test result is positive for tearing deficiency.
- Lower lip biopsy shows salivary gland infiltration by lymphocytes.

Skull fractures

- History includes recent head trauma.
- Skull X-ray shows fracture (minor vault fractures may not be visible).
- Neurologic examination evaluates cerebral function.
- Cerebral angiography reveals vascular disruption from internal pressure and injury.
- CT scan, echoencephalography, air encephalography, MRI, and radioactive scanning reveal cranial nerve injury or intracranial hemorrhage from ruptured blood vessels. These test results also help to localize subdural or intracerebral hematomas.

Sodium imbalance

- In hyponatremia:
  - Serum sodium level is decreased.
  - Urine sodium level is > 100 mEq/24 hours (SI, > 100 mmol/d).
  - Serum osmolality is low.
- In hypernatremia:
  - Serum sodium level is elevated.
  - Serum osmolality is high.

Spinal cord defects

- Examination reveals a protruding sac on the spine.
- Transillumination of sac reveals meningocele.
- Spinal X-ray shows bone defect (in spina bifida occulta).
- CT scan reveals hydrocephalus (in 90% of patients).

Spinal injuries without cord damage

- History includes trauma, metastatic disease, infection, or endocrine disorder.
- Physical examination reveals the location and level of injury.
- Spinal X-rays reveal fracture.
- Myelography reveals spinal mass.
- Lumbar puncture reveals increased CSF pressure, indicating spinal trauma or lesion.

Spinal neoplasms

- Lumbar puncture reveals clear yellow CSF with increased protein levels.
- X-rays show distortions of intervertebral foramina, changes in vertebrae or collapsed areas in the vertebral body, and localized enlargement of the spinal canal indicating an adjacent block.
- Myelography identifies the level of the lesion.
- CT scan and MRI show cord compression and tumor location.
- Radioisotope bone scan reveals evidence of metastatic invasion of the vertebrae by showing increased osteoblastic activity.
- Biopsy reveals malignant cells.

Sprains and strains

- History includes recent injury or chronic overuse of affected area.
- Examination reveals pain (local with a sprain, sharp and transient with a strain), swelling, and ecchymoses (rapid onset with a sprain; may take several days with a strain).
- X-ray of the affected body part doesn't indicate fracture.

Squamous cell carcinoma

- Examination reveals ulcerated nodule with indurated base.
- Biopsy reveals squamous cell carcinoma.

Staphylococcal scalded-skin syndrome

- Examination reveals three-stage progression of erythema, exfoliation, and desquamation.
- Skin lesions are positive for group 2 *Staphylococcus aureus*.

Stomatitis and other oral infections

- Examination reveals inflammation of the oral mucosa or surrounding area.
- Smear of ulcer exudate reveals fusiform bacillus or spirochete as the causative organism (in Vincent's angina).

Stroke

- Patient reports sudden onset of motor or sensory impairment.
- CT scan detects structural abnormalities, edema, and lesions, such as nonhemorrhagic infarction and aneurysms.
- Cerebral angiography reveals disruption or displacement of the cerebral circulation by occlusion or hemorrhage.
- Ultrasonography of carotid and cerebral arteries may reveal occlusion.
- Digital abstraction angiography evaluates the patency of the cerebral vessels and identifies their position in the head and neck. It also detects and evaluates lesions and vascular abnormalities.
- PET scan provides data on cerebral metabolism and cerebral blood flow changes, especially in ischemic stroke.
- Single-photon emission tomography identifies cerebral blood flow and helps diagnose cerebral infarction.
- EEG may detect reduced electrical activity in an area of cortical infarction.
- Transcranial Doppler studies examine the size of intracranial vessels and the direction of blood flow.
- MRI allows evaluation of the lesion's location and size.

Sudden infant death syndrome

- Autopsy reveals:
  - small or normal adrenal glands
  - petechiae over the visceral surface of the pleura, within the thymus, and in the epicardium
  - well-preserved lymphoid structures
  - pathologic changes suggesting chronic hypoxemia
  - edematous, congestive lungs fully expanded in the pleural cavities
  - liquid blood in the heart (not clotted)
  - curd from the stomach inside the trachea.

Syndrome of inappropriate antidiuretic hormone

○ History includes recent weight gain despite anorexia, nausea, and vomiting.
○ Serum osmolality is decreased.
○ Serum sodium level is decreased.
○ Urine sodium level is increased.

Syphilis

○ History includes sexual contact with partner who has syphilis.
○ Culture of lesion identifies *Treponema pallidum*.
○ The fluorescent treponemal antibody-absorption test identifies antigens of *T. pallidum* in tissue, ocular fluid, CSF, tracheobronchial secretions, and exudates from lesions.
○ Venereal Disease Research Laboratory (VDRL) slide test and rapid plasma reagin test are positive, detecting nonspecific antibodies.
○ In neurosyphilis:
  – CSF analysis reveals elevated total protein level.
  – VDRL slide test result is reactive.

Tay-Sachs disease

○ Family history includes Eastern European Jewish ancestry or history of the disease. Diagnostic screening may detect carriers of autosomal recessive gene.
○ Serum analysis shows hexosaminidase A deficiency.
○ Ophthalmic examination reveals optic nerve atrophy and a distinctive cherry-red spot on the retina.

Tendinitis and bursitis

○ History includes unusual strain or injury 2 to 3 days before onset of pain or heat-aggravated joint pain.
○ Examination reveals localized pain and inflammation at joint.
○ X-rays (in late stages) reveal bony fragments, osteophyte sclerosis, or calcium deposits.
○ Arthrography is usually normal, with occasional small irregularities on the undersurface of the tendon.

Testicular cancer

○ Physical examination reveals testicular mass.
○ Transillumination confirms tumor.
○ Biopsy reveals malignant cells.
○ Excretory urography reveals ureteral deviation (indicates node involvement).
○ Testosterone level is increased.
○ Urine testing indicates presence of hCG.
○ Serum AFP and beta-hCG levels are increased.

Testicular torsion

○ Physical examination reveals tense, tender swelling in the scrotum or inguinal canal and hyperemia of the overlying skin.
○ Doppler ultrasonography reveals testicular torsion.

Tetanus

○ History includes trauma and absence of tetanus immunization.
○ Meningitis, rabies, phenothiazine or strychnine toxicity, or other conditions that mimic tetanus are ruled out.
○ Cultures are positive for an anaerobic, spore-forming rod clostridium tetani.

Tetralogy of Fallot

○ Echocardiography reveals septal overriding of the aorta, the ventricular septal defect (VSD), and pulmonic stenosis, and detects hypertrophy of walls of the right ventricle.
○ Cardiac catheterization shows pulmonic stenosis, the VSD, and the overriding aorta and rules out other cyanotic heart defects.
○ Auscultation reveals a loud systolic heart murmur, which may diminish or obscure the pulmonic component of S_2.
○ Palpation may reveal a cardiac thrill at the left sternal border and an obvious right ventricular impulse.
○ ECG shows right ventricular hypertrophy, right-axis deviation, and, possibly, right atrial hypertrophy.
○ CXR reveals decreased pulmonary vascular marking (depending on the severity of pulmonary obstruction) and a boot-shaped cardiac silhouette.

Thalassemia

○ Thalassemia major reveals:
  – lowered RBC count and Hb level
  – elevated reticulocyte level
  – elevated bilirubin and urinary and fecal urobilinogen levels
  – low serum folate level
  – X-rays of the skull and long bones showing a thinning and widening of the marrow space
  – Hb electrophoresis revealing a significant rise in HbF and a slight increase in HbA_2
  – peripheral blood smear revealing extremely thin and fragile RBCs, pale nucleated RBCs, and marked anisocytosis.
○ Thalassemia intermedia reveals:
  – hypochromic and microcytic RBCs.
○ Thalassemia minor reveals:
  – hypochromic and microcytic RBCs
  – Hb electrophoresis revealing a significant increase in HbA_2 and a moderate rise in HbF.

Thoracic aortic aneurysm

○ CXR reveals widening of the aorta.
○ CT scan or MRI reveals location and size of aneurysm.
○ Aortography reveals the lumen of the aneurysm, its size and location, and, in dissecting aneurysm, the false lumen.

Thrombocytopenia

○ Platelet count is markedly decreased.
○ Bleeding time is prolonged.
○ PT and PTT are normal.
○ Bone marrow studies reveal an increased number of megakaryocytes (platelet precursors) and shortened platelet survival.

Thrombophlebitis

○ Homans' sign is positive.
○ Doppler ultrasonography reveals reduced blood flow to a specific area and obstruction to venous flow.
○ Plethysmography reveals decreased circulation distal to affected area.
○ Phlebography reveals filling defects and diverted blood flow.

Thyroid cancer
- History includes exposure to radiation therapy or a family history of thyroid cancer.
- Examination reveals an enlarged, palpable node in the thyroid gland, neck, lymph nodes of the neck, or vocal cords.
- Thyroid scan reveals a "cold," nonfunctioning nodule.
- Thyroid biopsy reveals a well-encapsulated, solitary nodule of uniform but abnormal structure.
- Serum calcitonin assay reveals an elevated fasting calcitonin and an abnormal response to calcium stimulation (with medullary cancer).

Thyroiditis
- Autoimmune thyroiditis reveals:
  - positive precipitin test
  - high titers of thyroglobulin
  - microsomal antibodies present in serum.
- Subacute granulomatous thyroiditis reveals:
  - elevated ESR
  - increased thyroid hormone levels
  - decreased thyroidal radioiodine uptake.

Tonsillitis
- Examination reveals generalized inflammation of the pharyngeal wall and swollen tonsils that project from between the pillars of the fauces and exude white or yellow follicles, with inflamed uvula.
- Purulent drainage appears when pressure is applied to the tonsillar pillars.
- Throat culture identifies infective organism, commonly beta-hemolytic streptococci.

Toxic shock syndrome
- Culture of vaginal discharge or lesions identifies *Staphylococcus aureus.*
- CK level is elevated.
- BUN level is elevated.
- Serum creatinine level is elevated.
- Platelet count is markedly decreased.

Toxoplasmosis
- History includes exposure to a cat or ingestion of uncooked meat.
- Blood, body fluid, or tissue tests positive for *Toxoplasma gondii* antibodies.
- *T. gondii* is identified in mice after their inoculation with specimens of patient's body fluids, blood, and tissue.

Tracheoesophageal fistula and esophageal atresia
- Examination reveals respiratory distress and drooling in a neonate.
- Catheter (#10 or #12 French) meets obstruction when passed through the nose at 4″ to 5″ (10 to 12.5 cm) distal from the nostrils.
- CXR demonstrates the position of the catheter and can show a dilated, air-filled upper esophageal pouch, pneumonia in the right upper lobe, or bilateral pneumonitis.
- Abdominal X-ray reveals gas in the bowel in a distal fistula (but none in a proximal fistula or atresia without fistula).
- Cinefluorography defines the upper pouch by allowing visualization on a fluoroscopic screen and differentiates between overflow aspiration from a blind end (atresia) and aspiration because of passage of liquids through a tracheoesophageal fistula.

Transposition of the great arteries
- Echocardiography reveals the reversed position of the aorta and the pulmonary artery and records echoes from both semilunar valves simultaneously because of the aortic valve displacement.
- Cardiac catheterization reveals decreased oxygen saturation in left ventricular blood and aortic blood; increased right atrial, right ventricular, and pulmonary artery oxygen saturation; and right ventricular systolic pressure equal to systemic pressure.
- Dye injection during catheterization reveals the transposed vessels and the presence of any other cardiac defects.
- CXR shows right atrial and ventricular enlargement causing the heart to appear oblong (within days to weeks) and increased vascular markings, except when pulmonic stenosis exists.
- ECG reveals right-axis deviation and right ventricular hypertrophy (may be normal in a neonate).
- ABG measurements reveal hypoxia and secondary metabolic acidosis.

Trichinosis
- History includes ingestion of raw or improperly cooked pork or pork products.
- Stool contains mature worms and larvae during the invasion stage.
- Skeletal muscle biopsy reveals encysted larvae 10 days after ingestion.
- Antibody titers are elevated during acute and convalescent stage.
- During acute stages, serum liver enzymes (AST, LD, and CK) are elevated.
- Eosinophil count is elevated.

Trichomoniasis
- History includes sexual contact with person who has trichomoniasis.
- Examination reveals vaginal erythema; edema; frank excoriation; a frothy, malodorous, greenish yellow vaginal discharge; and, rarely, a thin, gray pseudomembrane over the vagina.
- Cervical examination shows punctate cervical hemorrhages, giving the cervix a strawberry-like appearance.
- Microscopic examination of vaginal or seminal discharge identifies *Trichomonas vaginalis.*
- Culture of clear urine specimens may also reveal *T. vaginalis.*

Tricuspid insufficiency
- Cardiac catheterization shows markedly decreased cardiac output; mean right atrial and right ventricular end-diastolic pressures may be elevated.
- CXR reveals right atrial and ventricular enlargement.
- Echocardiography shows right ventricular dilation and paradoxical septal motion. It may also show prolapsing or flailing of the tricuspid valve leaflets. Doppler

echocardiography provides estimates of pulmonary artery and right ventricular systolic pressure.
○ ECG reveals right atrial hypertrophy and right or left ventricular hypertrophy. ECG may also reveal atrial fibrillation or incomplete right bundle-branch block.

Tricuspid stenosis
○ Cardiac catheterization shows increased right atrial pressure and decreased cardiac output; it may also show an increased pressure gradient across the tricuspid valve.
○ CXR reveals right atrial and superior vena cava enlargement.
○ Echocardiography reveals a thick tricuspid valve with reduced mobility and right atrial enlargement.
○ ECG shows right atrial hypertrophy and right ventricular hypertrophy. Atrial fibrillation may be present. Tall, peaked P waves are seen in lead II, and prominent, upright P waves are seen in lead V_1, indicating right atrial enlargement.

Trigeminal neuralgia
○ History includes pain in the superior mandibular or maxillary area, without sensory or motor impairment.
○ Examination reveals splinting on the affected side of the face while talking.
○ Skull X-rays, tomography, and CT scans rule out sinus or tooth infections and tumors.

Tuberculosis
○ Stains and cultures of sputum, CSF, urine, and abscess drainage reveal heat-sensitive, nonmotile, aerobic, acid-fast bacilli.
○ CXR shows nodular lesions, patchy infiltrates, cavity formation, scar tissue, and calcium deposits.
○ Auscultation reveals crepitant crackles, bronchial breath sounds, wheezes, and whispered pectoriloquy.
○ Chest percussion reveals dullness over the affected area.
○ Tuberculin skin test reveals that the patient has been infected with tuberculosis.

Typhus, epidemic
○ Weil-Felix reaction reveals a fourfold rise in agglutination titer 8 to 12 days after infection.
○ Complement fixation for group-specific typhus antigens is positive 8 to 12 days after infection.

Ulcerative colitis
○ History includes recurrent bloody diarrhea and GI disturbances.
○ Sigmoidoscopy shows increased mucosal friability, decreased mucosal detail, and thick inflammatory exudate.
○ Biopsy reveals histologic changes characteristic of ulcerative colitis.
○ Colonoscopy identifies the extent of the disease.
○ Barium enema identifies the extent of the disease and detects complications.
○ ESR increases, correlating with severity of attack.
○ Serum potassium and magnesium levels are decreased.
○ CBC shows decreased Hb level and leukocytosis.
○ Serum albumin level is decreased.
○ PT is prolonged.

Undescended testes
○ Examination of scrotum reveals impalpable testes, either unilateral or bilateral.
○ Buccal smear identifies genetic sex by showing a male sex chromatin pattern.
○ Serum gonadotropin levels confirm the presence of testes.

Urticaria and angioedema
○ History includes exposure to medications, food, and environmental influences.
○ Skin testing reveals specific allergens.
○ Serum complement 4 and complement 1 esterase inhibitor levels are decreased (confirming hereditary angioedema).
○ CBC, urinalysis, ESR, and CXR rule out inflammatory infections.

Uterine cancer
○ Endometrial, cervical, and endocervical biopsies reveal malignant cells.
○ Schiller's test shows cancerous tissues resisting stain.
○ Cervical biopsies and endocervical curettage identify degree of cervical involvement.
○ Barium enema reveals bladder or rectal involvement.

Uterine leiomyomas
○ History includes abnormal endometrial bleeding.
○ Pelvic palpation reveals round or irregular mass.
○ Ultrasonography shows a dense mass.
○ Hysterosalpingography reveals asymmetric uterus.
○ Laparoscopy reveals lumps on the uterus.
○ CBC reveals decreased RBC count, Hb level, and HCT.

Uveitis
○ Slit-lamp examination reveals a "flare and cell" pattern, which looks like light passing through smoke, and an increased number of cells over the inflamed area.
○ Examination with a special lens, slit-lamp, and ophthalmoscope identifies active inflammatory fundus lesions involving the retina and choroid.
○ Serologic tests indicate toxoplasmosis (in posterior uveitis).

Vaginal cancer
○ Pap test reveals abnormal cells.
○ Vaginal examination, aided by Lugol's solution, reveals lesion.
○ Lesion biopsy reveals malignant cells.
○ Gallium scan shows abnormal gallium activity.

Vaginismus
○ History and examination rule out physical disorders causing muscle constriction.
○ Pelvic examination reveals involuntary constriction of the musculature surrounding the outer portion of the vagina.
○ Detailed sexual history reveals involuntary spastic contraction of the lower vaginal muscles, possibly coexisting with dyspareunia, preventing intercourse.

Varicella

○ History includes exposure to person infected with chickenpox, although the patient may be unaware of contact.
○ Examination reveals crops of small, erythematous macules on the trunk or scalp progressing to papules and then clear vesicles on an erythematous base; vesicles become cloudy and break, and then form a scab.
○ Vesicular fluid tests positive for herpesvirus varicella-zoster.

Variola

○ History includes exposure to infected person.
○ Aspirate from vesicles and pustules reveals variola virus.
○ Complement fixation detects antibodies to variola virus.
○ Microscopic examination of smears from lesions shows variola virus.

Vascular retinopathies

○ In central retinal artery occlusion:
– Ophthalmoscopy (direct or indirect) shows emptying of retinal arterioles.
– Slit-lamp examination reveals, within 2 hours of occlusion, clumps or segmentation in the artery. Later examination shows a milky white retina around the optic disk (resulting from swelling and necrosis of ganglion cells caused by reduced blood supply). Other findings include a cherry-red spot in the macula (which subsides after several weeks).
– Ophthalmodynamometry measures approximate relative pressures in the central retinal arteries and indirectly assesses internal carotid artery blockage.
– Ultrasonography reveals blood vessel conditions in the neck.
– Digital subtraction angiography identifies carotid occlusion.
– MRI helps identify the reason for obstruction by revealing carotid or other obstruction.
– Contrast-enhanced CT scan discloses the diseased carotid artery.
○ In central retinal vein occlusion:
– Ophthalmoscopy (direct or indirect) reveals retinal hemorrhage, retinal vein engorgement, white patches among hemorrhages, and edema around the optic disk.
– Ultrasonography confirms or rules out occluded blood vessels.
○ In diabetic retinopathy:
– Slit-lamp examination shows thickening of retinal capillary walls.
– Indirect ophthalmoscopy demonstrates retinal changes, such as microaneurysms (earliest change), retinal hemorrhages and edema, venous dilation and beading, exudates, vitreous hemorrhage, proliferation of fibrin into vitreous from retinal holes, growth of new blood vessels, and microinfarctions of nerve fiber layer.
– Fluorescein angiography shows leakage of fluorescein from dilated vessels and differentiates between microaneurysms and true hemorrhages.
○ In hypertensive retinopathy:
– History reveals hypertension and decreased vision.

– Ophthalmoscopy (direct or indirect) in early disease discloses hard and shiny deposits, tiny hemorrhages, narrowed arterioles, nicking of the veins where arteries cross them (arteriovenous nicking), and elevated arterial blood pressure.
– Ophthalmoscopy in later disease shows cotton wool patches, exudates, retinal edema, papilledema caused by ischemia and capillary insufficiency, hemorrhages, and microaneurysms.

Vasculitis

○ In polyarteritis nodosa:
– History includes hypertension, abdominal pain, myalgia, headache, joint pain, and weakness.
– ESR is elevated.
– Leukocytosis, anemia, and thrombocytosis are present.
– C_3 complement is depressed.
– RF titer is $> 1:80$.
– Circulating immune complexes are present.
– Tissue biopsy shows necrotizing vasculitis.
○ In allergic angiitis and granulomatosis:
– History includes asthma.
– Eosinophilia is present.
– Tissue biopsy may show granulomatous inflammation with eosinophilic infiltration.
○ In polyangiitis overlap syndrome:
– History includes allergy.
– Eosinophilia is present.
– Tissue biopsy may show granulomatous inflammation with eosinophilic infiltration.
○ In Wegener's granulomatosis:
– Leukocytosis is present.
– Tissue biopsy reveals necrotizing vasculitis with granulomatous inflammation.
– ESR and IgA and IgG levels are elevated.
– RF titer is low.
– Circulating immune complexes are present.
○ In temporal arteritis:
– Hb level is decreased.
– ESR is elevated.
– Tissue biopsy shows panarteritis with infiltration of mononuclear cells, giant cells within vessel wall, fragmentation of internal elastic lamina, and proliferation of intima.
○ In Takayasu's arteritis:
– Hb level is decreased.
– Leukocytosis is present.
– Lupus erythematosus cell preparation is positive and ESR elevated.
– Arteriography shows calcification and obstruction of affected vessels.
– Tissue biopsy shows inflammation of adventitia and intima of vessels and thickening of vessel walls.
○ In hypersensitivity vasculitis:
– History includes exposure to an antigen, such as a microorganism or a drug.
– Tissue biopsy may show leukocytoclastic angiitis (usually in postcapillary venules), with infiltration of polymorphonuclear leukocytes, fibrinoid necrosis, and extravasation of erythrocytes.
○ In mucocutaneous lymph node syndrome:
– History and examination reveal fever, nonsuppurative cervical adenitis, edema, congested conjunctivae,

desquamation of fingertips, and erythema of oral cavity, lips, and palms.
- Tissue biopsy may show intimal proliferation and infiltration of vessel walls with mononuclear cells.

Velopharyngeal insufficiency
○ Examination reveals unintelligible speech.
○ Fiber-optic nasopharyngoscopy permits monitoring of velopharyngeal patency during speech and may identify the insufficiency.
○ Ultrasonography shows air-tissue overlap reflecting the degree of velopharyngeal sphincter incompetence; an opening of $> 20 \text{ mm}^2$ results in unintelligible speech.

Ventricular aneurysm
○ History includes persistent arrhythmias, onset of heart failure, or systemic embolization in a patient with left ventricular failure and a history of myocardial infarction.
○ CXR reveals an abnormal bulge distorting the heart's contour (with large aneurysm).
○ Left ventriculography reveals left ventricular enlargement, with an area of akinesia or dyskinesia and diminished cardiac function.
○ Echocardiography reveals abnormal motion in the left ventricular wall.

Ventricular fibrillation
○ ECG findings include:
 - Atrial rhythm isn't measurable.
 - Ventricular rhythm has no pattern or regularity.
 - Atrial and ventricular rates aren't measurable.
 - P wave and PR interval aren't measurable.
 - Duration of the QRS complex isn't measurable; configuration is wide and irregular.
 - T wave isn't measurable.

Ventricular septal defect
○ Echocardiography or MRI reveals a large defect and its location in the septum, estimates the size of a left-to-right shunt, suggests pulmonary hypertension, and identifies associated lesions and complications.
○ Cardiac catheterization determines the size and exact location of the defect, calculates the degree of shunting, determines the extent of pulmonary hypertension, and detects associated defects.
○ CXR is normal with small defects; in large defects, it shows cardiomegaly, left atrial and ventricular enlargement, and prominent pulmonary vascular markings.
○ ECG is normal with small defects; in large defects, it shows left and right ventricular hypertrophy.

Ventricular tachycardia
○ ECG findings include:
 - Atrial rhythm isn't measurable. Ventricular rhythm is usually regular but may be slightly irregular.
 - Atrial rate isn't measurable. Ventricular rate is usually rapid (140 to 220 beats/minute).
 - P wave is usually absent. It may be obscured by and is dissociated from the QRS complex. Retrograde and upright P waves may be present.
 - PR interval isn't measurable.

- QRS complex has a duration > 0.12 second, has a bizarre appearance, and usually has increased amplitude.
- T wave occurs in the opposite direction of the QRS complex.
- QT interval isn't measurable.

Vesicoureteral reflux
○ History includes symptoms of urinary tract infection.
○ Examination reveals hematuria or strong-smelling urine (in infants).
○ Palpation may reveal a hard, thickened bladder (if posterior urethral valves are causing an obstruction in male infants).
○ Cystoscopy reveals reflux.
○ Urinalysis reveals bacterial count $> 100,000$/ml; decreased specific gravity, and increased pH.
○ Excretory urography may show dilated lower ureter, ureter visible for its entire length, hydronephrosis, calyceal distortion, and renal scarring.
○ Voiding cystourethrography identifies and determines the degree of reflux, shows when reflux occurs, and may also pinpoint the cause.
○ Bladder catheterization identifies the amount of residual urine.

Vitamin A deficiency
○ History includes inadequate dietary intake of foods high in vitamin A.
○ Ocular examination reveals xerophthalmia, Bitot's spots, perforation, and scarring.
○ Serum vitamin A level is decreased.
○ Carotene level is decreased.

Vitamin B deficiency
○ History includes inadequate dietary intake of foods high in vitamin B.
○ Serum vitamin B_2 level is decreased.
○ A 24-hour urine test reveals:
 - thiamine deficiency
 - riboflavin deficiency
 - niacin deficiency
 - pyridoxine deficiency.

Vitamin C deficiency
○ History includes inadequate intake of ascorbic acid.
○ Serum ascorbic acid level is decreased.

Vitamin D deficiency
○ History includes inadequate dietary intake of preformed vitamin D.
○ Serum vitamin D_3 level is low or undetectable.
○ Serum calcium level is decreased.
○ Alkaline phosphatase level is decreased.
○ X-rays reveal characteristic bone deformities and abnormalities such as Looser's zones.

Vitamin E deficiency
○ History includes diet high in polyunsaturated fatty acids fortified with iron but not vitamin E.
○ Serum vitamin E level is decreased.
○ Serum CK level is increased.
○ Platelet level is increased.

Vitamin K deficiency

○ PT is 25% longer than the normal range of 10 to 20 seconds (in the absence of anticoagulant therapy or hepatic disease).
○ Capillary fragility test result is positive.

Volvulus

○ History includes sudden onset of severe abdominal pain.
○ Examination reveals palpable abdominal mass.
○ Abdominal X-rays reveal obstruction and abnormal air-fluid levels in the sigmoid and cecum (in midgut volvulus, abdominal X-rays may be normal).
○ Barium enema findings include:
 – In cecal volvulus, barium fills the colon distal to the section of cecum.
 – In sigmoid volvulus in children, barium may twist to a point; in adults, barium may take on an "ace of spades" configuration.
○ In midgut volvulus, upper GI series reveals obstruction and possibly a twisted contour in a narrow area near the duodenojejunal junction where barium won't pass.
○ WBC count is elevated, indicating strangulation or bowel infarction.

Von Willebrand's disease

○ History reveals family inheritance pattern.
○ Bleeding time is prolonged.
○ PTT is prolonged.
○ Factor VIII-related antigens are decreased and factor VIII activity level is low.
○ Clot retraction and platelet aggregation are normal.

Vulvovaginitis

○ Examination reveals vaginal discharge and inflammation of the vulva.
○ Culture of vaginal exudate identifies *Trichomonas vaginalis, Candida albicans, Gardnerella vaginitis, Neisseria gonorrhoeae,* or *Phthirus pubis.*

Whooping cough

○ Examination reveals forceful coughing that ends in a characteristic "whoop."
○ Nasopharyngeal swabs and sputum cultures identify *Bordetella pertussis* (in the early stages of illness).
○ WBC count is markedly elevated, with 60% to 90% lymphocytes.

Wilms' tumor

○ Examination reveals palpable abdominal mass in early childhood.
○ Gallium scan reveals abnormal activity.
○ Percutaneous renal biopsy reveals malignant cells.
○ Excretory urography doesn't indicate neoplasm or extrarenal mass.

Wilson's disease

○ Liver biopsy reveals excessive copper deposits and tissue changes indicative of chronic active hepatitis, fatty liver, or cirrhosis.
○ Slit-lamp ophthalmic examination reveals Kayser-Fleischer rings (in advanced disease).
○ Urine copper level is increased.

Wounds, open trauma

○ History includes injury.
○ Examination reveals open wound.
○ X-rays show bone damage, extent of injury to the area and surrounding tissue, and retention of injuring object.
○ EMG reveals isolated, irregular motor unit potentials with increased amplitude and duration indicating peripheral nerve injury.
○ Nerve conduction studies reveal abnormal nerve conduction time indicating peripheral nerve injury.
○ CBC reveals decreased Hb and HCT levels and increased WBC count.

Yellow fever

○ Blood culture reveals presence of arbovirus.
○ Urine albumin level is increased (in 90% of patients).
○ Antibody titer is elevated.

Zinc deficiency

○ History includes excessive intake of foods containing iron, calcium, vitamin D, and the fiber and phytates in cereals.
○ Serum zinc level is decreased.

Selected references

American Diabetes Association. "Diagnosis and Classification of Diabetes Mellitus," *Diabetes Care* 27(Suppl 1):S5-S10, January 2004.

Bickley, L.S., and Szilagyi, P.G. *Bates' Guide to Physical Examination and History Taking,* 8th ed. Philadelphia: Lippincott Williams & Wilkins, 2003.

Bolotin G, et al. "Use of Intraoperative Epiaortic Ultrasonography to Delineate Aortic Atheroma," *Chest* 127(1):60-65, January 2005.

Chernyshev, O.Y., et al. "Yield and Accuracy of Urgent Combined Carotid/Transcranial Ultrasound Testing in Acute Cerebral Ischemia," *Stroke* 36(1):32-37, January 2005.

Chojnowski, D. "The Latest in Cardiac Care," *Nursing Management* Suppl.:16-18, 2004.

Durston, S. "The ABCs and More of Hepatitis," *Nursing Made Incredibly Easy* 2(4), 22-31, July-August 2004.

Edelman, D., et al. "Utility of Hemoglobin A1c in Predicting Diabetes Risk," *Journal of General Internal Medicine* 19(12):1175-180, December 2004.

Fischbach, F.T. *A Manual of Laboratory and Diagnostic Tests,* 7th ed. Philadelphia: Lippincott Williams & Wilkins, 2004.

Hoffman, R., et al. *Hematology Basic Principles and Practice,* 4th ed. New York: Churchill Livingstone, Inc, 2005.

Kasper, D.L., et al., eds. *Harrison's Principles of Internal Medicine,* 16th ed. New York: McGraw-Hill Book Co., Inc., 2005.

Kozier, B., et al. *Fundamentals of Nursing Concepts, Process, and Practice,* 7th ed. Upper Saddle River, N.J.: Prentice Hall Health, 2004.

Min, R.J., et al. "Duplex Ultrasound Evaluation of Lower Extremity Venous Insufficiency," *Journal of Vascular & Interventional Radiology* 14(10):1233-241, October 2003.

Nursing Procedures, 4th ed. Philadelphia: Lippincott Williams & Wilkins, 2004.

Pagana, K.D., and Pagana, T.J. *Mosby's Diagnostic and Laboratory Test Reference,* 6th ed. St. Louis: Mosby–Year Book, Inc., 2003.

Pelikan, D.M., et al. "Quantification of Fetomaternal Hemorrhage: A Comparative Study of the Manual and Automated Microscopic Kleihauer-Betke Tests and Flow Cytometry in Clinical Samples," *American Journal of Obstetrics & Gynecology* 191(2):551-57, August 2004.

Phipps, W.J., et al. *Medical Surgical Nursing: Health and Illness Perspectives,* 7th ed. St. Louis: Mosby–Year Book, Inc., 2003.

Professional Guide to Diagnostic Tests. Philadelphia: Lippincott Williams & Wilkins, 2005.

Pruitt, W.C., and Jacobs, M. " Interpreting Arterial Blood Gases: Easy as ABC," *Nursing2004* 34(8), 50-53, August 2004.

Rakel, R., and Bope, E.T. *Conn's Current Therapy 2004.* Philadelphia: W.B. Saunders Co., 2004.

Rapid Assessment A Flowchart Guide to Evaluating Signs & Symptoms. Philadelphia: Lippincott Williams & Wilkins, 2004.

Rempher, K.J., and Little, J. "Assessment of Red Blood Cell and Coagulation Laboratory Data," *AACN Clinical Issues* 15(4):622-37, October-December 2004.

Roch, A., et al. "Usefulness of Ultrasonography in Predicting Pleural Effusions > 500 mL in Patients Receiving Mechanical Ventilation," *Chest* 127(1): 224-232, January 2005.

Tierney, L., et al. *Current Medical Diagnosis and Treatment,* 43rd ed. New York: McGraw-Hill/Appleton & Lange, 2004.

Waugh, J.J., et al. "Accuracy of Urinalysis Dipstick Techniques in Predicting Significant Proteinuria in Pregnancy," *Obstetrics & Gynecology.* 103(4):769-77, April 2004.

Woods, S., et al. *Cardiac Nursing,* 5th ed. Philadelphia: Lippincott Williams & Wilkins, 2005.

Yueh, B., et al. "Screening and Management of Adult Hearing Loss in Primary Care," *JAMA* 289(15):1976-985, April 2003.

Index

A

Abdomen
  computed tomography of, 103
  flat plate of, 241
  magnetic resonance imaging of
    urinary tract for masses in,
    270
Abdominal aorta ultrasonography,
  441
Abdominal pain evaluation
  percutaneous transhepatic
    cholangiography in, 307
  proctosigmoidoscopy in, 336
  serum amylase in, 23
Abdominal trauma
  blunt and penetrating, 495
  celiac and mesenteric
    arteriography in, 82
  computed tomography of abdomen
    and pelvis in, 103
  liver-spleen scanning in, 252
  paracentesis in, 300
  peritoneal fluid analysis in, 310
  splenic ultrasonography in, 447
ABO blood typing, 2
Abortion
  homocysteine in, 221
  hysterosalpingography in, 230
  transvaginal ultrasound in, 427
  urine human chorionic
    gonadotropin in, 223
Abruptio placentae, 490
Acceleration-deceleration cervical
  injuries, 490
Acetaminophen, serum drug levels,
  488t
Acetylcholine receptor antibodies, 3
Acid mucopolysaccharides, 4
Acid perfusion (Bernstein) test, 5
Acid phosphatase, 6
Acid-base balance disorders
  arterial blood gas analysis in, 40
  metabolic acidosis, 510
  metabolic alkalosis, 510
  respiratory acidosis, 519
  respiratory alkalosis, 519
  serum calcium in, 72
  serum chloride in, 89
  serum potassium in, 334
  serum sodium in, 390
  total carbon dioxide content in,
    419
  urine sodium in, 391

Acid-fast stain, 7
Acidified serum lysis test, 203
Acidosis
  metabolic, 510
  anion gap in, 27
  respiratory, 519
Acoustic admittance, 8
Acoustic reflex testing, 8
Acquired immunodeficiency
    syndrome, 490
  human immunodeficiency virus
    antibodies in, 225
  lymphocyte assays in, 400
Acromegaly
  growth hormone suppression in,
    202
  serum human growth hormone in,
    224
Actinomycosis, 491
Activated clotting time, 9
Acute tubular necrosis, 491
Addison's disease
  plasma cortisol in, 324
  urine 17-ketogenic steroids in, 463
Adrenal function evaluation
  insulin tolerance test in, 235
  plasma corticotropin in, 118
  plasma cortisol in, 324
  rapid corticotropin in, 356
  serum aldosterone in, 12
  serum sodium in, 390
  urine 17-hydroxycorticosteroids in,
    461
  urine 17-ketogenic steroids in, 463
  urine chloride in, 90
  urine free cortisol in, 188
  urine sodium in, 391
  urine vanillylmandelic acid in, 468
Adrenal hypofunction, 491
Adrenal tumors
  nephrotomography in, 285
  plasma catecholamines in, 322
Adult respiratory distress syndrome,
  519
  pulmonary artery catheterization
    in, 344
Age-related macular degeneration,
  491
Alanine aminotransferase, 10
Albumin, 11, 422-423
Alcohol detection, gamma
  glutamyltransferase in, 194

Alcoholism, 491
Aldosterone
  serum, 12
  urine, 13
Aldosteronism, 505
  plasma renin activity in, 328
  serum aldosterone in, 12
  urine aldosterone in, 13
Alkaline phosphatase, 14
Alkalosis
  metabolic, 510
  respiratory, 519
Allergic angiitis and granulomatosis,
  526
Allergic rhinitis, 491
Allergies, radioallergosorbent test in,
  351
Alpha-1 globulin, 15, 422-423
Alpha-2 globulin, 16, 422-423
Alpha-fetoprotein, 17
Alpha-subunit of pituitary
  glycoprotein hormones, 18
Alport's syndrome, 491
Alveolar-to-arterial oxygen gradient,
  19
Alzheimer's disease, 492
  cerebrospinal fluid analysis in, 84
  soluble amyloid beta protein
    precursor in, 392
Ambiguous genitalia, sex
    chromosome tests for, 379
Amenorrhea
  estrogen in, 166
  plasma luteinizing hormone in, 327
  serum follicle-stimulating hormone
    in, 186
  serum prolactin in, 338
  sex chromosome tests in, 379
Amikacin, serum drug levels, 488t
Amino acid disorders
  amniotic fluid analysis in, 21
  plasma amino acid screening in,
    320
  urine amino acid screening in, 457
Ammonia, plasma, 20
Amniocentesis
  alpha-fetoprotein screening and,
    17
  pelvic ultrasonography guidance of,
    446
Amniotic fluid analysis, 21
Amputation, traumatic, 492
Amsler's grid, 22, 22i

i refers to an illustration; t refers to a table.

i refers to an illustration; t refers to a table.

i refers to an illustration; t refers to a table.

i refers to an illustration; t refers to a table.

i refers to an illustration; t refers to a table.

i refers to an illustration; t refers to a table.

i refers to an illustration; t refers to a table.

Epilepsy, 500
  electroencephalography in, 149
Epistaxis, 500
Epstein-Barr virus antibodies, 160
Erythema infectiosum, parvovirus
      B-19 antibodies in, 305
Erythroblastosis fetalis, 500
Erythrocyte sedimentation rate, 161
Erythropoietin, 162
Esophageal acidity test, 163
Esophageal cancer, 500
Esophageal disorders
  acid perfusion (Bernstein) test in,
      5
  atresia, 524
  barium swallow in, 52
  diverticula, 500
  endoscopic ultrasound in, 156
  esophageal acidity test in, 163
  esophagogastroduodenoscopy in,
      164
  Mallory-Weiss syndrome, 510
Esophagogastroduodenoscopy,
      164-165
Estradiol, 166
Estriol, 166
Estrogen, 166
Ethosuximide, serum drug levels,
      488t
Evoked potential studies, 167
Excessive daytime sleepiness, sleep
      studies in, 386
Exchange transfusion, serum
      bilirubin for, 57
Excretory urography, 168
Exercise echocardiography, 144-145
Exercise electrocardiography, 147
Exercise prescription
  dobutamine stress
      echocardiography for, 143
  exercise echocardiography for, 144
  exercise electrocardiography for,
      147
Exophthalmos, 500
  exophthalmometry in, 169
  orbital computed tomography in,
      294
  thyroid-stimulating
      immunoglobulin in, 414
Expiratory reserve volume, 346
External auditory canal, otoscopy of,
      298
External fetal monitoring, 170-171
External sphincter electromyography,
      151
Extracellular cation-anion balance,
      serum chloride in, 89
Extractable nuclear antigen
      antibodies, 172

Eye disorders or injuries
  corneal abrasion, 497
  corneal staining in, 117
  exophthalmometry in, 169
  fluorescein angiography in, 182
  handheld ophthalmoscopy in, 291
  orbital computed tomography in,
      294
  orbital radiography in, 295
  slit-lamp examination in, 387
  ultrasonography in, 289

F

Failure to thrive, homocysteine in,
      221
Fallopian tube
  cancer of, 500
  hysterosalpingography of, 230
Fasting plasma glucose, 173
Fat metabolism disorders
  phospholipids in, 319
  total cholesterol in, 420
  triglycerides in, 428
Fatty liver, 501
Febrile agglutination, 174-175
Fecal lipids, 176
Fecal occult blood, 177
Fecal passage of mucus, blood, or
      pus, proctosigmoidoscopy for,
      336
Fecal test for *Helicobacter pylori,*
      206
Fecal urobilinogen, 469
Femoral aneurysm, 501
Ferritin, 178
Fetal assessment
  amniotic fluid analysis in, 21
  chorionic villi sampling in, 94, 94i
  contraction stress test in, 116,
      170-171
  estrogen in, 166
  external fetal monitoring in,
      170-171
  human placental lactogen in, 227
  internal fetal monitoring in, 236,
      237i
  pelvic ultrasonography in, 446
  transvaginal ultrasound in, 427
  understanding fetal monitoring
      terminology, 171
Fetal death, urine human chorionic
      gonadotropin in, 223
Fetal gender determination, amniotic
      fluid analysis in, 21
Fetal hemoglobin, 179, 209t
Fetal-maternal erythrocyte
      distribution, 180
Fever of unknown origin
  blood culture in, 60
  febrile agglutination in, 174
  gallium scanning in, 192

Fibrin split products, 181
Fibrinogen, plasma, 325
Fibrinogen abnormalities
  plasma fibrinogen in, 325
  plasma thrombin time in, 330
Fibrinolysis, D-dimer in, 133
Flexible sigmoidoscopy, 381
Fluid status evaluation
  blood urea nitrogen in, 61
  hematocrit in, 207
  pulmonary artery catheterization
      in, 344
  serum chloride in, 89
  serum sodium in, 390
  urine chloride in, 90
  urine sodium in, 391
Fluid-retaining conditions, beta
      globulin in, 55
Fluorescein angiography, 182
Fluorescent treponemal antibody
      absorption, 183
Fluoroscopy, thoracic, 184
Folic acid, 185
Folic acid deficiency, 501
  folic acid in, 185
  homocysteine in, 221
Follicle-stimulating hormone, serum,
      186
Forced expiratory volume, 346
Forced vital capacity, 346
Foreign body detection or removal
  chest radiography in, 88
  direct laryngoscopy in, 245
  esophagogastroduodenoscopy in,
      164
  ocular ultrasonography in, 289
  otoscopy in, 298
  pelvic ultrasonography in, 446
  ultrasonography in, 440
Fractionated erythrocyte porphyrins,
      187
Fracture
  arm or leg, 493
  bone scan of, 65
  computed tomography of bone in,
      104
  jaw, 498
  orbital computed tomography in,
      294
  orbital radiography in, 294
  skull, 522
  vertebral radiography in, 473
Free cortisol, urine, 188
Free thyroxine, 189
Free triiodothyronine, 189
Functional residual capacity, 346
Fungal serology, 190

G

Galactorrhea, serum prolactin in, 338

i refers to an illustration; t refers to a table.

i refers to an illustration; t refers to a table.

i refers to an illustration; t refers to a table.

i refers to an illustration; t refers to a table.

i refers to an illustration; t refers to a table.

i refers to an illustration; t refers to a table.

i refers to an illustration; t refers to a table.

i refers to an illustration; t refers to a table.

i refers to an illustration; t refers to a table.

i refers to an illustration; t refers to a table.

i refers to an illustration; t refers to a table.

i refers to an illustration; t refers to a table.

i refers to an illustration; t refers to a table.